MEDICAL RADIOLOGY
Diagnostic Imaging

Editors:
A. L. Baert, Leuven
M. Knauth, Göttingen
K. Sartor, Heidelberg

Royal Liverpool University Hospital – Staff Library

Please return or renew, on or before the last date below. Items may be renewed **twice**, if not reserved for another user. Renewals may be made in person, by telephone: 0151 706 2248 or email: library.service@rlbuht.nhs.uk. There is a charge of 10p per day for late items.

Goetz Benndorf

Dural Cavernous Sinus Fistulas

Diagnostic and Endovascular Therapy

Foreword by

K. Sartor

With 178 Figures in 755 Separate Illustrations, 540 in Color and 19 Tables

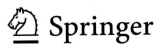 Springer

Goetz Benndorf, MD, PhD
Associate Professor, Department of Radiology
Baylor College of Medicine
Director of Interventional Neuroradiology
Ben Taub General Hospital
One Baylor Plaza, MS 360
Houston, TX 77030
USA

Medical Radiology · Diagnostic Imaging and Radiation Oncology
Series Editors:
A. L. Baert · L. W. Brady · H.-P. Heilmann · M. Knauth · M. Molls · C. Nieder · K. Sartor

Continuation of Handbuch der medizinischen Radiologie
Encyclopedia of Medical Radiology

ISBN 978-3-540-00818-7   e-ISBN 978-3-540-68889-1

DOI 10.0007 / 978-3-540-68889-1

Medical Radiology · Diagnostic Imaging and Radiation Oncology ISSN 0942-5373

Library of Congress Control Number: 2004116221

© 2010, Springer-Verlag Berlin Heidelberg

Cover-Design and Layout: PublishingServices Teichmann, 69256 Mauer, Germany

Printed on acid-free paper – 21/3180xq
9 8 7 6 5 4 3 2 1 0

springer.com

Dedicated to my parents,

Dorothea
and Eberhard Benndorf

Foreword

Of the dural venous sinuses, the cavernous sinus is anatomically the most complex. It has an intimate topographical relationship with the internal carotid artery and the sixth cranial nerve (both of which pass through its meshwork) and houses the cranial nerves III, IV and V1-2 in its lateral wall. Medially it abuts the pituitary gland, while laterally it nears the temporal lobe; Meckel's cave with the trigeminal ganglion lies immediately posterior to it. Located essentially at the center of the skull base, the cavernous sinus connects with numerous dural sinuses and veins of all three cranial fossae, as well as the orbit. Furthermore, there is an abundance of dural arteries in the sellar region that are interconnected and derive from the carotid system.

Due to its specific vascular anatomy, the cavernous sinus is a common site of various types of arteriovenous (AV) fistulas, which are essentially benign lesions but which may endanger both vision and cranial nerve function. These fistulas, including their largely endovascular interventional treatment, are the topic of Götz Benndorf's monograph. After describing the relevant anatomy of the cavernous sinus in great detail, the author continues by explaining the anatomic and hemodynamic classifications of AV fistulas of the cavernous sinus. This is followed by important information on etiology, pathogenesis and prevalence of the various lesions. Before embarking on the main part of his book, diagnostic and therapeutic radiology of AV cavernous fistulas, Benndorf devotes an entire chapter to clinical, largely neuro-ophthalmological symptoms and signs. The radiological chapters, all beautifully illustrated and containing a treatise on hemodynamics, will undoubtedly convince readers of the immense diagnostic and therapeutic experience of the author in his chosen topic. The treatment focuses on transvenous embolization rather than the transarterial approaches.

I am unaware of any publication that covers the diagnostic and interventional radiology of AV fistulas of the cavernous sinus in such a clear, systematic and complete way as Benndorf's book. Any interventional neuroradiologist dealing with skull base lesions needs a copy, as does any skull base surgeon. In addition, the book would not look out of place on a neurologist's bookshelf.

Heidelberg   KLAUS SARTOR

Preface

This volume of Medical Radiology is based to a large degree on my Ph.D. Thesis at Charité, Humboldt University (Berlin, 2002) and contains most of the original text and imaging material. During my subsequent years (2003 to 2009) at the departments of radiology, Baylor College of Medicine (BCM) and The Methodist Hospital (TMH) in Houston, this work grew substantially, and thus required more time to complete than anticipated. Nevertheless, I hope, the result represents a happy ending that was worth waiting for. The monograph stands for more than 13 years of personal experience in performing endovascular treatment and clinical management of patients with various types of intracranial arteriovenous shunting lesions, in particular fistulas of dural origin involving the cavernous sinus. It is intended as a practical guide and reference for those involved in the diagnosis and treatment of these lesions. Completing this book would have been impossible without the motivation, help and support from my teachers, colleagues and friends.

Acknowledgements:
I am very thankful to Christiane Kagel (University Greifswald) and Christiane Poehls (Helios Klinikum Berlin-Buch), who between 1989 and 1991, taught me the basic principles of diagnostic cerebral angiography and vascular interventional radiology. Horst Peter Molsen (Charité, Berlin), my INR fellowship director from 1991 to 1993, introduced the techniques of transvenous catheterization and embolization to me while we were treating the first CSF patients together. My most sincere gratitude goes to Jacques Moret (Foundation Rothschild, Paris) for his generous permission to use some of his material for my thesis. During his numerous visits and lectures at the Benjamin Franklin Hospital, Free University Berlin from 1992 to 1997, Pierre Lasjaunias (†, Kremlin Bicetre, Paris) was not only a brilliant teacher, but also a great inspirer in the studies of the vascular anatomy of the cavernous sinus region. I am very much indebted to Wolfgang Lanksch (Charité, Berlin), chair of the department of neurosurgery, who was my clinical mentor and a steady supporter of my work from 1991 to 2003.

I owe many special thanks to the entire INR team at Rudolf-Virchow-Hospital, Charité, but mostly to two nurses, Angelika Wehner and Petra Schlecht, whose loyal devotion and outstanding assistance over many years played a key role in the successful performance of complex endovascular procedures. Christof Barner, immensely experienced and dedicated neuroanesthesiologist at Charité, became an indispensable colleague for achieving good clinical outcomes. I also wish to thank Horst Menneking (maxillo-facial surgeon, Charité) for his exceptionally skillful surgical work in those cases, where transophthalmic SOV approaches became necessary. My colleague and friend, Andreas Bender (Charité until 1998), one of the most talented interventional neuroradiologists I had the good fortune to meet, helped me to master the treatment challenges of several of my early patients. Stephanie Schmidt, ophthalmologist at Charité until 2003, was an outstanding clinician and a most pleasant colleague to work with.

The majority of presented case reports are of patients, for whom staff members from the departments of neurosurgery, neurology and ophthalmology at Charité provided excellent care.

The following colleagues and friends contributed additional interesting and valuable imaging material: Jacques Moret (Foundation Rothschild, Paris), Alessandra Biondi (Pitié-Salpêtrière University Hospital, Paris); Gyula Gal (University Hospital Odense); Michel Mawad (BCM, Houston); Jacques Dion (Emory University Hospital, Atlanta); Richard Klucznik (TMH, Houston); Maria Angeles De Miquel (Hospital Universitari de Bellvitge, Barcelona); Michael Soederman (Karolinska University Hospital, Stockholm); Winston Lim (Singapore General Hospital); Adriana Campi (Ospedale San Raffaele, University of Milan); Rob De Keizer (University Hospital, Leiden); Charbel Mounayer (Foundation Rothschild, Paris); Raimund Parsche (Ruppiner Kliniken); Bernhard Sander (MRI Praxis, Berlin) and Ullrich Schweiger (Ullsteinhausklinik, Berlin).

Special credit goes to Alessandra Biondi, Gyula Gal, Stefanie Schmidt, Diane Nino (BCM Houston), Phillip Randall (TMH Houston) and Mia Carlson (MDA, Houston) for review, suggestions and corrections of the text.

The superb clinical photographs were taken by Franz Haffner and Peter Behrend (Charité, Berlin); David Gee (Houston) produced the high-quality dry skull pictures. Corinna Naujok (Charité, Berlin), Charlie Thran (TMH, Houston) and Scott Weldon (BCM, Houston) helped to create the nicely colored illustrations. Dirk Emmel (Charité, Berlin) provided invaluable support for the digital storage of the image material. Richard Klucznik (TMH, Houston) was very helpful in acquiring high-resolution 3D-data for the imaging studies of the cavernous sinus.

Last, but not least, I am truly grateful to Ursula Davis (Heidelberg), Christine Schaefer (Hemsbach), Kurt Teichmann (Mauer) and Klaus Sartor (Heppenheim), whose endless patience and understanding allowed me to produce and finish this volume.

Houston   GOETZ BENNDORF

Contents

Glossary

ACC	Anterior condylar confluens
ACT	Angiographic computed tomography (contrast enhanced DynaCT; based on C-arm mounted Flat panel technology)
ACV	Anterior condylar vein
AFR	Artery of the foramen rotundum
AMA	Accessory meningeal artery
APA	Ascending pharyngeal artery
AVM	Arteriovenous malformation
BP	Basilar plexus
BSC	Boston Scientific Corporation
CCF(s)	Carotid cavernous fistula (direct fistula)
CN(s)	Cranial nerve(s)
CS(s)	Cavernous sinus(es)
CSF(s)	Cavernous sinus fistula(s) (AV shunt involving the cavernous sinus in general)
CTA	Computed tomographic angiography (based on conventional CT technology)
CVD	Cortical venous drainage
DAVF(s)	Dural arteriovenous fistula
DAVS	Dural arteriovenous shunt
DCCF	Dural carotid cavernous fistula
DCSF(s)	Dural cavernous sinus fistula(s) (indirect fistula)
DSA	Digital subtraction angiography
DynaCT	Siemens term for cross sectional (CT-like) imaging using rotating C-arms
ECA	External carotid artery
F	French (Charrière; 1 french = 1/3 mm)
FLP	Foramen lacerum plexus
FrV	Frontal vein
FV	Facial vein
i.a.	Intraarterial
i.v.	Intravenous
ICA	Internal carotid artery
ICAVP	Internal carotid artery venous plexus
ICS	Intercavernous sinus
IJV	Internal jugular vein
ILT	Inferolateral trunk
IMA	Internal maxillary artery
IOF	Inferior orbital fissure (infraorbital)
IOV	Inferior ophthalmic vein
IPCV	Inferior petroclival vein
IPS	Inferior petrosal sinus
IPV	Intrapetrosal vein

JB	Jugular bulb
LCS	Laterocavernous sinus
LCV	Lateral condylar vein
LVD	Leptomeningeal venous drainage
MHT	Meningohypophyseal trunk
MIP	Maximum Intensity projections
MMA	Middle meningeal artery
MPR	Multiplanar reconstructions
MRA	Magnetic resonance angiography
MTA	Marginal tentorial artery (medial tentorial artery)
MTV	Middle Temporal vein
NBCA	N-butyl-cyanoacrylate
OA	Ophthalmic artery
PCP	Posterior clinoid process
PCV	Posterior condylar vein
PP	Pterygoid plexus
PPF	Pterygopalatine fossa
PVP	Prevertebral plexus
RAFL	Recurrent artery of the foramen lacerum
SMCV	Superficial middle cerebral vein
SOF	Superior orbital fissure (supraorbital)
SOV	Superior ophthalmic vein
SPPS	Sphenoparietal sinus
SPS	Superior petrosal sinus
SS	Sigmoid sinus
SSD	Surface shaded Display
STA	Superficial temporal artery
TAE	Transarterial embolization
TVO	Transvenous occlusion
UV	Uncal vein
VA	Vertebral artery
ViA	Vidian artery
VRT	Volume rendering technique

Introduction

In reference to cavernous sinus fistulas (CSFs) causing pulsating exophthalmos, WALTER DANDY (1937) wrote: *"The study of carotid-cavernous aneurysm – the clinical ensemble – the variation and capricious results of treatment – have been told and retold, and most admirably. Medical literature can scarcely claim more accurate and thorough studies than upon this subject."*

More than 70 years later, a similar statement can be made relating to a subgroup of CSFs, the arteriovenous shunts between small dural branches arising from the external and internal carotid arteries and the cavernous sinus, also called dural cavernous sinus fistulas (DCSFs). Indeed much has been written about these fistulas, which were recognized relatively late as a separate entity among CSFs, and which can be clinically perplexing and sometimes quite difficult to diagnose or to treat. The cure of patients, on the other hand, is one of the most rewarding in the spectrum of modern neuroendovascular treatments.

The initial angiographic descriptions by CASTAIGNE et al. (1966), NEWTON and HOYT (1970) and DJINDJAN et al. (1968) focused mainly on their peculiar arterial supply, which later became the basis for a widely used anatomic classification (BARROW et al. 1985).

The cavernous sinus itself represents a rather complex venous reservoir, embedded in the base of the skull and traversed by the cavernous carotid artery and four cranial nerves. It functions as a confluens, receiving multiple cerebral and intracranial afferent veins (tributaries) and drains into various efferent veins or dural sinuses.

Despite numerous studies, etiology, pathophysiology and clinical course of these fistulas are to date only partially understood.

Because the arteriovenous shunts develop within the dural walls of the cavernous sinus (CS), their flow is usually directed towards the superior ophthalmic vein (SOV), causing signs and symptoms very similar, albeit milder, to those observed in patients with direct high-flow carotid cavernous fistulas (CCFs).

Significant improvements in angiographic imaging technology over the last 15 years, such as the introduction of three-dimensional digital subtracted angiography (3D-DSA), have resulted in better understanding of the specific arterial and venous anatomy, opening the doors for novel treatment options. In combination with the advances made in endovascular tools and devices, transvenous occlusion using various transfemoral or percutaneous access routes has become increasingly popular.

Numerous case reports and small case series have been published, creating a wealth of information in the medical literature. However, the data scattered through journals of various clinical disciplines namely neuroradiology, neurosurgery, neurology and ophthalmology.

Regarding therapeutic options for patients with CSFs, HAMBY (1966) stated: *"The best possibility theoretically would be to induce thrombosis that would close the sinus completely. This appears to be hardly possibly, by currently known techniques, in the face of the tremendous arterial inflow of blood"*. This concept was reiterated by MULLAN (1974), and 40 years later, transvenous occlusion (TVO) techniques play a dominant role in the management of patients with DCSFs. Because TVO of DCSFs can often be performed successfully today with high efficacy and low morbidity, it has widely replaced microneurosurgery. On the other hand some controversy about its proper indication, associated complication rates and the use of therapeutic alternatives persists.

The purpose of this monograph was to collect and discuss much of the radiological and imaging information available. It aims to summarize and facilitate access to currently existing knowledge on these complex, incompletely understood, and sometimes challenging lesions.

Views and opinions stated below reflect personal experience in clinical and endovascular management of patients with DCSFs, demonstrating the evolution of minimal invasive techniques, particularly the increasing use of transvenous approaches to the CS.

Insights into all aspects of these interesting cerebrovascular lesions, including their anatomy, etiology, classification, clinical presentation, imaging techniques and hemodynamics, are provided. Various current treatment options and their role in patient management are described, such as conservative management, manual compression, controlled hypotension, radiosurgery, surgery, but foremost endovascular therapy.

Percutaneous catheterization techniques are covered in greater detail with great emphasis on transvenous access routes and the progress that has been made since HALBACH et al. (1989) published the first relevant series.

This volume is intended as a reference and a guide for neuroradiologists, neurosurgeons, neurologists and ophthalmologists, who see patients with DCSFs in their practice.

References

Dandy W (1937) Carotid-cavernous aneurysms (pulsating exophthalmos). Zentralbl Neurochir 2:77–206

Castaigne P, Laplane D, Djindjian R, Bories J, Augustin P (1966) Spontaneous arteriovenous communication between the external carotid and the cavernous sinus. Rev Neurol (Paris) 114:5–14

Newton TH, Hoyt WF (1970) Dural arteriovenous shunts in the region of the cavernous sinus. Neuroradiology 1:71–81

Djindjian R, Cophignon J, Comoy J, Rey J, Houdart R (1968) Neuro-radiologic polymorphism of carotido-cavernous fistulas. Neurochirurgie 14:881–890

Djindjian R, Manelfe C, Picard L (1973) External carotid-cavernous sinus, arteriovenous fistulae: angiographic study of 6 cases and review of the literature. Neurochirurgie 19:91–110

Newton TH, Hoyt WF (1968) Spontaneous arteriovenous fistula between dural branches of the internal maxillary artery and the posterior cavernous sinus. Radiology 91:1147–1150

Barrow DL, Spector RH, Braun IF, Landman JA, Tindall SC, Tindall GT (1985) Classification and treatment of spontaneous carotid-cavernous sinus fistulas. J Neurosurg 62:248–256

Hamby W (1966) Carotid-cavernous fistula. Springfield

Mullan S (1974) Experiences with surgical thrombosis of intracranial berry aneurysms and carotid cavernous fistulas. J Neurosurg 41:657–670

Halbach VV, Higashida RT, Hieshima GB, Hardin CW, Pribram H (1989) Transvenous embolization of dural fistulas involving the cavernous sinus. AJNR Am J Neuroradiol 10:377-383

Historical Considerations

2.1
Arteriovenous Fistula and Pulsating Exophthalmos

William Hunter in 1757, is credited with recognizing an arteriovenous aneurysm as direct communication between the artery and vein, while previous observers having interpreted the lesion as a simple aneurysm (HUNTER 1762). He studied two patients in whose arms the vessels had been injured by phlebotomy, an operation extensively practiced at that time not only by physicians but also charlatans and barbers. His first accurate appraisal of an arteriovenous communication, described not only the bruit and the palpable thrill at the site of communication but also the marked dilatation and tortuosity of the artery at the site of the fistula:

"In a former paper upon aneurysm, I took notice of a species of that complaint, which, so far as I know, had not been mentioned by any other author; where there is an anstomosis or immediate connection between the artery and the vein at the part where the patient let blood in consequence of the artery being wounded through the vein; so that blood passes immediately from the trunk of the artery into the trunk of the vein and so back into the heart. It will differ in its symptoms from the spurious aneurysm principally thus. The vein will be dilated or become vari-cose and it will have a pulsatile jarring motion on account of the stream from the artery. It will make a hissing noise, which will be found to correspond with the pulse for the same reason. The blood of the tumor will be altogether or almost entirely fluid because of its constant motion".

CLEGHORN (1769) suggested the name "aneurismal varix" for the direct communication. Without postmortem evidence for his conclusions, Benjamin TRAVERS in 1809 described first pulsating exophthalmos and designated it as "Aneurysma per anstomosin" or "cirsoid aneurysms of the orbit" (Fig. 2.1) (TRAVERS 1811).

Three years later on April 7, 1813, DALRYMPLE (1815) operated a second, similar case of pulsating exophthalmos and followed Travers' explanation for its etiology, as did the majority of subsequent writers until 1823.

In these years the French anatomist BRESCHET (1829) studied in detail the vascular anatomy of the brain and skull, as well as the head and neck area and provided color plates in most outstanding quality (Fig. 2.2).

GUTHRIE (1827) recorded during the same period the first necropsy of a patient with pulsating exophthalmos and found instead of a "cirsoid aneurysm" an aneurysm of the ophthalmic artery: "On the death of the patient an aneurism of the ophthalmic artery was discovered on each side, of about the size of a large nut". Thus, he was led to believe erroneously that it was the usual lesion in pulsating exophthalmos and advocated this as etiology of all reported cases of pulsating exophthalmos. This was supported by BUSK's (1839) autopsy findings of another case.

However, in France, four years prior to the BUSK report, it was BARON (1835) who is given credit for being the first to discover a direct communication between the internal carotid and the cavernous sinus. Even though his report was so brief that it was

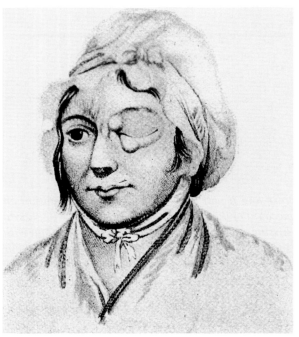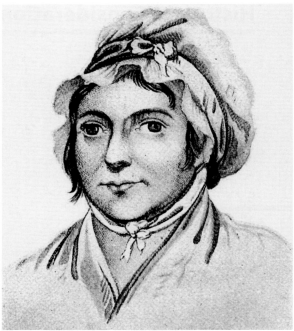

Fig. 2.1. The first description of a pulsating exophthalmos. Engravings of Travers' patient before and after operation. (From Med Chir Trans 1813)

not noticed by many of his colleagues, he in fact established very early on the most important aspect in the etiology of pulsating exophthalmos, namely its intracranial cause. GENDRIN (1841) found the same communication, and in 1856, Nelaton (HENRY 1959) reported the similar finding.

In 1851, NELATON (1857) also described the conversion of an arteriovenous aneurysm into a simple aneurysm due to thrombophlebitis and reported that the simple aneurysm was cured by proximal ligation. BROCA (1856) applied the name "varicose aneurysm" to the direct communication by way of a false aneurysm sac interposed between artery and vein. GUATTANUS (1785) is given credit for the first cure of a brachial aneurysmal varix by a combination of direct and indirect methods of compression. In 1833, BRESCHET described two cases of arteriovenous fistula treated by ligation of the artery proximal to the opening, followed in each instance by gangrene of the limb beyond the fistula.

BARON (1835) first showed that the essential defect of a carotid cavernous sinus fistula was an opening between the internal carotid artery and the cavernous sinus.

DELENS (1870) found in cadavers that the carotid artery, injected under pressure, ruptured most often in the segment coursing within the cavernous sinus. It was also found that, in certain cases, pre-existing aneurysms of the ICA had ruptured into the CS either spontaneously or as result of trauma. Direct trauma to the carotid cavernous sinus area by knitting needles, bullets, umbrella staves and similar sharp-pointed objects was also reported to have produced the lesion.

Interestingly, the concept of ruptured carotid artery in its course through the cavernous sinus, as supported by Delens, Nelaton and other French authors, was only reluctantly accepted in England. Travers, Dalrymple, and after them many English physicians, considered pulsating exophthalmos caused by an intraorbital aneurysm. This was in part due to HULKE (1859) and BOWMAN (1860), who observed a case in which they found all signs of pulsating exophthalmos including a dilated ophthalmic vein on autopsy, but no alterations in the carotid artery. Thus, they continued to suggest the theory of ophthalmic artery aneurysms based on the earlier observation of GUTHRIE (1827). Nunneley, Chief Surgeon of the Leeds Eye and Ear Infirmary, was the first English author who accepted that pulsating exophthalmos might indeed have an intracranial origin NUNNELEY (1864).

The excellent thesis of DELENS (1870), and the lectures of Timothy Holmes (HOLMES 1873) before the

a

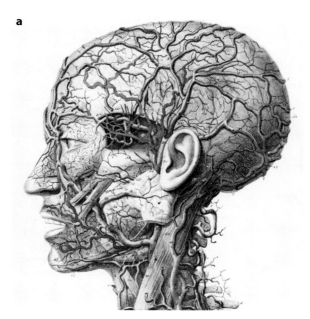

b

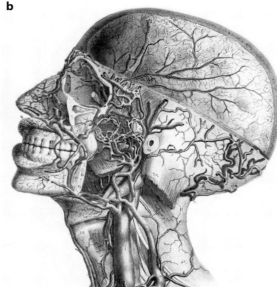

c

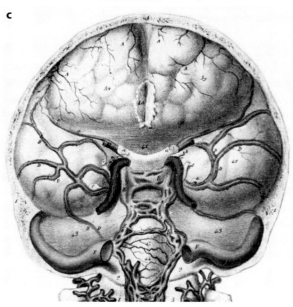

Fig. 2.2a–c. Vascular anatomy of the head and neck area as seen by Breschet in 1829, from *"Recherches Anatomique, Physiologique sur le Systeme Veineux et Specialment sur le Canaux Veineux des Os"*. **a** Superficial veins of the head and neck. Shown is the extensive network of scalp veins, mainly the superficial and middle temporal vein, frontal veins, angular vein, and facial vein draining into the external jugular vein. **b** Deep veins of the head and neck and their connection to the intraorbital veins. The pterygopalatine fossa is shown with the pterygoid plexus that drains via the retromandibular vein into the external jugular vein. The internal jugular vein, markedly larger in caliber, lies underneath and anterior to the external jugular vein. **c** Cerebral veins and intracranial sinuses. The ICA is shown with the cavernous sinus, intercavernous sinus, the inferior petrosal sinus and basilar plexus. The drawing also shows the communication between jugular bulb, intraspinal veins and vertebral plexus. Note the more plexiform appearance of both, the CS and the IPS

Royal College of Surgeons in England between 1872–1875 on the "The Surgical Treatment of Aneurism in Its Various Forms" helped the slow acceptance of the intracranial cause for an orbital symptomatology as arteriovenous aneurysm within the cavernous sinus (Fig. 2.3).

Sattler, Professor of Ophthalmology in Erlangen, provided the first detailed review of 106 cases collected to that date (SATTLER 1880). He was opposed to the reports of Guthrie, Busk and Hulke and supported the etiology of an arteriovenous communica-tion that in his opinion must have been frequently overlooked in previous descriptions. One of the interesting findings in his work is that in some cases significant thrombosis of the cavernous sinus or the superior ophthalmic vein was found. Nevertheless, he never assumed this per se could cause or trigger the typical symptoms of pulsating Exophthalmos. Most reports and studies of the following 50 years (including Dandys work) are based on the initial material provided by SATTLER (1920, 1930), who continued his work and reported on 322 patients.

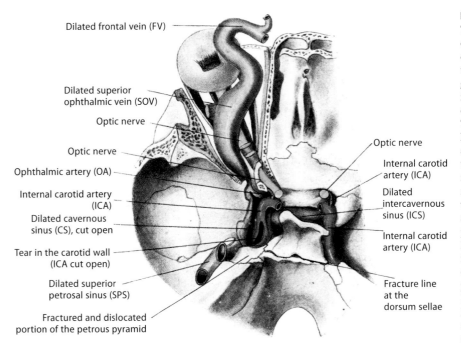

Dilated frontal vein (FV)

Dilated superior
ophthalmic vein (SOV)

Optic nerve

Optic nerve

Ophthalmic artery (OA)

Internal carotid artery
(ICA)

Dilated cavernous
sinus (CS), cut open

Tear in the carotid wall
(ICA cut open)

Dilated superior
petrosal sinus (SPS)

Fractured and dislocated
portion of the petrous pyramid

Optic nerve

Internal carotid
artery (ICA)

Dilated
intercavernous
sinus (ICS)

Internal carotid
artery (ICA)

Fracture line
at the
dorsum sellae

Fig. 2.3. Delens' (1870) case. The second illustrated case of a traumatic CCF from the clinic of Nelaton after an autopsy report of a 17-year-old girl who developed a "pulsating exophthalmos" after a fall out of a carriage in July 1864. The patient presented 6 months later and died 7 days following an unsuccessful operation due to pyemia. A fracture line running through the posterior and middle cranial fossa is seen, as well as a portion of the petrous apex that is detached and likely penetrated the carotid artery. Drainage into the enlarged intercavernous sinus, superior ophthalmic vein and superior petrosal sinus. (From Sattler 1920, 1930: Pulsierender Exophthalmus. In: Handbuch der Gesamten Augenheilkunde, Springer, pp 114–115)

de Schweinitz and Holloway (1908) in an analysis of 313 previously reported cases found that an abnormal communication between the internal carotid and cavernous sinus was the most frequent cause of unilateral exophthalmos, but that an aneurysm of the ophthalmic, or carotid arteries or even a tumor of the orbit could produce the same symptoms (Fig. 2.4).

Locke (1924) comprehensively reviewed 588 cases of pulsating exophthalmos, of which 126 occurred spontaneously and 418 were of traumatic origin. Conducting careful necropsies, he also found among 33 spontaneous cases that only 16 were caused by a communication between the artery and sinus. Seven cases occurred due to tumor, three due to aneurysm of the ICA, and three due to aneurysm of the ophthalmic artery. In one case no lesion was found. In 17 cases of traumatic origin, autopsies showed that 16 were due to direct communication between the carotid artery and the cavernous sinus and only one case was caused by an aneurysm.

Dandy (1935) and others found in reviews of postmortem examinations that the opening between the artery and sinus had varied in size from 1 mm to 10 mm and (Loehr 1937) that in a few instances the artery had been completely severed, the two ends lying within the sinus but separated by a centimeter or more. In some cases the carotid wall appeared to have weakened by arteriosclerosis and "given way, as do vessels in the brain".

2.2
Angiography

Only one year after the invention of X-rays by Conrad Roentgen in 1895, Hascheck and Lindenthal (1896) performed the first angiogram on an amputated hand using chalk as contrast agent. On the 28th of June, 1927 during his ninth attempt, Egaz Moniz (Moniz 1927) performed the first cerebral angiogram ever, using strontium bromide in a 20-year-old boy who was blind because of a tumor in the sellar region. This procedure required direct contrast injection after surgical exposure and temporary ligation of the carotid artery. It was the first in vivo radiogram of the cerebral arteries showing displacement and stretching of the vessels by the tumor and represents a milestone in the development of diagnostic radiology.

Terry and Mysel (1934) performed the first angiogram in a patient with pulsating exophthalmos by injecting thorium dioxide sol. They were able to demonstrate the AV fistula between the internal carotid artery and the internal jugular vein in the upper part of the neck.

In the same year, Ziedses des Plantes (1934) presented a thesis in which he introduced two major elements of the twentieth century radiology, film tomography and film subtraction angiography. The latter, which was the predecessor to X-ray digital subtraction angiography (DSA), was an important step forwards since it allowed for separating the relevant vessel information from superimposing osseous background. Some of the first angiographic images of patients with pulsating exophthalmos were presented by LOEHR (1936) and TOENNIS et al. (1936) in Berlin.

LOEHR (1936) initially did not express much enthusiasm when he stated: "Contrary to genuine aneurysms, the traumatic forms at the base of the cranium cannot be demonstrated so well by arteriography, since the blood and with it the contrast substance can pass into the sinus cavernous without coming into the hemisphere."

DANDY (1937) who felt the clinical signs of pulsating exophthalmos are so striking that confirmation by another diagnostic procedure is not required, was initially very reluctant to see the need for cerebral angiography. Referring to the work of Terry and Mysel he stated "Since the clinical picture of these aneurysms is unmistakable, one cannot be justified in unnecessary procedures merely to display them more graphically".

There has been a noteworthy contribution to the subject by WOLFF and SCHMID (1939) from Wuerzburg in 1939, who carefully studied the venous drainage pattern of carotid cavernous fistulas and developed the first classification for CCFs (Figs. 2.5 and 4.2) that brought more acceptance to cerebral angiography. LIST and HODGES (1945) confirmed this work and were followed by others (RAMOS and MOUNT 1953; RANEY et al. 1948; ALPERS et al. 1951). RANEY and RANEY (1948) recognized the value of arteriography in carotid cavernous fistulas for assessment of the collateral circulation through the circle of Willis; in cases where no dye would fill cerebral vessels, a trapping procedure could probably be performed safely.

FALCONER and HOARE (1951) reported on a patient with a traumatic carotico-cavernous fistula that was maintained through the external carotid

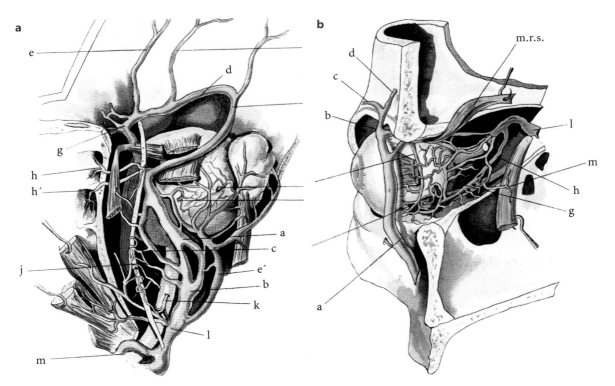

Fig. 2.4a,b. Veins of the orbit after Festal: *"Recherches anatomiques sur les veines de l'orbite, leurs anastmoses avec les veines des regiones voisins"*, Thesis, Paris 1878. In *"Die Erkrankungen der Orbita"*, Birch-Hirschfeld, 1930. The illustrations show nicely the intraorbital anatomy and the relationship between eye bulb, muscles and veins. The communications of the superior ophthalmic vein with the angular vein and facial vein, frontal and supraorbital vein are demonstrated. In addition, the superior and inferior root of the superior ophthalmic vein, as discussed in more detail later (Chap. 3), is shown

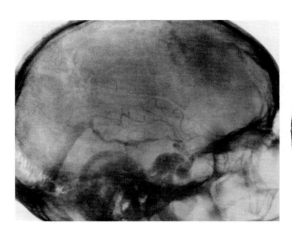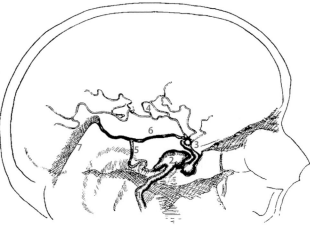

Fig. 2.5. Probably one of the first angiograms of a cavernous sinus fistula, obtained and published in 1939 (Wolff and Schmidt 1939). The authors described the leptomeningeal drainage via the basal vein of Rosenthal (6) and an anastomotic vein (5) which they were unable to identify as lateral (or anterior?) mesencephalic vein, probably filled via the SPS

artery. They were able to demonstrate angiographic evidence of cerebral arteries filled via the internal maxillary and ophthalmic artery anastomoses.

Parsons et al. (1954) reported the first spontaneous occlusion of a CSF following angiography.

Higazi and El-Bahanwy (1963) demonstrated the value of cerebral angiography for differential diagnosis in cases where other diseases may present the typical clinical picture of a classical carotid cavernous fistula. The authors emphasized its value in several aspects: the presence of a fistula, its exact site, the differentiation between unilateral and bilateral fistula etc.

Hayes (1958) suggested the differentiation in high-flow and low-flow fistulas. It became more obvious that angiography had significant value not only as a new diagnostic tool but also as a measure for efficacy of treatment methods and for development of new strategies. A few years later (Hayes 1963) he showed angiographic evidence in several cases of carotid cavernous fistula that reoccurred after ligation due to collateral flow through external carotid branches.

Possibly the first who observed a DCSF angiographically was Lie in 1961, when he performed an angiogram in a patient with "non-pulsating" exophthalmos (Lie 1968, Fig. 28 there). He noted a bilateral abnormal network near the sellar region, supplied by branches of the internal maxillary and middle meningeal artery. Although he could not identify a fistula to the CS he commented this must have been an "abnormal form of carotid cavernous shunt".

Castaigne et al. (1966) were probably the first to recognize and demonstrate the angiographic characteristics of a dural cavernous sinus fistula.

By 1939, Steinberg (1939) and Castellanos et al. (1937) had already investigated the possibility of performing iodine-enhanced angiography using intravenous injection. In the 1970s the development of real-time digital fluoroscopic image processors was begun and led to the introduction of three systems in 1980 (Mistretta and Grist 1998). Because intravenous DSA provided inconsistent image quality and often required repeated injection to overcome artery-vein overlap, a radiologist recognized that digital real time subtraction capabilities could be used with intra-arterial injections (intra-arterial DSA). Intra-arterial DSA has advanced and improved remarkably since, and despite significant technological efforts and investments in non-invasive imaging technique, is still the gold standard for vascular diagnosis due to its superior spatial resolution, unmatched time resolution and overall image quality. The development of three-dimensional DSA in the late 1990s has opened a wide range of new possibilities for visualization of cerebral vascular anatomy. Recently, the introduction of FD technology pushes again the limits of high quality vascular imaging (see more detail in Sect. 7.2.5).

2.3

Therapeutic Measures

When Travers was a demonstrator of anatomy at Guys Hospital in London in 1811, he ligated successfully the left common carotid artery for a carotid cavernous sinus fistula. Thus he became not only the first to describe the condition but also the first to describe its therapy even before the discovery of anesthesia.

France of Guys Hospital, in 1853 was the first to describe spontaneous thrombosis of the fistula (FRANCE 1855) without digital compression or ligation.

GIOPPI (1858) of Padua suggested intermittent digital compression of the carotid artery in 1856, and he is credited with being the first to use it successfully. VANZETTI (1858) very shortly afterward described this method in more detail.

Brainard, Professor of Surgery at Rush Medical School in Chicago in 1852 attempted as one of the first to cure an "erectile tumor of the orbit" by injecting "lactate of iron" and "puncture with hot needles" in a 35-year-old patient (BRAINARD 1853) in whom ligation a year earlier had failed (KOSARY et al. 1968). Similar attempts were made at the same time in Europe by GIRALDES (1853-1854) and PRAVEZ et al. (1853), who used "perchloride of iron" for injection, which was, however, followed by gangrene. These attempts represented a different therapeutic approach, namely ignoring the inflow tracts and attempting to obliterate the outflow tract of a carotid cavernous complex.

PETREQUIN (1846), BOURGUET (1855), and CINISELLI (1868) suggested electropuncture using acupuncture needles made of platinum with an iron tip.

LANSDOWN (1875), surgeon at Bristol General Hospital, attempted to cure a traumatic case with ligation and removal of the varicose ophthalmic veins. This technique was also performed and advocated by SATTLER (1880, 1905) (Fig. 2.6).

In Berlin, ZELLER (1911) questioned ligation of the carotid artery as a suitable treatment and opposed to the "dangerous" bilateral ligation in cases of retrograde filling of the fistula via collateral vessels through the circle of Willis or the external carotid system. He suggested a new approach namely the "voellige Ausschaltung des Arterienstueckes in dem das Loch sitzt, aus dem arteriellen Kreislauf durch proximale und distale Ligatur", the trapping of the fistulous carotid by proximal ligation in the neck and distal ligation proximal or immediately distal to the origin of the ophthalmic artery. After studies in cadavers he was able to demonstrate in 1908 that this procedure was effective. Even though his patient died due to intraoperative rupture of the ICA caused by an unfortunate mistake of his assistant, this approach was adopted later by HAMBY and GARDNER (1933), DANDY (1937) and others (TOENNIS 1937).

LOCKE (1924) described an apparatus for external compression of the large vessels in the neck, consisting of a wooden frame and a rubber band (Fig. 2.7).

BROOKS (1931), in discussing a paper by Noland and Taylor before the Southern Surgical Association, reported a unique method for obliteration of CCF: He opened the carotid and packed a strip of muscle between the clamps. The incision of the artery was then closed and the clamps removed so that the blood stream would force the muscle piece downstream into the fistula site. The patient lost vision but otherwise recovered. This procedure, although never really proven, has since been considered the first successful arterial embolization. Whether or not the muscle piece in fact plugged the fistula or just occluded the carotid remains unknown. Brooks himself discussed critically in his original description: "Owing to the marked curvature of the bony canal through which the carotid artery enters the intracranial cavity, it is of course, difficult to be sure that our attempt to obliterate the artery at the site of fistulous opening was successful. We believe however this was accomplished."

The procedure was modified by Gardner (HAMBY and GARDNER 1933) on May 15, 1931 who used a piece of muscle the size of a pea (5 mm) and attached a silver clip for radiographic localization. The idea here was to make the embolus small enough to enter the venous component (sinus) of the fistula where "it would be an active nucleus for the rapid production of thrombus that would close the opening". The bruit immediately ceased and proptosis improved until it reoccurred 8 days later and the patient underwent ligation.

In 1934, Dandy occluded the intracranial ICA with a silver clip (DANDY 1937), followed by WALKER and ALLEGRE (1956), ADSON (1942) and TOENNIS et al. (1937).

GURDJIAN (1938) reported a case in which external and internal carotid arteries were ligated and 2×0.25 cm muscle plugs were introduced to remove the carotid opening at the site of the lesion. This re-

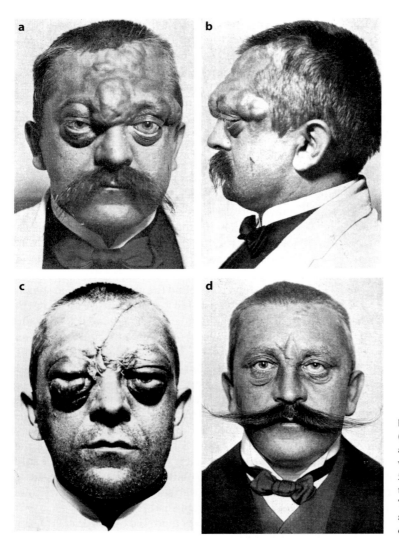

Fig. 2.6a–d. One of Sattler's patients (Case Wiesinger, 1903): Traumatic CCF in a 38-year-old male who presented in 1903 with bilateral pulsating exophthalmos of 5 years' standing. Extreme varicose dilation of frontal and supraorbital veins (**a,b**). Three weeks after bilateral ligation and resection of the SOV (**c**) and 17 months after cure of the fistula (**d**)

sulted in improvement of proptosis, ophthalmoplegia and vision.

JAEGER (1949) reported the successful combination of intracranial clipping of the internal carotid, muscle embolus and ligation of the carotid in the neck in a 12-year-old boy 7 years earlier. He was able to control the position of the embolus using X-ray identification of the silver clip at the carotid cavernous opening. The patient was immediately and completely cured when seen again for a 7-years follow-up. In 1959 he reported on six cases being successfully treated using the same technique.

PARKINSON (1963a,b) devised the direct surgical approach to the cavernous sinus using hyperthermia and cardiac arrest. Although his first patient died due to pulmonary complications, this new approach opened the door for microsurgical techniques in

the treatment of carotid cavernous fistulas, some of which are employed until today in intractable cases.

2.4
Embolization

On September, 25th in 1963, LANG and BUCY (1965) were able to successfully treat a case with free embolization of a muscle piece with silver clip and referred to several additional previous reports in the literature. While all of those had to undergo intracranial ligation because of persisting symptoms, the case of Lang and Bucy was cured by embolism

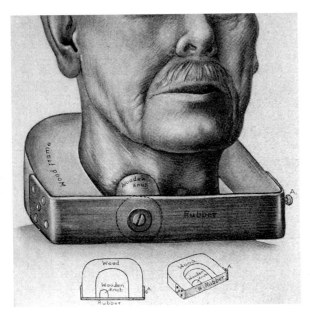

Fig. 2.7. Instrument employed to compress the common carotid artery against the transverse process of the cervical vertebrae, from LOCKE (1924): Intracranial arteriovenous aneurysm or pulsating exophthalmos. The frame was placed around the neck and the rubber band was then stretched over the screw

alone. The control angiogram confirmed complete thrombosis of the ipsilateral internal carotid while good cross flow was preserved from the contralateral territory. KOSARY et al. (1968) reported the successful embolization of a CCF using porcelain beads.

To avoid distal migration of the embolus, ARUTIUNOV et al. (1968) had developed a particular technique, consisting of a clipped muscle embolus attached to a nylon string. This allowed controlling of the embolus to the fistula site under X-ray, and securing it in place by anchoring it to the ICA ligation. This technique was performed in 13 patients with 100% success and can be considered the precursor of detachable balloons introduced a few years later. PROLO and HANBERY performed in October 1969 an occlusion of a CCF using a nylon balloon catheter through an arteriotomy in the common carotid artery achieving complete cure.

ISAMAT et al. (1970) ingeniously embolized the fistula and preserved the patency of the carotid artery using a previously magnetized metal clip on a muscle embolus. The authors thought of guiding the embolus by an electromagnet over the skin covering the superior-anterior part of the cavernous sinus of

the left zygoma, which was however not necessary because the pressure and flow was such as to conduct the embolus properly into the fistulous opening in its venous side without interfering the patency of the carotid.

In 1973, BLACK et al. followed this concept of "flow-directed" muscle embolization and were able to maintain the patency of the carotid artery.

SERBINENKO (1971) published an article about the use of detachable balloons for occlusion of cerebral vessels. This first and quite significant contribution was published only in the Russian literature and was initially missed by most Westerners. It was after his second report, this time published in the English literature (SERBINENKO 1974), that colleagues like CHERMET et al. (1977) followed in his footsteps.

PETERSON et al. (1969) deserves credit for the first retrograde venous passage through the SOV using a copper wire and positive current for electrocoagulation of a CCF.

KERBER et al. (1979) pioneered the use cyanoacrylate to occlude a carotid cavernous fistula with preservation of the carotid artery flow. He used a particular calibrated leak balloon microcatheter in three patients and was able to occlude the fistula but with persistent neurological complication in one.

These and other pioneering efforts opened the door to a new era of therapeutic management of carotid cavernous fistulas: endovascular treatment using arterial embolization. Minimal invasive management has been firmly established since, has continuously advanced over the following years, and has eventually been augmented by transvenous occlusion (TVO) techniques in the 1990s (more in Chap. 8).

References

Adson A (1942) Surgical treatment of vascular disease altering function of the eyes. Am J Ophthalmol 25:824

Alpers B, Schlezinger N, Tassman I (1951) Bilateral internal carotid aneurysm involving cavernous sinus, right carotid artery-cavernous fistula and left saccular aneurysm. Arch Ophthal 46:403–408

Arutiunov AI, Serbinenko FA, Shlykov AA (1968) Surgical treatment of carotid-cavernous fistulas. Prog Brain Res 30:441–444

Baron M (1835) Comptu rendu des travaux de la societe anatomique pendant l'annee 1835. Bull Acad Med. Paris 1:178

Black P, et al. (1971) Carotid-cavernous fistula: a technique for occlusion of fistula with preservation of carotid blood flow. Trans Am Neurol Assoc. 96:205–208.

Black P, et al. (1973) Carotid-cavernous fistula: a controlled embolus technique for occlusion of fistula with preservation of carotid blood flow. Technical note. J Neurosurg. 38(1):113-118.

Bourguet (1855). Note sur un cas d'anevrisme de l'artere ophthalmique et de ses principles branches gueri du moyen des injections de perchlorure de fer. Gaz. med. de Paris 49:772

Bowman (1860) Med Times Gaz II

Brainard (1853) Case of erectile tumor of the orbit, cured by iniltration with the solution of lactate of iron and puncture with hot needles after ligation of the carotid artery had failed etc. Lancet August 20th:162

Breschet G (1829) Recherches anatomique, physiologiques sur le systeme veineux et specialment sur les canaux veineux des os. Paris, Vileret et Rouen

Breschet, G. (1833) Memiore sur les aneurysmes. Mem Acad Roy Med (Paris). 3:101

Broca P (1856) Des anevrismes et de leur traitment. Paris, 1856

Brooks, B. (1930) The treatment of traumatic arteriovenous fistula. South. med. J. 23:100-106.

Brooks B (1931) Discussion of Noland L and Taylor AS. Trans South Surg Ass 43:176-177

Busk (1839) Med Chir Trans xxii:124

Castaigne P, Laplane D, Djindjian R, Bories J, Augustin P (1966) Spontaneous arteriovenous communication between the external carotid and the cavernous sinus. Rev Neurol (Paris) 114:5-14

Castellanos A, Pereiras R, Garcia A (1937) La angiocardiografia radiopaqua. Arch Habana 31:523-596

Chermet M, Cabanis EA, Debrun G, Haut J (1977) Carotidocavernous fistula treated with inflatable balloons. Bull Soc Ophtalmol Fr 77:903-908

Ciniselli (1868) Della electropunctura nell cura degli aneurismi dell' Aorta thoracica. Gaz Med Italiana Lombarda 39

Cleghorn G (1769) A case of aneurysmal varix. Med Obs Soc Phys (London) 3:110

Dalrymple W (1815) A case of aneurysm by anastomosis in the left orbit, cured by tying the common trunk of the left carotid artery. Trans Med Chir Soc Edinburg 6:111-112

Dandy W (1935) The treatment of carotid cavernous aneurysms. Ann Surg 102:916-920

Dandy W (1937) Carotid-cavernous aneurysms (pulsating exophthalmos). Zentral Bl Neurochir 2:77-206

Dandy WE. (1957) The treatment of carotid cavernous arteriovenous aneurysms. In: Selected writings of Walter E. Dandy, C.E. Troland and F.J. Otenasek, Editors. Charles Thomas: Springfield Ill. p. 521-522, 667-681

De Schweinitz G, Holloway T (1908) Pulsating Exophthalmos: its etiology, symptomatology, pathogenesis and treatment. Saunders, Philadelphia

Delens E (1870) De la communication de la carotide interne et du sinus caverneux. Paris

Falconer M, Hoare R (1951) Carotico-cavernous fistula causing pulsating exophthalmos with cerebral blood flow maintained through the external carotid artery. Proc R Soc Med 225-228

France J (1855) Case of pulsating swelling of the orbit. Guys Hosp Rep Series 3:58

Gendrin MAN (1841) Lecons sur la maladies du coeur. Bailliere (Paris) 1:240-260

Gioppi G (1858) Aneurisma dell' arteria oftalmica. Giornale d'oftalmol Italiana

Giraldes M (1853-1854) Presentation de malade. Bull Soc Chir (Paris) 4:22

Guattanus C (1785) De externis aneurysmatibus. Scriptorium Latinorum de Aneurysmatibus. Collectio. 101:234

Gurdjian ES (1938) Packing of the internal carotid artery with muscle in treatmentnt of carotid-cavernous arteriovenous aneurysms. Arch Ophthal 19:936-940

Guthrie (1827) Operative surgery of the eye, 2nd edn. Burgess and Hill, London

Hamby W, Gardner W (1933) Treatment of pulsating exophthalmos with report of 2 cases. Arch Surg 27:676-685

Hamby, WB, (1966) Carotid-cavernous fistula. Vol. III. Springfield: Charles C Thomas. 9-15; 59-62

Haschek E, Lindenthal T (1896) Ein Beitrag zur praktischen Verwertung der Photographie nach Roentgen. Wien Klin Wochenschr 9:63-64

Hayes GJ (1958) Carotid cavernous fistulas: diagnosis and surgical management. Am Surg 24:839-843

Hayes GJ (1963) External carotid-cavernous sinus fistulas. J Neurosurg 20:692-700

Henry (1956) Consideration sur l'anevrisme arteriosoveineux. Paris, p 13

Henry, J (1959) Contribution a l'etude de l'anatomie des vaisseaux de l'orbite et de la loge caverneuse par injection de matieres plastiques, du tendon de Zinn et de la capsule de Tenon. These. Paris: Typescript no. 638.

Higazi, I. and A. El-Banhawy (1964). The Value of Angiography in the Differential Diagnosis of Pulsating Exophthalmos; a Report of 3 Cases. J Neurosurg 21: 561-566.

Holmes T (1873) Holmes lectures. Lancet ii:142

Hulke (1859) All the capital signs of orbital aneurism present, in a marked degree, but independently of aneurism or any erectile tumor. Ophthalmic Hosp Rep II:6

Hunter W (1762) Further observations upon a particular species of aneurism. Med Observations Inquiries 2:390-440

Hunter, W (1757) The history of an aneurysm of the aorta, with some remarks on aneurysms in general. Med Observ Inquir. (1):323

Isamat F, Salleras V, Miranda AM (1970) Artificial embolization of carotid-cavernous fistula with post-operative patency of internal carotid artery. J Neurol Neurosurg Psychiatr 33:674-678

Jaeger R (1949) Intracranial aneurysms. South Surg 15:205-217

Kerber CW, Bank WO, Cromwell LD (1979) Cyanoacrylate occlusion of carotid-cavernous fistula with preservation of carotid artery flow. Neurosurgery 4:210-215

Kosary IZ, Lerner MA, Mozes M, Lazar M (1968) Artificial embolic occlusion of the terminal internal carotid artery in the treatment of carotid-cavernous fistula. Technical note. J Neurosurg 28:605-608

Lang ER, Bucy PC (1965). Treatment of Carotid-Cavernous Fistula by Muscle Embolization Alone: The Brooks Method. J Neurosurg 22:387-392

Lansdown F (1875) A case of varicose aneurism of the left orbit, cured by ligature of the diseased vessels. Brit Med J 1:736-846

Lie, T (1968) Congenital anomalies of the carotid arteries. An angiographic study and a review of the literature. Monograph. Excerpta Medical Foundation. Amsterdam: 35-51.

List C, Hodges F (1945) Intracranial angiography I. J Neurosurg 3:25–45

Locke C (1924) Intracranial arteriovenous aneurysm or pulsating exophthalmos. Ann Surg 80:1–24

Loehr (1937) Schlaefenlappentumoren, ihre Klinik und arteriographische Diagnostik. Zbl. Neurochir. 2: p. 1-7.

Loehr, W (1936) Hirngefaessverletzungen in arteriographischer Darstellung. Zbl. Chir. 63 2466-2482.

Loehr W, Jacobi W (1933) Die kombinierte Enzephalarteriographie. Fortschritte auf dem Gebiet der Roentgenstrahlen und Nuklearmedizin. 44

Mistretta CA, Grist TM (1998) X-ray digital subtraction angiography to magnetic resonance-digital subtraction angiography using three-dimensional TRICKS. Historical perspective and computer simulations: a review. Invest Radiol 33:496–505

Moniz E (1927) Radiografia das arterias cerebrais. J Soc Ciencias Med Lisboa XCL:8

Nelaton (1857) Cons. sur l'anevrsime arterio-veneux, These d'Henry, Paris

Nunnely (1864) On vascular protrusion of the eyeball, being a second series of three cases and two postmortem examinations of so-called aneurism by anastomosis of the orbit with some observations of the affection. Med Times Gaz 752:602

Parkinson D (1963a) Normal anatomy of cavernous carotid and its surgical significance. Presented at Annual Meeting of Harvey Cushing Society, Philadelphia

Parkinson D (1963b) Carotid cavernous fistula with pulsating exophthalmos: a fortuitous cure. Can J Surg 6:191–195

Parsons TC, Guller EJ, Wolff HG, Dunbar HS (1954) Cerebral angiography in carotid cavernous communications. Neurology 4:65–68

Peterson E, Valberg J, Whittingham D (1969) Electrically induced thrombosis of the cavernous sinus in the treatment of carotid-cavernous-fistula. Presented at Fourth International Congress of Neurological Surgery and Ninth International Congress of Neurology, Amsterdam, New York, London

Petrequin (1846) Memoire sur une nouvelle methode pour guerir certains anevrisme. Gaz Med Paris

Petrequin (1845) Anevrisme de l'artere opthalm. etc., in Comptes rendu de l'academie de science: Paris. 994.

Pravez M, Giraldes M, Debout M (1853) Revue Medico-Chirurgicale de Paris

Prolo DJ, Hanbery JW (1971) Intraluminal occlusion of a carotid-cavernous sinus fistula with a balloon catheter. Technical note. J Neurosurg. 35(2):237–242

Ramos M, Mount L (1953) Carotid cavernous fistula with signs on contralateral side. Case Report. J Neurosurg 10:178–182

Raney R, Raney AA, et al. (1949). The role of complete cerebral angiography in neurosurgery. J Neurosurg 6(3): 222–237.

Robb G, Steinberg I (1939) Visualization of the chambers of the heart, the pulmonary circulation, and the great blood vessels in man. AJR Am J Roentgenol 41:1–17

Sattler H (1880) Pulsierender exophthalmus. In: Graefe A, Saemisch T (eds) Handbuch der Gesamten Augenheilkunde. Engelmann, Leipzig, pp 745–948

Sattler H (1905) Ueber ein neues Verfahren bei der Behandlung des pulsierenden Exophthalmus. Klin Monatsbl Augenheilk 4:1–6

Sattler, H (1920) Pulsierender Exophthalmus, in Handbuch der Gesamten Augenheilkunde, A. Graefe and T. Saemisch, Editors. Julius Springer: Berlin. p 1–245.

Sattler, H (1930) Pulsierender Exophthalmus. In: Graefe A, Saemisch T (eds) Handbuch der Gesamten Augenheilkunde. Leipzig: Engelmann, p 1–241

Serbinenko F (1971) Catheterization and occlusion of major cerebral vessels and prospects for the development of vascular neurosurgery [in Russian]. Vopr Neirokhir 35:17–27

Serbinenko FA (1974) Balloon catheterization and occlusion of major cerebral blood vessels. J Neurosurg 41:125–145

Terry T, Mysel P (1934) Pulsating exophthalmos due to internal carotid-jugular aneurysm: the use of thorium dioxide sol in localization. JAMA 103:1036–1041

Toennis W (1936) Aneurysma arterio-venosusm, in Gefaessmissbildungen und Gefaessgeschwuelste des Gehirns, H. Bergstrand and H. Olivecrona, Editors. Thieme: Leipzig. p 88–134.

Toennis W (1961) Zur Entstehung der Rezidive bei der Behandlung der Carotis-Sinus-Cavernosus-Aneurysmen und ihre Verhuetung. Arch. klin. Chir. (295): p 186–191

Travers B (1811) A case of aneurysm by anastomosis in the orbit, cured by the ligature of the common carotid artery. Med Chir Tr 2:1–16

Vanzetti (1858) Secondo caso di aneurisma dell' arteria oftalmica guarito colla compressione digitali della carotide, e cenni pratici intorno a questo metodo di curare gli aneurismi. Padova, and Annali universali di medicina. CLXV:151

Walker AE, Allegre GF (1956) Carotid-cavernous fistulas. Surgery 39:411–422

Wolff H, Schmid B (1939) Das Arteriogramm des pulsierenden exophthamus. Zbl Neurochir 4:241–250

Zeller O (1911) Die chirurgische Behandlung des durch aneurysma arterio-venosum der carotis int. im Sinus cavernosus hervorgerufenen pulsirenden Exophthalmus – Ein neues Verfahren. Deutsche Ztschr Chir 111:1–39

Ziedses des Plantes B (1934) Planigrafie en Subtractie. Thesis. The University of Utrecht, The Netherlands

Anatomy of the Cavernous Sinus and Related Structures

3.1
Osseous Anatomy (Figs. 3.1, 3.2)

The cavernous sinus (CS) is closely related to the osseous structures of the middle cranial fossa such as the sphenoid bone and the sella turcica. The sphenoid bone is situated in the base of the skull and consists of a cuboid corpus containing the two sphenoid sinuses. The greater wings arise from the side of the corpus of the sphenoid bone and project transversely, bending superiorly in their anterior portion. The lesser wings are two thin triangular plates of bone arising from the anterior aspect of the sphenoid bone extending nearly horizontally and laterally. The lateral extremity of the smaller wing, slender and pointed, approaches the greater wing

but as a rule actually never touches it (TROTTER and PETERSON 1996). The superior surface is slightly smooth and concave forming the posterior part of the floor of the anterior fossa. The inferior surface constitutes a portion of the superior wall of the orbit and overhangs the superior orbital fissure (TROTTER and PETERSON 1996), the elongated opening between the wings. The posterior border of the lesser wings forms part of the boundary between the anterior and middle cranial fossa and is prolonged at its medial extremity to form the anterior clinoid process.

The superior surface of the sphenoid corpus contains the groove for the pituitary gland, Turkish saddle (sella turcica) ending anteriorly in the rounded elevation of the tuberculum sellae.

The posterior boundary of the sella turcica is formed by a quadrilateral plate of bone, the dorsum sellae; its posterior surface is sloped in continuation with the dorsal surface of the basilar part of the occipital bone and supports the pons and the basilar artery. The superior angles of the dorsum sellae are surrounded by the posterior clinoid process which give attachment to the tentorium cerebelli (TROTTER and PETERSON 1996).

On the lateral surface of the sphenoid, superior to the attachment of the greater wings is the carotid groove (sulcus caroticus), lodging the petrous and cavernous segment of the internal carotid artery (ICA). This sulcus is only posteriorly well formed where the artery enters from the apex of the petrous bone. Medially, the sulcus has a border, an osseous process, while laterally a bony projection, the lingula, continues posteriorly across the foramen lacerum (KELLER et al. 1997).

The middle clinoid processes are less well-defined and lie posterolateral to the optic canal.

An interclinoid osseous or fibrous bridge between the anterior and posterior clinoid processes can be found in 4%–9% (BORBA and AL-MEFTY 2000). A bony bridge between the anterior and middle clinoid process can form a so-called caroticoclinoid foramen (Henle). The ICA passes through this foramen during its course from the posterior to the anterior cavernous segment (C5 and C4 segment, see below) and to the supraclinoid portion. KELLER et al. (1997) found such foramen in 18 of 135 skulls (13%), of which 6 were bilateral. The interclinoid foramen, according to KEYES (1935), can be divided into complete type, contact type and incomplete type. These osseous details are mainly of interest for neurosurgeons when performing open surgical procedures for treatment of CS lesions. They are of minor importance in the context of endovascular treatment (EVT). More noteworthy instead is an understanding of the anatomic relationships between the CS and its connecting vascular structures, as well as of the related bony canals and foramina in the middle cranial fossa and the skull base. They may serve as potential routes for EVT of DCSF, and are described below in more detail.

The *foramen rotundum* is a short horizontal canal (canalis rotundus), located in the anteromedial portion of the greater sphenoid wing and is traversed by the maxillary nerve, the artery of the *foramen rotundum* and small emissary veins to the pterygoid fossa. It lies directly below the medial end of the superior orbital fissure and is intimately related to the lateral wall of the sphenoid sinus. The foramen is usually 3.4 mm long and has a size of 3 × 3 mm to 4×5 mm (LINDBLOM 1936). The foramen is best visible on radiographs (Figs. 7.17–7.20) in Caldwell and Waters projections (SHAPIRO and ROBINSON 1967). Asymmetric enlargement and communications with the superior orbital fissure are rarely seen. However, postnatal changes in its dimensions and shifts of its axis are described (LANG 1983). During postnatal life the width of the canal increases almost continuously from 2.06 mm in neonates to 3.34 mm in adults. The intracranial opening can be round or oval (SONDHEIMER 1971) and the *foramen rotundum* does not in fact form an almost circular shape, as initially stated by LUSCHKA (1967).

The *foramen ovale* is commonly an oval shaped hole in the greater sphenoid wing slightly lateral and posterior to the *foramen rotundum* (SHAPIRO and ROBINSON 1967). It transmits the mandibular division of the trigeminal nerve, the accessory meningeal artery and in the absence of the canaliculus innominatus, the lesser petrosal nerve. As stated by SHAPIRO and ROBINSON (1967), the *foramen ovale* also transmits emissary veins when the *foramen Vesalii* is not present. LINDBLOM (1936) found an average diameter of 5×8 mm. The distance from the midline averages 15–26 mm on the right and 17–30 mm on the left (LANG 1983). SHAPIRO and ROBINSON (1967) further pointed out that a wide range of variations exist, including absence and incomplete formation, which determines whether or not the vascular channels passing through them exist or not.

The sphenoidal emissary *foramen* (*foramen venosum Vesalii, sphenoid emissary foramen, foramen of Vesalius, canaliculus sphenoidalis*) is a small inconstant aperture in the greater wing, slightly anterior and medial to the *foramen ovale* and mediodorsal to the *foramen rotundum*. It transmits a small nerve (nervulus sphenoidalis lateralis) and a small vein (basal emissary vein) (LANG 1983) which connects the cavernous sinus with the pterygoid plexus (SHAPIRO and ROBINSON 1967). The foramen has an average diameter of 1.14 mm and was present in 49% on the right and 36% on the left (LANG 1983). Occasionally, the *foramen ovale* may communicate with the *foramen venosum (Vesalii)*. The venous segment may be separated from the remainder by a bony spur located anteriorly and medially, producing a duplicated foramen (LANG 1983).

The small circular *foramen spinosum* is situated directly lateral and posterior to the *foramen ovale* and gives passage to the middle meningeal artery (MMA), accompanying veins and a recurrent branch of the mandibular nerve. The *foramen spinosum* may be absent, asymmetric, incompletely formed or remain confluent with the *foramen ovale* (SHAPIRO and ROBINSON 1967). The *foramen spinosum* and the *foramen ovale* are separated by an average distance of 3.2 mm and they lie an average of 4.4 mm anterolateral to the carotid canal (BORBA and AL-MEFTY 2000). The distance from the midline ranges from 19–37 mm on the right and from 24–39 mm on the left (LANG 1983). Strictly speaking the *foramen spinosum*, like the *foramen rotundum*, is a bony canal with a length of about 7 mm.

The *foramen lacerum* is a short canal (actually not a true foramen) situated at the posterior end of the carotid groove, posteromedial to the *foramen ovale* bounded behind by the petrous apex, in front of the body and posterior border of the greater wing. It is approximately 1 cm long and contains the ICA, meningeal branches of the ascending pharyngeal artery and accompanying sympathetic and venous plexus. Some authors found, however, that no structures actually pass through the foramen (PAULLUS et al. 1977) and the carotid artery passes only through the upper half of it.

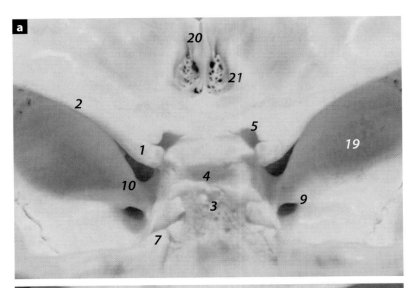

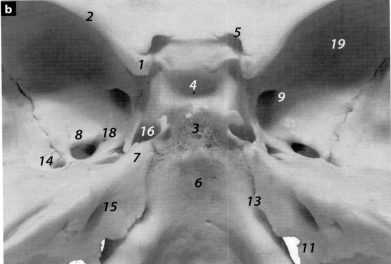

Fig. 3.1 a–c. Osseus anatomy of the parasellar region, the middle cranial fossa and the inner skull base. Cranial/posterior view.
a Most horizontal perspective from posterior showing the opening of the supraorbital fissure, the optic canal and the foramen rotundum. **b, c** More vertical views from above showing the foramen ovale, spinosum, lacerum and magnum.

1 Anterior clinoid process
2 Lesser wing of sphenoid
3 Posterior clinoid process and rough surfaced upper part of the clivus
4 Sella turcica
5 Optic canal (intracranial aperture)
6 Clivus
7 Pyramid apex
8 Foramen ovale
9 Foramen rotundum
10 Superior orbital fissure
11 Jugular foramen
12 Foramen magnum
13 Petroclival fissure (spheno-petrosal synchondrosis), groove for IPS
14 Foramen spinosum
15 Internal acoustic porus
16 Carotid canal, terminal portion of transverse petrosal part
17 Foramen lacerum
18 Foramen venosum (of Vesalius)
19 Greater wing of the sphenoid
20 Crista galli
21 Cribo-ethmoidal foramen

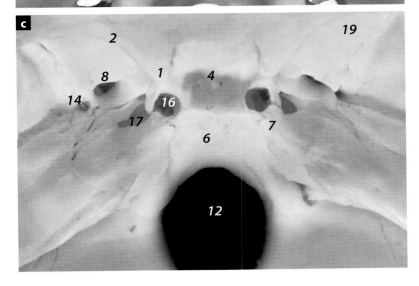

The *canaliculus innominatus* (canal of Arnold) is a minute canal, posterior to the *foramen ovale* and medial to the *foramen spinosum* (SHAPIRO and ROBINSON 1967).

The *foramen for the ophthalmomeningeal vein,* (*Hyrtl*) is situated in the greater wing, usually in the lateral half of the orbit (SHAPIRO and ROBINSON 1967). The ophthalmomeningeal vein connects orbital with cerebral veins and commonly drains into the CS. A meningolacrimal artery may also pass through this foramen and supply part of the lacrimal territory (LASJAUNIAS et al. 1975a).

The *jugular foramen* is a large aperture and lies posterolateral to the carotid canal between the petrous, temporal and occipital bones. The foramen is configured around the sigmoid sinus and the IPS. Traversing structures are the sigmoid sinus and jugular bulb, inferior petrosal sinus (IPS), meningeal branches of APA and occipital arteries, cranial nerves (CNs) IX–XI, tympanic branch of CN IX (Jacobson's nerve), auricular branch of CN X and the cochlear aqueduct. It is generally larger on the right than on the left side (68%) (KATSUTA et al. 1997), and may be subdivided into two compartments (INSERRA et al. 2004). The posterolateral pars venosa, which contains the jugular bulb and the CNs X and XI cranial nerves, is separated from the anteromedial pars nervosa, containing the IPS and CN IX, either by bone, fibrous tissue or thin connective tissue. More often, however, there is no septation and the jugular foramen exists as one compartment. The IPS, coursing from the cavernous sinus, empties into the medial aspect of the jugular bulb. The IPS often passes between the CN IX anteriorly and the CNs X and XI posteriorly.

3.1.1
Orbit (Fig. 3.2)

The orbit is shaped as a quadrilateral pyramid with its base in plane with the orbital rim. Seven bones conjoin to form the orbital structure. The orbital process of the frontal bone and the lesser wing of the sphenoid form the orbital roof. The orbital plate of the maxilla joins the orbital plate of the zygoma and the orbital plate of the palatine bones to form the floor. Medially, the orbital wall consists of the frontal process of the maxilla, the lacrimal bone, the sphenoid, and the thin lamina papyracea of the ethmoid. The lateral wall is formed by the lesser and greater wings of the sphenoid and the zygoma. The major nerves and vessels to the orbit and the globe enter through three openings.

The superior orbital fissure (SOF) represents the elongated opening between the wings and is situated between the orbits roof and lateral wall. In its medial part it is wide, but laterally it narrows and turns upwards. Its upper border is formed by the lower surface of the lesser wing. Its medial boundary is formed by the inferior root of the lesser wing and by part of the sphenoid body, while the inferior border of the SOF belongs to the greater wing of the sphenoid. It can be subdivided into a medial and lateral part by the spine of the lateral rectus muscle. The lateral boundary of the SOF is situated an average of 34 mm from the frontozygomatic suture. The greatest width of the fissure is usually found in the medial part (LANG 1983). The lesser wing of the sphenoid has a dural layer up to 3 mm thick, which covers it posteriorly together with the sphenoparietal sinus. The ramus communicans between the lacrimal artery and the frontal branch of the MMA is enclosed into this dural layer. Above the common tendinous ring, the trochlear nerve runs medially and forwards, laterally it is accompanied by the lacrimal and frontal nerves. The course of the SOV varies but is usually through the lateral part, occasionally piercing the tendinous ring. Arising from the frontal branch of the MMA, the communicating branch with the lacrimal artery runs in the lateral angle of the SOF or even through the greater wing. As a rule it anastomoses with the lacrimal artery immediately after the latter's origin from the ophthalmic artery (OA). This communicating branch can be absent or completely replace the OA, or the entire lacrimal artery can arise from the MMA. Not infrequently, a branch from this anastomotic region runs backwards through the SOF to take part in the blood supply of the nerves, bone and dura of the CS [anastomoses with the anteromedial branch of the inferolateral trunk (ILT), see Sect. 3.3.1.1.1].

The *inferior orbital fissure* (IOF) is formed by the greater wings of the sphenoid, the maxilla, and the palatines bones.

Inferior orbital fissure
- Infraorbital nerve
- Zygomatic nerve
- Parasympathetic nerves to lacrimal gland
- Infraorbital artery
- Infraorbital vein
- Inferior ophthalmic vein branch to pterygoid plexus

The *optic canal* is located at the apex of the orbit and formed by the sphenoid bone.

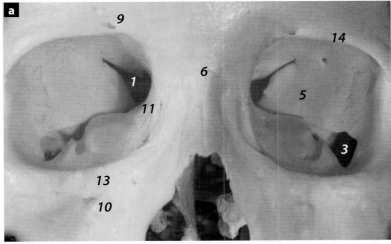

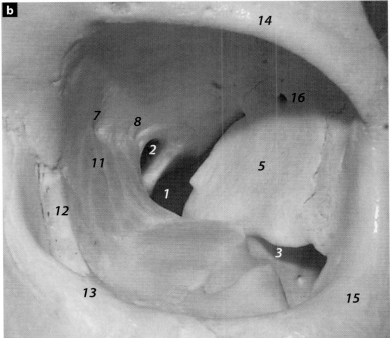

Fig. 3.2 a,b. Osseous anatomy of the orbit. Anterior view.

1 Superior orbital fissure
2 Optic canal
3 Inferior orbital fissure
4 Lesser sphenoid wing
5 Greater sphenoid wing
6 Nasion
7 Anterior ethmoidal foramen
8 Posterior ethmoidal foramen
9 Frontal foramen
10 Infraorbital foramen
11 Ethmoid
12 Lacrimal bone
13 Maxillary bone
14 Frontal bone
15 Zygoma
16 Lacrimal foramen (Hyrtl)

Optic canal
- Optic nerve
- Ophthalmic artery
- Central retinal vein

- Orbital branch of middle meningeal artery
- Recurrent branch of lacrimal artery
- Superior ophthalmic vein
- Inferior ophthalmic vein

The contents of these bony openings are as follows:
Superior orbital fissure
- Cranial nerves (CNs) III, IV, and VI
- Lacrimal nerve
- Frontal nerve
- Nasociliary nerve

As a rule the SOV runs lateral to the nerve group and lateral to the common tendinous ring and enters the CS from below (LANG 1983).

In the medial wall of the orbit along the fronto-ethmoidal suture line lie the anterior and posterior ethmoid foramina through which the anterior and posterior ethmoidal arteries pass.

3.2

Anatomy of the Dura Mater and the Cranial Nerves (Figs. 3.3, 3.4)

In most textbooks it is accepted that the CSs are located between the two layers of the dura mater: the periosteal (endosteal) layer forming the floor and most of the medial wall of the CS, and the dural layer forming its roof, lateral wall, and the upper part of the medial wall (UMANSKY and NATHAN 1987).

According to KELLER et al. (1997), only three surfaces are covered by dura mater: the superior, the lateral and the medial surface. The dura mater of the medial surface can be very thin or fenestrated.

The lower surface is covered by the periost of the floor of the middle cranial fossa. The roof of the CS is formed by the anterior extension of the tentorium and the lateral extension of the diaphragm sellae, while the lateral wall is formed by the dura propria of the middle cranial fossa.

Various concepts and contradictory descriptions of the lateral wall of the CS exist (UMANSKY and NATHAN 1987). While most classical textbooks (WARWICK and WILLIAMS 1973; CHRISTENSEN and TELFORD 1978) describe CNs III, IV and V1, V2 as being embedded in the lateral wall, others (PATURET 1964; ROUVIERE 1970) differentiate a deep and a superficial layer of the lateral wall, dividing the CS into two compartments by a "septum" and

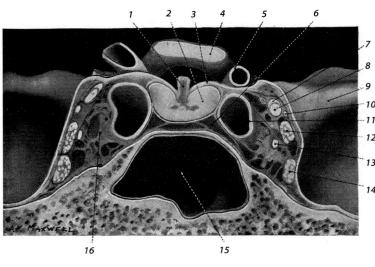

Fig. 3.3. From Professior Elliot Smiths *"Textbook of Anatomy"*, drawn from a dissection in the Moorfield Pathological Museum

1 Infundibulum
2 Hypophysis
3 Diaphragma sellae
4 Optic chiasm
5 Internal carotid artery
6 Intercavernous sinus
7 3rd cranial nerve (superior division)
8 3rd cranial nerve(inferior division)
9 Lesser sphenoid wing
10 Trochlear nerve
11 Internal carotid artery
12 1st division, 5th cranial nerve
13 6th cranial nerve
14 2nd division, 5th cranial nerve
15 Sphenoid sinus
16 Cavernous sinus

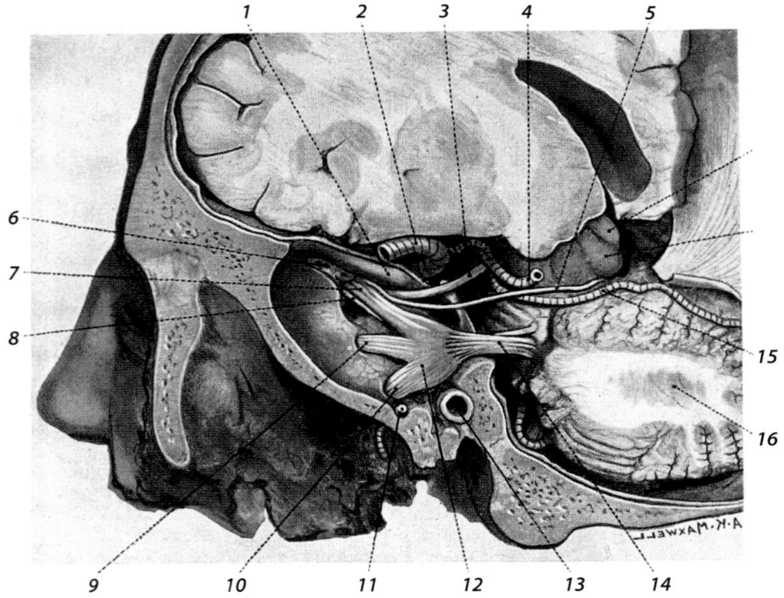

Fig. 3.4. Intracranial course of 3rd, 4th, and 5th cranial nerves (from a dissection of Wolff, E: *Anatomy of the Orbit*, 1940)

1 Anterior clinoid process
2 Middle cerebral artery
3 Third nerve
4 Posterior cerebral artery
5 Fourth nerve
6 Superior orbital fissure
7 1st division, 5th cranial nerve
8 6th cranial nerve
9 2nd division, 5th cranial nerve
10 3rd division, 5th cranial nerve
11 Middle meningeal artery
12 Gasserion ganglion
13 Internal carotid artery
14 Sensory and motor roots of 5th CN
15 Superior cerebellar artery
16 Cerebellum

containing the ICA and the sixth nerve in the deep and running the CNs III, IV and V1, V2 through this septum but not in the superficial layer. HARRIS and RHOTON (1976) found two dural layers of the lateral wall and the nerves III, IV and V1 running between them. UMANSKY and NATHAN (1982) studied the lateral wall of the CS in 70 specimens and found neither a septum dividing the CS, nor a single dural layer. They observed a superficial and a deep layer that were loosely attached to each other. The sheaths of the CNs III, IV and V1, V2 and an often incomplete reticular membrane extending between the sheaths, formed the deep layer.

The CN III penetrates the posterior CS via the oculomotor foramen (UMANSKY et al. 1994; INOUE et al. 1990) and courses anteriorly along the inferior surface of the anterior clinoid process to reach the SOF through the annulus of Zinn (KELLER et al. 1997).

The CN IV enters the CS in a dural opening between the anterior and posterior petroclinoid ligaments (UMANSKY and NATHAN 1982, 1987; UMANSKY et al. 1994) and crosses the III CN before entering the SOF without coursing through the Annulus of Zinn (KELLER et al. 1997).

The CN V1 courses from the Gasserian ganglion to the SOF inferior and lateral to CN IV and VI and lies at the level of the SOF lateral to CN VI (KELLER et al. 1997).

The CN VI exits the pontomedullary junction and courses through the subarachnoid space to reach Dorello's canal, a small triangular space formed beneath the petroclinoid ligament (Gruber's ligament) from the petrous apex to the posterior clinoid process (PCP) (KELLER et al. 1997). This canal contains the CN VI, usually lying laterally to the IPS and the dorsal meningeal artery from the meningohypophyseal trunk (MHT). The abducens nerve is considered the only true intracavernous nerve because of its course along the lateral surface of the ICA after leaving Dorellos canal (KELLER et al. 1997).

The arterial blood supply to these CNs is provided by multiple small branches mainly arising from the inferolateral trunk (ILT) and the MHT and in part arising from dural branches of the ECA territory (see below).

The development and increasing use of transarterial embolizations of DCSFs in the late 1980s and early 1990s required us to study in more detail the arterial blood supply of the CNs in the CS region (KNOSP et al. 1987b). At the present time this knowledge plays a minor role due to the introduction of transvenous occlusion techniques, being increasingly employed to treat DCSFs since 1990.

3.2.1
Autonomic Nervous System

A detailed knowledge of the sympathetic and parasympathetic nervous systems within the CS is still missing. It is known that the sympathetic fibers course along the extracranial ICA, through the carotid canal, to reach the petrous and cavernous portion where they form a plexus (KELLER et al. 1997; PAULLUS et al. 1997; MITCHEL 1953). Recently, parasympathetic fibers and ganglia have been found in the CS as well, probably connected with rami orbitalis arising from the sphenopalatine ganglion and coursing through the SOF (SUZUKI and HARDEBO 1993). BLEYS et al. (2001); while performing immunohistochemical studies in rats, found that the cavernous sinus ganglia, consisting of the pterygopalatine ganglion and small cavernous ganglia, contribute to parasympathetic cerebrovascular innervation and that the cavernous nerve plexus and abducens nerve are involved in the pathway from these ganglia to the cerebral arteries. It can be assumed that not only the sympathetic but also parasympathetic innervations play a role in the tone regulation of cerebral vessels (SUZUKI and HARDEBO 1993).

3.3
Vascular Anatomy

3.3.1
Arterial Anatomy (Figs. 3.5–3.7)

3.3.1.1
Internal Carotid Artery

The ICA provides the anterior circulation that supplies the largest part of the cerebrum, the eye and other intraorbital structures. The ICA also gives rise to the branches of the forehead and the nose. The artery begins at the bifurcation of the common carotid artery (CCA), usually at the level of the fourth cervical vertebra, where it is enlarged to form the so-called carotid sinus. FISCHER (1938) divided the ICA into four segments: the cervical, the petrous, the cavernous and the cerebral segment (Fig. 3.5).

The cervical segment extends almost vertically to the base of the skull to reach the Apertura externa (external aperture) of the Canalis caroticus (carotid canal) to enter the petrous bone. Just before entering

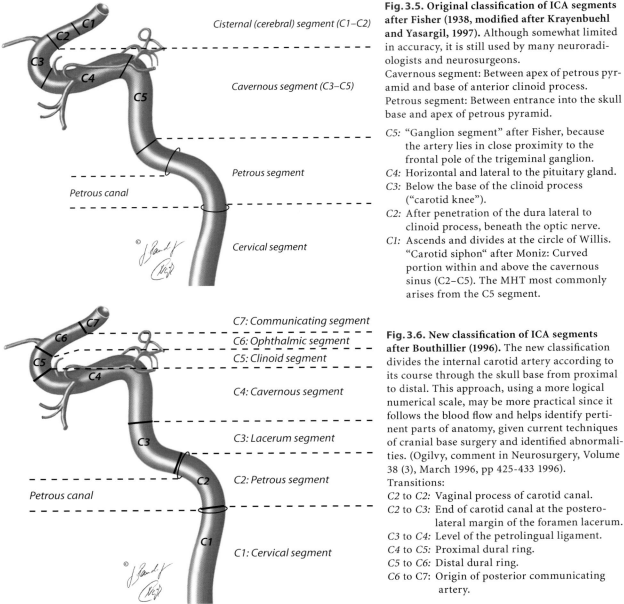

Cisternal (cerebral) segment (C1–C2)

Cavernous segment (C3–C5)

Petrous segment

Petrous canal

Cervical segment

C7: Communicating segment

C6: Ophthalmic segment

C5: Clinoid segment

C4: Cavernous segment

C3: Lacerum segment

C2: Petrous segment

Petrous canal

C1: Cervical segment

Fig. 3.5. Original classification of ICA segments after Fisher (1938, modified after Krayenbuehl and Yasargil, 1997). Although somewhat limited in accuracy, it is still used by many neuroradiologists and neurosurgeons.
Cavernous segment: Between apex of petrous pyramid and base of anterior clinoid process.
Petrous segment: Between entrance into the skull base and apex of petrous pyramid.

C5: "Ganglion segment" after Fisher, because the artery lies in close proximity to the frontal pole of the trigeminal ganglion.
C4: Horizontal and lateral to the pituitary gland.
C3: Below the base of the clinoid process ("carotid knee").
C2: After penetration of the dura lateral to clinoid process, beneath the optic nerve.
C1: Ascends and divides at the circle of Willis. "Carotid siphon" after Moniz: Curved portion within and above the cavernous sinus (C2–C5). The MHT most commonly arises from the C5 segment.

Fig. 3.6. New classification of ICA segments after Bouthillier (1996). The new classification divides the internal carotid artery according to its course through the skull base from proximal to distal. This approach, using a more logical numerical scale, may be more practical since it follows the blood flow and helps identify pertinent parts of anatomy, given current techniques of cranial base surgery and identified abnormalities. (Ogilvy, comment in Neurosurgery, Volume 38 (3), March 1996, pp 425-433 1996).
Transitions:
C2 to C2: Vaginal process of carotid canal.
C2 to C3: End of carotid canal at the posterolateral margin of the foramen lacerum.
C3 to C4: Level of the petrolingual ligament.
C4 to C5: Proximal dural ring.
C5 to C6: Distal dural ring.
C6 to C7: Origin of posterior communicating artery.

the canal, the ICA forms a medial convex curve. The cervical segment lies medial to the internal jugular vein (IJV), the vagus nerve usually between both vessels.

The ICA enters the cranium by passing through the carotid canal. This canal is lined by periosteum and is located in the petrous portion of the temporal bone. The posterior orifice of the canal opens onto the posterior wall of the foramen lacerum, adjacent to the jugular foramen. The anterior or internal orifice of the canal is located at the petrous apex (MILLER N 1998).

The petrous segment can be divided into a vertical and a horizontal portion with a course depending on the configuration and development of the skull base, particularly on the shape of the petrous bone. The total length of this segment is about 25–35 mm. The vertical portion courses 6–15 mm in the vertical direction then turns medially and anteriorly to form a genu and becomes the horizontal portion. The horizontal portion courses anteriorly and medially above the foramen lacerum to eventually leave the bony canal near the petrous apex. The petrous segment can give rise to two small arterial branches in 38% of the cases. The vidian artery, usually arising from the internal maxillary artery (see below), can also arise from the petrous ICA (30%) (PAULLUS et al. 1977). The small caroticotympanic artery, previously reported to be the most common branch, is thought to enter the tympanic cavity through a foramen in the wall of the carotid canal, was not found by PAULLUS et al. (1977), but often seen by LANG (1983). The latter also saw periosteal twigs ramifying in the periosteum of the carotid canal and the neighborhood of the foramen lacerum, which have been described only by LAZORTHES (1961). They may be responsible for retrograde filling of the petrous ICA in patients with ICA occlusions.

The cavernous segment begins at the superior margin of the petrolingual ligament at the posterior aspect of the CS and ends at the root of the anterior clinoid process. This segment lies within the CS, surrounded by its venous spaces and by some trabecular connective tissue. From the petrous apex medial and rostral towards the lateral side of the sphenoid bone, the ICA is separated from the Gasserian ganglion by a thin osseous or connective tissue septum. Because the posterior limits of the cavernous segment vary and are difficult to exactly define, this segment was also divided into a presellar and juxtasellar segment by some authors (DILENGE and HEON 1974).

Above the foramen lacerum the ICA courses almost perpendicularly cranial in a groove along the lateral side of the sphenoid bone and lies directly adjacent to the frontal pole of the Gasserian ganglion [C5 after FISCHER (1938) or ascending segment]. From here the ICA passes rostrally to reach the root of the anterior clinoid process, to which it lies laterally. Lateral to the pituitary fossa the ICA lies in a shallow groove of the lateral sphenoid bone (C4, or horizontal segment). The medial wall of the ICA lies within the CS, which is separated from the pituitary gland by a thin sheet of the dura mater. Underneath the root of the anterior clinoid process ,the ICA forms the so-called "knee of the carotid", a sharp, anteriorly convex curve (C3 or clinoid segment).

After piercing the dura and the arachnoid membrane at the medial margin of the anterior clinoid process, the ICA courses within the subarachnoid space (cerebral or cisternal segment, C2) upward and posteriorly underneath the optical nerve that enters the optic canal. Finally, the ICA ascends to reach its bifurcation into the middle and anterior cerebral artery (MCA and ACA) to form the circle of Willis (C1, terminal segment after Fischer). In this manner the segments C3–C5 form the cavernous and C1–C2

form the cerebral segment of the ICA. The double or S-shape curve of the ICA within and above the CS is, according to MONIZ (1927), called the "carotid siphon". After KRAYENBÜHL and YASARGIL (1997), the shape of this carotid siphon may differ remarkably: a U-shape, a V-shape, Arcus-shape and Omega-shape, a double siphon, a megasiphon or a dolichosiphon can be seen. The first three types are seen more frequently, while in older patients (51–74 years) the omega type occurs more often.

Today, Fischer's system is considered somewhat limited as it is anatomically inaccurate and numbers the ICA segments opposite the direction of blood flow. It has been modified or replaced by several others, e.g. by BOUTHILLIER et al. (1996), who divided the ICA into seven segments using a numerical scale in the direction of the blood flow: C1 = cervical, C2 = petrous, C3 = lacerum, C4 = cavernous, C5 = clinoid, C6 = ophthalmic and C7 = terminal segment (Fig. 3.6). LASJAUNIAS et al. (2001) have pointed out that the morphological continuity of the ICA obscures significant differences between various segments which can also be marked by the origins of embryonic vessels (see below). In clinical practice, however, the classification of Fischer is still widely used.

3.3.1.1.1
Branches of the ICA
Branches of the Cavernous Segment (Fig. 3.7 and Figures in Sects. 7.2.1–7.2.12)

Within the CS, the C5 segment usually gives rise to one (MHT), and the C4 segment gives rise to two small but important branches (ILT, capsular arteries).

Meningohypophyseal Trunk (MHT)

LUSCHKA (1860) first described the Arteria hypophysialis inferior. MC CONELL (1953) studied the arterial supply of the pituitary gland by a small arterial trunk, of which the inferior hypophyseal artery is the largest. Later on, SCHNÜERER and STATTIN (1963), PARKINSON (1965), and RHOTON and INOUE (1991) gave a more detailed description of these anatomic vascular relationships. Origin and branching of the small arteries vary significantly. Most frequently, a 0.75-mm meningohypophyseal ramus arises from the dorsal circumference of the C5 segment, just immediately before the vertical part turns into the horizontal part. This vessel is in the English literature commonly named the meningohypophyseal trunk (MHT) according to Parkinson (1965, 1990), the inferior hypophyseal artery according to Mc Connell (1953), the dorsal main stem artery according to Schuerer and Stattin (1963) or the posterior trunk according to Tran-Dinh (1987). The classification of Parkinson (1984) differentiated initially three main branches of the MHT, the radiological appearance of which was described by Pribam et al. (1966).

- The *marginal tentorial artery* (artery of the free margin of the tentorium cerebelli, tentorial artery, medial tentorial artery), first described by Bernasconi and Cassinari (1956) ascends to the roof of the CS, courses along the free edge of the tentorium and gives two branches for the third and fourth cranial nerve and to the roof of the CS. It supplies the medial third of the tentorium and may anastomose with a meningeal branch of the ophthalmic artery, with a corresponding contralateral branch and a meningeal branch of the ascending pharyngeal artery. This artery was found by Lasjaunias et al. (1977) to arise from the superior branch of the ILT in 8/20 cases (see below).
- The *lateral clival artery* (dorsal meningeal artery or dorsal clival artery) arose from the MHT in 90% of 50 studied cadavers (Harris and Rhoton 1976), supplies the sixth cranial nerve and anastomoses with the contralateral side and branches of the vertebral artery and the jugular ramus of the APA. This artery supplies the dura of the dorsum sellae and clivus and is most often involved in the arterial supply of DCSF (Barrow et al. 1985).
- The *inferior hypophyseal artery* (posteroinferior hypophyseal artery) crosses the CS medially, divides into superior and inferior branches, connects with the corresponding artery of the contralateral side and supplies the posterior lobe of the pituitary gland, the dura of the posterior clinoid process, the floor of the sella and parts of the posterior CS. According to Martins et al. (2005) this dural territory is supplied by a medial clival artery, which can also arise directly from the ICA and anastomoses with the hypoglossal ramus of the APA. The inferior hypophyseal artery is often superimposed on angiograms and difficult to identify (Lasjaunias et al. 2001).

Further described are:
- A *basal tentorial branch* (lateral tentorial artery) by Schnüerer and Stattin (1963) and Lasjaunias et al. (1978a) which can arise from a common trunk with medial tentorial artery (Martins et al. 2005).
- A *medial clival artery* has been described by Lasjaunias et al. (2001) and Martins et al. (2005) (see above).

It should be mentioned that Pribram et al. (1966) have already emphasized that the classic MHT arising as a single trunk is not constantly seen. The existence of a singular trunk was observed by Lasjaunias et al. (1978a) in only 10% of the cases. He suggested instead that these branches more often arise independently as single vessels corresponding to the remnants of two transient embryonic vessels, the primitive maxillary and the primitive trigeminal artery. The former gives rise to the inferior hypophyseal artery, the latter to the medial and lateral clival arteries as well as to the basal tentorial artery. Lasjaunias et al. (1978a) furthermore pointed out that the marginal tentorial artery of Bernasconi may originate from eight different pedicles, [including the accessory meningeal (Silvela and Zamarron 1978), middle meningeal, intraorbital ophthalmic and lacrimal arteries], of which the C5 siphon is only one.

The term MHT is nevertheless widely used, although it not only supplies the meninges and the pituitary gland but also the oculomotor, trochlear and abducens nerves. In over 200 cavernous carotid dissections it was identified in 100% of the cases (Parkinson 1965).

Martins et al. (2005) have recently provided a comprehensive review of the anatomy of dural arteries within the CS region and differentiate the MHT into the following components:

1. *Tentorial trunk*
   - Medial tentorial artery (marginal tentorial artery, Bernasconi)
   - Lateral tentorial artery (basal tentorial artery)
2. *Dorsal meningeal artery* (lateral clival artery)
   - Medial branch
   - Medial clival branch
   - Lateral branch
3. *Inferior hypophyseal artery*
   - Hypophyseal circle
   - Medial clival artery

The inferolateral trunk (ILT) according to Lasjaunias et al. (1977), also named artery of the inferior cavernous sinus (Miller 1998; Parkinson 1965), the lateral main stem (Schnüerer and Stattin 1963) or the lateral trunk (Tran-Dinh 1987) in the

Fig. 3.7.=Arterial anatomy in the cavernous sinus region (artist's drawing of small dural arteries arising from ICA and ECA, considered so-called "dangerous anastomoses", in the cavernosus sinus region, lateral view.) The dural arteries of the ICA and ECA connecting both territories in the cavernous sinus region are also referred to as "dangerous anastomoses". Because of their small caliber these branches are often not (or not completely) visualized in diagnostic arteriograms, unless they are enlarged due to increased flow caused by AV-shunting lesions, arterial occlusions or tumors. The numerous possibilities of inadvertent migration of embolic material into the cerebral circulation during transarterial embolization of ECA branches are obvious. However, it is not the vessel per se which is "dangerous", but lack of knowledge or negligence of the particular anatomy in this region. In cases of arteriovenous shunts developing within or adjacent to the cavernous sinus, these branches become supplying feeders and are recruited from ipsi- and contralateral ECA and ICA territory. Even in case of a successful positioning of a microcatheter in the ILT or MHT, reflux of embolic material such as particles or glue may easily occur and poses a risk for neurological complications.

1 Internal carotid artery (ICA, C5)	*16* Capsular arteries
2 Internal carotid artery (C4)	
3 Ophthalmic artery (OA)	*17* External carotid artery (ECA)
	18 Ascendending pharyngeal artery (APA)
4 Meningohypophyseal trunk (MHT)	*19* Superficial temporal artery (STA)
5 Inferior hypophyseal artery	*20* Internal maxillary artery (IMA)
6 Lateral clival artery	*21* Middle meningeal artery(MMA)
7 Medial clival artery	*22* Accessory meningeal artery (AMA)
8 Basal tentorial artery	*23* Sphenopalatine artery
9 Marginal tentorial artery	*24* Artery of the foramen rotundum (AFR)
	25 Recurrent artery of the foramen lacerum (RAFL)
10 Inferolateral trunk (ILT)	*26* Artery of the pterygoid canal (vidian artery)
11 Superior ramus	
12 Anteromedial ramus	*a* Supraorbital fissure
13 Anterolateral ramus	*b* Foramen rotundum
14 Posterolateral ramus	*c* Foramen ovale
15 Posteromedial ramus	*d* Foramen spinosum

English literature, corresponds to the remnant of the dorsal ophthalmic artery (Lasjaunias et al. 1977). It arises from the lateral aspect of the horizontal portion of the cavernous portion of the ICA distal to the origin of the MHT (C4 segment). It usually curves over the CN VI (96%) and divides into three main branches:

- The *superior ramus* (ramus tentorii marginalis, marginal tentorial artery) supplies the roof of the CS and the proximal part of CN III and IV. It can replace or anastomose with the tentorial artery of the MHT.

- The *anterior ramus* divides into a lateral and medial branch. The anteromedial ramus passes to the supraorbital fissure and supplies the distal parts of the CN III and IV. It ends as deep recurrent ophthalmic artery (or dorsal ophthalmic artery) and anastomoses with the intraorbital ophthalmic artery. The anterolateral ramus courses together with the second division of the trigeminal nerve (V/2) through the foramen rotundum and anastomoses with the artery of the foramen rotundum of the internal maxillary artery (IMA).

- The posterior ramus divides into a lateral and medial branch. The posteromedial ramus courses together with the third division of CN V towards the foramen ovale and anastomoses with the accessory meningeal artery (AMA) a branch of the IMA. It also supplies the CN VI, the medial third of the Gasserian ganglion and the motor roots of the CN V3. The posterolateral ramus reaches the foramen spinosum and supplies the middle and lateral third of the Gasserian ganglion and anastomoses with a branch of the middle meningeal artery (MMA).

PARKINSON (1965) was able to identify the ILT in 80% of the cases, others in 65%–84% (HARRIS and RHOTON 1976; TRAN-DINH 1987; LASJAUNIAS and BERENSTEIN 1987; RHOTON et al. 1979). Unlike the MHT, the ILT was not observed to show variants and always arose as a single trunk (TRAN-DINH 1987; WILLINSKY et al. 1987). According to LANG and SCHAFER (1976), the MHT is called Truncus carotico-cavernosus posterior and the ILT can be called Truncus carotico-cavernosus lateralis. As mentioned above, LASJAUNIAS et al. (1977, 1978a,b) and WILLINSKY et al. (1987) as well as BRASSIER (1987) have suggested a different concept that considers the intracavernous ICA branches embryological remnants, assuming that observed normal dispositions and variants rather represent various phases in the embryological development of the primitive maxillary and trigeminal arteries, possibly influenced by individual hemodynamic balance between ICA and ECA, right and left or anterior and posterior.

TRAN-DINH (1987) who studied the various classifications and terminology extensively proposed a simplification into primary and secondary branches. The fourth Nomenclatura Anatomica (1977) contains a list of intracavernous ICA branches but no systematic classification. Table 3.1 provides an overview of various terms used for the anastomotic branches of the C4 and C5 segment.

Capsular arteries according to MC CONNELL (1953) and PARKINSON (1965), and a medial group according to TRAN-DINH (1987) can angiographically be identified in less than 30% of cases (OSBORN 1991) and were seen in cadaver dissections in 28% of the cases (HARRIS and RHOTON 1976). The inferior capsular artery courses inferomedially to supply the floor of the sella turcica and anastomoses with the contralateral side and with branches of the inferior hypophyseal artery. The superior capsular artery passes along the roof of the sella. The capsular arteries may also arise from the inferior hypophyseal artery. They do not contribute to the supply of the CNs and usually play no role in the supply of DCSFs.

Recurrent artery of the foramen lacerum (RAFL), a small branch of the lateral surface of the vertical portion of the C5 segment, descends to the foramen lacerum and usually anastomoses with the carotid branch of the APA. It supplies the pericarotid autonomic nerve plexus and the carotid wall (MARTINS et al. 2005) and may connect with the posterior ramus of the ILT (cavernous branch of MMA) (LASJAUNIAS et al. 2001).

Ophthalmic Artery

The ophthalmic artery (OA) is the most proximal major intracranial branch of the ICA and arises just as this vessel is emerging from the cavernous sinus on the medial side of the anterior clinoid process, and enters the orbital cavity through the optic foramen, below and lateral to the optic nerve. The origin is intradural in about 90% and extradural in about 10% of the time, from either the cavernous or the clinoid segment of the ICA (PUNT 1979). The most commonly reported variants are the origins from the MMA (HEYRE 1974) and from the ACA (LASJAUNIAS et al. 2001). Other possible origins are the accessory meningeal artery and the basilar artery (LASJAUNIAS et al. 2001), the MMA, the anterior deep temporal artery or directly from the ECA (NEWTON and POTTS 1974).

The OA usually courses anterolaterally below the optic nerve and enters the optic canal where it pierces the dural sheath of the optic nerve, usually inferolateral but sometimes directly below the nerve (HAYREH 1962a). The intraorbital portion of the OA may be divided into three segments, the first extending from its entry to where the artery crosses under the nerve. The second segment crosses the nerve (in 80% from lateral to medial), and the third extends from here to its termination. The OA gives off a number of branches including the short and long posterior ciliary arteries and the central retinal artery (CRA). The central retinal artery has a diameter of about 200 microns and may have a tortuous course along the inferior surface of the optic nerve before it pierces the optic nerve sheaths 10–15 mm posterior to the globe and runs for 1–3 mm with

Table 3.1. Various terms for cavernous ICA branches (modified after TRAN-DINH 1987)

LUSCHKA 1860	Inferior hypophyseal artery		
MC CONNELL 1953	Inferior hypophyseal artery	–	Capsular arteries
BERNASCONI and CASSINARI 1956	Tentorial (marginal) artery		
SCHNURER and STATTIN 1963	Dorsal main stem (Basal tentorial branch, Clival branches, Inferior hypophyseal artery)	Lateral main stem (Marginal tentorial branch)	–
PRIBRAM et al. 1966	Meningohypophyseal trunk (Inferior hypophyseal artery, dorsal meningeal artery, tentorial artery)		
PARKINSON 1964, 1984	Meningohypophyseal trunk (Inferior hypophyseal artery, dorsal meningeal artery, tentorial (marginal) artery)	Artery of the inferior CS Artery to Meckel's Cave	Capsular arteries
LASJAUNIAS 1977, 1978	Primitive maxillary	Dorsal ophthalmic artery	Capsular arteries
WILLINSKY et al. 1987	(Posterior inferior hypophyseal artery) Trigeminal artery (Lateral clival artery) Medial clival artery Basal tentorial artery	(Inferolateral trunk)	
TRAN-DINH 1987	Posterior trunk	Lateral trunk	Medial group
MARTINS et al. 2005	MHT (Tentorial trunk, medial tentorial artery, lateral tentorial artery, medial clival artery)	ILT	Capsular arteries

the subarachnoid space of the optic nerve (MILLER 1998). The CRA gives numerous small branches to the optic nerve and finally passes through the retrolaminar portion of the nerve where it gives off its terminal branches to supply the inner layers of the retina (HAYREH 1963).

The intraorbital course of the OA and its branching pattern was studied in detail by HAYREH (1962b). He found major variations, depending on whether the OA crosses over or under the nerve. In the former case, the first major branch is the central retinal artery, followed by the lateral posterior ciliary artery, lacrimal artery, muscular arteries, medial posterior ciliary arteries, supraorbital artery, anterior and posterior ethmoidal arteries and medial palpebral artery. In the latter case, the OA sends small perforating branches to the optic nerve, followed by the lateral posterior ciliary, central retinal artery, muscular arteries, medial posterior ciliary arteries, lacrimal artery, posterior ethmoidal artery, supraorbital artery and anterior ethmoidal and medial palpebral artery (HAYREH 1962b). The OA also gives rise to small meningeal arteries of which

the anterior falx artery originates from the anterior ethmoidal artery. The terminal branches are the supratrochlear and the dorsal nasal arteries (MILLER N 1998). The posterior ciliary arteries vary in number and form the anastomosing ring, the Circle of Zinn and Haller (HAYREH 1962b). They are called short posterior ciliary arteries and give rise to the cilioretinal arteries which supply the retina in the region of the optic disc (RANDALL 1887). The long posterior ciliary arteries supply the internal structure of the anterior portion of the eye (DUCASSE et al. 1986). Important anastomoses are formed by the anterior and posterior ethmoidal arteries, the lacrimal artery and the deep and superficial recurrent ophthalmic arteries. The deep recurrent ophthalmic artery usually arises from the first part of the intraorbital OA, courses backwards through the SOF and consistently anastomoses with the anteromedial ramus of the ILT. The angiographic appearance of this vessel is characteristic when it projects below the C3 and C4 portion of the ICA (LASJAUNIAS et al. 1978b). The superficial recurrent ophthalmic artery may arise from the intraorbital OA or from the lacrimal artery and usually courses through the most lateral part of the SOF to supply the intradural parts of CN III and IV and continues as an artery of the free margin of the tentorium (LASJAUNIAS et al. 1978b). Two others can establish anastomoses between OA and MMA, the recurrent meningeal artery and the meningolacrimal artery (LASJAUNIAS et al. 1975b). The recurrent meningeal artery is an adult remnant of the common meningoorbital vascular system, courses through the SOF and connects the lacrimal artery with the anterior branch of the MMA. The meningolacrimal artery also arises from the anterior branch MMA to enter the orbit through the meningolacrimal foramen (foramen of Hyrtl, also called cranioorbital, meningoorbital, stapedial-ophthalmo-lacrimal foramen), which usually lies just lateral to the SOF (MORET et al. 1977).

Ethmoidal Arteries

The ethmoidal arteries arise from the ophthalmic artery and can be divided into an anterior and a posterior group. Their origin, course and supplied regions were studied on 30 injected adult heads by LANG and SCHAEFER (1979). After branching off, the anterior ethmoidal artery normally turns in a single loop by first coursing forwards and then, reversing towards the anterior ethmoidal foramen, it passes into the canal portion. Occasionally, a common ethmoidal artery or a common source for the ethmoidal arteries is present. As a rule, the smaller posterior ethmoidal artery arises from the ophthalmic artery; occasionally it is absent or can even very rarely arise from the MMA (LANG and SCHAFER 1979). The artery usually courses over the superior oblique muscle, passes through the posterior ethmoid canal, supplies the posterior ethmoidal cells and enters the cranium, the dura mater and gives off branches to descend to the nasal cavity through the cribriform plate where they anastomose with branches from the sphenopalatine artery (GRAY 1918). Before or while entering the olfactory fossa the artery usually gives off branches to supply the dura and bone of the planum sphenoidale, lesser wing of the sphenoid and adjacent dura of the anterior cranial fossa.

The anterior ethmoidal artery accompanies the nasociliary nerve through the anterior ethmoidal canal, supplying the anterior and middle ethmoidal cells and frontal sinus. It then enters the cranium to supply the dura mater with the anterior meningeal artery, which gives off the anterior falx artery and nasal branches to supply the lateral wall and the septum of the nose (GRAY 1918). The ethmoidal arteries

are usually involved in the arterial supply of DAVFs located on the floor of the anterior cranial fossa, but may also contribute to the arterial supply of DCSFs.

Table 3.2. ICA and ECA branches relevant for supply of DCSF and their main anastomoses to adjacent territories (modified after MARTINS et al. 2005)

MHT
- Tentorial trunk
  - Medial tentorial artery (to contralateral, lateral tentorial, dorsal meningeal, MMA, ILT)
  - Lateral tentorial artery (to medial tentorial, dorsal meningeal, posterior meningeal, mastoid)
- Dorsal meningeal artery (to contralateral, medial clival, tentorial, MMA, APA)
- Inferior hypophyseal artery (to contralateral, capsular)
- Medial clival artery (to contralateral, dorsal meningeal, medial tentorial)

ILT
- Superior ramus (to medial tentorial)
- Anterior Ramus
  - Anteromedial ramus (to deep recurrent ophthalmic)
  - Anterolateral ramus (to AFR)
- Posterior Ramus
  - Posteromedial ramus (to AMA)
- Posterolateral ramus (to MMA)

Ophthalmic artery
- Anterior ethmoidal arteries
- Posterior ethmoidal arteries
- Deep recurrent ophthalmic artery (to ILT)
- Superficial recurrent ophthalmic artery (to medial tentorial)
- Recurrent meningeal artery (to MMA)
- Recurrent artery of the foramen lacerum (to APA, ILT, vidian)

ECA
- Ascending pharyngeal artery
  - Carotid ramus (to RAFL)
  - Jugular ramus (to lateral clival)
  - Hypoglossal ramus (to medial clival)
- Maxillary artery
  - Artery of pterygoid canal (to AMA, APA, C5 segment, RAFL)
  - Pterygovaginal artery
- Middle meningeal artery (to ILT, AMA, OA)
- Accessory meningeal artery (to MMA, ILT, medial tentorial)

3.3.1.2
External Carotid Artery

The external carotid artery (ECA) gives off four major arteries, the branches of which contribute to the supply of the CS and the CNs.

3.3.1.2.1
Ascending Pharyngeal Artery

The ascending pharyngeal artery (APA), the smallest branch of the ECA, is a rather gracil, long vessel. It arises close to the origin of the ECA at its dorsal circumference and ascends between ICA and the pharyngeal wall to reach the base of the skull. Its meningeal branches are very small vessels, supplying the dura mater and have been described in detail by LASJAUNIAS and MORET (1976). One branch enters the skull through the foramen lacerum, another through the jugular foramen, and sometimes a third one through the hypoglossal canal.

The first, the carotid ramus (ramus caroticus), accompanies the ICA in its canal. It anastomoses at the level of the foramen lacerum with a small branch of the C5-portion (recurrent artery of the foramen lacerum).

The second, the jugular ramus (ramus jugularis), passes with CNs 9–11 through the jugular foramen and reaches the dura mater. It anastomoses within the sigmoid sinus with the dorsal branch of the occipital artery and within the inferior petrous sinus with the medial branch of the lateral clival artery.

The third, the hypoglossal ramus (ramus hypoglossus), accompanies and supplies the hypoglossal nerve. It branches further within the dura of the foramen magnum and anastomoses with the medial clival artery arising from the MHT (LASJAUNIAS and MORET 1976). This ramus does sometimes not exist, in which case a connection between the extradural course of the vertebral artery and a corresponding branch can be found.

3.3.1.2.2
Internal Maxillary Artery

The internal maxillary artery (IMA), or maxillary artery according to current terminology, is the largest terminal branch of the ECA consisting of a mandibular, a pterygoid and a pterygopalatine segment giving rise to at least 16 terminal branches. Because of their anastomoses with branches of the C4 segment of the ICA, the middle meningeal artery and the accessory meningeal artery (both arising from the second, the pterygoid segment), are of greater importance in the context of this monograph. The branches of the third portion leave the pterygopalatine fossa through corresponding foramina and fissures (ALLEN et al. 1973) which account for a relative constant angiographic pattern. Among the anteriorly directed branches are the posterior superior alveolar artery, the infraorbital artery and the greater (descending) palatine artery. The sphenopalatine artery is considered the terminal branch of the maxillary artery and leaves the pterygopalatine fossa through the sphenopalatine foramen (ALLEN et al. 1973). The posteriorly directed branches are from medial to lateral the pterygovaginal artery, the artery of the pterygoid canal (Vidian) and the artery of the foramen rotundum (see also Figs. 7.77–7.79).

The artery of the foramen rotundum (AFR), because of its connection with the ILT, has particular importance (DJINDJIAN and MERLAND 1973), lying within the pterygoid fossa and leaving it through the foramen rotundum as the most laterally coursing branch (ALLEN et al. 1973). It anastomoses with the anterolateral branch of the ILT (in older literature, artery of the inferior cavernous sinus). This very small artery has a diameter of about 150 microns (LANG 1979a) and is usually not visualized on standard angiograms, unless its diameter is increased (RIBEIRO et al. 1984; ALLEN et al. 1974). Its course is usually oblique, posterior and cranial through the canal. It represents one of the most prominent branches in the supply of DCSFs, and may also play a role as collateral supply to the circle of Willis in case of ICA occlusions or as tumor feeding vessel for meningiomas of the sphenoid wing (RIBEIRO et al. 1984).

The *vidian artery* (Arteria canalis pterygoidei Vidii, artery of the pterygoid canal) arising within the pterygopalatine fossa as a branch of the distal maxillary artery, courses within the vidian canal towards the foramen lacerum and may anastomose within the oropharyngeal roof with branches of the AMA and APA (LASJAUNIAS 1984). It can arise from the greater palatine artery and may continue and anastomose with the petrous segment of the ICA. The vidian artery is a remnant of the first aortic arch and has been demonstrated to arise from the inferior (55%) or anteroinferior (35%) aspect of the internal carotid artery within the petrous bone in 30% of anatomic specimens (PAULLUS et al. 1977; QUISLING and RHOTON 1979). It runs here for an average of 7 mm along the anterior wall of the carotid canal before it emerges from the skull through the cartilage of the foramen lacerum and enters the pterygoid canal and has an average diameter of less than 0.5 mm (Lang 1983). The vidian artery supplies the lateral pharyngeal recess, giving rise to branches supplying the auditory tube and the tympanic region (Allen et al. 1973). This artery can be involved in the arterial supply of DCSFs (Osborn 1980b).

In contrast the pterygovaginal artery arises from the distal part of the maxillary artery and passes posteriorly through the pterygovaginal canal along the roof of the nasopharynx and anastomoses with the inferomedial eustachian branch of the accessory meningeal artery, the Eustachian branch of the APA and the mandibular branch of the ICA (Lasjaunias et al. 2001). This most medial coursing branch is also called the pharyngeal artery and supplies the choanes, the pharynx and eustachian tube.

As mentioned by Allen et al. (1974), other collateral branches may traverse the lateral aspect of the superior orbital fissure and are called Aa. anastomoticae after Lie (1968). The latter erroneously described these branches as all passing through the supraorbital fissure and did not recognize the artery of the foramen rotundum.

Although neglected in several textbooks, modern high-resolution DSA and, in particular, 3D-DSA reveal that in some DCSFs these "Aa. anastomoticae", passing through the SOF, are indeed identifiable. They course more cranially above the artery of the foramen rotundum and often contribute to the supply of DCSFs (see Chap. 7).

3.3.1.2.3
Middle Meningeal Artery

The middle meningeal artery (MMA) is the second ascending branch of the IMA and the largest of the dural arteries. Its main branch courses through the foramen spinosum to enter the skull. Of the four groups of branches (extracranial, basal, anterior and posterior) the extracranial and basal arteries are of special interest. The extracranial branches supply local structures, in particular the AMA with a branch to the foramen ovale and the above lying meninges. The basal group supplies the cranial fossa (Lasjaunias and Theron 1976). Of the latter, the inferior meningeal branches supplying the middle cranial fossa, as well as their anastomotic branches to the extracranial arteries, are of importance: to the APA via the carotid canal and the foramen lacerum, to the vidian artery via the foramen lacerum, to the AMA via the foramen ovale and to the IMA via the

foramen rotundum. Other anastomotic vessel are medial branches to the Gasserian ganglion and to the cavernous segment and their anastomoses to the ICA and other branches supplying the CS; finally anterior branches supplying the superior orbital fissure and their anastomoses. Sometimes one larger branch of the temporal segment of the MMA curves posteriorly and medially and contributes to the supply of the CS or even the tentorium. The MMA usually has anastomoses with the posterolateral branch of the MMA and may also give rise to the medial (marginal) tentorial artery (Benndorf 2008).

3.3.1.2.4
Accessory Meningeal Artery

The accessory meningeal artery (AMA) supplies the pharynx and the eustachian tube, sometimes the meninges. According to Baumel and Beard (1961) it arises almost as frequently from the IMA as from the MMA, depending on if the latter is of the deep or superficial variant. It never originates before the MMA. In the superficial variation (IMA lateral to the lateral pterygoid muscle), the AMA originates from the MMA, in the deep variation (IMA medial to the lateral pterygoid muscle), it stems directly from the IMA (Lasjaunias and Theron 1976; Vitek 1989) in 60% of cases, immediately following the origin of the MMA, and in the remaining cases from the middle portion of the pterygoid segment. In 24% of the cases it consists of more than one vessel. The AMA courses parallel to the superior boundary of the medial pterygoid muscle in a fascial plane between the medial and lateral pterygoid muscles (Vitek 1989). The artery ascends through the interaponeurotic space and divides below the skull base into its anterior and posterior rami. The anterior ramus courses along the eustachian tube, the posterior meningeal ramus courses in circa 10% through the foramen ovale (Lang 1979a) or the foramen of Vesalius to supply the lateral wall of the CS, the Gasserian ganglion and the antero-superior surface of the petrous bone. It may also contribute to the supply of the sphenoid sinus. In case of a dominant supply of the CS region by transcranial branches of the IMA, the AMA may supply the entire area, giving rise to four branches usually belonging to the ILT in 20% of the cases (Lasjaunias et al. 2001). Lang (1979b) describes the AMA as a branch of the MMA, contributing to the rich vascular network on the surface of the dura mater that is provided mainly by the latter (Djindjian and Merland 1973). Other small arteries in the neighborhood may also be involved such as the APA and OA. Other small connections are provided by arterioles of the intracavernous and supracavernous portion of the ICA that supply the sella, the Gasserian ganglion and the tentorium. The arterioles also supply the lateral wall of the CS by AMA branches and branches of the vidian artery and of the artery of the foramen rotundum.

As already discussed by BAUMEL and BEARD (1961), there is a discrepancy between the nomenclature of this artery and the territory supplied is meningeal in only 10% (VITEK 1989). Therefore, VITEK (1989) suggested a more appropriate term, the pterygomeningeal artery. According to LASJAUNIAS and BERENSTEIN (1987), the AMA can have four branches, the posterior, inferomedial, inferopalatine and intracranial branch. The latter, also named the intracranial ascending ramus, courses through the foramen ovale and anastomoses with the posteromedial ramus of the ILT. BRASSIER et al. (1987) emphasized the importance of these arterial anastomoses in the region of the CS and the intracavernous ICA.

3.3.2
Venous Anatomy
(Figs. 3.8–3.12 and Figs. in Sects. 7.2.13–7.2.38)

3.3.2.1
The Cavernous Sinus, Receptaculum, Sinus Caroticus (Rektorzik), Confluens Sinuum Anterius, Sinus Spheno-Parietale (Cruveilhier), Cavernous Plexus, Lateral Sellar Compartment

3.3.2.1.1
Embryology

The role of the CS as a draining pathway changes during life. As described by PADGET (1956b), the CS forms during the 40-mm stage of embryonic development as a plexiform extension of the prootic sinus and the ventral myelencephalic vein. The primitive maxillary vein, initially draining into the prootic sinus, connects with the CS and becomes the superior ophthalmic vein. At the 60-mm embryonic stage, the CS is still not involved in the cerebral venous drainage and receives blood only from the ophthalmic veins draining it into the IJV via the IPS. During this time, the peri (internal) carotid venous plexus may participate instead, bringing blood from the CS through the carotid canal (KNOSP et al. 1987a). Padget considered the CS and the IPS, secondary sinuses and an intracra-

nial detour through the base of the skull between two extracranial veins, the SOV and the IJV. In a typical infant stage (3rd month) the CS and the IPS have no connection with cerebral veins, the superficial middle cerebral vein (SMCV) still drains through the embryonic tentorial sinus and the superior petrosal sinus (SPS) is still not conjoined, draining only cerebellar veins. Whereas only in a typical adult stage the CS may receive blood from the SMCV, the sphenoparietal sinus (SPPS) and the SOV and drains into the inferior petrosal sinus (IPS), pterygoid plexus (PP) and SPS (SUZUKI and MATSUMOTO 2000). The condition that the CS does not participate in the cerebral venous drainage may persist, but frequently the secondary anastomoses involving the CS occur before adult life (PADGET 1956b).

This concept is not in full agreement with more recent studies on fetal skull bases by KNOSP et al. (1987a) who found that in 20% the superficial middle cerebral vein drains into the CS, or the tentorial sinus has no connection to the CS. The authors further observed the SPS in 60% connected with the CS, however minor functional significance, demonstrating the prenatal existence of cerebral venous blood flow through the CS. A recent study on 270 patients using CT-angiography showed that in approximately 27% of the adult population the SMCV may not be connected to the CS (SUZUKI and MATSUMOTO 2000).

Based on this staged embryologic development and various possibilities of persistence in adult life, the pattern of venous tributaries and drainage of the CS seen on cerebral angiograms can vary considerably.

3.3.2.1.2
Anatomy and Topography

The cavernous sinus (CS) belongs to the group of the great dural sinuses (sinus durae matris) which, because of their particular anatomical structure, are not named veins. An endothelial tube is surrounded by firm connective collagenous tissue without valves, but numerous lacunes and trabeculae. The CS surrounds the sphenoid bone and the pituitary gland. It forms in the middle cranial fossa a central collector for the blood coming from the meningeal veins (MV), the sphenoparietal sinus (SPPS), the superficial middle cerebral vein (SMCV) and the ophthalmic veins. The CS is located at the lateral side of the sphenoid bone, is triangular in shape and its medial border is formed by a connective tissue layer of the hypophysis. The CS has a length of approximately

20 mm and a width of 29 mm (LANG 1979a), extends from the petrous apex to the basal roots of the lesser sphenoid wing and reaches the medial part of the superior orbital fissure.

Since its very first description, controversy concerning the true anatomic structure of the CS has repeatedly occurred and persists to some extent until today.

The cavernous sinus was probably first described by RIDLEY (1695) as follows: "Another I discovered by having these veins injected with wax, running round the pituitary gland on its upper side, forwardly within the duplicature of the dura mater, backwardly between the dura mater and pia mater, then somewhat loosely stretched over the subjacent gland itself and laterally in a sort of canal made up of the dura mater above and the carotid artery on each outside of the gland, which by being fastened to the dura mater above, and below at the basis of the skull, leaves only a little interstice betwixt itself

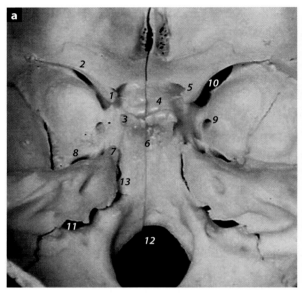 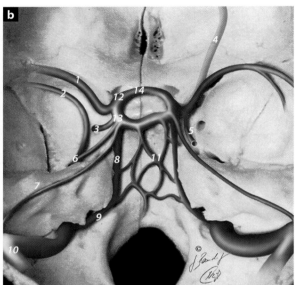

Fig. 3.8a,b. The complex anatomy of the cavernous sinus and its communicating venous structures can be appreciated. The main tributaries are the superior ophthalmic vein, sphenoparietal sinus, superficial middle cerebral vein and the uncal vein. The Sylvian vein drains into the sphenoparietal sinus or directly into the venous plexus of the foramen ovale (FOP). The most important draining vessels are the plexus of the forman ovale which is connected to the pterygoid plexus, the inferior petrosal sinus and the superior petrosal sinus. The course of the inferior petrosal sinus to the jugular foramen along the petroclival fissure and the course of the superior petrosal sinus to the sigmoid sinus along the petrous ridge are demonstrated. Because of its straight and short course, the inferior petrosal sinus represents the most suitable venous approach to the cavernous sinus in the majority of cases. **Note also:** The internal carotid artery venous plexus (ICAVP, Rektorzik) is not illustrated. The marginal sinus that receives the blood from the BP is not shown. The IPCV and the ACC would not be visible in this perspective.

a Osseus anatomy of the sellar region. Cranial and posterior view onto the middle cranial fossa and the inner skull base.

  1 Anterior clinoid process
  2 Sphenoid bone
  3 Posterior clinoid process
  4 Sella turcica
  5 Optic canal
  6 Clivus
  7 Pyramid apex
  8 Foramen ovale
  9 Foramen rotundum
10 Superior orbital fissure
11 Jugular foramen
12 Foramen magnum
13 Petroclival fissure

b Osseus and venous anatomy of the sellar region. Venous tributaries and drainage of the cavernous sinus (artist's drawing).

  1 Sphenoparietal sinus (SPPS)
  2 Superficial middle cerebral vein (SMCV)
  3 Emissary vein of the foramen rotundum
  4 Superior ophthalmic vein (SOV)
  5 Uncal vein (UV)
  6 Foramen ovale plexus (FOP)
  7 Superior petrosal sinus (SPS)
  8 Inferior petrosal sinus (Pars verticalis)
  9 Inferior petrosal sinus (Pars horizontalis)
10 Sigmoid sinus (SS)
11 Basilar plexus (BP)
12 Cavernous sinus (anterius)
13 Cavernous sinus (posterius)
14 Intercavernous sinus (ICS)

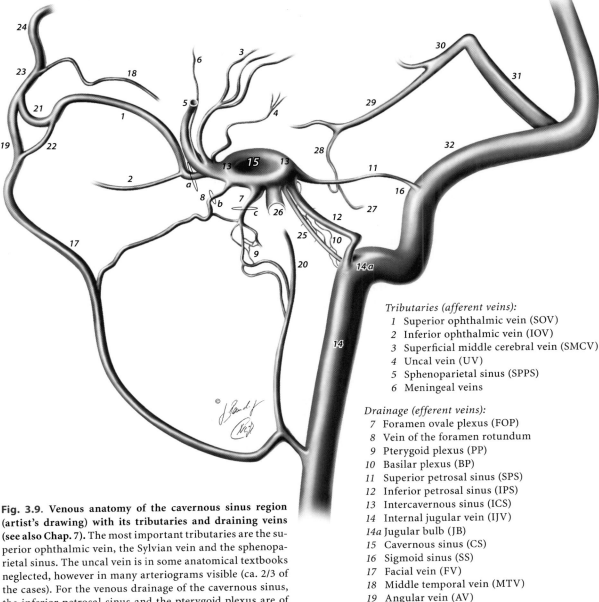

Fig. 3.9. Venous anatomy of the cavernous sinus region (artist's drawing) with its tributaries and draining veins (see also Chap. 7). The most important tributaries are the superior ophthalmic vein, the Sylvian vein and the sphenoparietal sinus. The uncal vein is in some anatomical textbooks neglected, however in many arteriograms visible (ca. 2/3 of the cases). For the venous drainage of the cavernous sinus, the inferior petrosal sinus and the pterygoid plexus are of major importance. In general, tributaries as well as draining veins, may serve as endovascular access routes to the cavernous sinus, depending on individual angioarchitecture of the fistula, hemodynamics and associated thrombosis causing occlusion. Note: the internal carotid artery venous plexus (ICAVP, Rektorzik) is usually not easily visible on 2D angiograms due to its very thin circular lumen in tangential projections. The inferior petroclival vein (IPCV) is in lateral angiographic views difficult to identify, because the sinus is often superimposed onto the IPS (see Figs. 7.85–7.91). Both veins are neglected in many textbooks. Furthermore, the anterior condylar confluens (ACC) lies anterior and medial to the jugular bulb, is a collector that anastomoses with the internal and external vertebral venous plexus and is not shown here (see Figure 3.12.).

Tributaries (afferent veins):
1 Superior ophthalmic vein (SOV)
2 Inferior ophthalmic vein (IOV)
3 Superficial middle cerebral vein (SMCV)
4 Uncal vein (UV)
5 Sphenoparietal sinus (SPPS)
6 Meningeal veins

Drainage (efferent veins):
7 Foramen ovale plexus (FOP)
8 Vein of the foramen rotundum
9 Pterygoid plexus (PP)
10 Basilar plexus (BP)
11 Superior petrosal sinus (SPS)
12 Inferior petrosal sinus (IPS)
13 Intercavernous sinus (ICS)
14 Internal jugular vein (IJV)
14a Jugular bulb (JB)
15 Cavernous sinus (CS)
16 Sigmoid sinus (SS)
17 Facial vein (FV)
18 Middle temporal vein (MTV)
19 Angular vein (AV)
20 Retromandibular vein
21 Superior root of SOV
22 Inferior root of SOV
23 Supraorbital vein
24 Frontal vein (FrV)
25 Inferior petroclival vein (IPCV)
26 Internal carotid artery venous plexus (ICAVP, Rektorzik)

Other:
27 Cerebellar vein
28 Lateral mesencephalic vein
29 Basal vein of Rosenthal
30 Vein of Galen   a Superior orbital
31 Straight sinus   b Foramen rotundum
32 Transverse sinus   c Foramen ovale

and the gland". WINSLOW (1732) found the internal carotid artery "bathed in the blood of the sinus together with the third, fourth, fifth and sixth pairs of nerves". It was Winslow who named the sinus "cavernous" because of its spongious (cavernous) structure that seemed to be formed by numerous fibers and septa of connective tissue. At the beginning of the last century, most anatomical textbooks (HUBER 1930; SOBOTTA 1928; SPALTEHOLZ 1933), as well clinical contributions (CAMPBELL 1933; PACE 1941) repeatedly emphasized that the lumen of the CS is crossed by numerous fibrous laminae, termed trabeculae. KNOTT (1882) observed that the CS "is crossed by fibrous trabeculae from some which villous process hang into the current of venous blood".

This so-called cavernous structure has been later on increasingly questioned. BUTLER (1957) found that only the extended cavernous sinus in adults contains minimal filaments and those are only found close to the connections with tributaries. He did not find trabeculae in fetal sinuses.

PARKINSON (1965, 1967) initially perpetuated the concept of the CS as one large venous space, but found in a later study using venous corrosion specimens that it represents an irregular plexus of varying sized venous channels, dividing and coalescing and incompletely surrounding the carotid artery (PARKINSON 1973).

Also BONNET (1957) expressed the opinion that the CS per se does not exist and the space between the dural sheets is filled by the carotid lumen, surrounded by a plexus of veins and nerves. The trabeculae seen in cadavers were probably cut walls of the small veins.

BEDFORD (1966) examined 34 cavernous sinuses and found in 80% an "unbroken" venous channel. She therefore proposed not to call this sinus cavernous but instead "sinus orbito-temporalis", or as already suggested by RIDLEY (1695) the "circular sinus". This concept was initially defended also by HARRIS and RHOTON (1976) after detailed studies on 50 cadavers. Later on, RHOTON et al. (1984) found the CS "not appearing" an unbroken cavern, but composed of several anastomosing venous channels formed by the convergence of multiple veins and dural venous sinuses. These venous channels would converge to form three main venous spaces, identified by their relationship to the ICA in medial, anteroinferior and posterosuperior compartments (INOUE et al. 1990; RHOTON et al. 1984; OKA et al. 1985). These three compartments are substantially larger than the space between the ICA and the lateral wall. The small lateral space can be so narrow that the CN VI "is adherent"

to the carotid wall medially and to the lateral sinus wall laterally (BEDFORD 1966).

BEDFORD (1966) further found that the internal carotid artery and the CN VI were outside the lumen of the sinus in 77% of the adult specimens. To consider the CS obstructive in nature and that it would predispose to thrombus formation was accordingly incorrect. Even though one may expect that thrombus formation would be seen more often in sinuses with dense trabeculae, TURNER and REYNOLDS (1926) found only a few trabeculae in their studies on CS thrombosis.

KNOSP et al. (1987a) focused in his studies on fetal cavernous sinus and preferred the term cavernous venous plexus referring to the CS as a network of distinct, individual veins.

There is otherwise no doubt that trabeculae have been found in some CS. Through the CS passes the ICA, surrounded by a plexus of sympathetic nerves. These structures are separated from the blood by a layer of endothelium. According to LANG (1979a), in an embryo there exists a venous plexus that is in 70% of the cases replaced by a single blood space, which can be traversed by 10–60 trabeculae. In 27% of the cases the CS consists of different large venous lakes that anastomose with each other. BROWDER and KAPLAN (1976) found the outer and inner walls of the CS relatively fixed by irregularly placed strands of fibrocollagenous tissues which did not form a recognizable pattern. They further emphasized that valve-like membranes were not observed at or near the orifice of any of the tributaries.

TAPTAS (1987) described the cavernous sinus as a network of small caliber extradural veins and not as a single trabeculated venous canal. He gave an excellent historical overview and compared the English and French literature of the last century with German authors, revealing the numerous discrepancies in reports and anatomic textbooks between LANGER (1884) and ROUVIERE (1985). It is astonishing, as it remains difficult to understand why for more than 100 years, particularly in the English and French literature, the concept of a large trabeculated sinus prevailed. As speculated by TAPTAS (1987), it may in part be due to the most convenient explanation of Nelaton's first observation of a pulsating exophthalmos by a ruptured carotid wall and shunting blood into a large single lumen cavern. The lack of precise angiographic imaging certainly contributed to this long-lasting misconception.

The controversial terminology is continued by others (KNOSP et al. 1987a; SARMA and TER BRUGGE

2003; Lasjaunias 1997), suggesting the term cavernous plexus because of its resemblance to other plexiform structures in the neighborhood, such as the retroclival (basilar) plexus, the venous plexus along the anterior margin of the foramen magnum (marginal sinus) and the spinal venous plexus (Brown et al. 2005).

Parkinson (2000) in a more recent communication emphasized that the term "cavernous sinus" remains one of the greatest obstacles to understanding the anatomy of the sellar and parasellar region. He suggests the term lateral sellar compartment as an enlarged segment of the extradural neural axis compartment (EDNAC). This extends from the coccyx to the orbit and contains valueless veins through which blood may run freely in either direction in addition to nervous, arterial and venous elements that may either leave or enter the compartment in its various segments.

The CS is probably neither an unbroken trabeculated venous cavern (Harris and Rhoton 1976; Inoue et al. 1990; Bedford 1966) nor a plexus of various-sized veins (Parkinson 1965, 1973; Bonnet 1957), but rather a complex venous compartment where numerous dural sinuses and veins converge to form larger venous spaces around the carotid artery which could be termed caverns (Rhoton et al. 1984).

This concept finds, at least in part, support in the angiographic pattern of the CS in normal carotid artery venograms and in the angioarchitecture of many DCSFs or CCFs. The angiographic pattern of the CS varies significantly in size and shape but is often one of a more or less single vascular space on each side of the sphenoid bone. In most direct high-flow carotid cavernous fistulas (CCFs), the blood seems to shunt into a single more or less enlarged cavity in which large detachable balloons may easily migrate after being detached. Finally, in the majority of low-flow DCSF with usually multiple feeders, the shunting zone often appears rather as a single communicating venous space which can often (although not always) be approached from both sides using various CS tributaries or draining channels. A true "anatomical compartmentalization" of the CS (Chaloupka et al. 1993) may occur, but remains seldom and likely represents often a misinterpreted thrombosed CS. Platinum coils, used for transvenous occlusions, usually take a configuration that resembles rather one single venous space than a true plexus of multiple veins.

Harris and Rhoton (1976) and others (Inoue et al. 1990; Oka et al. 1985) have described three or four main venous spaces within the CS, which they termed according to their relationship with the ICA as medial, anteroinferior, posterosuperior and lateral compartments. The medial compartment lies between the pituitary gland and the ICA, the anteroinferior compartment lies in the concavity below the first curve of the ICA, the posterosuperior compartment between the ICA and the posterior roof of the CS (Miller 1998).

The CSs communicate via *intercavernous sinuses* (ICSs), which have been described already by Winslow (1732) as the "inferior circular sinus" lying underneath the pituitary gland. Knott (1882) reported these connections in 6 of 44 specimens and described two intercavernous sinuses, located anteriorly and posteriorly to the hypophysis. This intrasellar venous connection through the midline has been further studied by Renn and Rhoton (1975) who concluded that an intrasellar communication between both CS may or may not be present. Typical are the anterior and posterior ICS (see below), which are named by other authors as coronary sinuses (Rabischong et al. 1974).

It is noteworthy that San Millan Ruiz et al. (1999) recently described a venous channel separate from the CS but enclosed in its lateral wall, which was found in 24% of the cases. This so-called laterocavernous sinus was found to drain the SMCVs in 22% of the cases and was separated from the CS anatomically and angiographically (Gailloud et al. 2000). Knowledge of this laterocavernous sinus may become crucial in case of a DCSF that may be not accessible. employing common transvenous approaches via the IPS or the SOV because communications between CS and laterocavernous sinus seem to be rare (3 cases in 58 specimens) (San Millan Ruiz et al. 1999).

Besides the SMCVs, the ophthalmic veins and some inferior veins of the brain are connected with the CS. The sphenoparietal sinus (SPPS) at the lower surface of the sphenoid wing, after receiving blood from several small veins of the dura mater and the anterior trunk of the middle meningeal vein (MMV), also drains into the CS. The CS communicates with the transverse sinus via the superior petrosal sinus, with the IJV via the inferior petrosal sinus (IPS), with the basilar plexus (BP), internal carotid artery venous plexus (ICAVP) and pterygoid plexus (PP) via veins through the sphenoid emissary foramen, thin veins of the canalis rotundis, larger veins of the foramen ovale, lacerum, and foramen venosum (Vesalii), and with the facial vein (FV) via the superior ophthalmic vein (SOV). In addition, communications with the IJV via the ICAVP can be found.

The venous vessels, connected with the CS, may be divided into tributaries and draining veins, of which their functions may be changed under pathological conditions such as thrombosis, tumors or arteriovenous shunts (MILLER N 1998).

The SOV, IOV, SMCV, small hypophyseal veins, and occasionally the uncal vein are considered afferent veins (tributaries). The efferent veins are the emissary veins, the IPS, and the petro-occipital sinus (if present) (DOYON et al. 1974). The SPS can drain into both the sigmoid sinus (SS) and the CS, depending on the hemodynamic balance. It is believed that the ICA pulsations support indirectly the venous flow in the CS. In case of a carotid artery occlusion this flow is slowed down and the flow in the CS may become more continuous (DOYON et al. 1974).

Table 3.3. Cavernous sinus and its main afferent (tributaries) and efferent (draining) veins CS

Afferent veins
- Orbital veins
  - Superior ophthalmic vein
  - Inferior ophthalmic vein
  - Central retinal vein (to SOV, CS)
- Angular vein (to SOV)
- Superficial middle cerebral vein (SMCV)
- Uncal vein (UV)
- Sphenoparietal sinus (SPPS)
- Intracavernous sinus (ICS)
- Meningeal veins
- Veins of the foramen rotundum

Efferent veins
- Superior petrosal sinus (SPS)
- Inferior petrosal sinus (IPS)
- Basilar plexus (BP)
- Pterygoid plexus (PP)
- Inferior petroclival vein (IPCV)
- Petro-occipital sinus
- Internal carotid venous plexus
- Foramen ovale plexus (FOP)
- Foramen lacerum plexus
- (Transverse occipital sinus)

3.3.2.2
Tributaries of the Cavernous Sinus (Afferent Veins)

Orbital Veins

The orbit is drained by the superior and inferior ophthalmic veins. These veins and their tributaries are unusual in that they are without valves and are markedly tortuous with many plexiform anastomoses (DOYON et al. 1974). The complex anatomy of the orbital veins, their numerous tributaries, anastomoses and drainage pathways has been studied early on by both detailed anatomic dissections (HENRY 1959),and a specifically developed radiographic technique, orbital phlebography. The latter, a major diagnostic method for intraorbital tumors and infectious diseases in the "pre CT MRI" era provided highly detailed anatomic knowledge, that still cannot be obtained today even when using high-resolution MRI or DSA (DOYON et al. 1974; FISCHGOLD et al. 1952; HANAFEE et al. 1968; LOMBARDI and PASSERINI 1967, 1968, 1969; CLAY and VIGNAUD 1974; CLAY et al. 1976; VIGNAUD and CLAY 1974; VIGNAUD et al. 1972, 1974; THERON 1972; GOZET et al. 1974).

In 1755, Zinn described the superior ophthalmic vein, its course through the superior orbital fissure, and its venous anastomoses in the orbit. According to that author, Vesalius was the first to describe the ophthalmic vein as beginning at the medial angle of the eye and Fallopian was the first to describe its anastomoses with the facial vein. Walter first correctly described the anatomic relation of the superior ophthalmic vein, inferior ophthalmic vein and facial veins in 1775. In their reports, GURWITSCH (1883) and, in 1887, Festal described fairly accurately the orbital veins and their relation with the cavernous sinus, the ocular muscles, the optic nerve and the ophthalmic artery. By dissection of the veins in ten orbits that had been injected previously with gelatin, HENRY (1959) described the orbital veins most accurately (DOYON et al. 1974).

Superior Ophthalmic Vein (Fig. 3.10)
The superior ophthalmic vein (SOV) is connected with all other intraorbital veins through numerous direct and indirect collaterals. The vein originates at the junction of its inferior and superior roots, also described as inferior and superior tributaries (DOYON et al. 1974). The vein measures 2 mm anteriorly and approximately 3.5 mm posteriorly, and increases in diameter at the junction of each tributary. As described by DOYON et al. (1974), the inferior root can be considered the true initial segment of the SOV belonging to the angular vein, while the superior root represents a continuation of the frontal vein. Some authors (DUTTON 1994) consider the superior root the supratrochlear vein and the true SOV emerging at the junction between the infratrochlear and the supraorbital vein. As stressed by BIONDI et al. (2003), this particular anatomy may

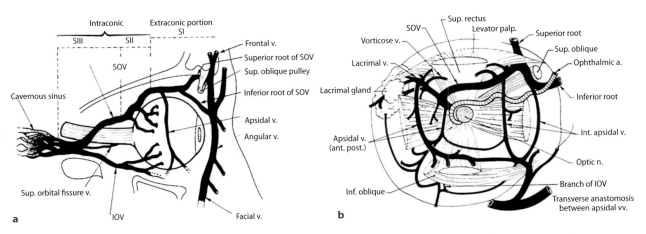

Fig. 3.10a,b. Segments of the superior ophthalmic vein. (From Doyon et al., 1974). Note the particular arrangment of superior and inferior roots of the SOV, not demonstrated in all textbooks. Being aware of this particular anatomy can become important when navigating a microcatheter through the angular vein during facial vein/superior ophthalmic vein approach (Biondi et al. 2003) (see also Fig. 7.31 a–d)

become important when performing transfacial or transophthalmic approaches. Sesemann (1869) as well as Gurwitsch (1883) divided the SOV into two or three branches that unify later on. The SOV enlarges during their course and narrows after passing the SOF, indicating that drainage is mainly posterior towards the CS. The slight enlargement before entering the CS is sometimes described as the ophthalmic sinus (Sinus ophthalmicus). Hanafee et al. (1968) and others (Doyon et al. 1974) made the suggestion to classify the SOV into three segments.

The anterior segment (first segment, Doyon et al. 1974) forms underneath the superior oblique muscle by unification of two branches, of which one comes from the supraorbital vein (often larger) and passes through the supraorbital incisura (superior root). The other originates from the angular vein (inferior root) and passes along the medial orbital wall. The anterior part of the SOV lies initially adjacent to the orbital roof, lies outside the muscle cone but is fixed by its relation to the superior oblique muscle.

The vein then enters the muscle cone about 5 mm behind the posterior pole of the globe and courses as the middle (second) segment lateral and below the superior rectus muscle and the levator palpebrae muscle dorsally to reach the superior orbital fissure (SOF). As the vein approaches the lateral wall of the orbit, it crosses the underlying optic nerve and ophthalmic artery and receives the lacrimal vein. In this segment the vein is not fixed and can be easily displaced by intraorbital masses.

The posterior (third) segment begins when the vein turns medially, posteriorly and slightly down-

wards. The SOV leaves the muscle cone, courses between the tendinous portions of the superior rectus and levator muscles and the lateral rectus muscle inferiorly. It leaves the orbit by following the lateral edge of the annulus of Zinn and then descending along the inferior edge of the superior portion of the SOF (Doyon et al. 1974). When the vein passes the fissure and enters the anterior CS its lumen is usually narrowed. On angiograms, this segment is best visible in lateral projections, starting where the vein turns downwards, and then passes through the fissure and ending at the CS (Hanafee et al. 1968; Brismar 1974).

The SOV has connections with the veins of the face and forehead (angular vein, facial vein, frontal and temporal veins) and receives blood from the territory of the ophthalmic artery (four vortex veins of the globe, ciliary veins, central retinal veins) when passing through the orbit. The diameter of the SOV varies considerably and asymmetrical arrangement of the vein is frequently seen without underlying pathology (Brismar 1974). The SOV receives blood mainly from two large ethmoidal veins, four vortex veins and a large lacrimal vein, which may occasionally drain into the CS separately (Miller N 1998).

Inferior Ophthalmic Vein

The inferior ophthalmic vein (IOV) is much smaller and often not visible on angiograms. It courses over the floor of the orbit, takes off branches from the inferior oblique muscle as well as from the inferior rectus muscle, drains veins of the lacrimal sac and the lower eye lid and two lower vortex veins, and then passes with the inferior rectus muscle backwards through the orbit. It drains in the orbit into the SOV or gives off a connecting branch and empties after passing the SOF into the CS (LOMBARDI and PASSERINI 1967, 1968). According to HANAFEE et al. (1986), the IOV drains directly into the PP. BROWDER and KAPLAN (1976) found the SOV was the largest venous trunk joining the CS. According to GURWITSCH (1883) this vein may be absent in one-third of the cases and is usually an inconspicuous structure that is has been given numerous other names (LANG 1983). The existence of a third intraorbital vein, the middle ophthalmic vein, is doubtful (LOMBARDI and PASSERINI 1967).

Central Retinal Vein (No Direct CS Tributary)

The central retinal vein (CRV) drains the retina and the intraorbital parts of the optic nerve and is of special clinical significance. Formed by the union of various retinal veins at the level of the lamina cribrosa, it runs through the core of the optic nerve in company with the central retinal artery. Within the lamina cribrosa the central retinal vein anastomoses through lateral twigs with the choroidal venous plexus. In patients with occlusion or chronic compression of the CRV (MILLER N 1998), these small anastomotic channels may enlarge to become optociliary veins that shunt blood from the retinal to the choroidal circulation The CRV exits from the optic nerve about 10 mm posterior to the globe, usually in company with the CRA. The vein normally courses for 4–8 mm through the vaginal spaces surrounding the nerve before it pierces the dura to exit the nerve 1–2 mm dorsal to the point of entry of the artery. The CRV may drain into the SOV, into some other orbital veins or directly into the CS (LANG 1983). It is believed that the CRV has no functionally adequate collaterals within the eyeball. Occlusion of the vein will therefore result into serious circulatory disorders with retinal venous infarcts or hemorrhages and subsequently secondary glaucoma.

Superficial Middle Cerebral Vein, Sylvian Vein

The superficial middle cerebral vein (SMCV), also called the superficial Sylvian vein (SYLVII) (GALLIGIONI et al. 1969), originates in the posterior segment of the lateral fissure, and courses along the fissure downwards and anteriorly to reach the regio pterionalis. According to traditional views, the vein penetrates the dura and becomes a venous sinus (the sphenoidal part of the Breschet` sinus, sphenopari-

etal sinus) which courses medially along the lesser sphenoid wing to the anterior part of the CS. The existence of this connection was recently questioned by RUIZ et al. (2004) who studied the cranial venous system of 15 nonfixed human specimens. These authors could not find a connection between the SMCV and the sphenoparietal sinus in their series and, referring to the original work of Breschet, stress that this connection was in fact never illustrated in his work (see below).

Though the connection of the SMCV with the CS is not developed at birth, it forms in a later stage of life. Typically, at infant stage the vein drains posteriorly into the tentorial sinus to reach the transverse sinus. Under normal conditions and after complete development, the SMCV drains the insula, the cortex on both sides of the lateral fissure, as well as parts of the occipital and frontal lobes. It anastomoses with the deep venous system via the uncal vein, the insular vein and the basilar veins and other superficial cerebral and dural veins. It communicates also with the facial veins via the venous circulation of the orbit (GALLIGIONI et al. 1969). It may further take off blood from the middle meningeal veins, which are connected with diploic veins and the superior sagittal sinus. The drainage system of the SMCV may show numerous variations. As a rule the SMCV as a vein of dural origin usually does not drain into the basal vein of Rosenthal, since the latter and its tributaries are derived from veins of pial origin (HUANG and WOLF 1974). It may however be joined by the first or second segment of the basal vein and continue into a dural sinus.

BISARIA (1985). who studied the course of the SMCV in 140 human cadavers, found the following variations in its drainage: 51% into both SPPS, 6% into SPPS and CS, 13% in SPPS and middle meningeal veins. In 14% the vein drained into the CS alone, in 5% into the CS and meningeal veins. In one case it drained into a vein in the foramen lacerum and the SPPS, in one case into the SPPS and the SPS, in another into the middle meningeal vein on either side. The authors found one unusual drainage into the SSS and emphasize that prior to their study, the majority of the work on the termination of the SMCV was based on roentgenographic findings rather than on dissections.

Based on CT angiograms, SUZUKI and MATSUMOTO (2000) found seven different types of drainage of which the most frequent were the sphenoparietal sinus (54%), the cavernous sinus (7%) and an emissary vein of the foramen ovale

(12%). The superficial and deep SMCVs may also drain directly into the laterocavernous sinus (SAN MILLAN et al. 1999). This work was recently complemented by Tanoue et al. 2006 who, by means of MRI examinations, simply classified the SMCV into four main types of variation. A direct connection with the SPPS and anterior CS was found in 39%, a connection with the lateral aspect of the CS independently in 30%, direct communication with the PP in 11% and a posterior course across the petrous ridge to drain into the SPS or transverse sinus in 8% of their cases.

Uncal Vein, Uncinate Vein

The uncal vein (UV) is a small, but important vein that can be angiographically identified in two out of three cases (GOZET et al. 1974). Surprisingly, this vein however, is neglected in schematic drawings of many textbooks. It passes the medial temporal lobe along the anterior margin of the uncus and drains either in the SMCV, the SPPS or directly in the CS. According to WOLF et al. (1955) this vessel marks the medial aspect of the temporal lobe and therefore has diagnostic importance. BISARIA (1985) found it in only 5% of the specimens pointing to the fact that this vein has been not described hitherto in many anatomical textbooks. The uncal vein is a derivate of the deep telencephalic vein, one of three primitive veins forming the basal vein of Rosenthal (HUANG and WOLF 1974; PADGET 1956a) by longitudinal anastomoses, and joins the SMCV in the neonate state, both draining into the CS. Failure of these longitudinal anastomoses is most frequent between the first and second segments of the basal vein resulting into a common stem formed by tributaries of the striate veins and posterior insular veins that drain anteroinferior into the SPPS, CS or PCS (HUANG and WOLF 1974). This vein has been designated the uncal vein (WOLF et al. 1963) and may be responsible for redirection of cortical venous drainage causing intracerebral venous hemorrhage in a DCSF (TAKAZAWA et al. 2005). Various secondary anastomoses between the SMCV, SPPS, SOV, CS and the uncal vein can occur (HUANG and WOLF 1974).

Sphenoparietal sinus (Breschet), Sinus alae parvae, Sinus sphenoidales superior (Sir C. Bell)

The sphenoparietal sinus (SPPS) is the largest of the meningeal veins, usually coursing with the anterior branch of the MMA above the level of the pterion (OKA et al. 1985). The classic description of the SPPS is an antero-inferior continuation of the meningeal sinus following the arc of the sphenoid wing and reaching the anterior CS. The term sphenoparietal sinus was introduced originally by BRESCHET (1829) and has been widely used in anatomical textbooks. According to him, the anterior branch of the middle meningeal vein joins a small dural sinus, the sinus of the lesser sphenoid wing (RUIZ et al. 2004). In many textbooks (GRAY 1918; LANG 1979a; OSBORN 1980a) and early original papers (WOLF 1963), this sinus is considered the main drainage of the SMCV to reach the cavernous sinus which is probably due to the close anatomical relationship of both vessels while coursing along the sphenoid wing. As pointed out by Padget, this sinus is not clearly defined and readily confused with a conspicuous remnant of the tentorial sinus draining the SMCV while following the lesser sphenoid wing. A true constant connection between the SMCV and the SPPS was also questioned in a recent study of RUIZ et al. (2004) who suggested instead that both veins pass next to each other but independently under the sphenoid wing to reach the cavernous sinus. This is supported by a reevaluation of original descriptions of the French anatomists BRESCHET (1829), TROLARD (1890) and others. The authors suggest that the parietal portion of the SPPS should be rather considered a continuation of the anterior middle meningeal vein whereas the sphenoidal portion of SPPS would represent a distinct dural sinus coursing under the lesser sphenoid wing with its own tributaries. This arrangement would be more appropriately termed sinus of the lesser sphenoid wing as earlier suggested by WOLF et al. (1963).

The SPPS may join the sphenoidal emissary veins to reach the PP, or pass further posteriorly to reach the SPS or the transverse sinus (TS; lateral sinus, LS). The former variant is called sphenobasal sinus, the latter sphenopetrosal sinus. Because both are remnants of the embryonic tentorial sinus, the SMCV may also empty into these sinuses when the SPPS is absent (OKA et al. 1985). The course of the SMCV laterally over the middle cranial fossa is also named paracavernous sinus (SAN MILLAN RUIZ et al. 1999).

Intercavernous Sinus, Sinus intercavernosus, Sinus circularis (Ridley), Sinus ellipticus, Sinus coronarius, Sinus clinoideus (Sir C. Bell), Sinus transversus sellae equinae (Haller)

The two cavernous sinuses are connected by means of one or more transverse vessels, intercavernous sinuses (ICS) which cross the pituitary fossa

(Knott 1882). There are usually two ICS with a diameter of up to 8 mm (Lang and Weigel 1983), connecting the CS anteriorly and posteriorly to the hypophysis and forming a venous circle (elliptic sinus, circular sinus, clinoid sinus). The anterior ICS is larger; the posterior can be completely absent. Knott (1882) found its absence in 26/44 cases (anatomical studies). In two cases he found the posterior ICS was larger and in one case it was the only one present. He found 3 transverse ICS in 15/44 cases. Small irregular venous sinuses coursing beneath the pituitary gland and draining into the ICS were already described by Winslow as so-called inferior circular sinus. Knott (1882) found this arrangement in only 6 cases, whereas in 12 others he found a single intercavernous vein beneath the pituitary body. In addition to the two ICS, Doyon et al. (1974) and others (Lasjaunias et al. 2001) have described a posterior communication via an occipital transverse sinus which probably corresponds to the basilar plexus.

Yasuda et al. (2004, 2005) in his recent study of the medial wall of the CS also described an inferior intercavernous sinus that connects the paired CS. These ICS extend across the midline between the meningeal dural layer covering the inferior aspect of the pituitary gland and the endosteal layer covering the floor of the sella.

Meningeal Veins

The meningeal veins (MV) are often developed as pairs, enclosed by dura sheets. Commonly, they accompany meningeal arteries and provide venous drainage for the cranial dura mater and are considered meningeal sinuses by some authors (Oka et al. 1985). They course between the arteries and the overlying bone which lead to a compression of their lumen and the typical radiographic appearance of parallel channels (Oka et al. 1985). They communicate with the superior sagittal sinus and unify to form two trunci anteriorly and posteriorly, which accompany the branches of the meningeal arteries. At the base of the skull they pass through the foramen spinosum and ovale to connect with the pterygoid plexus. The veins accompanying the anterior branch of the MMA drain into the SPPS, the CS or emissary veins (Oka et al. 1985).

Veins of the Foramen Rotundum, Emissary Vein

Knott (1882) observed in 2 cases (2/44) an additional small tributary in the form of an emissary vein passing through the canalis rotundus accompanying the maxillary division of the trigeminal nerve. It is connected with the extracranial pterygoid plexus and is considered by Browder and Kaplan (1976) a draining vein (rarely several small veins). Knott (1882) found in 23/44 subjects an inconstant vein lying in the dura mater on the inner surface of the greater sphenoid wing.

On rare occasions, the basal vein or the inferior ventricular vein was found to anastomose with the lateral wall of the CS (Lang 1983).

3.3.2.3
Drainage of the Cavernous Sinus (Efferent Veins)

Superior Petrosal Sinus, Sinus petrobasilaris (Langer), Sinus tentorii lateralis (Weber), Sinus petrosus superficialis

The superior petrosal sinus (SPS) courses between the layers of the tentorium cerebelli over the superior aspect of the petrous bone and connects the posterior superior angle of the CS with the proximal sigmoid sinus or the transverse sinus (Oka et al. 1985). It receives blood from the cerebellar veins, the lateral mesencephalic vein, the petrosal vein, the paracavernous sinus, the basal vein and the arcuate vein. Although often considered a channel draining the CS, the SPS may actually not drain blood from the CS. The blood flow is frequently directed from posterior to anterior, towards a confluence at the petrous apex, which is formed by the posterior part of the CS, a (transverse) communicating sinus, connecting the posterior CS and the IPS, draining the blood towards the IJV (Krayenbühl and Yasargil 1997). In contrast to Theron (1972), in our experience the posterior CS is relatively often visible in vertebral angiograms, which is explained by this direction of the flowing blood within the SPS. Knott (1882) found a complete absence of this sinus in 3/45 cases.

Inferior Petrosal Sinus, Sinus petrosus profundus, Sinus petro-occipitalis superior (Trolard)

The inferior petrosal sinus (IPS), shorter but larger than the SPS, represents the main posterior drainage of the CS towards the bulb of the internal jugular vein. It courses along the lower edge of the petrous bone and the petro-occipital suture, lying between the petrous pyramid and the clivus in the petroclival fissure. It reaches the jugular foramen and passes together with the glossopharyngeal, vagus and accessory nerve to enter the internal jugular vein (IJV). It receives blood from veins of the labyrinth, the cochlear aqueduct, medulla, pons and cerebellum. The IPS has a close relationship with the abducens nerve, which is imbedded in the wall of its sagittal segment.

According to BOSKOVIC et al. (1963) this sinus has a diameter of 7–10 mm in 93% of cases and has horizontal and sagittal parts. According to LANG (1983) it enters the posterior fossa 2–6 mm medial to the trigeminal pore (Dorello's canal) with a diameter of 7–10 mm in its longitudinal and 0.5–5 mm in its transverse part. The actual entry is usually situated below the superior sphenopetrosal ligament and also contains the sixth CN in its lateral angle.

SHIU et al. (1968) studied 346 patients undergoing petrosal sinus sampling and described 4 different types of junction between the IPS and the IJV (Fig. 3.11):

- Type I: 45% directly into the IJV
- Type II: 24% into a vein, which connects the deep cervical plexus with the IJV
- Type III: 24% via a plexus into the IJV
- Type IV: 7% directly into the cervical plexus

MILLER et al. (1993) modified this classification and added an incomplete type IV which is characterized by a small vein between the IJV and the point at which the IPS anastomoses with the vertebral venous plexus. It needs to be remembered, however, that these descriptions are exclusively based on retrograde venous angiograms and therefore may, due to variable venous hemodynamics, thrombosis of the IPS and suboptimal image quality, not fully reflect the true anatomy in this area. Thus, some vascular details like the IPCV was not recognized as such, although opacified in some of the figures (Fig. 2C therein).

KNOTT (1882) and others (LABALETTE 1891; SAPPEY 1888; THEILE 1843) described in the nineteenth century a connection between the IPS and the IJV below the skull base (3/8 of an inch). LANG and WEIGEL (1983) found such a variant in 10% of their specimens. The authors describe in addition an inferior petrosal sinus canal in 2%–3% of the cases. Surprisingly, this variant is not included in the classical description of SHIU et al. (1968). Recent studies have shown that the IPS, as an anatomical variant, may also enter the IJV far below the skull base (up 4–5 cm) (GAILLOUD et al. 1997). GAILLOUD et al. (1997) have named this deep termination of the IPS as the accessory jugular vein. We have observed this situation in three patients with a vascular lesion of the CS (see Fig. 7.37) and were able to successfully catheterize

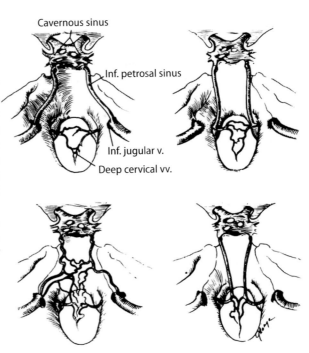

Fig. 3.11. Four main types of IPS-IJV connections as described by Shiu (from Shiu et al., 1968). This widely used classification is based on 2D angiograms from the pre-DSA era. It does not display all anatomic details in this area, which is in part due to the technique used for the cavernous sinus venography. Retrograde opacification of the IPS and CS can be limited by local hemodynamics and thrombotic processes. Furthermore, modern bi-plane DSA imaging provides significanly better spatial resolution (see Chap. 7). The inferior petroclival vein and the internal carotid artery venous plexus are not illustrated, although visualized in modern high-quality phlebograms. In AP view the vein lies next to the IPS and follows an almost parallel course. Neither the fact that the IPS may be thrombosed and thus only partially filled, nor the possibility of an abberant inferior petrosal sinus (deep termination below the skull base) was known or taken into account at that time

this aberrant inferior petrosal sinus (BENNDORF and CAMPI 2001). According to KATSUTA et al. (1997) the IPS, in its course along the petroclival fissure, also has connections with the CVP through the intrapetrosal veins and with the venous channel, called the inferior petroclival vein (IPCV, see below) which courses along the extracranial surface of the petroclival fissure [probably identical to the petro-occipital sinus described by AUBIN et al. (1974) and others (CLAY and VIGNAUD 1974)]. The IPS forms within the jugular foramen a venous confluens of 2–3 mm diameter, receiving blood from the venous plexus of the hypoglossus canal, the inferior petroclival vein and tributaries from the vertebral venous plexus and the posterior condylar vein. Sometimes two main channels connect the petrosal confluens with the jugular bulb (KATSUTA et al. 1997).

Venous Plexus of the Hypoglossal Canal, Anterior Condylar Vein

This plexus is also referred to as the anterior condylar vein (ACV), which connects the marginal sinus with the JB. It is crossed by trabeculae and may empty into the lower end of the IPS or directly into the IJV. Occasionally it drains into the lower end of the sigmoid sinus and may communicate with the posterior condylar vein and the vertebral plexus (KATSUTA et al. 1997).

Posterior Condylar Vein

The posterior condylar vein (PCV) passes through the posterior condylar foramen and courses in the posterior condylar canal to connect the vertebral venous plexus with the junction of the sigmoid sinus and the JB. The posterior condylar foramen opens into the posteromedial junction of the sigmoid sinus and the JB. It has communications with the confluens at the lower end of the IPS and via a bony channel with the anterior condylar vein (venous plexus of the hypoglossal canal) (KATSUTA et al. 1997).

Lateral Condylar Vein

The lateral condylar vein (LCV) runs between the inferior aspect of the external orifice of the hypoglossal canal (anterior condylar canal) and the suboccipital cavernous sinus as described by SAN MILLAN RUIZ et al. (2002) and ARNAUTOVIC et al. (1997).

Inferior Petroclival Vein

The inferior petroclival vein (IPCV) (Fig. 3.12, see also Figs. 7.85–7.90) is, according to KATSUTA et al. (1997), a "mirror image" to the IPS coursing along the extracranial surface of the petroclival fissure and empties into the confluens at the lower end of the IPS (RHOTON 2000). This vein is in some studies, probably erroneously called inferior petro-occiptal vein (SAN MILLAN RUIZ et al. 2002).

Petro-occipital Sinus, Sinus petro-occipitalis inferior, petro-occipital vein (Padget)

This very small sinus, described by TROLARD (1890), also originates from the CS, courses parallel to the IPS, but outside the skull, along the petro-occipital suture, enters the IPS just before

its connection with the IJV and can be seen in phlebograms of the jugular vein (AUBIN et al. 1974) or in orbital phlebograms (CLAY and VIGNAUD 1974). Because of its small caliber and its proximity to the IPS it may be easily superimposed and is best visualized in the projection after AUBIN et al. (1974) and can be missed on standard angiographic projections (see Chap. 7). The projection is called after Hirtz and was suggested by Aubin. Both, the petro-occipital sinus and the inferior petroclival vein are possibly referring to the same vascular structure.

Transverse Occipital Sinus (Doyen)

DOYEN et al. (1974), while reviewing the ophthalmic veins, described a sinus as transverse occipital sinus that connects both posterior CSs horizontally along the upper surface of the clivus. In another figure (Fig. 7.64 therein) this sinus travels caudally to reach the foramen magnum. I have not be able to find this sinus mentioned elsewhere other than in AUBIN et al. (1974) who describe it as the communication of the two posterior CS with the anterior segments of the IPS and the SPS.

Basilar Plexus (Virchow)

The basilar plexus (BP) consists of several communicating venous channels between the dural sheets above the dorsum sellae of the sphenoid bone and the bony skull base. The largest and most constant connection across the midline between the CS (RENN and RHOTON 1975) extends from the dorsum sellae and the pars basilaris of the sphenoid bone downwards, to become the marginal sinus. Its upper part, lying over the rostral end of the clivus, is connected with the posterior CS and both SPS. Its lower part is connected with both IPS and with the anterior internal vertebral venous plexus. According to LANG (1979a) it regularly contains clival rami of the MHT.

Marginal Sinus

This sinus lies between the layers of the dura mater adjacent to the anterior inner surface of the foramen magnum. It receives blood from the basilar plexus and communicates with the occipital sinus and the anterior internal venous plexus. TUBBS et al. (2006) recently studied further the anatomy and found significant communication between the marginal sinus and the veins of the hypoglossal canal, and that the vertebral artery was noted to pierce this sinus in the majority of the cases.

Internal Carotid Artery Venous Plexus, Sinus Venous Caroticus (Haike), Carotid Sinus, Pericarotid Plexus

The internal carotid artery venous plexus (ICAVP) was first described by Rektorzik in 1858 as pars intracanalem sinus caroticus, and descends from the inferior cavernous sinus enclosing the carotid artery more or less completely at the lower part of the carotid canal (KNOTT 1882) (Fig. 3.12). This plexus converges to form one or more trunks which open finally into the IJV and was found by KNOTT (1882) in each case of his series. HAIKE (1902) found that the sinus resembles the architecture of the CS, consisting of numerous small vascular spaces in children that confluent to larger lacunes with age. To him it appeared in some cases more like a plexus, in others more like a sinus. KNOSP et al. (1987a) considers the plexus in many cases a very important drainage system and found it more prominent in the fetus when compared to the adult condition. LANG (1983) found this plexus running together with the artery, sympathetic nerves and tissue of the arterial sheath to form two longitudinal veins at the external aperture of the carotid canal which originate near the bend of the ICA. The initial part of the plexus communicates with the IPS via a medial intrapetrosal vein in about 46% and via a lateral intrapetrosal vein in 50% of the cases. The former terminates about 11 mm above the jugular foramen, the latter terminates in the vicinity of the foramen (LANG and WEIGEL 1983). PAULLUS et al. (1977) found this (periarterial venous) plexus in 76% of the cases, in 24% it was poorly developed or absent. It extended an average of 7.6 mm into the canal and was located between the floor of the middle cranial fossa and the artery in only 4%. A fistula between the ICA and this plexus could mimic a true CCF. This sinus is difficult to identify on angiograms or phlebograms and may be superimposed by the IPS or IPCV, and thus is not shown by several authors investigating the angiographic anatomy in the CS–IPS region (HANAFEE et al. 1968; SHIU et al. 1968; MILLER DL et al. 1993). AUBIN (1974) demonstrated its visibility in axial projections, although it may be superimposed by the petro-occipital sinus (IPCV). Modern high-resolution DSA and three-dimensional DSA proves valuable in visualizing Rektorzik plexus (Chap. 7).

Foramen Ovale Plexus (Trigeminal Sinus), Sphenoid Emissary, "Rete" of the Foramen Ovale

Nuhn (in KNOTT 1882) described a pair of small veins, which pass through the foramen ovale to reach the pterygoid plexus. Knott found this plexus quite variable: in 18/45 cases he found a pair of veins on both sides, in 10 cases he found a pair on one side and a single vein on the other, in 11 cases there was a single vein on each side and in 5/45 cases a total absence on one side. HENDERSON (1966) called this sinus trigeminal sinus. BROWDER and KAPLAN (1976) found a number of veins draining the pachymeninx of the inferior part of the cerebral hemispheres converging to the middle cranial fossa and coursing to the foramen ovale, where channels from the ventrolateral aspect of the CS join them. PADGET (1956b) assumed that this plexus may not necessarily be concerned with the venous drainage, especially in the young. In adults, however, we see this plexus often drains the SMCV directly, bypasses the CS and may reach a diameter of up 6 mm (roughly the diameter of the foramen).

Vein of the Sphenoid Foramen (Foramen Venosum, Foramen of Vesalius)

A very small, inconstant vein supplementing the foramen ovale plexus when passing through the foramen venosum the margins of which are usually not ossified at birth (PADGET 1956b).

Foramen Lacerum Plexus

KNOTT (1882) constantly found a varying number of small veins passing through the foramen lacerum and always being connected with the cavernous sinus. The emissary veins connect with the pterygoid plexus but also with the inferior petroclival vein.

Pterygoid Plexus

The pterygoid plexus (PP) is an extensive network of small venous channels in the neighborhood of the IMA and lies lateral and medial to the lateral pterygoid muscle and is connected with the CS via sphenobasal emissary channels passing through the foramina in the middle cranial fossa. It receives blood from the transbasal veins (middle meningeal veins, foramen ovale plexus, carotid venous plexus, vein of the foramen rotundum, vein of the foramen venosum). The pterygoid plexus also communicates with the ophthalmic veins through the inferior orbital fissure, with the anterior facial vein via a deep facial branch and receives tributaries corresponding to branches of the pterygopalatine maxillary artery segment (OSBORN 1981). It usually drains posteriorly into the maxillary vein, which forms together with the superficial temporal vein the retromandibular vein. Although the latter vessel is usually a major tributary of the external jugular vein (EJV) the pterygoid plexus may also drain via posterior and common facial veins into the IJV (Osborn 1981; Goss 1966). In some cases, the SMCV drains not via the CS but directly into the PP, a disposition identified by Osborn (1981) as the sphenobasal pattern and found in 34% of the cases. This pattern was differentiated from the sphenopetrosal pattern via the sphenopetrosal vein into the transverse sinus (13%) or a combination of both (24%).

3.3.2.4
Other Veins of Importance for the CS Drainage or for Transvenous Access to the CS

Facial Vein

The anatomy of the facial vein (FV) has been described in part above (see under SOV) and has some importance for retrograde transvenous approaches. This vein drains the anterior portion of the scalp and the soft tissue of the face and begins at the medial palpebral angle as a direct continuation of the angular vein (Osborn 1981). The FV receives the supratrochlear and supraorbital veins and descends obliquely downwards crossing the face and the masseteric muscle behind the facial artery and until it reaches the body of the mandible. Slightly inferior and anterior to the angle of the mandible, it is joined by the anterior portion of the retromandibular vein and forms the common facial vein, which usually drains into the internal jugular vein (Peuker et al. 2001). In some cases it may also drain into the EJV (Osborn 1981) and under rare circumstances even into the superficial temporal vein (Peuker et al. 2001). The FV receives blood from the ala nasi, the deep facial vein (connection to the pterygoid plexus), inferior palpebral, superior and inferior labial, buccinator, parotid and masseteric veins. Under the mandible the submental and the submandibular veins join the FV.

Frontal Vein

The frontal vein (FrV) begins on the forehead in a venous plexus which communicates with the frontal branches of the superficial temporal vein (Gray 1918). The veins converge to form a single trunk, which runs downward near the middle line of the forehead parallel with the vein of the opposite side. The two FrVs are joined at the root of the nose by a transverse branch, called the nasal arch, which receives some small veins from the dorsum of the nose. At the root of the nose the veins diverge and at the medial angle of the orbit each of them joins the supraorbital vein to form the angular vein. Occasionally, the frontal veins join to form a single trunk, which bifurcates at the root of the nose into the two angular veins. The main stem of the FV usually forms the superior tributary to the angular vein (AV) (Doyon et al. 1974) consisting of two parts: the superior root of the SOV and the internal frontal vein. The former is accompanied by the supraorbital nerve and artery, which pass through the supraorbital notch (incisura supraorbitalis) and penetrate the orbital septum above the trochlea of the superior orbital muscle. The latter is a direct superior extension of the angular vein and has been used as a common approach to perform orbital phlebography (Doyon et al. 1974). Therefore, in case of a DCSF with prominent anterior venous drainage, it can also be used as a percutaneous approach for catheterization of the SOV and CS (Venturi et al. 2003).

Angular Vein

The angular vein (AV) represents an anastomosis between the facial vein and the SOV and is formed by the confluence of the supraorbital and frontal veins. Its subcutaneous course is down the side of the nose, lateral to the angular artery. The vein then crosses the nasal edge of the medial palpebral ligament approximately 8 mm from the internal canthus. The angular vein is continuous below with the facial vein (Doyon et al. 1974). The angular vein has three main tributaries: a medial or prenasal arch, the inferior root of the SOV and the internal frontal vein (Doyon et al. 1974).

Middle Temporal Vein

The middle temporal vein (MTV) arises near the eye, has an almost horizontal course above the zygomatic process and is connected with palpebral veins, the supraorbital vein and the facial vein. The vessel joins the superficial temporal vein to form the retromandibular vein. According to Hyrtl (1885) this vein is often found as a plexus. On angiograms it usually occurs as a single vein that has a typical acute angle when it passes over the zygomatic arch.

Because it anastomoses with the angular vein, this vessel may also be involved in the drainage of a DCSF and can be used as an approach for EVT (Cheng et al. 2003).

Internal Jugular Vein

The internal jugular vein (IJV) is the major drainage pathway for the cerebrovascular system, collecting blood from the brain, the superficial part of the face, and from the neck (GRAY 1918). The IJV begins in the posterior compartment of the jugular foramen, at the base of the skull, being continuous with the sigmoid sinus. Its origin is somewhat dilated, called the jugular bulb (JB, or superior bulb) (GRAY 1918). It runs down the side of the neck, lying at first lateral to the ICA and then lateral to the CCA. Above it lies the rectus capitis lateralis, behind the ICA and the nerves passing through the jugular foramen. Lower down, the IJV and ICA lie in the same plane, the CNs IX and XII passing forward between them. The CN X descends between and behind the vein and the artery in the same sheath and the CN XI runs obliquely backward, superficial or deep to the vein. At the base of the neck the right IJV is located at a little distance from the CCA and crosses the first part of the subclavian artery while the left IJV usually overlaps the CCA. The left IJV is usually smaller and each vein contains a pair of valves approximately 2.5 cm above their termination. The most important superficial relationship of the IJV is the sternomastoid muscle, which is lateral to the vein in its upper part and covers it in its lower part. The IJV unites at the base of the neck with the subclavian vein to form the innominate vein with a little second dilatation above, called the inferior bulb.

The IJV receives blood from the sigmoid sinus, inferior petrosal sinus, facial, lingual, pharyngeal superior thyroid, middle thyroid veins and sometimes the occipital veins. In a clinical sense the most crucial relationship is with the VA and CCA/ICA because inadvertent puncture (usually of the ICA) can be a serious complication (see below).

The External Jugular Vein

The external jugular (EJV) vein drains the greater part of the blood from the exterior of the cranium and the deep parts of the face. It is formed by the junction of the posterior division of the posterior facial vein and the posterior auricular vein. This vessel originates in the substance of the parotid gland at the level of the angle of the mandible and runs perpendicularly down the neck to end in the subclavian vein (GRAY 1918). It usually takes the retromandibular vein as major tributary, which is formed by the maxillary vein (draining the PP, see above) and the superficial temporal vein. There appears to be an inverse correlation between the size of the external and internal jugular vein – thus the presence of a large EJV may be an indicator of a small IJV and therefore of a potentially more difficult IJV puncture (STICKLE and MCFARLANE 1997).

Vertebral Vein, Vertebral Artery Venous Plexus

The vertebral vein is formed in the sub-occipital angle, from numerous small tributaries of the internal vertebral venous plexuses, mainly by the confluences of the anterior and posterior condylar veins (roots) which join to form the plexus of the vertebral vein, the supply functions of which can be modified by the presence of the mastoid anastomotic emissary veins (BRAUM and TOURNADE 1977). The anterior root of the vertebral vein originates at the level of the junction of the anterior and middle thirds of the occipital venous plexus from the anterior condylar vein (venous plexus of the hypoglossal canal). It follows an oblique, outward and forward course, crossing the anterior condylar canal before it joins the posterior root of the vertebral vein. The posterior root originates at the level of the posterior third of the occipital venous plexus, crosses the atlanto-occipital membrane and terminates by joining the anterior root to form the vertebral vein (BRAUN and TOURNADE 1977). The veins form a dense plexus around the vertebral artery, which descends in the canal formed by the foramina transversaria of the sixth cervical vertebrae. This vertebral artery venous plexus ends in a single trunk which emerges from the foramen transversarium of the sixth vertebra and empties into the back part of the innominate vein with a pair of valves (GRAY 1918). In the sub-occipital angle the vein communicates with the anterior internal vertebral venous plexuses with the deep cervical, and occipital veins, and is joined by veins coming from the recti and oblique muscles and from the pericranium. ARNAUTOVIC et al. (1997) studied the venous anatomy of the suboccipital region in particular around the third segment (V3) of the vertebral artery and found an astonishing resemblance with the cavernous sinus, naming it accordingly suboccipital cavernous sinus.

Deep Cervical Vein

The deep cervical vein, larger than the vertebral vein, passes down the neck posterior to the cervical transverse processes. It corresponds to the deep cervical artery from which it is separated by the semispinalis cervicis muscle. It begins in the posterior vertebral venous plexus and receives tributaries from the deep muscles of the neck. It communicates or entirely drains the occipital vein by a branch that perforates the trapezius muscle. The deep cervical vein then passes forward beneath the transverse process of the seventh cervical vertebra to open into the innominate vein near the vertebral vein, or into the latter its termination. Its orifice is guarded by a pair of valves (Gray 1918).

Anterior Condylar Confluent (Confluens Condyloideum Anterius, Trolard 1868)

The anterior condylar confluent (ACC) (Fig. 3.12) was initially observed by Trolard (1868), but was to a large extent ignored in the literature. San Millan Ruiz et al. (2002) recently "rediscovered" this short, venous structure located extracranially in front of the aperture of the hypoglossal canal at the level of the skull base. It provides a communication between the cerebral venous system and the internal and external vertebral venous plexus via six main channels: the anterior condylar vein, the lateral condylar vein, the IJV, the IPS, the venous plexus of Rektorzik, and the prevertebral plexus. Knott (1882) saw a venous plexus surrounding the hypoglossal nerve as it passes through the inner part of the anterior condyloid foramen, (the circellus venosus hypoglossi after Luschka) and found two veins proceeding from this plexus, one of which communicates with the vertebral plexus, the other with the IPS. He did not observe a consistent confluent. Katsuta et al. (1997), however, described in their study on microsurgical anatomy of the jugular foramen (see therein) a confluens that connects the anterior condylar vein, the posterior condylar vein, the IPS, the inferior petroclival and the vertebral venous plexus vein with the JB. This channel likely corresponds to the ACC illustrated by San Millan Ruiz et al. (2002).

Detailed knowledge of the complex and variant anatomy in this region is important, not only to understand of basic physiology of the venous circulation in the cranio-cervical region but also to perform petrosal sinus sampling. It certainly facilitates transvenous catheterizations for transvenous occlusion of a DCSF. The ACC may form anastomoses with the IPS at a variable distance from its termination into the IJV. In some cases the direct communication between IPS and IJV may be small or non-existent and the route through the ACC is the alternative. See more details in Chap. 7.

References

Allen WE III, Kier EL, Rothman SL (1973) The maxillary artery: normal arteriographic anatomy. Am J Roentgenol Radium Ther Nucl Med 118:517–527

Allen WE III, Kier EL, Rothman SL (1974) The maxillary artery in craniofacial pathology. Am J Roentgenol Radium Ther Nucl Med 121:124–138

Arnautovic KI, Al-Mefty O, Pait TG, Krisht AF, Husain MM (1997) The suboccipital cavernous sinus. J Neurosurg 86:252–262

Aubin ML, Paleirac R, Traserra J (1974) Radioanatomy of the jugular sinus and its anterior collaterals. Ann Radiol (Paris) 17:247–252

Barrow DL, Spector RH, Braun IF, Landman JA, Tindall SC, Tindall GT (1985) Classification and treatment of spontaneous carotid-cavernous sinus fistulas. J Neurosurg 62:248–256

Baumel JJ, Beard D (1961) The accessory meningeal artery of man. J Anat 95:356–402

Bedford MA (1966) The "cavernous sinus". Brit J Ophthal 50:41–46

Benndorf G, Campi A (2001) The aberrant inferior petrosal sinus: an unusual approach to the cavernous sinus. Neuroradiology DOI 10.1007/s002340100659

Benndorf G (2008) Anomalous origin of the marginal tentorial artery: detection by contrast-enhanced angiographic computed angiography. Clin Neurorad 4:1–4

Bernasconi V, Cassinari V (1956) Un sengo carotidografico tipico di meningioma del tentorio. Chirurgia 11:568–588

Biondi A, Milea D, Cognard C, Ricciardi GK, Bonneville F, van Effenterre R (2003) Cavernous sinus dural fistulae treated by transvenous approach through the facial vein: report of seven cases and review of the literature. AJNR Am J Neuroradiol 24:1240–1246

Bisaria KK (1985) The superficial sylvian vein in humans: with special reference to its termination. Anat Rec 212:319–325

Bleys RL, Thrasivoulou C, Cowen T (2001) Cavernous sinus ganglia are sources for parasympathetic innervation of cerebral arteries in rat. J Cereb Blood Flow Metab 21:149–156

Bonnet P (1957) Les syndromes de la loge caverneuse. Rev Oto-Neuro-Ophth 65–80

Borba LAB, Al-Mefty O (2000) Normal anatomy of the cavernous sinus. In: Eisenberg MB, Al Mefty O (eds) The cavernous sinus. Lippincott Williams &Williams, Philadelphia, pp 21–33

Boskovic M, Savic V, Josifov J (1963) Über die Sinus petrosi und ihre Zuflüsse. Gegenbaurs Morphol Jahrb 104:420–429

Bouthillier A, van Loveren HR, Keller JT (1996) Segments of the internal carotid artery: a new classification. Neurosurgery 38:425–432; discussion 432–423

Brassier G, P. Lasjaunias, et al. (1987) Microsurgical anatomy of collateral branches of the intracavernous internal carotid artery. In: Dolenc VV (ed) The cavernous sinus: a multidisciplinary approach to vascular and tumorous lesions. Springer: Wien-New York, pp 81–103.

Braun JP, Tournade A (1977) Venous drainage in the cranio-cervical region. Neuroradiology 13:155–158

Breschet G (1829) Recherches anatomique, physiologiques sur le systeme veineux et specialment sur les canaux veineux des os. Paris, Vileret et Rouen

Brismar J (1974) Orbital phlebography. II. Anatomy of superior ophthalmic vein and its tributaries. Acta Radiol Diagn (Stockh) 15:481–496

Browder J, Kaplan H (1976) Cerebral dural sinuses and their tributaries. Charles C. Thomas, Springfield

Brown RD Jr, Flemming KD, Meyer FB, Cloft HJ, Pollock BE, Link ML (2005) Natural history, evaluation, and management of intracranial vascular malformations. Mayo Clin Proc 80:269–281

Butler H (1957) The development of certain human dural venous sinuses. J Anat Lond 91:510

Campell E (1933) Ann Otol (St Louis) 42:51

Chaloupka JC, Goller D, Goldberg RA, Duckwiler GR, Martin NA, Vinuela F (1993) True anatomical compartmentalization of the cavernous sinus in a patient with bilateral cavernous dural arteriovenous fistulae. Case report [see comments]. J Neurosurg 79:592–595

Cheng KM, Chan CM, Cheung YL (2003) Transvenous embolisation of dural carotid-cavernous fistulas by multiple venous routes: a series of 27 cases. Acta Neurochir (Wien) 145:17–29

Christensen J, Telford I (1978) Synopsis of gross anatomy, with clinical correlations. Harper and Row, New York

Clay C, Vignaud J (1974) Orbital vessels supplying the cavernous plexus. Ann Radiol (Paris) 17:237–246

Clay C, Vignaud J, et al (1976) Recent contribution of neuroradiography to the study of the orbital regions and the sinus cavernosus. Bull Mem Soc Fr Ophtalmol 223–226

Dilenge D, Heon M (1974) The internal carotid artery. Radiology of the Skull and Brain: Angiography. T. Newton and D. Potts. St. Louis, The C.V. Mosby Company. 2, Arteries, pp 1202–1246.

Djindjian R, Merland JJ (1973) Super-selective arteriography of the external carotid artery. Springer, Berlin Heidelberg New York

Doyon D, Aaron-Rosa D, et al. (1974). Orbital veins and cavernous sinus. Radiology of the Skull and Brain: Angiography. T. Newton and D. Potts. St. Louis, The C.V. Mosby Company, pp 2220–2254

Ducasse A, Segal A, Delattre JF (1986) Macroscopic aspects of the long posterior ciliary arteries. Bull Soc Opthalmol Fr 86:845–848

Dutton J (1994) The venous system of the orbit. In: Dutton J (ed) Clinical and surgical orbital anatomy. W.B. Saunders, Philadelphia, pp 81–92

Fischer E (1938) Die Lageabweichungen der vorderen Hirnarterie im Gefäßbild. ZblNeurochir 3:300–313

Fischgold H, Bregeat P, David M (1952) Premiers essais d'opacification du sinus caverneux chez l'homme par phlebographie orbitaire. Presented at Congres International d'Oto-Neuro-Ophthalmologie, Lisbon

Gailloud P, Fasel JH, Muster M, Desarzens F, Ruefenacht DA (1997) Termination of the inferior petrosal sinus: an anatomical variant. Clin Anat 10:92–96

Gailloud P, San Millan Ruiz D, Muster M, Murphy KJ, Fasel JH, Rufenacht DA (2000) Angiographic anatomy of the laterocavernous sinus [In Process Citation]. AJNR Am J Neuroradiol 21:1923–1929

Galligioni F, Bernardi R, Pellone M, Iraci G (1969) The superficial sylvian vein in normal and pathologic cerebral angiography. Am J Roentgenol Radium Ther Nucl Med 107:565–578

Goss C (1966) Anatomy of the human body. Lea & Febiger, Philadelphia

Gozet G, Clarisse J, Franck JP, Bonte G, Delandsheer JM (1974) Anatomie radiologique de la vein uncinee. Ann Radiol 17:253–257

Gray H (1918) Anatomy of the human body

Gurwitsch M (1883) Über die Anastomosen zwischen den Gesichts-und Orbitavenen. Albrecht v. Graefes. Arch Ohthalm 29:31

Haike H (1902) Zur Anatomie des Sinus caroticus (Plexus venous caroticus) und seine Beziehungen zu Erkrankungen des Ohres. Archiv f. Ohrenheilkunde 17–22

Hanafee WN, Shiu PC, Dayton GO (1968) Orbital venography. Am J Roentgenol Radium Ther Nucl Med 104:29–35

Harris FS, Rhoton AL (1976) Anatomy of the cavernous sinus. A microsurgical study. J Neurosurg 45:169–180

Hayreh S (1962a) The ophthalmic artery. II Intra-orbital course. Br J Ophthalmol 46:165–185

Hayreh S (1962b) The ophthalmic artery. III Branches. Br J Ophthalmol 46:212–247

Hayreh S (1963) The central artery of the retina – its role in the blood supply of the optic nerve. Br J Ophthalmol 47:651–663

Henderson W (1966) A note on the relationship of the human maxillary nerve to the cavernous ssinus and to and emissary vein passing through the foramen ovale. J Anat 100:905–908

Henry J (1959) Contribution a l'etude de l'anatomie des vaisseaux de l'orbite et de la loge caverneuse par injection de matieres pastiques, du tendon de Zinn et de la capsule de Tenon. These. Paris: Typescript no. 638.

Huang Y, Wolf BS (1974) The basal cerebral vein and its tributaries. In: Newton TH, Potts DG (eds): Radiology of the skull and brain: angiography. C.V. Mosby, St. Louis, pp 2111–2154

Huber G (1930) Piersol`s human Anatomy. Lippincott, Philadelphia

Hyrtl J (1885) Lehrbuch der Anatomie des Menschen mit Ruecksicht auf die physiologische Begruendung und praktische Anwendung. Braumueller, Wien

Inoue T, Rhoton AL Jr, Theele D, Barry ME (1990) Surgical approaches to the cavernous sinus: a microsurgical study. Neurosurgery 26:903–932

Inserra MM, Pfister M, Jackler RK (2004) Anatomy involved in the jugular foramen approach for jugulotympanic paraganglioma resection. Neurosurg Focus 17:E6

Katsuta T, Rhoton AL Jr, Matsushima T (1997) The jugular foramen: microsurgical anatomy and operative approaches. Neurosurgery 41:149–201; discussion 201–142

Keller JT, Tauber M, Loveren HR (1997) The cavernous sinus: anatomical considerations. In: Tomsick TA (ed) Carotid cavernous fistula. Digital Educational Publishing

Keyes J (1935) Observation on four thousand optic foramina in human skulls of known origin. Arch Ophthalmol 13:538–568

Knosp E, Mueller G, Perneczky A (1987a) Anatomical remarks on the fetal cavernous sinus and on the the veins of the middle cranial fossa. In: Dolenc VV (ed) The cavernous Sinus. Springer, Berlin Heidelberg New York

Knosp E, Mueller G, Perneczky A (1987b) The blood supply of the cranial nerves in the lateral wall of the cavernous sinus. In: Dolenc VV (ed) The cavernous sinus. Springer, Berlin Heidelberg New York, pp 67–79

Knott J (1882) On the cerebral sinuses and their variations. The journal of anatomy and physiology. G. Humphry, W. Turner and J. M'Kendrick. London and Cambridge, Macmillan and Co. XVI.

Krayenbühl H, Yasargil MG (1997) Zerebrale Angiographie in Klinik und Praxis. Thieme, Stuttgart

Labalette F (1891) Les veines de la la tet et du cou. These de Lille, pp 1–91

Lang J (1979a) Kopf, Teil A, Übergeordnete Systeme, vol 1. Springer, Berlin Heidelberg New York

Lang J (1979b) Kopf, Teil B, Gehirn und Augenschädel, vol 1. Springer, Berlin Heidelberg New York

Lang J (1983) Clinical anatomy of the head: neurocranium-orbit-craniocervical regions. Springer, Berlin Heidelberg New York

Lang J, Schafer K (1976) The origin and ramifications of the intracavernous section of the internal carotid artery. Gegenbaurs Morphol Jahrb 122:182–202

Lang J, Schafer K (1979) Ethmoidal arteries: origin, course, regions supplied and anastomoses. Acta Anat (Basel) 104:183–197

Lang J, Weigel M (1983) Nerve-vessel relation in jugular foramen region. Anat Clin 5:1–16

Langer C (1884) Der Sinus cavernosus. CR Acad Sci Vienne

Lasjaunias P (1984) Arteriography of the head and neck: Normal functional anatomy of the external carotid artery. Head and neck imaging excluding the brain. R. Bergeron, A. Osborn and P. Som. St Louis, CV Mosby: 344–354.

Lasjaunias P (1997) Angioarchitecture and natural history of dural arteriovenous shunts. Interventional Neuroradiol 3:313–317

Lasjaunias P, Berenstein A (1987) Surgical neuroangiography, vol 1. Springer, Berlin Heidelberg New York

Lasjaunias P, Moret J (1976) The ascending pharyngeal artery: normal and pathological radioanatomy. Neuroradiology 11:77–82

Lasjaunias P, Theron J (1976) Radiographic anatomy of the accessory meningeal artery. Radiology 121:99–104

Lasjaunias P, Michotey P, Vignaud J, Clay C (1975a) Vascularization of the orbit. II. Radio-anatomy of the arterial vascularization of the orbit with the exception of the trunk of the ophthalmic artery. Ann Radiol (Paris) 18:181–194

Lasjaunias P, Vignaud J, Hasso AN (1975b) Maxillary artery blood supply to the orbit: normal and pathological aspects. Neuroradiology 9:87–97

Lasjaunias P, Moret J, Mink J (1977) The anatomy of the inferolateral trunk (ILT) of the internal carotid artery. Neuroradiology 13:215–220

Lasjaunias P, Moret J, Doyon D, Vignaud J (1978a) C5 collaterals of the internal carotid siphon: embryology, angiographic anatomical correlations, pathological radioanatomy (author's transl). Neuroradiology 16:304–305

Lasjaunias P, Brismar J, Moret J, Theron J (1978b) Recurrent cavernous branches of the ophthalmic artery. Acta Radiol Diagn (Stockh) 19:553–560

Lasjaunias P, Berenstein A, Ter Brugge K (2001) Clinical vascular anatomy and variations. Springer, Berlin Heidelberg New York

Lazorthes G (1961) Vascularisation et circulation cerebrales. Masson, Paris

Lie T (1968) Congenital anomalies of the carotid arteries. An angiographic study and a review of the literature. Monograph. Excerpta Medical Foundation. Amsterdam, pp 35–51.

Lindblom K (1936) Roentgenographic study of vascular channels of skull with special reference to intracranial tumors and arteriovenous aneurysms. Acta Radiol 30:1–146

Lombardi G, Passerini A (1967) The orbital veins. Am J Ophthalmol 64:440–447

Lombardi G, Passerini A (1968) Venography of the orbit: technique and anatomy. Br J Radiol 41:282–286

Lombardi G, Passerini A (1969) Venography of the orbit: pathology. Br J Radiol 42:184–188

Luschka H (1860) Die Hirnanhang und die Steissdrüse des Menschen. Reimer 97

Luschka H (1867) Der Kopf. Tuebingen, H Laupp, 1867, vol III/2

Martins C, Yasuda A, Campero A, Ulm AJ, Tanriover N, Rhoton A Jr (2005) Microsurgical anatomy of the dural arteries. Neurosurgery 56:211–251; discussion 211–251

Mc Connell EM (1953) The arterial supply of the human hypophysis cerebri. Anat Rec 115:175–201

Miller DL, Doppman JL, Chang R (1993) Anatomy of the junction of the inferior petrosal sinus and the internal jugular vein. AJNR Am J Neuroradiol 14:1075–1083

Miller N (1998) Anatomy and physiology of the cerebral vascular system. In: Miller N, Newmann N (eds) Walsh and Hoyt's clinical neuro-opthalmology. Williams & Wilkins, pp 2869–2889

Mitchel GAG (1953) Anatomy of the autonomous nervous system. The sympathic component. Edinburgh, E.S. Livingstone, pp 201–221.

Moniz E (1927) La radiographie cerebrale. Bull Acad Med Paris 98:40–45

Moret J, Lasjaunias P, Theron J, Merland JJ (1977) The middle meningeal artery. Its contribution to the vascularisation of the orbit. J Neuroradiol 4:225–248

Newton TH, Potts DG (1974) The ophthalmic artery. In: Newton T, Potts D (eds) Radiology of the Skull and Brain. Angiography. 1333-1350.

Oka K, Rhoton AL Jr, Barry M, Rodriguez R (1985) Microsurgical anatomy of the superficial veins of the cerebrum. Neurosurgery 17:711–748

Osborn AG (1980a) Introduction to cerebral angiography. Harper & Row, Philadelphia

Osborn AG (1980b) The vidian artery: normal and pathologic anatomy. Radiology 136:373–378

Osborn AG (1981) Craniofacial venous plexuses: angiographic study. AJR Am J Roentgenol 136:139–143

Osborn AG (1991) Diagnostic cerebral angiography. Lipincott, Philadelphia

Pace E (1941) Arch Otolaryng (Chicago) 33:216

Padget D (1956a) Development of cranial venous system in man in reference to development, adult configuration andrealation to arteries. Am J Anat 98:307–350

Padget DH (1956b) The cranial venous system in man in reference to development, adult configuration, and relation to the arteries. Am J Anat 98:307–355

Parkinson D. (1964) Collateral circulation of the cavernous carotid artery: anatomy. Can J Surg 1964;7:251–268.

Parkinson D (1965) A surgical approach to the cavernous portion of the carotid artery. Anatomical studies and case report. J Neurosurg 23:474–483

Parkinson D (1967) Transcavernous repair of carotid cavernous fistula. Case report. J Neurosurg 26:420–424

Parkinson D (1973) Carotid cavernous fistula: direct repair with preservation of the carotid artery. Technical note. J Neurosurg 38:99–106

Parkinson D (1984) Arteries of the cavernous sinus. J Neurosurg 61:203

Parkinson D (1990) Surgical anatomy of the lateral sellar compartment (cavernous sinus). Clin Neurosurg 36:219–239

Parkinson D (2000) Extradural neural axis compartment. J Neurosurg 92:585–588

Paturet G (1964) Traite d'anatomie humaine, vol 4. Systeme nerveux. Masson, Paris

Paullus WS, Pait TG, Rhoton AI (1977) Microsurgical exposure of the petrous portion of the carotid artery. J Neurosurg 47:713–726

Peuker ET, Fischer G, Filler TJ (2001) Facial vein terminating in the superficial temporal vein: a case report. J Anat 198:509–510

Pribram HF, Boulter TR, McCormick WF (1966) The roentgenology of the meningohypophyseal trunk. Am J Roentgenol Radium Ther Nucl Med 98:583–594

Punt J (1979) Some observations on aneurysms of the proximal internal carotid artery. J Neurosurg 51:151–154

Quisling RG, Rhoton AL Jr (1979) Intrapetrous carotid artery branches: radioanatomic analysis. Radiology 131:133–136

Rabischong P, Vignaud J, Paleirac R, Clay C (1974) Serial anatomy of the cavernous sinus. Ann Radiol (Paris) 17:219–224

Randall B (1887) Cilioreatinal or aberrant vessels. Trans Am Ophthalmol Soc 4:511–517

Renn WH, Rhoton AL Jr (1975) Microsurgical anatomy of the sellar region. J Neurosurg 43:288–298

Rhoton AL Jr (2000) Jugular foramen. Neurosurgery 47: S267–285

Rhoton AL Jr, Inoue T (1991) Microsurgical approaches to the cavernous sinus. Clin Neurosurg 37:391–439

Rhoton AL Jr, Hardy DG, Chambers SM (1979) Microsurgical anatomy and dissection of the sphenoid bone, cavernous sinus and sellar region. Surg Neurol 12:63–104

Rhoton A, Harris F, Fujii K (1984) Anatomy of the cavernous sinus. In: Kapp J, Schmidek H (eds) The cerbral venous system and its disorders. Grune & Stratton, Orlando, pp 61–91

Ribeiro C, Goulao A, Evangelista J, Evangelista P, Correia G, Mauricio JC (1984) The foramen rotundum artery–angiographic characterization and clinical significance. Acta Med Port 5:127–132

Ridley (1695) The anatomy of the brain. Smith and Walford, London

Rouviere H (1970) Anatomie humaine. Descriptive et topographique. Masson, Paris

Rouviere H, Delmas A (1985) Anatomie humaine. Masson, Paris

Ruiz DS, Fasel JH, Rufenacht DA, Gailloud P (2004) The sphenoparietal sinus of breschet: does it exist? An anatomic study. AJNR Am J Neuroradiol 25:112–120

San Millan Ruiz D, Gailloud P, de Miquel Miquel MA, Muster M, Dolenc VV, Rufenacht DA, Fasel JH (1999) Laterocavernous sinus. Anat Rec 254:7–12

San Millan Ruiz D, Gailloud P, Rufenacht DA, Delavelle J, Henry F, Fasel JH (2002) The craniocervical venous system in relation to cerebral venous drainage. AJNR Am J Neuroradiol 23:1500–1508

Sappey PC (1888) Traite d'anatomie descriptive. Tome 2. Delahaye et Lecvrsonier, p 692

Sarma D, ter Brugge K (2003) Management of intracranial dural arteriovenous shunts in adults. Eur J Radiol 46:206–220

Schnürer LB, Stattin S (1963) Vascular supply of intracranial dura from internal carotid artery with special reference to its angiographic significance. Acta Radiol (Diagn) 58:441–450

Sesemann E (1869) Die Orbitalvenen des Menschen und ihr Zusammenhang mit den oberflächlichen Venen des Kopfes. Arch Anat Physiol 2:154

Shapiro R, Robinson F (1967) The foramina of the middle fossa: a phylogenetic, anatomic and pathologic study. Am J Roentgenol Radium Ther Nucl Med 101:779–794

Shiu PC, Hanafee WN, Wilson GH, Rand RW (1968) Cavernous sinus venography. Am J Roentgenol Radium Ther Nucl Med 104:57–62

Silvela J, Zamarron MA (1978) Tentorial arteries arising from the external carotid artery. Neuroradiology 14:267–269

Sobotta J (1928) Atlas of human anatomy. Stechart, New York

Sondheimer (1974). Basal foramina and canals. Radiology of the skull and brain. T. Newton and T. Potts. St. Louis, Mosby. 1: 287–356

Spalteholz W (1933) Hand atlas of human anatomy, vol 2. Lippincott, Philadelphia

Stickle BR, McFarlane H (1997) Prediction of a small internal jugular vein by external jugular vein diameter. Anaesthesia 52:220–222

Suzuki N, Hardebo JE (1993) The cerebrovascular parasympathetic innervation. Cerebrovasc Brain Metab Rev 5:33–46

Suzuki Y, Matsumoto K (2000) Variations of the superficial middle cerebral vein: classification using three-dimensional CT angiography. AJNR Am J Neuroradiol 21:932–938

Tanoue S, Kiyosue H et al. (2006) Para-cavernous sinus venous structures: anatomic variations and pathologic conditions evaluated on fat-suppressed 3D fast gradient-echo MR images. AJNR Am J Neuroradiol 27(5):1083–1089

Takazawa H, Kubo M, Kuwayama N, Hasegawa S, Horie Y, Hirashima Y, Endo S (2005) Dural arteriovenous fistula involving the cavernous sinus as the cause of intracerebral venous hemorrhage: a case report. No Shinkei Geka 33:143–147

Taptas J (1987) Must we still call cavernous sinus the parasellar vascular and nervous crossroads? The necessity of a definete topographical description of the region. In: Dolenc VV (ed) The cavernous sinus: a multidisciplinary approach to vascular and tumorous lesions. Springer: Wien–New York, pp 30–40

Theile (1843) Sinus de la dure-mere. Encyclopedie Anatomique. Tome 3

Theron J (1972) Cavernous plexus affluents. Neurochirurgie 18:623–638

Tran-Dinh H (1987) Cavernous branches of the internal carotid artery: anatomy and nomenclature. Neurosurgery 20:205–210

Trolard P (1868) Anatomie du systeme veineux de l'encephale et du crane. These de la Faculte de Medicine de Paris, pp 1–32

Trolard P (1890) Les veins meningees moyennes. Rev Sci Biol 485–499

Trotter M, Peterson R (1996) Osteology. In: Anson B (ed) Morris' human anatomy. The Blakiston Co, Philedelphia, pp 161–200

Tubbs RS, Ammar K, Liechty P, Wellons JC III, Blount JP, Salter EG, Oakes WJ (2006) The marginal sinus. J Neurosurg 104:429–431

Turner AL, Reynolds F (1926) J Larynyng 41:73

Umansky F, Nathan H (1982) The lateral wall of the cavernous sinus. With special reference to the nerves related to it. J Neurosurg 56:228–234

Umansky F, Nathan H (1987) The cavernous sinus. An anatomical study of its lateral wall. In: Dolenc VV (ed) The cavernous sinus: a multidisciplinary approach to vascular and tumorous lesions. Springer: Wien–New York, pp 81–103

Umansky F, Valarezo A, Elidan J (1994) The superior wall of the cavernous sinus: a microanatomical study. J Neurosurg 81:914–920

Venturi C, Bracco S, Cerase A, Gennari P, Lore F, Polito E, Casasco AE (2003) Endovascular treatment of a cavernous sinus dural arteriovenous fistula by transvenous embolisation through the superior ophthalmic vein via cannulation of a frontal vein. Neuroradiology 45:574–578

Vignaud J, Clay C (1974) Opacification technics using the venous approach to the cavernous plexus. Ann Radiol (Paris) 17(3):229–236

Vignaud J, Doyon D, Aubin ML, Clay C (1972) Opacification of the cavernous sinus by the posterior approach. Neurochirurgie 18:649–664

Vignaud J, Hasso AN, Lasjaunias P, Clay C (1974) Orbital vascular anatomy and embryology. Radiology 111:617–626

Vitek JJ (1989) Accessory meningeal artery: an anatomic misnomer. AJNR Am J Neuroradiol 10:569–573

Warwick R, Williams P (1973) Gray's anatomy. Longman, Edinburgh

Willinsky R, Lasjaunias P, Berenstein A (1987) Intracavernous branches of the internal carotid artery (ICA). Comprehensive review of their variations. Surg Radiol Anat 9:201–215

Winslow JB (1732) Exposition Anatomique de la Structure du Corpus Humain, vol 2. Pervost, London

Wolf BS, Newman CM, Schlesinger B (1955) The diagostic value of the deep cerebral veins in cerebral angiography. Radiology 64:161–171

Wolf BS, Huang YP, et al. (1963) The superficial sylvian venous drainage system. Am J Roentgenol Radium Ther Nucl Med 89:398–410

Wolff E (1940) The anatomy of the eye and orbit. 2nd Edition. The Blakiston Company, Philadelphia. p 286

Yasuda A, Campero A, Martins C, Rhoton AL Jr, Ribas GC (2004) The medial wall of the cavernous sinus: microsurgical anatomy. Neurosurgery 55:179–189; discussion 189–190

Yasuda A, Campero A, Martins C, Rhoton AL Jr, Oliveira E, Ribas GC (2005) Microsurgical anatomy and approaches to the cavernous sinus. Neurosurgery 56:4–27; discussion 24–27

Classification of Cavernous Sinus Fistulas (CSFs) and Dural Arteriovenous Fistulas (DAVFs)

4

CONTENTS

Introduction

Cavernous sinus fistulas (CSF), like other arteriovenous fistulas, represent abnormal communications between the arterial and venous blood circulation, either directly between the ICA lumen and the CS or indirectly between branches of the ICA and/or ECA and the CS. The vascular anomalies involving the cavernous sinus and the internal carotid artery are accordingly named carotid cavernous fistulas (CCFs) (PARKINSON 1987), carotid cavernous sinus fistulas (CCSF) (BARROW et al. 1985), cavernous-carotid fistulas (Yoo and KRISHT 2000), or carotid artery cavernous fistulas (PHATOUROS et al. 2000). Likewise, communications linking the cavernous sinus and dural arterial supply are aptly named, dural cavernous sinus arteriovenous malformations (HOUDART et al. 1993), dural carotid cavernous fistulas (dural CCF) (MEYERS et al. 2002), cavernous sinus dural arteriovenous malformation (CSDAVM) (STIEBEL-KALISH et al. 2002; BARCIO-SALORIO et al. 2000), cavernous sinus dural arteriovenous fistulae (CSDAVF) (SATOMI et al. 2005; SUH et al. 2005) or dural cavernous sinus fistulas (DCSFs) (PEETERS and KROGER 1979). This inconsistent terminology reflects a need to elucidate further the etiology, pathophysiology and natural history of these fistulas to standardize and simplify their classification. In this monograph, the term CSF is used for all arteriovenous fistulas involving the CS regardless of their anatomy, etiology, prognosis or hemodynamic characteristics.

In general, CSFs are classified anatomically, based on their etiology, or according to their specific hemodynamic characteristics.

4.1
Anatomic Classification

4.1.1
Dural Arteriovenous Fistulas (DAVFs)

Because of their vascular supply by dural arteries, Type B–D fistulas are categorized by some authors into the large group of dural arteriovenous fistulas (DAVF) (MALEK et al, 2000; CHUNG et al. 2002; KLISCH et al. 2003; TSAI et al. 2004; MIRONOV 1995; COGNARD et al. 1995; SARMA and TER BRUGGE 2003; DAVIES et al. 1997), which are located at the great cerebral sinuses such as the sigmoid, transverse, superior sagittal, inferior and superior petrosal sinus. DAVFs have been anatomically classified according either to their specific location, or according to their anatomic features seen on cerebral angiograms (Table 4.1). The severity or aggressiveness of DAVFs has been outlined previously using several classification schemes (COGNARD et al. 1995; DAVIES et al. 1996; BORDEN et al. 1995; LALWANI et al. 1993; MIRONOV 1995). All DAVF classifications are based on specific angiographic features of the venous drainage pattern including venous stenosis, occlusions or cortical (leptomeningeal) drainage.

One of the first attempts to classify these lesion was made by AMINOFF et al. (1973) who divided them

Table 4.1. Anatomic classifications of DAVFs

Author	Type/ grade/ group	Type of venous drainage
CASTAIGNE (1975)	1	Sinus, direct or indirect (SSS, SPS, CS)
	2	Sinus via venous ectasia
	3	Cortical vein
DJINDJIAN (1978)	1	Into a sinus or meningeal vein
	2	Sinus drainage with reflux into cerebral veins
	3	Solely into cortical veins
	4	With supra- or infratentorial venous lakes
LALWANI (1993)	1	Anterograde sinus, no venous restriction, no cortical drainage
	2	Anterograde and retrograde sinus, no venous restriction, no cortical drainage
	3	Retrograde and cortical drainage without antegrade venous drainage
	4	Cortical venous drainage only
BORDEN (1995)	I	Sinus only
	II	Sinus and subarachnoid veins
	III	Subarachnoid veins only
COGNARD (1995)	I	Sinus, without reflux
	IIa	Sinus with reflux (insufficient antegrade flow)
	IIb	Sinus with reflux into cortical veins
	IIa+b	Reflux into sinus and cortical veins
	III	Cortical vein without ectasia
	IV	Cortical vein with venous ectasias (>5 mm, 3×>draining vein)
	V	Spinal perimedullary veins

Author	Type/ grade/ group	Location of the AV-shunt
AMONOFF (1973)	1	Anterior-inferior (cavernous sinus)
	2	Superior-posterior (transverse and signoid sinus)
PICARD (1987)	1	Lateral sinus
	2	Cavernous sinus
	3	Superior sagittal sinus
	4	Other: tentorial, falcine, convexity
AWAD (1990)	1	Transverse sigmoid sinus (62%)
	2	Cavernous sinus (11.9%)
	3	Tentorial incisures (8.4%)
	4	Convexity – superior sagittal sinus (7.4%)
	5	Orbital – anterior flax (5.8%)
	6	Sylvian middle cranial fossa (3.7%)
	7	Others: marginal sinus
MIRONOV (1995)	1	Dural sinuses (40.6%)
	2	Cavernous sinus (30.2%)
	3	Galen's system (10.4%)
	4	Venous plexus at the base of the skull (9.3%)
	5	Parasinusal cortical veins (9.3%)
MORET (2006)	1	Osteo – Dural
	2	Duro – Dural
	3	Duro – Arachnoidal
	4	Duro – Pial
GEIBPRASERT (2008)	1	Anterior epidural (includes CS region)
	2	Dorsal epidural
	3	Lateral epidural

Note that many anatomical classifications include the cavernous sinus region into two groups, anterior and posterior, depending on their venous drainage into the cavernous sinus or into the lateral sinus.

CASTAIGNE et al. (1976) studied 13 cases of meningeal arteriovenous fistulas with venous and cortical drainage and suggested dividing them into three groups: Group 1 would drain directly or via a meningeal vein into the sinus, Group 2, rarely seen would drain into a large venous sac, and Group 3 would drain into a cortical vein. Group 3 represented a special entity because only these fistulas would produce neurological symptoms.

DJINDJIAN and MERLAND (1978) extended this classification and subdivided DAVFs into four types: (1) fistulas draining into a sinus or a meningeal vein (most frequent), (2) fistulas draining directly into a sinus without significant reflux into cortical veins, (3) fistulas draining into cortical veins, and (4) fistulas with large supra- or infratentorial lakes. Type 2 fistulas, although possibly developing from the preceding Type 1, were considered a separate group because of their potential to cause neurological complications. Type 3 fistulas were considered a specific group because of their constant production of neurological signs.

According to CASTAIGNE et al. (1975), more than 42% and according to MALEK et al. (2000) 33% of the fistulas with cortical venous drainage were associated with intracranial hemorrhage.

The classification of COGNARD et al. (1995) was based on 205 patients and a modification of the one provided by DJINDJIAN and MERLAND (1978). The authors subdivided Grade II DAVFs and further specified the drainage into cortical veins with and without ectasias. They found that in their group, venous ectasias and cortical drainage represent significant risk factors. It has recently been suggested that patients who develop a reversible dementia due to bilateral venous hypertension should receive a Type VI classification; however, the usefulness has not been established yet (HOUDART 2005).

MIRONOV (1995) divided DAVFs into five groups: Type 1–DAVFs of the dural sinuses; Type 2–DAVFs of the cavernous sinus; Type 3–DAVFs of Galen's system; Type 4–DAVFs of the venous plexus at the base of the skull; Type 5–DAVFs of the parasinusal cortical veins. He studied angiograms in 96 patients and found that the documentation of a causal sinus thrombosis depends on the location of the DAVF: in 72% of the cases with Type 1 DAVFs there was a thrombosis at the time of the investigation, but no thrombosis was proven in cases with Type 4 DAVFs.

Mironov concluded that the morphological development of DAVFs seems to depend on the flow volume of the venous recipient. A pronounced development of pathological AV shunts takes place at the level of the large basal dural sinuses. A delayed development of pathological AV shunts with a low shunt volume occurs in a venous recipient with a low AV pressure gradient.

LALWANI et al. (1993) and MALEK et al. (2000) proposed a grading system for DAVFs in four grades: fistulas of grade 1 show no venous restriction and a normal antegrade drainage, grade 2 show antero- and retrograde drainage with or without cortical component. Grade 4 fistulas show exclusively cortical venous drainage. They were able to demonstrate that patients with grade 3 or grade 4 fistulas have a significantly higher risk for intracranial hemorrhage or visual symptoms. Table 4.1 shows several classifications based on venous drainage and associated risk of intracranial hemorrhage. However, this classification has limited application to DCSFs, because most of the latter are Type 1–2 and cortical drainage is not often seen (10%–31%) (HALBACH et al. 1987; COGNARD et al. 1995; TOMSICK 1997; MEYERS 2002). Even when cortical drainage is present, associated intracranial hemorrhage seems to occur less frequently than DAVFs. On the other hand, in clinical practice most groups consider cortical draining veins in a DCSF an indication for endovascular treatment.

MORET et al. (2006) have proposed a new anatomical classification, dividing DAVFs without DCSFs, according to their relationship to the adjacent tissue components into four types. The osteo-dural and duro-dural fistulas are caused by pathology of the dura mater while the duro-arachnoidal and duro-pial fistulas are caused by a pathology of the perivascular space. In their series of more than 200 DAVFs, the osteo-dural type of DAVF is the most frequently seen and can be cured in up to 94% of the cases. Duro-dural or mural type fistulas are relatively rare in comparison. Typical of the duro-archnoidal type is the frequent hemorrhagic complications (up to 50%). Attempts to categorize and classify DAVFs continue as is demonstrated by the recent effort of GEIBPRASERT et al. (2008), who divided, based on embryological aspects, dural arteriovenous shunts (DAVS) into three groups: anterior epidural, posterior epidural and lateral epidural shunts. It is suggested that this classification allows a prediction of the venous drainage and possibly facilitates treatment decisions that still depend on the presence of cortical or leptomeningeal venous drainage (CVD, LVD). It is interesting to note that DCSFs would be grouped into the anterior epidural shunts in which reflux into cortical/leptomeningeal veins usually does not occur, unless there is venous outflow restriction due to thrombosis or a high-flow condition. DAVFs of the anterior fossa, such as ethmoidal DAVFs are anatomically closely related to DCSFs but are grouped into the lateral epidural shunts. They drain in up to 100% into cortical veins and are associated with a bleeding rate of 61% (AGID 2009). This corresponds with aggressive symptoms seen in 86% of these fistulas, versus 92% benign symptoms observed in anterior epidural shunts. Whether or not DCSFs with present CVD/LVD have to be treated with the same urgency remains unclear, and the fact that they actually rarely bleed, even when reflux into cerebral veins is present (up to 31%, MEYERS 2002) is still not explained. Although the reference to embryology provides new insights into potential mechanisms of development and morphological and clinical presentations of DAVFs, the usefulness of this classification for clinical practice needs to be proven.

4.1.2
Cavernous Sinus Fistulas (CSFs)

The particular anatomic arrangement in the cavernous region causes the patho-anatomical sequelae of CSFs. While the venous component of the fistulous connection is invariably provided by the cavernous sinus, the arterial supply and the venous drainage exiting from the CS may differ remarkably resulting in various angiomorphologies of the fistulas. The original clinical presentation characterized by DANDY (1937), as the trias of exophthalmos, chemosis and bruit is caused by a single defect in the wall of the internal carotid artery during its course through the cavernous segment (C5–C4-portion). Depending on the size of this tear, a smaller or larger AV shunt volume develops within a short period of time. This type of AV fistula occurs either after trauma (car accident, blunt injury etc.) or develops spontaneously after rupture of a cavernous carotid aneurysm or a preexisting weakness of the arterial wall (Ehlers Danlos Type IV, Fibromuscular dysplasia). It is therefore called direct CSF or CCF (cavernous carotid fistula).

Although widely ignored in the recent literature, WOLFF and SCHMIDT (1939) made the first effort to identify various forms of CSFs. Based on their own observations in three patients with pulsating exophthalmos (mostly posttraumatic CCFs) undergoing cerebral angiography, as well as existing angiographic descriptions in the literature, they were able to identify four main types of venous drainage: anterior via the SOV, posterior to the IPS, superficial cortical to the vein of Trolard and deep cortical via the lateral mesencephalic and basal vein of Rosenthal (Fig. 4.1). If one considers the limited knowledge of cerebral angiography only 5 years after its first introduction by MONIZ (1927), this detailed analysis is quite remarkable.

It was PARKINSON (1965) in his early work on traumatic carotid cavernous fistulas who made the distinction between direct and indirect fistulas. He considered the first type a single fistula resulting from a tear in the wall of the carotid and the second type resulting from a tear across one of the small dural branches within the cavernous sinus. A few years later, NEWTON and HOYT (1970) subdivided DCSFs into two types. The first was characterized by a shunt adjacent to or within the wall of the CS and the second by a shunt involving more distant dural sinuses that communicate with the CS.

Patients with an indirect arteriovenous shunt involving the CS may present with similar, but usually less dramatic and progressive symptoms. In some patients the signs and symptoms, generally considered characteristic of CSFs, are conspicuously absent (NEWTON and HOYT 1970). Because the AV shunting develops between the network of the small dural arteries of the ICA and ECA or their branches and the CS, they are properly named dural cavernous sinus fistulas (DCSFs).

DJINDJIAN and MERLAND (1973) reported on six cases of fistulas between the ECA and the CS and classified them into three types: (1) fistulae that develop after ineffective trapping or embolization of a direct CCF; (2) fistulas that are supplied by both ICA and ECA branches, or (3) true ECA-CS fistulas. Whether Type 1 can be considered a separate fistula remains questionable because it represents the residual or secondary supply of an incompletely occluded direct high-flow AV shunt as described by HAYES (1963).

In addition, PEETERS and KROEGER (1979) suggested a classification of CSFs into direct, indirect or dural fistulas (Figs. 4.2 and 4.3). The authors studied 19 patients and found 9 indirect and 10 direct fistulas of three different types: (1) direct internal carotid – cavernous sinus fistula, (2) dural internal

Fig. 4.1a–d. Classification of CCFs (Zbl Neurochir, 1939). The first angiographic classification of CSFs by Wolff and Schmid. Based on angiographic observations in three patients with "pulsating exophthalmus" and reported cases in the literature at that time, they identified four main types of venous drainage. Type A, anterior drainage via the SOV; Type B, posterior drainage via the IPS and SPS; Type C, cortical drainge via the superior anastomotic vein of Trolard; and Type D, deep venous draiange via the perimesencephalic vein and basal vein of Rosenthal. (Note: the perimesencephalic vein as such was not identified by the authors, who discussed an "unknown vein" instead.)

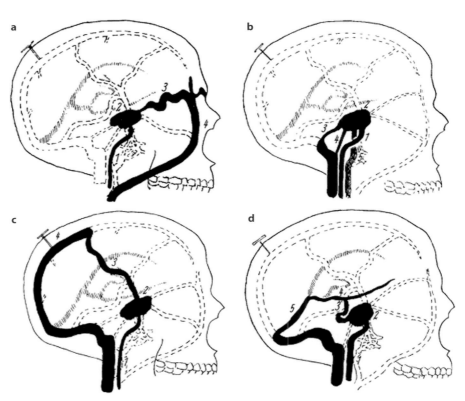

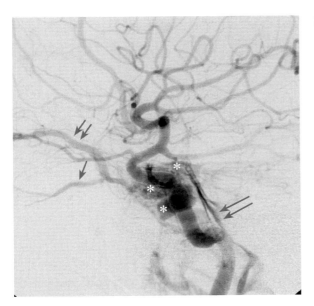

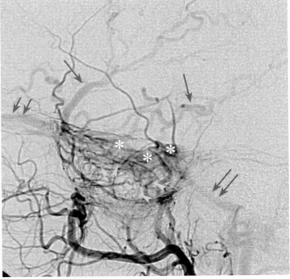

Fig. 4.2. Type A fistula (direct, traumatic), in principle identical to the spontaneous Type A after Barrow. The wall of the carotid artery has a defect and blood shunts directly into the cavernous sinus (*asterices*) draining via the SOV (*short double arrow*), the IOV (*single arrow*) and the IPS (*double arrow*). Note that saccular structures are sometimes visible in traumatic cases; they may represent venous outpouchings and can mimic cavernous aneurysms

Fig. 4.3. Type D (indirect, dural) fistula. The wall of the carotid artery is intact and the AV shunt is indirectly supplied by either a few or a network of multiple small dural branches (*arrowheads*) arising from the APA, AMM, MMA and distal IMA and draining from the CS (*asterisk*) via the SOV (*short double arrow*) and the IPS (*double arrow*) as well as multiple cortical veins (*arrows*). For Type B fistula and Type C fistula see Figs. 8.14 a–d and 8.19 a–b, respectively)

carotid – cavernous sinus fistula and (3) dural external carotid – cavernous sinus fistula (Table 4.2).

FERMAND (1982) and MORET et al. (1978) classified the indirect fistulas further into two types: Type I fistulas, fed by a complex network of feeders whose systematization is impossible and Type II fistulas in which all the feeders can be precisely identified.

PICARD et al. (1983) differentiated fast-flow and slow-flow fistulas, emphasizing that the latter with multiple feeders actually represent the true DCSFs. Fast-flow fistulas, exhibited a single communication. Since they were not dural fistulas, they did not require the same treatment as traumatic CCF, regardless if they occurred spontaneously or due to a ruptured cavernous aneurysm.

Based on these anatomical differences, BARROW et al. (1985) developed a more detailed classification for spontaneous cavernous sinus fistulas. This schemata, until recently was the mainstay of classification, allowing differentiation of fistulas according to the type of arterial supply (Fig. 4.4). He defined

Type A fistulas as direct fistulas as described in preceding paragraphs. Type B–D fistulas depict various fistulas, depending on whether the small dural arteries arise from the ICA, ECA or both. Thus, these Type B–D fistulas are called dural cavernous sinus fistulas (DCSFs). Type B fistulas are solely supplied by ICA-branches (ILT, MHT, Fig. 7.45) and Type C fistulas only by the dural branches of the ECA (MMA, AMA, APA, IMA, Fig. 7.44). Type D fistulas are supplied by both territories. This classification provided prognostic value and had some impact on therapeutic decision making. Type A fistulas are usually treated by transarterial approach using detachable balloons. Type B–D fistulas, on the other hand, are effectively treated by transarterial or transvenous embolization, or a combination therein. Posttraumatic CCFs, not included in Barrow's classification, represent morphologically, hemodynamically and with regard to their treatment options, a Type A fistula.

DE KEIZER (2003) emphasized the following additional fistula types: (a) presentation of clinical signs

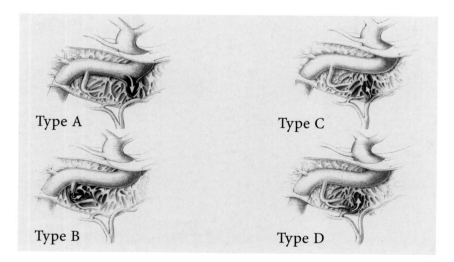

Fig. 4.4. Classification of spontaneous CSFs after Barrow (J Neurosurg, 1985).
Type A, direct fistula through a defect in the wall of the ICA (high-flow)
Type B, DCSF, indirect fistula supplied by ECA-feeder (low-flow)
Type C, DCSF, indirect fistula supplied by ICA-feeder (low-flow)
Type D, DCSF, indirect fistula supplied by ECA and ICA-feeder (low-flow)
Type A fistula develops either spontaneously or due to ruptur of an intracavernous ICA aneurysm. They can be anatomically and hemodynamically identical to traumatic direct fistulas.
Indirect fistulas are also referred to as dural cavernous sinus fistulas (DCSFs), because they are supplied by dural branches of ECA and ICA. The most frequent type is the Type D fistula (90%), often supplied by numerous branches from both territories, sometimes bilaterally. This classification does not take into account the venous drainage and does not differentiate between uni- and bilateral supply fistulas. With the increasing use of transvenous occlusions for treatment of DCSFs, this classification is today of less importance, although still widely used. Type B or D fistulas, in the past usually considered "difficult to treat lesions" (by transarterial embolization), can be transvenously occluded with the same success rate as Type C fistulas. The latter although rare, were thought to be "easy to treat lesions", because ECA feeders are less difficult to reach with a microcatheter

Table 4.2. Classifications of CSF and (CCF and DCSF)

Author	Type	Type of arterial supply
WOLFF and SCHMIDT (1939)	1	Anterior into SOV
	2	Posterior into IPS
	3	Into superficial cortical veins
	4	Into deep pial veins
PARKINSON (1965)	1	"Direct" fistula: tear in the carotid wall
	2	"Indirect" fistula: tear across MHT or ILT branch
NEWTON (1970)	1	Dural supply adjacent or within wall of the CS
	2	Dural supply distant to the CS
DJINDJIAN (1973)	1	Persistent "dural" AV shunt after trapping or embolization of CCF
	2	Supply from ICA and ECA (mixed DCSF)
	3	Supply from ECA only
PEETERS (1979)	1	Direct internal carotid cavernous sinus fistulas
	2	Dural internal carotid cavernous sinus fistulas
	3	Dural external carotid cavernous sinus fistula
MORET (1982)[a]	I	By complex network of feeders (cannot be systematized)
	II	Feeder identifiable
PICARD (1983)	I	Fast flow (single communication)
	II	Slow flow (multiple feeders, "true dural fistulas")
BARROWS (1985)		Spontaneous carotid cavernous sinus fistulas
	A	Direct fistula from ICA (non-traumatic)
	B	ECA supply only
	C	ICA supply only
	D	ECA and ICA supply
LARSON (1995)	1	Direct (traumatic)
	2	Direct (rupture of intracavernous aneurysm)
	3	Indirect (ICA and ECA supply)
	4	Combined direct and indirect characteristics
TOMSICK (1997)		Barrows Types A–D
	D1	Unilateral ICA and ECA supply
	D2	Bilateral ICA and ECA supply
BARCIA-SOLARIO (2000)		Barrows Types A–D
	T	Traumatic Type A (AT)
	1	Supply ipsilateral
	2	Supply bilateral
STIEBEL-KALISH (2002)		DCSFs (venous drainage)
	1	Flow reversal into anterior CS and SOV
	2a	Ophthalmic vein thrombosis
	2b	Stagnant ophthalmic vein flow
	3	IPS
	4	SPS
SUH (2005)		DCSFs (angiographic pattern)
	1	Proliferative
	2	Restrictive
	3	Late Restrictive
SATOMI (2005)	1	Anterior and posterior drainage open
	2	Posterior drainage closed, posterior open
	3	Anterior and posterior drainage route closed

[a] This classification from Moret is mentioned in the paper of FERMAND (1982)

on the contralateral side, (b) connection of a primitive trigeminal artery; although rare, and intraorbital connections between the ophthalmic artery and ophthalmic vein or its branches. The latter are in some series not considered separately and may cause similar symptoms, thus mimicking a cavernous sinus dural arteriovenous malformation (Huna-Baron et al. 2000). As observed by Huna-Baron et al. (2000), even high resolution MRI may fail and show an enlarged SOV without abnormality of the CS. Only superselective angiography may allow identification of these small slow-flow intraorbital AV shunts. Deguchi et al. (2005) recently reported a purely intraorbital arteriovenous fistula that was successfully embolized using transvenous approach via facial and angular vein.

I have observed the case of a young man, who presented with symptoms typical for a DCSF, caused by a small AV fistula of the intraorbital SOV (Fig. 4.5).

Barrow's classification (Barrow et al. 1985) specifically proposed for spontaneous lesions is based only on the arterial angioarchitecture and does not reflect the venous drainage pattern. It allows differentiation with regard to technical difficulties anticipated during transarterial catheterization, which was the most common endovascular approach in the 1980s. Under those aspects, Type C lesions were usually considered "easier to treat" because catheterization of ECA feeders was technically less difficult and injecting liquid embolic agents was clinically less risky. Types B and D fistulas were, on the other hand, seen as more challenging lesions (and still are by some authors), and are often considered "difficult to treat lesions" or "intractable fistulas". Picard et al. (1987) stated: "The slow flow fistulas with multiple pedicles are true dural fistulas. Their treatment is always limited to the embolization of the external carotid branches; embolization of the internal carotid artery branches should never be attempted. Therefore, it is important to classify these fistulas according to the respective participation of the internal and of the external carotid artery, even if in most cases both are involved".

In the era of transarterial embolizations, the majority of Type D fistulas have been partially occluded or were completely cured only when adjunctive more aggressive techniques or complementary treatment options such as microneurosurgery or radiosurgery were applied. Because of the increasing experience and technical advancement in using transvenous techniques in the 1990s, the technical challenges of transarterial embolizations are meanwhile of little

importance. Thus, the type of arterial supply (B, C or D) has only minor impact on whether or not to perform a transvenous occlusion.

Today, the pattern of venous drainage, either anteriorly via ophthalmic veins, or posteriorly via petrosal sinuses, is certainly of greater significance because these draining veins can be used as endovascular routes to the CS.

Some fistulas are located only on one side, but are supplied by bilateral feeders from the ICA and the ECA. Because of the usually associated higher flow, these fistulas have been considered by Tomsick (1997) and Barcia-Salorio et al. (2000) as more complex and more difficult to treat and were classified as Type D1 and Type D2 fistulas. However, not only the bilateral fistulous communication is of significance for the size of the AV-shunt, but also the capacity of the draining veins.

Furthermore, in my experience it is more important to decide whether or not a uni- or bilateral AV-shunt is present: the latter case occurs less frequently, but may be overlooked and can result in an incomplete occlusion. It is certainly of major importance for planning and performing a transvenous occlusion to decide whether to occlude the CS on one or on both sides. Whether or not a bilateral supply

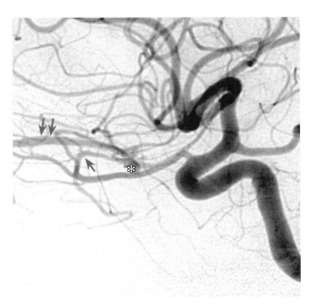

Fig. 4.5. "Para-cavernous" intraorbital AVF. A 35-year-old male presenting with double vision and eye redness. ICA injection, lateral view shows a moderately enlarged OA that suplies a small AV shunt (*asterisk*) at the proximal segment of the SOV (*double arrow*) with a recurrent dural branch (*arrow*). This fistula is in fact not a true DCSF, but an intraorbital communication between OA and SOV

is present appears less crucial than if a true bilateral AV shunt is present. Both these constellations can easily be mistaken due to insufficient angiographic image quality. In order to avoid occluding the wrong side, fistulas draining via the contralateral CS and SOV should be recognized before occluding the sinus.

Some fistulas, despite bilateral supply, can be angiographically low-flow fistulas, when the venous outflow is restricted due to a thrombosed SOV or IPS. Whether or not cortical or leptomeningeal venous drainage is present, constitutes an important factor for clinical decision-making. Even though DCSFs with cortical drainage seem to bleed less frequently than DAVF in general (30%), based on the same concept, they are often aggressively treated to prevent neurological deficits or hemorrhagic complications. In order to block such venous exit and to minimize the risk of procedure-related intracranial bleeding, precise localization of its origin is crucial.

STIEBEL-KALISH et al. (2002) have studied the venous drainage pattern and differentiated into four types. 1. Venous outflow into anterior CS and SOV was present in 77/85 patients. In this group cortical veins were present in 25%, IPS in 21% and SPS in 12%. 2. Abnormal ophthalmic venous flow with ophthalmic vein thrombosis was seen in 11/85 among which cortical veins were found in 73%, IPS in 27% and SPS in 27% of the cases. 3. IPS drainage was seen in 22 cases with 41% of cortical drainage, 18% SPS drainage and paraspinal veins (4.5%). 4. SPS drainage was seen in 11 cases with cortical drainage in all of them (100%).

SUH et al. (2005) have recently suggested angiographic differentiation of DCSFs into three types:

1. *The Proliferative type (PT):*
   - Numerous arterial feeder to the CS (network)
   - Large AV shunt with rapid filling of CS, afferent and efferent veins
   - Both CSs completely filled and bulging into the sinus wall
2. *The Restrictive type (RT):*
   - Less arterial feeders than PT, each identifiable
   - Obliteration of flow in IPS, increased flow in SOV and cortical veins
   - Less AV shunt than in PT
   - CS margins less well defined (loss of normal contour)
3. *The Late Restrictive type (LRT):*
   - Few arterial feeders
   - With sluggish retrograde venous flow
   - Constrictive changes of the veins
   - CS stasis

The authors were able to correlate presented symptoms in 58 patients with these three drainage patterns. Patients with a PT fistula would mostly present with a cavernous pattern such as ptosis, diplopia, anisocoria and ophthalmoplegia caused by CN deficits. Patients with a RT fistula presented with a cavernous symptom pattern or with an orbital (chemosis, exophthalmos, periorbital pain, eyelid swelling) or ocular pattern (decreased vision, increased IOP, severe ocular pain, glaucoma and retinal hemorrhage). Patients with a fistula of the LRT presented mostly with ocular pattern. A cerebral pattern with infarction in the basal ganglia or brainstem caused by reflux into cortical veins was seen in 5% of the patients with RT and LRT fistulas. Although this approach seems appealing, the study showed a progression from one type to another in only 7/58 patients (12%). Angiograms could only be compared in 11 patients and many (unknown number) patients were embolized either by the transarterial or transvenous approach. Therefore, changes of the venous drainage pattern in these patients cannot be simply related to the natural course of the disease. In 4/11 patients no change from RT to LRT was documented. Only some patients with the LRT presented with serious cerebral complications. In my opinion, the results leave several unanswered questions, including whether a patient with RT or LRT requires endovascular treatment.

A similar, but more simple approach to the problem has been proposed by SATOMI et al. (2005). Based on 65 patients, seen over a period of 29 years, the authors staged the progression of the disease into three phases based on the venous drainage pattern. Stage 1 fistulas drain predominantly posteriorly via the IPS and to a lesser degree anteriorly, producing mainly tinnitus. Stage 2 fistulas are characterized by closed (thrombosed) IPS and PP redirecting the flow into the SOV and the IOV and to a lesser degree into the Sylvian vein. In this stage the patients present not with bruit but with increased ophthalmological symptoms. Stage 3 is defined as a fistula that drains exclusively into either the Sylvian vein or the SPS due to the occlusion of initially anterior and posterior draining veins. In this study, a relatively small number of patients, 11/65 (17%) demonstrated indeed a chronological change of the venous drainage pattern. One patient (9%) developed a cortical reflux. Because half of the patients underwent transarterial embolization, the observed changes do not allow referring

to the natural history of DCSFs either, even though all 11 cases showed a change in one direction: from 1 to 2 or 3 associated with a reduction of draining venous channels. A relatively small number of four patients were categorized as Stage 3 fistulas with cortical venous drainage all of which were directed anteriorly towards the Sylvian vein. Only a single case showed the development of this type of drainage during angiographic FU studies. Interestingly, none of the stage 3 cases showed leptomeningeal venous drainage towards the mesencephalic and cerebellar veins even though the SPS remained patent. Thus, the progression of these changes seems not always predictable and the value of the staging for future treatment strategy is uncertain.

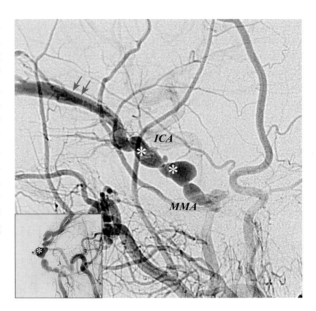

Fig. 4.6. Traumatic "Type C" fistula: Motorcycle accident 15 years previously. External carotid arteriogram shows a fistulous comunication between the MMA and the CS that results in a high-flow AV shunt, draining only anteriorly into the SOV (*short double arrow*). Note: This fistula could also be considered a traumatic AV-fistula of the MMA

4.2
Etiologic Classification

According to their etiology, CSFs can mainly be classified into spontaneous and traumatic fistulas. Most traumatic fistulas are anatomically Type A fistulas with a direct communication between ICA and CS. However, in some cases, a ruptured dural artery may cause the arteriovenous shunting into the CS leading to identical symptoms (Fig. 4.6). A dural artery may also contribute to a persisting direct AV shunt (Fig. 4.7), or become the only remaining supply of a previously treated CCF, e.g. after ineffective trapping procedure as described by Hayes (1963). The great majority of indirect CSFs represent dural arteriovenous shunting lesions and correspond to Type B–D fistulas as classified by Barrow. It becomes obvious that, in some cases, etiological and anatomical classification may overlap (see more about etiology in Chap. 5).

4.3
Hemodynamic Classification

Hemodynamics have long been used as a means to characterize AV shunting lesions with regard to their clinical prognosis. Lacking correct data on pressure and flow in these fistulas, arteriograms have often been used to estimate when a shunt is low-flow or high-flow. Hayes (1958) was the first in attempting to identify different types based on the AV-shunting flow. He identified fistulas draining all blood from the ICA into the CS and those draining only a part of it to the venous side. He classified them accordingly as high- and low-flow fistulas. Experience has shown that most Type A fistulas are high-flow fistulas, the majority of which are represented by posttraumatic fistulas (76%). Some high-flow fistulas may also be supplied by meningeal branches (Phelps et al. 1982). Usually, (indirect) Types B–D fistulas are associated less with AV-shunting flow than (direct) Type A fistulas and are called low-flow fistulas. However, the clinical signs may appear similar during a protracted course of the disease to the ones caused by Type A fistulas except for the pulsating exophthalmos and the audible bruit (see Chap. 6). They frequently consist of a red-eye syndrome, which is characterized by dilated, tortuous episcleral veins, elevated intraocular pressure and often a less prominent exophthalmos (Phelps et al. 1982). The term low-flow fistula is to some degree confusing because it implies a mild clinical course. Some DCSFs, however, despite low-flow

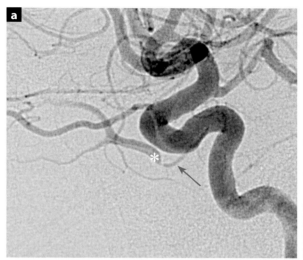

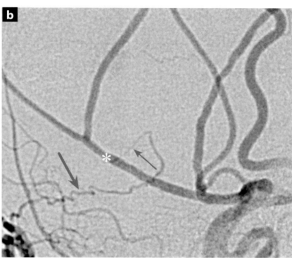

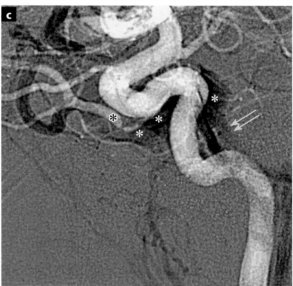

Fig. 4.7a–c. Type B or Type D fistula? a Filling of the anterior compartment of the CS (*asterisk*) through the anteromedial ramus (*thin arrow*) of the ILT that courses through the supraorbital fissure. **b** The same fistulous connection (*asterisk, thin arrow*) filled by the artery of the foramen rotundum (*thick arrow*) through its connection with the anterolateral ramus of the ILT. This example shows another limitation of Barrow's classification besides the lacking consideration of venous drainage. From an endovascular point of view, classifying into Type B or D fistula might be of pure academic interest. The ipsilateral IPS and CS are opacified, widely open and can be accessed easily. The angiographic separation between the anterior compartment involved in the fistula and the remaining compartments draining the cerbral venous blood flow is most likely not anatomic but rather pathophysiologic or hemodynamic due to intracavernous thrombosis. **c** Arterio-venogram: Moving the mask into the early arterial phase allows to better identify that the fistulous compartment (*black asterisk*) is indeed imbedded (although angiographically not communicating) within the anterior CS (*white asterices*)

condition and small AV-shunt volume, may cause considerably elevated intravenous pressure resulting in severe ophthalmological symptoms. This venous hypertension is often caused by venous outflow restriction usually due to stenosis or thrombosis of the CS or the SOV. Reliable data on intracavernous pressure and flow in DCSFs is lacking which makes a proper hemodynamic classification difficult (see also Chap. 10).

NORNES (1972) studied the hemodynamic aspects of five carotid cavernous fistulas, four traumatic and one occurring spontaneously. He performed intraoperative blood flow measurements and was able to document the amount of "fistula steal" ranging from 90 to 975 ml and stated that the ratio reverse flow/forward flow is assumed to give an indication of the collateral capacity of the cerebral vasculature and of the tolerance to occlusion of the ICA by trap ligation. There was no attempt to classify fistulas according to their hemodynamics and no dural CSF was included.

BRASSEL (1983) aimed to classify direct CCFs with regard to their hemodynamic effects on the cerebral circulation. Based on their angiographic appearance, he divided patients into three classes: small, moderate and large. While small fistulas cause no reduction of arterial pressure or flow in the ipsilateral intracranial circulation, moderate fistulas do, and consequently "steal" some supply from the cerebral circulation via the circle of Willis. Large CCFs shunt completely into the CS without remaining antegrade carotid flow distal to the fistula site.

He concluded that the latter group requires treatment, while moderate and small fistulas may not. This classification has rather limited value for clinical practice, because many patients with moderate or small AV shunts may still need treatment because they suffer from "non-cerebral" symptoms. In addition, DCSFs are not considered.

Much later LIN et al. (1994) applied duplex carotid sonography criteria such as flow volume and resistance index (RI) for a classification of CSFs (see also Sect. 7.1.2.). The authors were able to separate three groups of fistulas: (1) small RI and increased flow volume in the ICA: direct (Type A) CCF; (2) normal RI and flow volume in the ICA and ECA: dural branch of ICA-cavernous sinus fistulas (Type B); (3) small RI with or without increased flow volume in the ECA: dural branch of ECA-cavernous sinus fistulas (Type C) or dural branches of ICA- and ECA-cavernous sinus fistulas (Type D). This approach has not found a wider acceptance.

Some dural CSFs may recruit a large number of feeding pedicles causing a large AV shunting volume and may have an angiographic appearance that resembles an AVM. They are therefore erroneously called high-flow fistulas. Because quantitative data on flow are lacking so far, only direct AVF should be named as such.

Based on the various aspects discussed above, a truly consequent classification of DCSFs with or without etiological aspects would require incorporating the arterial and venous patterns as well as hemodynamic parameters. Such an approach, however, would necessarily result in a confusingly large number of different types of fistulas without significant impact on prognosis or therapy. Although a proper classification for DCSFs is of prime importance, it seems for the time being an aim difficult to accomplish. Because these fistulas represent a relatively infrequent disease, it may be practical to simplify or not a cortical drainage is present, whether the AV-shunt is located uni- or bilateral, and which transvenous route is accessible.

Today the majority of DCSFs are treated by transvenous occlusion techniques and transarterial embolization is mainly reserved for Type A fistulas, regardless of their etiology spontaneous or traumatic. From an endovascular therapy point of view, the differentiation of B–D fistulas appears no longer very useful and is more of academic interest. While it has little prognostic value, for the purpose of endovascular strategy, the old classification in direct and indirect fistulas still seems suitable.

References

Agid R, et al. (2009) Management strategies for anterior cranial fossa (ethmoidal) dural arteriovenous fistulas with an emphasis on endovascular treatment. J Neurosurg 110(1):79–84.

Aminoff MJ (1973) Vascular anomalies in the intracranial dura mater. Brain 96:601–612

Awad IA, et al. (1990) Intracranial dural arteriovenous malformations: factors predisposing to an aggressive neurological course. J Neurosurg 72(6):839–850.

Barcia-Salorio, J.L, Barcia JA, Soler F (2000). Radiosurgery for Carotid-Cavernous Fistulas. In: The Cavernous Sinus. E. M.B. and O. Al-Mefty EMB, Al-Mefty O (eds). Philadelphia, Lipincott: 227-240

Barrow DL, Spector RH, Braun IF, Landman JA, Tindall SC, Tindall GT (1985) Classification and treatment of spontaneous carotid-cavernous sinus fistulas. J Neurosurg 62:248–256

Borden JA, Wu JK, Shucart WA (1995) A proposed classification for spinal and cranial dural arteriovenous fistulous malformations and implications for treatment. J Neurosurg 82:166–179

Brassel F (1983) Haemodynamik und Therapie der Karotis-Kavernosus Fistel, in Radiology. Bonn, pp 1–89

Castaigne P, Bories J, Brunet P et al. (1975) Fistules de la dure-mere, etude clinique et radiologique de 13 observations. Ann Med Interne 126:813–817

Castaigne P, Bories J, et al. (1976) Meningeal arterio-venous fistulas with cortical venous drainage. Rev Neurol (Paris) 132:169–181

Chung SJ, Kim JS, Kim JC, Lee SK, Kwon SU, Lee MC, Suh DC (2002) Intracranial dural arteriovenous fistulas: analysis of 60 patients. Cerebrovasc Dis 13:79–88

Cognard C, Gobin YP, Pierot L, Bailly AL, Houdart E, Casasco A, Chiras J, Merland JJ (1995) Cerebral dural arteriovenous fistulas: clinical and angiographic correlation with a revised classification of venous drainage. Radiology 194:671–680

Dandy W (1937) Carotid-cavernous aneurysms (pulsating exophthalmos). Zentralbl Neurochir 2:77–206

Davies M, TerBrugge K, Willinsky R, Coyne T, Saleh J, Wallace MC (1996) The validity of classification for the clinical presentation of intracranial dural arteriovenous fistulas. J Neurosurg 85:830–837

Davies M, Saleh J, Ter Brugge K, Willinsky R, Wallace MC (1997) The natural history and management of intracranial dural arteriovenous fistulae. Part 1: Benign lesions. Intervent Neuroradiol 3

de Keizer R (2003) Carotid-cavernous and orbital arteriovenous fistulas: ocular features, diagnostic and hemodynamic considerations in relation to visual impairment and morbidity. Orbit 22:121–142

Deguchi J, Yamada M, Ogawa R, Kuroiwa T (2005) Transvenous embolization for a purely intraorbital arteriovenous fistula. Case report. J Neurosurg 103:756–759

Castaigne P, et al. (1975) Arteriovenous fistulae of the dura mater. Clinical and radiological study of 13 cases. Ann Med Interne (Paris) 126(12):813–817

Castaigne P, Bories J, et al. (1976). Meningeal arterio-venous fistulas with cortical venous drainage. Rev Neurol (Paris) 132(3):169–181.

Djindjian R, Merland JJ (1973) Super-selective arteriography of the external carotid artery. Springer, Berlin Heidelberg New York

Djindjian R, Merland JJ (1978) Super-selective arteriography of the external carotid artery. Springer, Berlin Heidelberg New York

Fermand M (1982) Les fistules durales de la loge caverneuse. Thesis, St. Antoine. Paris

Geibprasert S, et al (2008) Dural arteriovenous shunts: a new classification of craniospinal epidural venous anatomical bases and clinical correlations. Stroke 39(10):2783–2794.

Halbach VV, Higashida RT, Hieshima GB, Reicher M, Norman D, Newton TH (1987) Dural fistulas involving the cavernous sinus: results of treatment in 30 patients. Radiology 163:437–442

Hayes GJ (1958) Carotid cavernous fistulas: diagnosis and surgical management. Am Surg 24:839–843

Hayes GJ (1963) External carotid-cavernous sinus fistulas. J Neurosurg 20:692–700

Houdart E (2005) Classification and new endovascular approaches in intracranial DAVF. Presented at WFITN, Venice

Houdart E, Gobin YP, Casasco A, Aymard A, Herbreteau D, Merland JJ (1993) A proposed angiographic classification of intracranial arteriovenous fistulae and malformations. Neuroradiology 35:381–385

Huna-Baron R, Setton A, Kupersmith MJ, Berenstein A (2000) Orbital arteriovenous malformation mimicking cavernous sinus dural arteriovenous malformation. Br J Ophthalmol 84:771–774

Klisch J, Huppertz HJ, Spetzger U, Hetzel A, Seeger W, Schumacher M (2003) Transvenous treatment of carotid cavernous and dural arteriovenous fistulae: results for 31 patients and review of the literature. Neurosurgery 53:836–856

Larson, JJ, et al. (1995) Treatment of aneurysms of the internal carotid artery by intravascular balloon occlusion: long-term follow-up of 58 patients. Neurosurgery 36(1):26–30; discussion 30.

Lalwani AK, Dowd CF, Halbach VV (1993) Grading venous restrictive disease in patients with dural arteriovenous fistulas of the transverse/sigmoid sinus. J Neurosurg 79:11–15

Lin HJ, Yip PK, Liu HM, Hwang BS, Chen RC (1994) Noninvasive hemodynamic classification of carotid-cavernous sinus fistulas by duplex carotid sonography. J Ultrasound Med 13:105–113

Malek AM, Halbach VV, Higashida RT, Phatouros CC, Meyers PM, Dowd CF (2000) Treatment of dural arteriovenous malformations and fistulas. Neurosurg Clin N Am 11:147–166, ix

Meyers PM, et al. (2002) Dural carotid cavernous fistula: definitive endovascular management and long-term follow-up. Am J Ophthalmol 134:85–92

Mironov A (1995) Classification of spontaneous dural arteriovenous fistulas with regard to their pathogenesis [see comments]. Acta Radiol 36:582–592

Moniz E (1927) Radiografia das arterias cerebrais. J Soc Ciencias Med Lisboa XCL:8

Moret J (2006) Dural arteriovenous fistulae: classification and endovascular management. Presented at LINC, Houston

Moret J, Lasjaunias P, Vignaud J, Doyon D (1978) The middle meningeal blood supply to the posterior fossa (author's transl). Neuroradiology 16:306–307

Newton TH, Hoyt WF (1970) Dural arteriovenous shunts in the region of the cavernous sinus. Neuroradiology 1:71–81

Nornes H (1972) Hemodynamic aspects in the management of carotid-cavernous fistula. J Neurosurg 37:687–694

Parkinson D (1965) A surgical approach to the cavernous portion of the carotid artery. Anatomical studies and case report. J Neurosurg 23:474–483

Parkinson D (1987) Carotid cavernous fistula, history and anatomy. In: Dolenc VV (ed) The cavernous sinus: a multidisciplinary approach to vascular and tumorous lesions. Springer, Berlin Heidelberg New York, pp 3–29

Peeters FL, Kroger R (1979) Dural and direct cavernous sinus fistulas. AJR Am J Roentgenol 132:599–606

Pereira, VM, et al. (2008) Pathomechanisms of symptomatic developmental venous anomalies. Stroke 39(12):3201–3215.

Phatouros CC, Meyers PM, Dowd CF, Halbach VV, Malek AM, Higashida RT (2000) Carotid artery cavernous fistulas. Neurosurg Clin N Am 11:67–84, viii

Phelps CD, Thompson HS, Ossoinig KC (1982) The diagnosis and prognosis of atypical carotid-cavernous fistula (redeyed shunt syndrome). Am J Ophthalmol 93:423–436

Picard L, Roland J, Bracard S, Lepoire J, Montaut J (1983) Spontaneous dural fistulas: classification, diagnosis, endovascular treatment. Springer, Berlin Heidelberg New York

Picard L, Bracard S, Moret J, Per A, Giacobbe H, Roland J (1987) Spontaneous dural arteriovenous fistulas. Sem Intervent Radiol 4:219–241

Sarma D, ter Brugge K (2003) Management of intracranial dural arteriovenous shunts in adults. Eur J Radiol 46:206–220

Satomi J, Satoh K, Matsubara S, Nakajima N, Nagahiro S (2005) Angiographic changes in venous drainage of cavernous sinus dural arteriovenous fistulae after palliative transarterial embolization or observational management: a proposed stage classification. Neurosurgery 56:494–502; discussion 494–502

Stiebel-Kalish H, Setton A, Nimii Y, Kalish Y, Hartman J, Huna Bar-On R, Berenstein A, Kupersmith MJ (2002) Cavernous sinus dural arteriovenous malformations: patterns of venous drainage are related to clinical signs and symptoms. Ophthalmology 109:1685–1691

Suh DC, Lee JH, Kim SJ, Chung SJ, Choi CG, Kim HJ, Kim CJ, Kook M, Ahn HS, Kwon SU, Kim JS (2005) New concept in cavernous sinus dural arteriovenous fistula: correlation with presenting symptom and venous drainage patterns. Stroke 36:1134–1139

Tomsick TA (1997) Typ B,C, & D CCF: Etiology, prevalence & natural history. In: Tomsick TA (ed) Carotid cavernous fistula. Digital Educational Publishing, pp 59–73

Tsai LK, Jeng JS, Liu HM, Wang HJ, Yip PK (2004) Intracranial dural arteriovenous fistulas with or without cerebral sinus thrombosis: analysis of 69 patients. J Neurol Neurosurg Psychiatr 75:1639–1641

Willinsky, R, et al. (1990) Angiography in the investigation of spinal dural arteriovenous fistula. A protocol with application of the venous phase. Neuroradiology 32(2):114–116.

Wolff H, Schmid B (1939) Das Arteriogramm des pulsierenden Exophthalmus. Zbl Neurochir 4:241–250, 310–319

Yoo K, Krisht AF (2000) Etiology and classification of cavernous-carotid fistulas. In: Eisenberg MB, Al Mefty O (eds): The cavernous sinus. Lippincott Williams & Wilkins, Philadelphia, pp 191–200

Etiology, Prevalence and Natural History of Dural Cavernous Sinus Fistulas (DCSFs)

CONTENTS

Introduction

Although the clinical phenomenon of the "pulsating exophthalmos" has been known since BENJAMIN TRAVERS (1811) observation, the discussion about its underlying pathophysiological substrate remained controversial for a long time. He assumed early on that the pathological anatomy of the pulsating exophthalmos would be a carotid-cavernous fistula, while other reports in the nineteenth century on "intraorbital aneurysms", causing similar signs and symptoms, interpreted those as the main cause. It was mostly the English school that assumed an intraorbital pathology as underlying mechanism, whereas in France the cavernous sinus was considered the true source of the pulsating exophthalmos. This was to a large extent due to the popular work of NELATON (1876), physician of Napoleon and Garibaldi, who was able to demonstrate post mortem a direct arteriovenous communication between carotid artery and cavernous sinus in two patients with a pulsating exophthalmos after trauma (see also Chap. 2). Inspired by this, BARTHOLOW (1872) published more clinical observations on pulsating exophthalmos. But it was not until RIVINGTON (1875) and SATTLER (1880) presented their extensive monographs that the anatomical concept of (direct) carotid cavernous fistula found broader acceptance. The term "pulsating exophthalmos" was nonetheless used throughout the following 70 years (LOCKE 1924; SATTLER 1920; SUGAR and MEYER 1940; WOLFF and SCHMID 1939; DANDY 1937; HAMBY and GARDNER 1933; NOLAND and TAYLOR) until it was eventually replaced by "carotid cavernous fistula" (POTTER 1954; ECHOLS and JACKSON 1959; HAYES 1958; WALKER and ALLEGRE 1956; PARKINSON 1967; HAMBY 1966).

Although indirect fistulas frequently may cause symptoms similar to direct fistulas, they represent in terms of etiology and pathogenesis entirely different lesions. Reports on pulsating or non-pulsating exophthalmos in the pre-angiography era did not differentiate between indirect and direct fistulas. Even after introduction of cerebral angiography by MONIZ (1927) at the beginning of the last century, it took decades until diagnostic arteriograms in a quality allowing for detailed analysis of angiomorphology became available. Only when the fine, minute network of dural arteries could be angiographically visualized, did separating Type A from Types B–D fistulas become possible (CASTAIGNE et al. 1966b; LIE 1968; NEWTON and HOYT 1970). Thus, it can be assumed that because of the lacking suitable imaging tools such as selective external and internal carotid arteriography, in many of the historic series some "spontaneous" or "idiopathic" fistulas were in fact dural cavernous sinus arteriovenous fistulas. NEWTON and HOYT (1970) described and characterized clinical, etiological and angiographic features of dural arteriovenous shunts in the CS region.

5.1

Etiology and Pathogenesis of Type A Fistulas

Direct communications between ICA and CS can be considered Type A fistulas, regardless of their etiology. The clinical picture of a spontaneous fistula (true Type A fistulas according to Barrows classification) is usually indistinguishable from a traumatic CCF. Since very early on, it was believed that an inherent weakness of the intracavernous portion of the ICA is a predisposing factor to the formation of a CSF. DELEN (1870) found that if the carotid artery is cannulated and liquid is injected with force, the vessel will rupture within the CS: *"Aussi, en injectant le système carotidien, avon-nous constater que la carotide interne se rompt facilement dans le sinus si l'on pousse un peu fortment l'injection. Sur un sujet auquel nous avions lié les deux vertebrales et la carotide primitive droite en poussant par la carotide primitive gaunche une injection solidifiable, nous avons obtenu la rupture de la carotide interne dans le sinus caverneux. La matière à injection pénétrant dans le sinus passa dans la veine opthalmique et les veines de la face, realising ainsi, sur le cadaver, les conditions anatomiques de l'anévrysme artérioveineux."*

In some early series, fistulas of traumatic origin represent 69%–77% of all CSFs (LOCKE 1924; SATTLER 1920) and usually develop following severe head trauma with sharp or blunt head injuries. In the past, they were seen most frequently in men, being more often involved in wars, and industrial or traffic accidents. The modern environment with a high prevalence of automobile accidents may have erased this gender difference (HAMBY 1966; DEBRUN et al. 1988b; VINUELA et al. 1984). On the other hand, improved head protection for motorcycle riders seem to have decreased the number of traumatic CCFs. Only large populations riding bicycles and still being exposed to frequent severe head trauma in some areas of the world, like South-East Asia, may explain the relatively high rate of traumatic CCFs there.

A characteristic morphologic feature of traumatic CCFs is a tear of the carotid wall allowing a high-flow arteriovenous shunt to develop directly and rapidly. Patients often present with dramatic ophthalmic symptoms developing within a few days and usually require emergency treatment. In some cases, however, a delay of several months may occur before symptoms, such as a bruit or an exophthal-

mos, become evident. The size of the tear can vary from 1 to 5 mm and it may occur as single or multiple laceration or in some cases as complete transsection. Bilateral Type A fistulas, although rare, may occur and have been observed even among the earliest reported cases (SATTLER 1930). They have a less favorable prognosis and may present with delayed clinical deterioration (AMBLER et al. 1978). Angiographically, Type A fistulas show a rapid AV shunting with venous drainage into efferent and afferent veins, often significant cortical or leptomeningeal drainage, and sometimes associated with complete arterial steal. In some cases, the traumatic rupture of an intracavernous branch of the ICA or a dural branch of the ICA can cause a Type A fistula that may present with only little arteriovenous shunting (OBRADOR et al. 1974; PARKINSON 1973). Under rare circumstances traumatic CSFs occur due to a rupture of a trigeminal artery (BERGER and HOSOBUCHI 1984; KERBER and MANKE 1983; DEBRUN et al. 1988a; FLANDROY et al. 1987; GUGLIELMI et al. 1990; TOKUNAGA et al. 2004). Whether unrecalled microtrauma may be an etiologic factor for spontaneous CCFs is uncertain (TOMSICK 1997a).

The etiology of spontaneous CSFs is more difficult to ascertain (HAMBY 1966). Spontaneous rupture of an intracavernous aneurysm can cause Barrow's Type A fistula that may result in a high-flow arteriovenous shunt, clinically and angiographically indistinguishable from a traumatic direct fistula (BARROW et al. 1985). DANDY (1937) reported on an 18-year-old male who complained about progressive exophthalmos over 6 years with no history of an injury and he considered a congenital intracavernous aneurysm being the only possible cause. LOCKE (1924) observed in his autopsy series 7 traumatic and 33 spontaneous cases. FROMM et al. (1967) demonstrated angiographically the existence of a saccular aneurysm of the cavernous carotid artery (C4-C5-segment) in a patient who spontaneously developed a direct CCF. TAPTAS (1950) found in his series a true communication between ICA and CS in only 50% of cases. DEBRUN et al. (1988b) reported 5 spontaneous Type A fistulas in 132 patients, among whom 3 had a ruptured cavernous aneurysm, 1 developed after pregnancy and another was seen in a 5-year-old child. TAKI et al. (1994) saw 2 out of 44 patients with spontaneous direct shunts without any clinical angiographic evidence of congenital disorder, and thus considered them caused by rupture of an infraclinoid aneurysm.

Nonetheless, the true incidence of Type A fistulas due to a ruptured cavernous sinus aneurysm is difficult to assess because small aneurysms can be obscured angiographically or mimicked by a rapidly filled and outpouched CS (Tokunaga et al. 2004). Image acquisition using high frame rate may help to identify an aneurysm as documented in some reports (van Rooij et al. 2006). To what degree a true association between intracavernous aneurysms and spontaneous CCFs exists, is controversial. Only a few reports on cases of CCFs, developing on the basis of previously known cavernous aneurysms, exist (Barrow et al. 1985; Lesoin et al. 1984; Horton et al. 1991). Among Barrow's 14 cases (Barrow et al. 1985) was a 51-year-old woman presenting with large bilateral intracavernous aneurysms, of which one was treated using gradual occlusion with a Crutchfield clamp. The patient developed a contralateral Type A fistula following carotid occlusion. Vinuela et al. (1984) reported on two such cases in a group of 20 patients.

Klisch et al. (2003) more recently reported on a series of 17 patients with CSFs, among whom one presented with a ruptured cavernous carotid aneurysm. Kobayashi et al. (2003) treated six cases of direct CCF caused by an intracavernous aneurysm. Overall, intracavernous aneurysms account for 1.9%–9.0% of intracranial aneurysms and 6%–9% of them are complicated by a CCF (Linskey et al. 1990, 1991; Polin et al. 1996). van Rooij et al. (2006) reported on 10 patients with ruptured cavernous sinus aneurysms causing a direct CCF. However, based on the figures shown in their paper, only one out of three (Fig. 3 there) shows convincingly enough a characteristic saccular structure in the very early arterial phase, before complete filling of the fistula. The same may be true for Klisch's case (Fig. 4 there) (Klisch et al. 2003). The true nature of any aneurysm-like shaped structure within the CS remains necessarily uncertain and some of these cases may instead represent an arterial pseudoaneurysm or a venous pouch.

Such skepticism seems justified because, according to some studies, the incidence of spontaneous direct CCFs based on intracavernous aneurysm is rather low (Kupersmith et al. 1992; Inagawa 1991). Tomsick (1997a), despite a large number of cavernous aneurysms and a large number of spontaneous CCFs in the institution, did not observe a single case where a known cavernous aneurysm had subsequently caused a CCF. And surprisingly, in some large series like the one of Higashida et al. (1989) reporting on a group of 234 direct CCFs, no spontaneous fistula due to a ruptured aneurysm was noted. Autopsy proven cases like the one of Rosso et al. (1999), who reported recently on a postmortem examination of a direct CCF, are rare. The authors demonstrated a smooth-edged wall defect that was completely occluded by the detachable balloon. Microscopy at this site showed a thin-walled aneurysm with a deficient internal elastic lamina and muscularis media.

Non-traumatic Type A fistulas may also occur in association with connective tissue disorders such as Ehlers Danlos Type IV (Dany et al. 1986; Desal et al. 2005; Chuman et al. 2002; Purdy 2002; Mitsuhashi et al. 2004; Halbach et al. 1990; Debrun et al. 1996; Kanner et al. 2000), fibromuscular dysplasia (Sattler 1920; Taki et al. 1994; Zimmerman et al. 1977), or osteogenesis imperfecta (Okamura et al. 1995; de Campos et al. 1982), pseudoxanthoma elasticum (Koh et al. 1999), neurofibromatosis (Lasjaunias and Berenstein 1987), hemorrhagic teleangiectasia (von Rad and Tornow 1975) and hereditary choriocarcinoma (Chen et al. 1993), lymphoid granulomatosis treated with cytotoxic therapy (Rosenthal and Rowe 1987), syphilitic arteritis (Sugar and Meyer 1940), and fungal arteritis (Saff et al. 1989). Hypertension leading to weakness of the arterial wall has been suggested as a cause early on (Wolff and Schmid 1939). Rupture of microaneurysms that develop due to dilatation and thinning of the carotid vessel wall cause most likely CSFs fistulas in these patients.

5.2
Etiology and Pathogenesis of Type B–D Fistulas

Due to initially limited anatomic information obtained by angiography, DCSFs have been recognized relatively late as a separate entity (Lie 1968, Castaigne 1966). For a long time, pulsation of the eyeball was described characteristic for CCFs but was a actually found in only one-third of the patients (Hamby 1966). It appears obvious that some of the remaining two-thirds with "non-pulsating" exophthalmos were likely caused by DCSFs. Although in 1961 Lie (1968) observed such a case that had in retrospective a DCSF, he was unable to identify exactly the fistula type due to poor image quality and lack of subtraction technique at that time. Even in the work of PALESTINE et al. (1981), who 20 years later reported on 74 CSF patients, nothing is mentioned with regard to angioarchitecture of the fistulas. This is somehow surprising, as CASTAIGNE et al. (1966a) had already noted various anatomic characteristics of the arterial supply in DCSFs. They also emphasized the need for selective ECA injections. A few years later, NEWTON and HOYT (1968) undertook their detailed study of clinical symptomatology and angioarchitecture in 11 patients with dural arteriovenous fistulas of the CS. They described precisely the small dural arteries as feeding pedicles of the fistulas and explained the development of these fistulas with tears in the walls of these small arteries or rupture, possibly caused by distension of the vessel wall in predisposed or diseased vessel walls or by direct trauma. Although a number of studies investigated etiology and pathogenesis of DCSFs, the exact mechanisms of their development are still unknown. Various factors and predispositions seem to contribute, some of them because of their similar pathogenetic role in DAVFs. Although most older series necessarily mix causes for direct (mostly pulsating) and indirect (commonly non-pulsating) AV shunts, some of them may also apply to DCSFs.

5.2.1
Pregnancy

Pregnancy and childbirth have long been known predisposing factors for CSFs since their descriptions by DANDY (1937) and others (WALKER and ALLEGRE 1956; SATTTLER 1920, 1930). SATTLER (1880), in his first review of cases reported up to 1880, had already collected 32 idiopathic cases, among which 23 were women, 6 of whom were pregnant,while 1 developed the fistula during delivery. Six of these women had been repeatedly pregnant and five had been in a late stage of pregnancy. In all cases the symptoms developed rather quickly. Sattler also described cases that occurred under certain circumstances during physical stress such as coughing, at passing stool, stenuous work or severe vomiting: *"A woman returned from a walk and was bending over to take her shoes off when the process developed."* (author's translation). Many years later he found that 28% of women had developed their idiopathic exophthalmos (17/61) during pregnancy or within the first weeks after delivery (SATTLER 1920, 1930). WALKER and ALLEGRE (1956) found pregnancy an important precipitating fac-

tor for about 25%–30 % of the afflicted women, who would develop the fistula during the latter half of the pregnancy or during delivery. More recent statistics show that only 28% of the fistulas occur during puerperium, whereas 54% develop during menopause (TOMSICK 1997b). Physical stress during delivery may cause rupture of small dural vessels and development of DCSFs. In the largest series published so far, the onset of symptoms was associated in 6% of cases with pregnancy (MEYERS et al. 2002). Due to lack of imaging, it remains unclear how many patients in these early series were suffering from dural AV shunts.

5.2.2
Hormonal Factors

TANAGUCHI et al. (1971) confirmed Newton's observations of the predisposition in women not only during but also after pregnancy. The higher incidence of DCSFs in women during menopause and in men over 50 years of age also supports the theory of a tear of an arteriosclerotic altered vessel wall. On the other hand, it indicates that hormonal factors may contribute and possibly represent an important etiological factor for DCSFs occurring more frequently in elderly women.

The exact underlying mechanisms remain unclear. Endogenous estrogen is responsible for inhibiting the progression of arteriosclerosis in women, while exogenous estrogen may promote thrombosis. It is possible that lack of endogenous estrogen affects the integrity of the dural micro shunt regulation and can promote the development of macro shunts (SUZUKI and KOMATSU 1981). Interestingly, estrogen injections into the ECA for embolization of DAVFs and meningeomas resulted in total disappearance of the nidus in six out of eight patients (SUZUKI and KOMATSU 1981). This could be due to either aggregation of blood platelets, damage of smooth muscle cells and fibroblasts or activation of extrinsic and intrinsic clotting cascade. Infusion of the estrogen compound into mesenteric arteries of rats caused local spherocytosis and severe rapid degeneration of endothelial cells, followed by injury to the underlying muscle cells and fibroblasts (SHIMIZU et al. 1987).

The concept that oestrogen has a direct angiogenic effect and may stimulate fibroblast growth factor that is thought to be one of the inducing factors of dural AVF was tested by TERADA et al. (1998).

The authors administered oestrogen to rats in a dose similar to that used in women in the postmenopausal period. However, they could not prove that oestrogen in fact induces dural AVFs with a higher incidence.

5.2.3
Thrombosis

It was Tanaguchi et al. (1971) who recognized early on the potential of the minute vascular dural network when reacting to a thrombosing fistula between ICA and CS. They suggested fresh thrombus as initial stimulus for building a fistula, a concept widely accepted today. That thrombosis in sinuses involved by DCSFs occurs, was observed by Voigt and coworkers and was reported by Brismar and Brismar (1976) who documented the presence of thrombus in six patients using orbital phlebography. The thrombus was considered secondary to the fistula and not as a source or trigger of the developing AV-shunt. Seeger et al. (1980) reported on six patients with DCSFs, who showed a thrombosed CS in their follow-up angiograms. I have observed similar phenomena in two patients: one patient showed a spontaneous thrombosis of a dural AVF involving the inferior petrosal sinus diagnostic arteriogram (Case Illustration in Sect. 9.1). In another patient, I noticed a change in the venous drainage within 3 weeks (Fig. 5.1), due to ongoing thrombosis in the CS, possibly aggravated by the initial diagnostic angiography. In a third patient with a sigmoid sinus DAVF, a diagnostic arteriogram showing a partially stenosed sinus due to thrombus and was followed by another within less than 24 h which demonstrated complete occlusion of the AV shunt (Fig. 5.2).

Rather little attention has been paid for long time to a possible causal relationship between thrombus in the CS and the development of a CSF, which is somewhat surprising when one considers that several related observations were made in the nineteenth century. Sattler (1880) reviewed autopsies of several cases in which *"no arterial disease, but enlargement and occlusion of the cavernous sinus and the circular sinus and the superior ophthalmic vein by clotted blood was found"* (authors translation).

A similar case was observed by Hulke (1860), who wrote: *"the thrombosis of the cavernous sinus and the ophthalmic vein at its entrance has been the cause of pulsating exophthalmos"*.

Sattler (1880), however, disagreed and was convinced it would be impossible that *"a thrombus in the CS is capable to produce the group of symptoms of pulsating exophthalmos"* (author's translation). Later on, (Sattler 1920, 1930) provided a more detailed report on nine cases among which four were spontaneous fistulas without evidence for a ruptured ICA. He, however, critically stated that those carotid arteries might have not been fully examined.

Kerber and Newton (1973) studied the vascularization of the dura mater and observed arteriovenous AV-shunts adjacent to the superior sagittal and lateral sinus. In an attempt to recanalize a thrombosed sinus, a functional enlargement of these shunts would occur. Houser et al. (1979) suggested that a DCSF might develop subsequently to a thrombus in the CS that induces an "arteriolar neoformation" and represents the trigger for the development of an arteriovenous shunt. Most authors share this opinion today. Although angiographically sometimes difficult to identify with certainty, a thrombus in the CS has been observed by some authors in up to 85% of the cases (Theaudin et al. 2006).

Chaudhary et al. (1982) considered thrombosis or thrombophlebitis of the recipient venous system the primary event in the formation of four patients with DAVF in the sigmoid, lateral and superior sagittal sinus. Mironov (1994) has provided the largest body of work on this subject so far. He studied extensively the pathogenesis in 96 DAVFs in all locations and found overall concomitant phlebothrombus in more than 50%, while thrombus was seen in 62% of the 29 DCSFs. He discusses the chronological relation between phlebothrombosis and DAVFs, for which not enough angiographic evidence exists. Not all DAVFs develop on the ground of thrombosis and not all patients with SVT develop DAVFs. Only a few cases provide angiographic evidence of thrombosed sinus preceding a fistula (Houser et al. 1979; Chaudhary et al. 1982; Pierot et al. 1993) with an interval between 6 months and 9 years. It is assumed that thrombus undergoes organization and recanalization, which triggers the opening of latent preexisting AV communications. When a fistula shunts into the sinus, it will increase the venous pressure and open more AV shunts, by some authors being considered a vicious cycle (Nishijima et al. 1992). Mironov suggested a disturbance of the myogen autoregulation of the physiological micro AV-shunts of the parasinusal and basal, probably caused by phlebothrombosis. He also discussed the relationship between the size of an AV shunt and the pressure gradient in the venous recipient. According to his concept, fistulas with a small shunt volume would

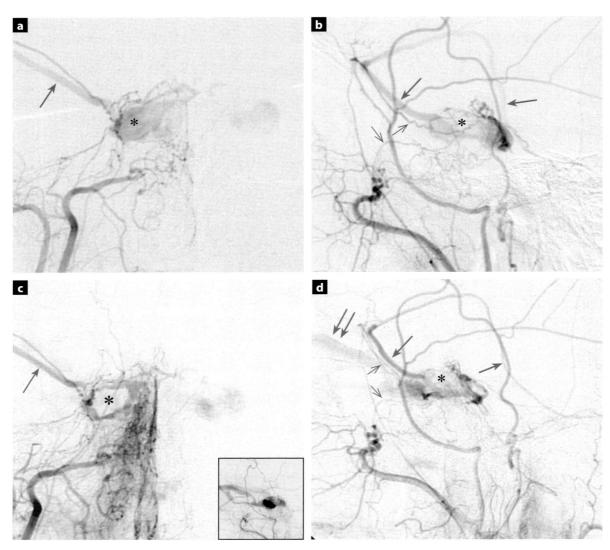

Fig. 5.1 a–d. Dynamics in a DCSF: Ongoing thrombosis in the CS reroutes the venous drainage anteriorly towards the SOV demonstrating the dynamic process of the AV shunting in a DCSF. **a–b** Initial diagnostic angiogram, 26th August 1999, right ECA injection, AP and lateral views: Filling of a dural AV shunt at the right CS supplied by MMA, AMA and IMA branches. Drainage predominantly via the right SPPS (*arrow*) into a paracavernous sinus (*thin arrow*); Sylvian vein not involved; no IPS opacified. **c–d** On the 15th September (21 days later), the patient was rescheduld for treatment. The repeated DSA in almost identical projections shows a large filling defect within the right CS, indicating ongoing thrombosis, possibly triggered by the initial arteriogram. The thrombus is not easily identifiable in lateral views, although some of the feeding branches from the IMA and MMA appear less prominent and seem to have regressed (*small arrows*). Note that the SOV is meanwhile opacified, showing a change in the venous drainage pattern and explaining the slight aggravation of the patient's symptoms within these 3 weeks. Note also that the left ECA supply fills almost exclusively the right SOV, but not the SSPS, indicating not only a bilateral AV shunt, but also (angiographic) compartmentalization (*inset*). (For treatment, see Case Report IV)

occur in venous recipients with low pressure, such as at the level of the skull base, e.g. the CS as low-flow fistulas.

Tsai et al. (2004) studied more recently 69 patients with DAVF in different locations and found in 39% associated cerebral sinus thrombosis. Thrombosis was found always in the sinuses around to the fistula in the sinuses downstream to the fistulas which supports the two main hypothesis, that (1) venous outflow obstruction (by thrombus) may cause opening of physiologic arteriovenous shunts or (2) venous hypertension causes ischemia and angiogenesis (see below). Third, the theory that thrombosis may be caused or augmented by the turbulent fistula flow as suggested

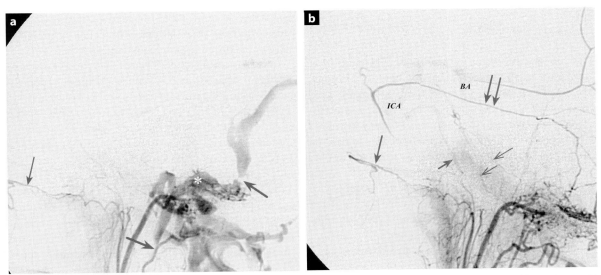

Fig. 5.2 a,b. Dynamics in a DAVF: Spontaneous thrombosis of a sigmoid sinus DAVF in less than 24 h observed in a 56-year-old female presenting with bruit and headaches in January 2003. **a** Left APA injection, lateral view shows a dural AV shunt (*asterisk*) involving the jugular bulb and the sigmoid sinus. Note the stenoses and the restricted outflow (*thick arrows*), proximal in the IJV, and distal in the sigmoid sinus, indicating ongoing thrombosis. **b** Control injection before endovascular treatment the next morning no longer shows AV shunting due to thrombosis of the involved sinus segment, probably triggered by the angiography on the previous afternoon. Note the filling of the vidian artery (*single arrow*) via pharyngeal arteries, communicating with the IMA, and the retrograde opacification of MMA branches (*double arrows*). Due to changed hemodynamics, the small extra-intracranial anastomses become better visible: Carotid branch of the ICA filling the vertical carotid segment (*short arrow*), clival branches (*thin arrows*) anastomosing with the C5 segment (TMH). Faint blush of the carotid siphon (ICA) and basilar artery (BA)

by some authors (CHAUDHARY et al. 1982; NISHIJIMA et al. 1992; LAWTON et al. 1997; LASJAUNIAS et al. 1986) is supported as well. Areas of low flow velocity or flow stagnation found in sinuses where two parts of flow anterograde cerebral blood flow and retrograde fistula flow meet, could create such hemodynamic condition. Although this potential mechanism is not well studied, it may play a role as a trigger for sinus stenosis. It is corroborated by observation of acquired stenoses due to a longstanding AV shunt flow seen in "non-dural" AV fistulas (see Fig. 6.2).

A number of more recent studies focusing on the role of the coagulation system may add valuable insights in the etiology of DAVFs (KRAUS et al. 1998, 2000; GERLACH et al. 2003; SINGH et al. 2001). KRAUS et al. (1998) reported resistance to activated protein C (APCR) in three out of seven patients with DAVFs (non-CS locations). APCR has been shown to be a cause of familial thrombophilia and considered the most common genetic risk factor for venous thrombosis. It also impairs the recanalization of sinus thrombosis, and thus may further contribute to the development of a DAVF. In a larger group of patients, the same authors found evidence that the incidence of sinus thrombosis, underlying DAVFs, is higher in patients with FV Leiden (KRAUS et al. 1986). SINGH

et al. (2001) reported on a 30-year-old woman with thrombosis and a DAVF of the sigmoid sinus who also had a prothrombin gene mutation. WENDEROTH and PHATOUROS (2003) accidentally discovered a dural arteriovenous fistula in a 58-year-old patient with APCR, concluding that these patients have an initial predisposition to dural sinus thrombosis and thus to pathophysiological conditions, possibly leading to the development of a DAVF. GERLACH et al. (2003) recently studied 15 patients with DAVFs (one case of DCSF) and found a surprisingly high incidence (33%) of genetic thrombophilic abnormalities (mutation of prothrombin gene in 26% and FV Leiden mutation in 6.7%). Although the number of patients in this study is relatively small, there is increasing evidence that genetic thrombophilic abnormalities may contribute to the development of DAVFs. These results need to be confirmed by studies on larger groups of patients, but they support the theory of an inherent association between DAVFs (and DCSFs) and sinus thrombosis. To what degree thrombotic changes trigger the formation of a dural arteriovenous shunt may further depend on geographic and ethnic differences. It was shown in a recent survey in Japan (SATOMI 2008), that dural sinus thrombosis might play a less important role than generally assumed.

5.2.4
Venous Hypertension

The concept of venous hypertension, being another key factor in the etiology of DAVFs, is encouraged by results of animal experiments conducted by Terada et al. (1994), who demonstrated that increased venous pressure can cause newly acquired AVFs, even in absence of thrombosis. It can be suspected that a similar mechanism may also play a role in humans (Phatouros et al. 2000). Kusuka et al. (2001) recently reported the development of a DCSF remotely from a previously thrombosed lateral sinus that developed another DAVF, emphasizing the role of venous hypertension. The authors conclude that the thrombosis caused venous hypertension not only within the superior sagittal and right transverse/sigmoid sinus, but also in the CS, causing here micro AV shunts within the dura mater to open and eventually to trigger the DCSFs. This is an interesting interpretation, but raises some questions. First, there was no direct evidence that the CS was in fact exposed to an increased venous pressure. Second, one would probably expect another fistula to develop in the neighborhood of the thrombosed lateral sinus where most likely the venous pressure was elevated. The hemodynamic effects associated with dural arteriovenous shunts in the sigmoid/transverse sinus area may be more complex than assumed and our knowledge on this subject is still limited.

The role of venous hypertension as etiological factor is reassured by another observation. A possible causal relationship between hypertension and arteriovenous shunts at the CS has already been assumed by Potter (1954) as well as by Echols and Jackson (1959), who suggested that creating hypotension might be beneficial for causing spontaneous thrombosis of a CCF. There are anecdotal reports that symptoms and signs caused by a CSF have disappeared after air travel (Debrun et al. 1988a; Kupersmith 1988). I have seen one patient who noticed his bruit, caused the first time by a sigmoid DAVF immediately after landing in an airplane. Another more recent patient with a DCSF reported a drastic increase in eye swelling and redness following a 3-h flight. Changes of atmospheric pressure seem to interfere with pressure in the cerebral venous system. They may have a bidirectional effect on the arteriovenous shunt flow, causing either an increase, or a decrease with spontaneous occlusion.

Ornauqe et al. (2003) have successfully applied this concept to treat patients with DAVFs and DCSFs using controlled hypotension (see also Sect. 9.3).

Lawton et al. (1997) were able to demonstrate a causal relationship between venous hypertension and angiogenic activity and DAVF formation. The authors suggested that venous hypertension is induced by a venous outflow obstruction due to a thrombus and may initiate the pathogenesis of a DAVF. Venous hypertension can cause ischemia and tissue hypoxia that may stimulate angiogenesis. This "aberrant" angiogenic activity of dural vessels could lead to arteriovenous shunting and formation of a DAVF. The subsequent arterialization will increase venous pressure and outflow obstruction and thereby create the vicious cycle mentioned above that may enlarge the AV shunt and aggravate a DAVF into a progressive lesion.

5.2.5
Trauma

Trauma, although reported in some anecdotal cases (Newton and Hoyt 1970), is probably less likely a cause of a DCSF (Tomsick 1997b). Sattler (1920) had doubts that minor trauma can indeed cause a pulsating exophthalmos and if so only if the vessel is *diseased already or in case of pregnancy* (author's translation). Tomsick (1997b) observed two patients with a spontaneous fistula after blunt head trauma, and one patient with a Type D fistula following rhizotomy. He emphasized the development of DCSFs following severe head trauma makes it difficult to define the exact etiology. The early series of Halbach et al. (1987) contained 1 patient while later, the same group reported on 234 traumatic carotid and vertebral artery lesions in which they observed 7 indirect fistulas. Berenstein et al. (1986) reported on 11 patients with DCSFs of which 1 was a traumatic fistula supplied by the MMA. Jacobson et al. (1996) described in detail two cases in which a ruptured AMA solely supplied a CSF.

True traumatic indirect fistulas represent possibly a specific entity of DCSFs since their angioarchitecture with a "single artery to single vein or sinus" pattern is distinctly different from the usual Type D fistula with a complex network of numerous feeders emptying into the CS. This typical angioarchitecture, on the other hand, can hardly be explained by trauma. Revascularization of a thrombus (or more than one) in the CS with subsequent neovascularization and opening of multiple micro AV-shunts will most likely lead to a network of feeding vessels. Trauma and rupture will most certainly affect only one (or a few) of them, but will not create a network of vessels. A case of traumatic DCSF following craniectomy has been reported (WATANABE et al. 1984). FIELDS et al. (2000) described a 46-year-old patient who after sustaining a gunshot wound to his face developed a CSF supplied by dural ICA branches that completely disappeared 11 days after diagnostic angiography. Some iatrogenic CS fistulas may appear as single artery-CS shunts.

AMINOFF (1973) considered the close anatomical relationship between dural arteries and veins a predisposition for the development of an AVF following head trauma. Moreover, the absence of trauma in the history would not exclude the possibility of minor head traumas causing an AVF in particular in children and young adults as a cause of DAVF.

Otherwise, many cases of DAVFs have no history of trauma and, even if they do, then there is usually an interval of several weeks or months before symptoms of an AV shunt appear. Thus, direct trauma seems unlikely to be a major cause for the development of DCSFs (CHAUDHARY et al. 1982). Tomsick (1997b) gave an overview that revealed approximately 3% of DCSFs are related to trauma. He observed an asymptomatic DCSF during diagnostic angiography for other indications, including one CCF on the contralateral side and concludes that major head trauma can cause DCSF. None of the patients with DAVFs or DCSFs in my own material could clearly be related to a relevant trauma. Despite justified skepticism on the role of trauma in the etiology of DAVFs and lack of sufficient proof, it should be considered that minimal trauma might be very difficult to evaluate as many patients will not recall minor events that could have resulted in the formation of an abnormal AV shunt.

Iatrogenic vessel injury during endovascular procedures may lead to AV shunts involving the CS and can be caused by transsphenoidal surgery of pituitary adenomas (TAPTAS 1982; BAVINZSKI et al. 1997). I have seen three iatrogenic direct CCFs in my practice, two patients after hypophysectomy and one patient who underwent septoplasty and presented with a high-flow CCF (Fig. 5.3). Catheterization of cavernous dural ICA branches for embolization of meningeomas may cause rupture and lead to an "indirect" CSF as well (BARR et al. 1995). Figure 5.4 illustrates such a case in which microcatheter manipulation into the marginal tentorial artery resulted in extravasation that fortunately resolved without clinical consequences.

5.2.6
Embolization

The de novo development of a DAVF in a sigmoid or transverse sinus in association with embolization of a DCSF has been reported several times and is explained by transvenous catheter manipulations with subsequent injury or by venous turbulence initiating thrombus and recanalization as a trigger (NAKAGAWA et al. 1992; YAMASHITA et al. 1993; MAKIUCHI et al. 1998; KUBOTA et al. 1999; KAWIGUCHI et al. 1999). Gupta et al. (2005) recently reported a case where 4 months after transarterial embolization of a DCSF a new AV shunt at the ipsilateral sigmoid sinus developed. Strangely enough, the opposite order of events, namely development of a dural CSF following embolization of a DAVF in other location, has to my knowledge not been reported.

5.2.7
Congenital

Although LIE (1968) proposed a congenital origin in some of the spontaneous CSFs, this etiology remains speculative. DAVFs in general, and DCSFs in particular are rare in childhood, and if they occur represent probably a separate entity (BIGLAN et al. 1981; YAMAMOTO et al. 1995). BIGLAN et al. (1981) observed a 7-week-old infant with a non-traumatic fistula between the external carotid artery and the cavernous sinus. KONISHI et al. (1990) reported a case of a 2-month-old boy with a congenital fistula of the dural carotid-cavernous sinus. SKOLNICK and MCDONNELL (2000) recently reported on a 9-year-old boy who presented with proptosis, conjunctival congestion and decreased vision caused by spontaneous "dural cavernous sinus fistula". Among other reasons, the fact that the cavernous sinus is not fully developed at birth and only partially participates in the cerebral venous drainage may explain why a typical dural CSF, as encountered in the adult population, is unlikely to occur in the pediatric age group.

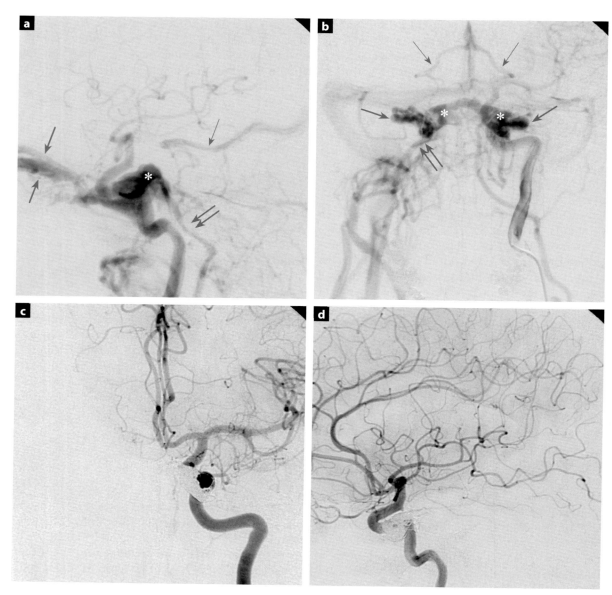

Fig. 5.3 a–d. Iatrogenic direct CCF following septoplasty in a 57-year-old patient. This patient was referred with exophthalmos, diplopia and eye-redness for 4 weeks following surgery to correct a septal deviation in August 1996. **a–b** Direct fistula of the left CS (*asterisk*) with drainage into the right CS, both SOVs (*short arrows*), both basal veins of Rosenthal (*thin arrow*) and leptomeningeal veins of the posterior fossa. The fistulous opening was too small to be passed with a detachable balloon. Thus, transvenous embolization was performed using the right IPS (*double arrow*). Tight packing with GDC®s resulted in complete occlusion of the AV shunt that remained stable over the next 5 years (**c–d** FU in 2001). The patient recovered completely.

5.2.8
Other Potential Factors

Recently, the role of basic fibroblast growth factor (bFGF) and vascular endothelial growth factor (VEGF) has been studied (TERADA et al. 1996; SHIN et al. 2003). bFGF, considered a powerful angiogenic growth stimulator associated with the endothelial cell, was found with strong immunoreactivity in sinuses of patients with DAVFs (MALEK et al. 2000). URANISHI et al. (1999) examined histologically dural AVFs that were surgically resected in nine patients and found that the thick wall of the dural sinus stained strongly

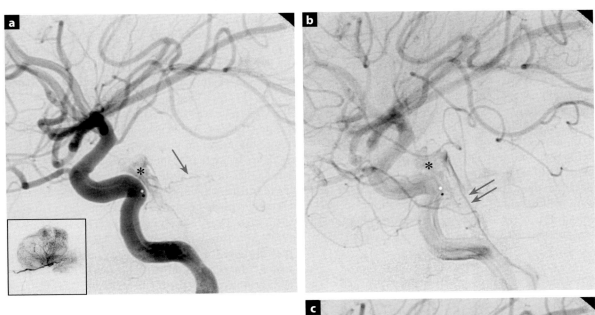

Fig. 5.4a–c. Iatrogenic "DCSF" due to microcatheter manipulation during embolization of a tentorial meningeoma in June 2001. a–b The ruptured branch of the MHT fills the posterior CS (*asterisk*) and the IPS (*double arrow*). **c** The fistulous communication disappeared after 10 min and the patient woke up without sequelae. *Arrow:* marginal tentorial artery (Bernasconi and Cassinari), *double arrow:* inferior petrosal sinus. *Inset:* Tentorial meningeoma

for bFGF, mainly in the subendothelial layer and media. VEGF was expressed in the endothelium of the sinus in all nine cases indicating that angiogenetic growth factors may play a role in the pathogenesis of DAVFs. This angiogenetic process could be associated with loss of venular surface properties and contribute to venous thrombosis (SARMA and TER BRUGGE 2003).

LAWTON et al. (1997) were able to prove that angiogenic activity measured by the rabbit cornea assay was significantly greater in animals with venous hypertension, suggesting that the venous hypertension and sinus thrombosis may alter the balance

of proangiogenic and antiangiogenic substances (FOLKMAN 1995).

5.2.9
Various

The higher incidence of DCSFs in women during menopause and in men over 50 years indicates a potential role of vessel wall weakening over time due to arteriosclerotic changes. Arterial hypertension and diabetes are considered predisposing factors as well, but correlative data are lacking so far.

In summary, despite major advances in diagnosis and management, the etiology and pathogenesis of DAVFs and DCSFs remains a matter of controversy and is far from being fully understood. The development of dural arteriovenous shunts must be seen in close relation with thrombotic processes and venous hypertension in the cerebral sinuses. Therefore, the term "venous diseases" appears suitable. To what extend other factors trigger or contribute to the development of dural AV shunts, remains to be investigated by further experimental and clinical studies. Better understanding of mechanisms of molecular pathogenesis in the development of dural AVFs might aid in the establishment of new therapeutic measures for this unique vascular disease.

5.3
Prevalence

Epidemiologic data regarding the overall incidence of both DAVFs as well as of DCSFs are limited. Large autopsy series have found 46 AVMs among 3200 brain tumors (1.4%) (OLIVECRONA and RIIVES 1948). Population-based data showed an incidence of 1.84 per 100,000 person years during 1965–1992; the incidence of symptomatic cases was 1.22 per 100,000 person years (BROWN et al. 1996). The detection rate in a more recent study was 0.29 per 100,000 adults (SATOMI 2008).

According to older literature, DAVF comprise 10%–15% of all intracranial arteriovenous malformations. Most recent authors refer to the work of NEWTON and CRONVIST (1969) who reported on a total of 129 patients among whom 94 had pure pial, 20 had mixed pial-dural and 15 (12%) had pure dural supply. One recent review on natural history of intracranial vascular malformation does not provide new numbers on incidence and prevalence of DAVFs (BROWN et al. 2005).

Most patients with DAVFs are more than 40 years of age (82%) and women (71%) (MIRONOV 1995). Because similar diagnostic and therapeutic measures apply to all dural fistulas, DCSFs and DAVF can be considered as one epidemiologic group of disease. For both, the association with menopause (54%) and puerperium (18%) and lower incidence in men is typical (NEWTON and HOYT 1970; TOMSICK 1997b; TOYA et al. 1981).

In a metaanalysis published by AWAD et al. (1990), with an additional 17 cases, the incidence of AVFs in the CS among all DAVFs was 11.9%, whereas the relationship of "aggressive" to "non-aggressive" cases was 1:6.5 (Table 5.1). In his review of 322 cases, published up to 1920, SATTLER (1920, 1930) found a frequency of traumatic vs idiopathic fistulas of 3:1. As elucidated above, this distribution changed towards the end of the twentieth century, and traumatic CSFs were less frequently seen in the western world. This trend is likely due to improved safety standards for traffic vehicles, in particular motorcycles and bicycles. Even large cities in Asia with a high percentage of motorcycle and bicycle riders have a decreased incidence, as recently reported from the Queen Elizabeth Hospital in Hong Kong, where among 80 patients with CSF, 76 (95%) were spontaneous and only 4 (5%) were of traumatic origin (CHENG 2006). Among all CSFs, approximately 10%–15% account for indirect or dural fistulas (BARCIO-SALORIO et al. 2000) and Type D is by far the most frequent (TOMSICK 1997b).

The true prevalence of DCSFs is difficult to assess due to the fact that many patients present with mild symptoms, may undergo spontaneous resolution and are never diagnosed. According to series of several major endovascular centers, Type B–D DCSFs occur five times more frequently than Type A fistulas (TOMSICK 1997b).

Another difficulty in obtaining accurate numbers lies in the fact that many DCSFs patients are studied as different groups, either included in DAVFs, CCFs or evaluated as a separate entity. The series of COGNARD et al. (1995) contained 205 cases of DAVF of which 33 were DCSF (16%). KLISCH et al. (2003) reported on 17 CSFs, including 11 DCSFs. SATOMI et al. (2002) reported on 117 cases of benign DAVF (without cortical venous drainage) with DCSF representing the largest group (42.7%). TSAI et al. (2004) investigated 69 patients with DAVFs among whom 30% involved

Table 5.1. Frequency of DCSFs in large series of DAVFs

References	DAVFs	CS
AWAD et al. 1990 [a]	377	45 (11.9%)
COGNARD et al. 1995	205	33 (16%)
MIRONOV 1995	96	29 (30.2%)
SATOMI et al. 2002 [b]	117	50 (42.7%)
TSAI 2004	69	(30%)
MALEK et al. 2000	366	122 (34%)
CHUNG et al. 2002	60	(57%)
LING 2001	121	38 (69.1%)

[a] 17 cases and metaanalysis   [b] Cases of benign DAVF

the CS. Chung et al. (2002) found the CS as the most common (57%) location for the DAVF in 60 patients. Cheng et al. (2003) reported on 27 patients who were assessed based on Cognard's classification.

Tomsick (1997b) observed Type B–D fistulas in 68% of all spontaneous CSF and discusses the influence of the referring praxis. Table 5.2 provides an overview on published series of spontaneous, traumatic and dural fistulas involving the CS. It reveals that the distribution of various fistula types differs considerably among the groups. While Andoh et al. (1991) reports an incidence of Type D fistulas of 25% and Liu et al. (2001) noted 54%, this type is observed by Vinuela et al. (1984) and Takahasi and Nakano (1980) in 100%.

As discussed above, diagnostic quality of cerebral angiography as major tool for identifying, classifying and understanding etiology and natural history of CSFs has significantly improved over the last 25 years. This must be considered when looking at data in older series using angiographic assessments. Today, high-resolution DSA provides more morphological information than was available in the past and helps to further develop theories and new etiological concepts. Thus, it happened probably not completely by chance that in several recent studies, categorization of DCSFs as groups with different arterial supply (Types B–D) has no longer been applied (see Table 5.2) (Meyers et al. 2002; Cheng et al. 2003; Stiebel-Kalish et al. 2002).

Table 5.2. Prevalence of DCSFs related to either trauma or spontaneous occurrence. Modified after Tomsick (1997b)

References	Years	Types B–D (s)	Types B–D (t)	Type B	Type C	Type D
Newton	1962–1969	10	1	2	3	6
Taniguchi	1971	11	0	-	-	-
Takahashi	1979	9	2	0	0	11
Seegher	1977	5	1	0	1	5
Halbach	1978–1986	29	1	-	-	-
Vinuela	1978–1982	18	0	0	0	16
Kupersmith	1982–1986	26	-	-	0	-
Barrow	1978–1984	13	0	5	3	5
Debrun	1988	32	0	0	4	28
Andoh	1991	15	0	5	6	4
Kurata	1974–1992	12	0	2	2	7
Saski	1974–1992	26	?	-	-	-
Kinugasa	1994	24	0	1	4 (C1/C2)	19 (D1/D2)
Taki	1994	35	2	-	-	-
Tomsick	1978–1994	48	2	-	5	38 (D1/D2)
Liu	2001	121	?	30	26	65
Meyer	2002	133	NP	NP	NP	NP
Cheng	2002	27	[a]	[a]	[a]	[a]
Stiebel-Kalish	2002	85	NP	NP	NP	NP
Klisch	2003	11	-	3[a]	-	
Suh	2005	58	N/A	N/A 23 PT	N/A 23 RT	8[a]
Wakhloo	2005	14	N/A	4	2, C2 = 1	
Theaudin	2006	27	N/A	NP	NP	
Kim	2006	65	NP	NP	NP	N/A 12 LRT

D2 = bilateral
C2 = bilateral
NP = not provided
[a] According to Cognard's classification
? = Not identified by authors

5.3.1
Natural History

DCSFs, in general, are referred to as "benign" or "non-aggressive" fistulas because of their tendency to occlude spontaneously, usually caused by CS thrombosis. Although these spontaneous occlusions seem to occur more frequently than in other AV shunting lesions, they can be accompanied by serious clinical deteriorations. Neither such a course nor a neurological deficit caused by venous ischemia or intracranial hemorrhage, both rare events, can in fact be considered "benign". But even though such a clinical course may be progressive or in some cases fulminant, terms like "aggressive", "malignant" or "benign", widely used by neuroradiologists, appear unsuitable and rather imprecise to characterize a dural arteriovenous shunting lesion. They should be reserved for diseases for which they were defined, i.e. tumors.

As true for prevalence and incidence of DCSFs, exact data on natural history do not exist, which is in part due to the fact that a large number of fistulas is discovered relatively late in their course. Furthermore cases undergoing diagnostic angiography are necessarily affected by the angiographic procedure itself as contrast injection can accelerate thrombosis of the CS and "spontaneous occlusion" (Newton and Hoyt 1970; Seeger et al. 1980; Voigt et al. 1971; Phelps et al. 1982). In some recent series the natural course is additionally influenced by particulate arterial embolization (Satomi et al. 2005; Suh et al. 2005).

The number of reported "spontaneous" occlusions reported in the literature may lie between 11% and 90% (Vinuela et al. 1984; Kupersmith et al. 1988) and is on average 35% according to Tomsick (1997b). When looking at rates of spontaneous occlusion after angiography one has to consider the number of patients reported. For example, frequently quoted, Phelps et al. (1982) observed a "43%" (in Meyers et al. 2002) occlusion rate in 3 out of 7 patients undergoing angiography in a group of 19 patients with atypical signs of a carotid cavernous fistula! This rate is lower in larger series. Only one case in my own material developed a spontaneous occlusion, a patient with an IPS fistula, draining via the CS and causing diplopia (see also Sect. 9.1 and Case illustration XII).

Throughout the process of spontaneous occlusion the progress of thrombosis in the CS and its effects on the venous drainage is uncertain. In many patients regression of ophthalmological symptoms is preceded by an exacerbation of ophthalmologi-cal symptoms. CS thrombosis, spontaneous or triggered by embolization, may involve the ophthalmic veins and can cause significant deterioration of symptoms due to sudden increase of venous pressure (Seeger et al. 1980). This phenomenon has been described by Sergott et al. (1987) as "paradoxical worsening". In some cases even vision loss may occur (Sergott et al. 1987; Bianchi-Marsoli et al. 1996; Suzuki et al. 1989; Knudtzon 1950; Miki et al. 1988). Because it may accentuate intrinsic thrombotic effects on the central retinal vein, an embolization procedure in a patient with worsening of symptoms might be contraindicated (Tomsick 1997b). If increased intraocular pressure occurs, additional anticoagulation may be advisable. Subcutaneous use of low-molecular heparin has improved clinical signs in four patients as reported by Bianchi-Marsoli et al. (1996).

Suh et al. (2005) have retrospectively studied the evolution of fistulas over a mean follow-up period of 23 months. They found that seven (30%) of their patients, angiographically classified as proliferative type (PT), showed chronological progression to the late restrictive type (LRT). Unfortunately, it is not clear from their description how many of these patients underwent treatment by embolization which makes it presumptuous to apply the results to the natural history.

This is similarly true for the study of Satomi et al. (2005) who categorized patients according to their changes in venous drainage but included embolized patients as well.

As for DAVFs, presence of leptomeningeal drainage is a main indicator for risk assessment and decision-making in patients with DCSFs by most authors. The number for cortical or leptomeningeal reflux varies from 10% to 31% (Table 5.3). Nevertheless, the associated risk of intracranial hemorrhage (around 2%) seems, however, relatively low compared to patients with DAVFs in other locations, especially at the tentorial sinus or in the anterior cranial fossa (Agid 2009). For example, none of the DCSF patients in the study in Cognard's series (Cognard et al. 1995) showed an "aggressive" course and in another large study no case with such behavior was found (Awad et al. 1990). Consequently, cortical or leptomeningeal drainage in DCSFs must not necessarily be seen an indicator of a progressive or "malignant" course or nature, as in DAVFs. Yet today, most operators will probably agree to treat these fistulas as early as possible even though they may pose a lesser risk than direct CCFs with cortical drainage.

Table 5.3. Frequency of cortical/leptomeningeal venous drainage and associated hemorrhage

Authors	DCSFs	C/LVD	Hemorrhage
HALBACH et al. 1987	30	3 (10%)	
AWAD et al. 1990[a]	45	n/a	n/a
COGNARD et al. 1995	33	4 (12%)	0
TOMSICK 1997	50	8 (16%)	0
SATOMI et al. 2005[b]	65	17 (26.1%)	1 (1.5%)
THEAUDIN et al. 2006	27	5 (18.5%)	0
STIEBEL-KALISH et al. 2002	88	22 (26%)	2 (2.2%)
MEYERS et al. 2002	135	41 (31%)	2 (1.5%)

[a] 17 cases and metaanalysis   [b] Cases of benign DAVF

In summary, lacking accurate data, only limited knowledge on prevalence and natural history in patients harboring DCSFs exist. Larger studies with long-term follow-up of patients, not undergoing any sort of treatment including manual compression therapy, will be needed to obtain reliable information on the natural course of the disease. The term "benign" fistula, referring to a generally milder clinical course, does not appear suitable and should be reserved for diseases of that biological nature.

References

Agid R, et al. (2009) Management strategies for anterior cranial fossa (ethmoidal) dural arteriovenous fistulas with an emphasis on endovascular treatment. J Neurosurg. 110(1):79–84.

Ambler MW, Moon AC, Sturner WQ (1978) Bilateral carotid-cavernous fistulae of mixed types with unusual radiological and neuropathological findings. J Neurosurg 48:117–124

Aminoff MJ (1973) Vascular anomalies in the intracranial dura mater. Brain 96:601–612

Andoh T, Nakashima T, Araki Y, Sakai N, Yamada H, Kagawa Y, Hirata T, Tanabe Y, Takada M (1991) Spontaneous carotid-cavernous sinus fistula; analysis of 16 cases. No Shinkei Geka 19:831–839

Awad IA, et al. (1990) Intracranial dural arteriovenous malformations: factors predisposing to an aggressive neurological course. J Neurosurg 72:839–850

Barcio-Salorio JL, Barcia JA, Soler FM (2000) Radiosurgery for carotid-cavernous fistulas. In: Eisenberg MB, Al Mefty O (eds) The cavernous sinus. Lippincott Williams & Williams, Philadelphia, pp 227–242

Barr JD, Mathis JM, Horton JA (1995) Iatrogenic carotid-cavernous fistula occurring after embolization of a cavernous sinus meningioma. AJNR Am J Neuroradiol 16:483–485

Barrow DL, Spector RH, Braun IF, Landman JA, Tindall SC, Tindall GT (1985) Classification and treatment of spontaneous carotid-cavernous sinus fistulas. J Neurosurg 62:248–256

Bartholow R (1872) Aneurysms of the arteries of the base of the brain-their symptomatology diagnosis and treatment. Ann J Med Sci 64:375–386

Bavinzski G, Killer M, Knosp E, Ferraz-Leite H, Gruber A, Richling B (1997) False aneurysms of the intracavernous carotid artery–report of 7 cases. Acta Neurochir (Wien) 139:37–43

Berenstein A, Scott J, Choi IS, Persky M (1986) Percutaneous embolization of arteriovenous fistulas of the external carotid artery. AJNR Am J Neuroradiol 7:937–942

Berger MS, Hosobuchi Y (1984) Cavernous sinus fistula caused by intracavernous rupture of a persistent primitive trigeminal artery. Case report. J Neurosurg 61:391–395

Bianchi-Marsoli S, Righi C, Ciasca P (1996) Low dose heparin therapy for dural cavernous sinus fistulas. Neuroradiology Suppl:15

Biglan AW, Pang D, Shuckett EP, Kerber C (1981) External carotid-cavernous fistula in an infant. Am J Ophthalmol 91:351–356

Brismar G, Brismar J (1976) Spontaneous carotid-cavernous fistulas: phlebographic appearance and relation to thrombosis. Acta Radiol Diagn (Stockh) 17:180–192

Brown RD Jr, Wiebers DO, Torner JC, O'Fallon WM (1996) Incidence and prevalence of intracranial vascular malformations in Olmsted County, Minnesota, 1965 to 1992. Neurology 46:949–952

Brown RD Jr, Flemming KD, Meyer FB, Cloft HJ, Pollock BE, Link ML (2005) Natural history, evaluation, and management of intracranial vascular malformations. Mayo Clin Proc 80:269–281

Castaigne P, Blancard P, Laplane D, Djindjan R, Sorato M (1966a) Spontaneous arteriovenous communication between the external carotid and the cavernous sinus. Bull Soc Ophtalmol Fr 66:47–49

Castaigne P, Laplane D, Djindjian R, Bories J, Augustin P (1966b) Spontaneous arteriovenous communication between the external carotid and the cavernous sinus. Rev Neurol (Paris) 114:5–14

Chaudhary MY, Sachdev VP, Cho SH, Weitzner I Jr, Puljic S, Huang YP (1982) Dural arteriovenous malformation of the major venous sinuses: an acquired lesion. AJNR Am J Neuroradiol 3:13–19

Chen MN, Nakazawa S, Hori M (1993) A case of primary intracranial choriocarcinoma with a carotid-cavernous fistula. No Shinkei Geka 21:1031–1034

Cheng K (2006) Neuro-endovascular therapy of carotid cavernous fistula. Hong Kong Med Diary 11

Cheng KM, Chan CM, Cheung YL (2003) Transvenous embolisation of dural carotid-cavernous fistulas by multiple venous routes: a series of 27 cases. Acta Neurochir 145:17–29

Chuman H, Trobe JD, Petty EM, Schwarze U, Pepin M, Byers PH, Deveikis JP (2002) Spontaneous direct carotid-cavernous fistula in Ehlers-Danlos syndrome type IV: two case reports and a review of the literature. J Neuroophthalmol 22:75–81

Chung SJ, Kim JS, Kim JC, Lee SK, Kwon SU, Lee MC, Suh DC (2002) Intracranial dural arteriovenous fistulas: analysis of 60 patients. Cerebrovasc Dis 13:79–88

Cognard C, Gobin YP, Pierot L, Bailly AL, Houdart E, Casasco A, Chiras J, Merland JJ (1995) Cerebral dural arteriovenous fistulas: clinical and angiographic correlation with a revised classification of venous drainage. Radiology 194:671–680

Dandy W (1937) Carotid-cavernous aneurysms (pulsating exophthalmos). Zentralbl Neurochir 2:77–206

Dany F, Fraysse A, Priollet P, Brutus P, Bokor J, Catanzano G, Bernard P, Christides C, Beylot C (1986) Dysmorphic syndrome and vascular dysplasia: an atypical form of type IV Ehlers-Danlos syndrome. J Mal Vasc 11:263–269

de Campos JM, Ferro MO, Burzaco JA, Boixados JR (1982) Spontaneous carotid-cavernous fistula in osteogenesis imperfecta. J Neurosurg 56:590–593

Debrun GM, Davis KR, Nauta HJ, Heros RE, Ahn HS (1988a) Treatment of carotid cavernous fistulae or cavernous aneurysms associated with a persistent trigeminal artery: report of three cases. AJNR Am J Neuroradiol 9:749–755

Debrun GM, Vinuela F, Fox AJ, Davis KR, Ahn HS (1988b) Indications for treatment and classification of 132 carotid-cavernous fistulas. Neurosurgery 22:285–289

Debrun GM, Aletich VA, Miller NR, DeKeiser RJ (1996) Three cases of spontaneous direct carotid cavernous fistulas associated with Ehlers-Danlos syndrome type IV. Surg Neurol 46:247–252

Delens E (1870) De la communication de la carotide interne et du sinus caverneux (anevrysme arterio-veineux). Paris

Desal HA, Toulgoat F, Raoul S, Guillon B, Bommard S, Naudou-Giron E, Auffray-Calvier E, de Kersaint-Gilly A (2005) Ehlers-Danlos syndrome type IV and recurrent carotid-cavernous fistula: review of the literature, endovascular approach, technique and difficulties. Neuroradiology 47:300–304

Echols DH, Jackson JD (1959) Carotid-cavernous fistula: a perplexing surgical problem. J Neurosurg 16:619–627

Fields CE, Cassano AD, Dattilo JB, Yelon JA, Ivatury RR, Broderick TJ (2000) Indirect carotid-cavernous sinus fistula after shotgun injury. J Trauma 48:338–341

Flandroy P, Lacour P, Marsault C, Stevenaert A, Collignon J (1987) The intravascular treatment of a cavernous fistula caused by rupture of a traumatic carotid trigeminal aneurysm. Neuroradiology 29:308–311

Folkman J (1995) Seminars in medicine of the Beth Israel Hospital, Boston. Clinical applications of research on angiogenesis. N Engl J Med 333:1757–1763

Fromm H, Habel J, Halama H (1967) On the diagnostic significance of the Bernasconi and Cassinari artery in the cerebral angiogram. Nervenarzt 38:220–222

Gerlach R, Yahya H, Rohde S, Bohm M, Berkefeld J, Scharrer I, Seifert V, Raabe A (2003) Increased incidence of thrombophilic abnormalities in patients with cranial dural arteriovenous fistulae. Neurol Res 25:745–748

Guglielmi G, Vinuela F, Dion J, Duckwiler G, Cantore G, Delfini R (1990) Persistent primitive trigeminal artery-cavernous sinus fistulas: report of two cases. Neurosurgery 27:805–808; discussion 808–809

Gupta R, Horowitz M, Tayal A, Jovin T (2005) De novo development of a remote arteriovenous fistula following transarterial embolization of a carotid cavernous fistula: case report and review of the literature. AJNR Am J Neuroradiol 26:2587–2590

Halbach VV, Higashida RT, Hieshima GB, Reicher M, Norman D, Newton TH (1987) Dural fistulas involving the

cavernous sinus: results of treatment in 30 patients. Radiology 163:437–442

Halbach VV, Higashida RT, Dowd CF, Barnwell SL, Hieshima GB (1990) Treatment of carotid-cavernous fistulas associated with Ehlers-Danlos syndrome. Neurosurgery 26:1021–1027

Hamby WB (1966) Carotid-cavernous fistula, vol III. Springfield: Charles C Thomas

Hamby W, Gardner W (1933) Treatment of puslating exophthalmos with report of two cases. Arch Surg 27:676

Hayes GJ (1958) Carotid cavernous fistulas: diagnosis and surgical management. Am Surg 24:839–843

Higashida RT, Halbach VV, Tsai FY, Norman D, Pribram HF, Mehringer CM, Hieshima GB (1989) Interventional neurovascular treatment of traumatic carotid and vertebral artery lesions: results in 234 cases. AJR Am J Roentgenol 153:577–582

Horton JA, Jungreis CA, Stratemeier PH (1991) Sharp vascular calcifications and acute balloon rupture during embolization. AJNR Am J Neuroradiol 12:1070–1073

Houser OW, Campbell JK, Campbell RJ, Sundt TM Jr (1979) Arteriovenous malformation affecting the transverse dural venous sinus–an acquired lesion. Mayo Clin Proc 54:651–661

Hulke (1860) All the capital signs of orbital aneurism present, in a marked degree, but independently of aneurism or any erectile tumor. Ophthalmic Hosp Rep 2:6

Inagawa T (1991) Follow-up study of unruptured aneurysms arising from the C3 and C4 segments of the internal carotid artery. Surg Neurol 36:99–105

Jacobson BE, Nesbit GM, Ahuja A, Barnwell SL (1996) Traumatic indirect carotid-cavernous fistula: report of two cases. Neurosurgery 39:1235–1237; discussion 1237–1238

Kanner AA, Maimon S, Rappaport ZH (2000) Treatment of spontaneous carotid-cavernous fistula in Ehlers-Danlos syndrome by transvenous occlusion with Guglielmi detachable coils. Case report and review of the literature. J Neurosurg 93:689–692

Kawaguchi T, Kawano T, Kaneko Y, Tsutsumi M, Ooigawa H, Kazekawa K (1999) Dural arteriovenous fistula of the transverse sigmoid sinus after transvenous embolization of the carotid cavernous fistula. No To Shinkei 51:1065–1069

Kerber CW, Manke W (1983) Trigeminal artery to cavernous sinus fistula treated by balloon occlusion. Case report. J Neurosurg 58:611–613

Kerber CW, Newton TH (1973) The macro and microvasculature of the dura mater. Neuroradiology 6:175–179

Kim DJ, et al. (2006). Results of transvenous embolization of cavernous dural arteriovenous fistula: a single-center experience with emphasis on complications and management. AJNR Am J Neuroradiol 27(10):2078–2082

Klisch J, Huppertz HJ, Spetzger U, Hetzel A, Seeger W, Schumacher M (2003) Transvenous treatment of carotid cavernous and dural arteriovenous fistulae: results for 31 patients and review of the literature. Neurosurgery 53:836–856

Knudtzon A (1950) A remarkable case of pulsating exophthalmos in an old patient who recovered spontaneoulsly after bilateral aseptic thrombosis of the cavernous sinus. Acta Ophthalmol 28:363–369

Kobayashi N, Miyachi S, Negoro M, Suzuki O, Hattori K, Kojima T, Yoshida J (2003) Endovascular treatment strategy for direct carotid-cavernous fistulas resulting from rupture of intracavernous carotid aneurysms. AJNR Am J Neuroradiol 24:1789–1796

Koh JH, Kim JS, Hong SC, Choe YH, Do YS, Byun HS, Lee WR, Kim DK (1999) Skin manifestations, multiple aneurysms, and carotid-cavernous fistula in Ehlers-Danlos syndrome type IV. Circulation 100:e57–58

Konishi Y, Hieshima GB, Hara M, Yoshino K, Yano K, Takeuchi K (1990) Congenital fistula of the dural carotid-cavernous sinus: case report and review of the literature. Neurosurgery 27:120–126

Kraus JA, Stuper BK, Berlit P (1998) Association of resistance to activated protein C and dural arteriovenous fistulas. J Neurol 245:731–733

Kraus JA, Stuper BK, Nahser HC, Klockgether T, Berlit P (2000) Significantly increased prevalence of factor V Leiden in patients with dural arteriovenous fistulas. J Neurol 247:521–523

Kubota Y, Ueda T, Kaku Y, Sakai N (1999) Development of a dural arteriovenous fistula around the jugular valve after transvenous embolization of cavernous dural arteriovenous fistula. Surg Neurol 51:174–176

Kupersmith MJ, Berenstein A, Choi IS, Warren F, Flamm E (1988) Management of nontraumatic vascular shunts involving the cavernous sinus. Ophthalmology 95:121–130

Kupersmith MJ, Hurst R, Berenstein A, Choi IS, Jafar J, Ransohoff J (1992) The benign course of cavernous carotid artery aneurysms. J Neurosurg 77:690–693

Kusaka N, Sugiu K, Katsumata A, Nakashima H, Tamiya T, Ohmoto T (2001) The importance of venous hypertension in the formation of dural arteriovenous fistulas: a case report of multiple fistulas remote from sinus thrombosis. Neuroradiology 43:980–984

Lasjaunias P, Berenstein A (1987) Dural arteriovenous malformation, vol 1. Springer, Berlin Heidelberg New York

Lasjaunias P, Chiu M, ter Brugge K, Tolia A, Hurth M, Bernstein M (1986) Neurological manifestations of intracranial dural arteriovenous malformations. J Neurosurg 64:724–730

Lawton MT, Jacobowitz R, Spetzler RF (1997) Redefined role of angiogenesis in the pathogenesis of dural arteriovenous malformations. J Neurosurg 87:267–274

Lesoin F, Rousseau M, Petit H, Jomin M (1984) Spontaneous development of an intracavernous arterial aneurysm into a carotid-cavernous fistula. Case report. Acta Neurochir (Wien) 70:53–58

Lie T (1968) Congenital anomalies of the carotid arteries. Excerpta Med 35–51

Ling F, Wu J, Zhang H (2001). Classification of intracranial dural arteriovenous fistula and its clinical signification. Zhonghua Yi Xue Za Zhi 81(23):1439–442.

Linskey ME, Sekhar LN, Hirsch WL Jr, Yonas H, Horton JA (1990) Aneurysms of the intracavernous carotid artery: natural history and indications for treatment. Neurosurgery 26:933–937; discussion 937–938

Linskey ME, Sekhar LN, Horton JA, Hirsch WL Jr, Yonas H (1991) Aneurysms of the intracavernous carotid artery: a multidisciplinary approach to treatment. J Neurosurg 75:525–534

Liu HM, Wang YH, Chen YF, Cheng JS, Yip PK, Tu YK (2001) Long-term clinical outcome of spontaneous carotid cavernous sinus fistulae supplied by dural branches of the internal carotid artery. Neuroradiology 43:1007–1014

Locke C (1924) Intracranial arteriovenous aneurysm or pulsating exophthalmos. Ann Surg 80:1–24

Makiuchi T, Takasaki W, Oda H et al. (1998) A case of sigmoid sinus dural arteriovenous fistual after treated cavernous dural arteriovenous fistula. Intervent Neuroradiol 4:219–222

Malek AM, Halbach VV, Higashida RT, Phatouros CC, Meyers PM, Dowd CF (2000) Treatment of dural arteriovenous malformations and fistulas. Neurosurg Clin N Am 11:147–166, ix

Meyers PM, Halbach VV, Dowd CF, Lempert TE, Malek AM, Phatouros CC, Lefler JE, Higashida RT (2002) Dural carotid cavernous fistula: definitive endovascular management and long-term follow-up. Am J Ophthalmol 134:85–92

Miki T, Nagai K, Saitoh Y, Onodera Y, Ohta H, Ikoma H (1988) Matas procedure in the treatment of spontaneous carotid cavernous sinus fistula: a complication of retinal hemorrhage. No Shinkei Geka 16:971–976

Mironov A (1994) Pathogenetical consideration of spontaneous dural arteriovenous fistulas (DAVFs). Acta Neurochir (Wien) 131:45–58

Mironov A (1995) Classification of spontaneous dural arteriovenous fistulas with regard to their pathogenesis see comments. Acta Radiol 36:582–592

Mitsuhashi T, Miyajima M, Saitoh R, Nakao Y, Hishii M, Arai H (2004) Spontaneous carotid-cavernous fistula in a patient with Ehlers-Danlos syndrome type IV–case report. Neurol Med Chir (Tokyo) 44:548–553

Moniz E (1927) La radiographie cerebrale. Bull Acad Med. Paris 98:40–45

Nakagawa H, Kubo S, Nakajima Y, Izumoto S, Fujita T (1992) Shifting of dural arteriovenous malformation from the cavernous sinus to the sigmoid sinus to the transverse sinus after transvenous embolization. A case of left spontaneous carotid-cavernous sinus fistula. Surg Neurol 37:30–38

Nelaton H (1876) Carotid cavernous fistula. Lancet 2:142

Newton TH, Cronqvist S (1969) Involvement of dural arteries in intracranial arteriovenous malformations. Radiology 93:1071–1078

Newton TH, Hoyt WF (1968) Spontaneous arteriovenous fistula between dural branches of the internal maxillary artery and the posterior cavernous sinus. Radiology 91:1147–1150

Newton TH, Hoyt WF (1970) Dural arteriovenous shunts in the region of the cavernous sinus. Neuroradiology 1:71–81

Nishijima M, Takaku A, Endo S, Kuwayama N, Koizumi F, Sato H, Owada K (1992) Etiological evaluation of dural arteriovenous malformations of the lateral and sigmoid sinuses based on histopathological examinations. J Neurosurg 76:600–606

Noland L, Taylor AS (1931) Pulsating exophthalmos the result of injury. Trans South surg Ass 43:171–177

Obrador S, Gomez-Bueno J, Silvela J (1974) Spontaneous carotid-cavernous fistula produced by ruptured aneurysm of the meningohypophyseal branch of the internal carotid artery. Case report. J Neurosurg 40:539–543

Okamura T, Yamamoto M, Ohta K, Matsuoka T, Takahashi M, Uozumi T (1995) A case of ruptured cerebral aneurysm associated with fenestrated vertebral artery in osteogenesis imperfecta. No Shinkei Geka 23:451–455

Olivecrona H, Riives J (1948) Arteriovenous aneurysms of the brain: their diagnosis and treatment. Arch Neurol Psychiatr 59:567–602

Ornaque I, Alonso P, Marti Valeri C, de Miquel MA, Cambra

R, Gabarros A, Conesa G (2003) Spontaneous closure of a intracraneal dural arteriovenous fistula by controlled hypotension during a general anesthesia procedure. A case report. Neurologia 18:746–749

Palestine AG, Younge BR, Piepgras DG (1981) Visual prognosis in carotid-cavernous fistula. Arch Ophthalmol 99:1600–1603

Parkinson D (1967) Transcavernous repair of carotid cavernous fistula. Case report. J Neurosurg 26:420–424

Parkinson D (1973) Carotid cavernous fstula: direct repair with preservation of the carotid artery.Technical note. J Neurosurg 38:99–106

Phatouros CC, Meyers PM, Dowd CF, Halbach VV, Malek AM, Higashida RT (2000) Carotid artery cavernous fistulas. Neurosurg Clin N Am 11:67–84

Phelps CD, Thompson HS, Ossoinig KC (1982) The diagnosis and prognosis of atypical carotid-cavernous fistula (red-eyed shunt syndrome). Am J Ophthalmol 93:423–436

Pierot L, Chiras J, Duyckaerts C, Jason M, Martin N (1993) Intracranial dural arteriovenous fistulas and sinus thrombosis. Report of five cases. J Neuroradiol 20:9–18

Polin RS, Shaffrey ME, Jensen ME, Braden L, Ferguson RD, Dion JE, Kassell NF (1996) Medical management in the endovascular treatment of carotid-cavernous aneurysms. J Neurosurg 84:755–761

Potter JM (1954) Carotid-cavernous fistula; five cases with spontaneous recovery. Br Med J 4891:786–788

Prolo, DJ, Hanbery JW (1971) Intraluminal occlusion of a carotid-cavernous sinus fistula with a balloon catheter. Technical note. J Neurosurg. 35(2):237–242

Purdy PD (2002) Managing carotid-cavernous fistulas in Ehlers-Danlos syndrome type IV. J Neuroophthalmol 22:73–74

Rivington (1875) Med Chir Trans lviii:191

Rosenthal AK, Rowe JM (1987) Lymphomatoid granulomatosis associated with a carotid sinus fistula: response to cytotoxic therapy. Am J Med 83:381–382

Rosso D, Hammond RR, Pelz DM (1999) Cavernous aneurysm rupture with balloon occlusion of a direct carotid cavernous fistula: postmortem examination. AJNR Am J Neuroradiol 20:771–773

Saff G, Frau M, Murtagh FR, Silbiger ML (1989) Mucormycosis associated with carotid cavernous fistula and cavernous carotid mycotic aneurysm. J Fla Med Assoc 76:863–865

Sarma D, ter Brugge K (2003) Management of intracranial dural arteriovenous shunts in adults. Eur J Radiol 46:206–220

Satomi J, van Dijk JM, Terbrugge KG, Willinsky RA, Wallace MC (2002) Benign cranial dural arteriovenous fistulas: outcome of conservative management based on the natural history of the lesion. J Neurosurg 97:767–770

Satomi J, Satoh K (2008). Epidemiology and etiology of dural arteriovenous fistula. Brain Nerve 60(8):883–6.

Satomi J, Satoh K, Matsubara S, Nakajima N, Nagahiro S (2005) Angiographic changes in venous drainage of cavernous sinus dural arteriovenous fistulae after palliative transarterial embolization or observational management: a proposed stage classification. Neurosurgery 56:494–502; discussion 494–502

Sattler H (1880) Pulsirender exophthalmus. In: Graefe A, Saemisch T (eds) Handbuch der Gesamten Augenheilkunde. Leipzig, Engelmann, pp 745–948

Sattler H (1920) Pulsierender exophthalmus. In: Graefe A, Sae-

misch T (eds) Handbuch der Gesamten Augenheilkunde. Springer, Berlin Heidelberg New York, pp 1–245

Sattler H (1930) Pulsierender exophthalmus. In: Graefe A, Saemisch T (eds): Handbuch der Gesamten Augenheilkunde. Springer, Berlin Heidelberg New York, pp 1–245

Seeger JF, Gabrielsen TO, Giannotta SL, Lotz PR (1980) Carotid-cavernous sinus fistulas and venous thrombosis. AJNR Am J Neuroradiol 1:141–148

Sergott RC, Grossman RI, Savino PJ, Bosley TM, Schatz NJ (1987) The syndrome of paradoxical worsening of dural-cavernous sinus arteriovenous malformations. Ophthalmology 94:205–212

Shimizu Y, Nagamine Y, Fujiwara S, Suzuki J, Yamamoto T, Iwasaki Y (1987) An experimental study of vascular damage in estrogen-induced embolization. Surg Neurol 28:23–30

Shin Y, Uranishi R, Nakase H, Sakaki T (2003) Vascular endothelial growth factor expression in the rat dural arteriovenous fistula model. No To Shinkei 55:946–952

Singh V, Meyers PM, Halbach VH, Gress DR, Higashida RT, Dowd CF, Smith WS (2001) Dural arteriovenous fistula associated with prothrombin gene mutation. J Neuroimaging 11:319–321

Skolnick KA, McDonnell JF (2000) Spontaneous dural cavernous sinus fistula in a child. J Aapos 4:383–385

Stiebel-Kalish H, Setton A, Nimii Y, Kalish Y, Hartman J, Huna Bar-On R, Berenstein A, Kupersmith MJ (2002) Cavernous sinus dural arteriovenous malformations: patterns of venous drainage are related to clinical signs and symptoms. Ophthalmology 109:1685–1691

Sugar HS, Meyer SJ (1940) Pulsating exophthalmos. Arch Ophtalmol Rev Gen Ophthalmol 64:1288–3121

Suh DC, Lee JH, Kim SJ, Chung SJ, Choi CG, Kim HJ, Kim CJ, Kook M, Ahn HS, Kwon SU, Kim JS (2005) New concept in cavernous sinus dural arteriovenous fistula: correlation with presenting symptom and venous drainage patterns. Stroke 36:1134–1139

Suzuki J, Komatsu S (1981) New embolization method using estrogen for dural arteriovenous malformation and meningioma. Surg Neurol 16:438–442

Suzuki Y, Kase M, Yokoi M, Arikado T, Miyasaka K (1989) Development of central retinal vein occlusion in dural carotid-cavernous fistula. Ophthalmologica 199:28–33

Takahashi M, Nakano Y (1980) Magnification angiography of dural carotid-cavernous sinus fistulae with emphasis on clinical and angiographic evolution. Neuroradiology 19:249–256

Taki W, Nakahara I, Nishi S, Yamashita K, Sadatou A, Matsumoto K, Tanaka M, Kikuchi H (1994) Pathogenetic and therapeutic considerations of carotid-cavernous sinus fistulas. Acta Neurochir (Wien) 127:6–14

Taniguchi RM, Goree JA, Odom GL (1971) Spontaneous carotid-cavernous shunts presenting diagnostic problems. J Neurosurg 35:384–391

Taptas JN (1950) Etiology and pathogenesis of exophthalmias of vascular origin, called pulsatile exophthalmias. Arch Ophthalmol Rev Gen Ophtalmol 10:22–50

Taptas JN (1982) Cavernous carotid artery. J Neurosurg 56:312–313

Terada T, Higashida RT, Halbach VV, Dowd CF, Tsuura M, Komai N, Wilson CB, Hieshima GB (1994) Development of acquired arteriovenous fistulas in rats due to venous hypertension. J Neurosurg 80:884–889

Terada T, Tsuura M, Komai N, Higashida RT, Halbach VV, Dowd CF, Wilson CB, Hieshima GB (1996) The role of angiogenic factor bFGF in the development of dural AVFs. Acta Neurochir (Wien) 138:877–883

Terada T, Higashida RT, Halbach VV, Dowd CF, Hieshima GB (1998) The effect of oestrogen on the development of arteriovenous fistulae induced by venous hypertension in rats. Acta Neurochir (Wien) 140:82–86

Theaudin M, et al. (2006) Diagnosis and treatment of dural carotid-cavernous fistulae: a consecutive series of 27 patients. J Neurol Neurosurg Psychiatry

Tokunaga K, Sugiu K, Kameda M, Sakai K, Terasaka K, Higashi T, Date I (2004) Persistent primitive trigeminal artery-cavernous sinus fistula with intracerebral hemorrhage: endovascular treatment using detachable coils in a transarterial double-catheter technique. Case report and review of the literature. J Neurosurg 101:697–699

Tomsick TA (1997) Typ A (direct) CCF: etiology, prevalence and natural history. In: Tomsick TA (ed) Carotid cavernous fistula. Digital Educational Publishing, Philadelphia, pp 59–73

Tomsick TA (1997) Typ B,C, and D CCF: etiology, prevalence and natural history. In: Tomsick TA (ed) Carotid cavernous fistula. Digital Educational Publishing, Philadelphia, pp 59–73

Toya S, Shiobara R, Izumi J, Shinomiya Y, Shiga H, Kimura C (1981) Spontaneous carotid-cavernous fistula during pregnancy or in the postpartum stage. Report of two cases. J Neurosurg 54:252–256

Travers B (1811) A case of aneurysm by anastomosis in the orbit, cured by the ligature of the common carotid artery. Med Chir Tr 2:1–16

Tsai LK, et al. (2004) Intracranial dural arteriovenous fistulas with or without cerebral sinus thrombosis: analysis of 69 patients. J Neurol Neurosurg Psychiatry 75:1639–1641

Uranishi R, Nakase H, Sakaki T (1999) Expression of angiogenic growth factors in dural arteriovenous fistula. J Neurosurg 91:781–786

van Rooij WJ, Sluzewski M, Beute GN (2006) Ruptured cavernous sinus aneurysms causing carotid cavernous fistula: incidence, clinical presentation, treatment, and outcome. AJNR Am J Neuroradiol 27:185–189

Vinuela F, Fox AJ, Debrun GM, Peerless SJ, Drake CG (1984) Spontaneous carotid-cavernous fistulas: clinical, radiological, and therapeutic considerations. Experience with 20 cases. J Neurosurg 60:976–984

Voigt K, Sauer M, Dichgans J (1971) Spontaneous occlusion of a bilateral caroticocavernous fistula studied by serial angiography. Neuroradiology 2:207–211

von Rad M, Tornow K (1975) Spontaneous carotid cavernous fistula in a case of hereditary hemorrhagic telangiectasia (Osler-Rendu) (author's transl). J Neurol 209:237–242

Walker AE, Allegre GF (1956) Carotid-cavernous fistulas. Surgery 39:411–422

Watanabe A, Takahara Y, Ibuchi Y, Mizukami K (1984) Two cases of dural arteriovenous malformation occurring after intracranial surgery. Neuroradiology 26:375–380

Wenderoth JD, Phatouros CC (2003) Incidental discovery of a dural arteriovenous fistula in a patient with activated protein C resistance. AJNR Am J Neuroradiol 24:1369–1371

Wolff H, Schmid B (1939) Das Arteriogramm des pulsierenden Exophthalmus. Zbl Neurochir 4:241–250, 310–319

Yamamoto T, Asai K, Lin YW, Suzuki K, Ohta S, Ohta K, Yamamoto M, Ichioka H (1995) Spontaneous resolution of symptoms in an infant with a congenital dural caroticocavernous fistula. Neuroradiology 37:247–249

Yamashita K, Taki W, Nakahara I, Nishi S, Sadato A, Kikuchi H (1993) Development of sigmoid dural arteriovenous fistulas after transvenous embolization of cavernous dural arteriovenous fistulas. AJNR Am J Neuroradiol 14:1106–1108

Zimmerman R, Leeds NE, Naidich TP (1977) Carotid-cavernous fistula associated with intracranial fibromuscular dysplasia. Radiology 122:725–726

Neuro-Ophthalmology in

Dural Cavernous Sinus Fistulas (DCSFs)

CONTENTS

Introduction

Hemodynamic dysregulation in AV-shunting lesions of the CS lead in 80% of cases to elevated pressure in peri- and intraorbital veins. This results in interstitial edema and increased caliber of the orbital veins and the CS, which causes in turn mechanical compression and ischemia. Spectrum and progression of resulting neuroophthalmological deficits in patients with a DCSF are determined by individual hemodynamics and angioarchitecture of the fistulas drainage (Table 6.1).

Most DCSFs drain via the superior ophthalmic vein into the angular, supraorbital and facial veins. Such anterior drainage is usually associated with more impressive clinical symptoms. It may cause ipsilateral CN deficits and damage to orbital organs. The posterior drainage via IPS or SPS instead rarely causes ophthalmologic symptoms, but may be responsible for oculomotor deficits due to ischemic, or less frequently, mechanical disturbance of CN functions. Fistulas with posterior drainage may also cause trigeminal neuropathy or facial nerve paresis (EGGENBERGER 2000; RIZZO 1982).

Association with local thrombosis of the CS or IPS is often found. It may lead to a rapid deterioration caused by acute elevation of the intravenous and intraocular pressures and can be the reason for slow recovery later on. Bi- or contralateral symptoms occur in 10% of the patients with DCSFs and can be due to thrombotic occlusions of ipsilateral draining veins and involvement of intracavernous and /or basilar sinuses as well as of the contralateral CS in the fistulas drainage. It remains unclear whether venous thrombosis, often seen on angiograms, has developed secondarily on the basis of hemodynamic turbulences, or as a residuum of the initial thrombotic processes considered a triggering factor in the pathogenesis of DCSFs (GROVE 1984). Complications and unfavorable long-term outcomes in the natural course of the disease mainly involve the eye. The spontaneous occlusion rate of DCSFs in the literature may lie between 11% and 90%, depending on observations made by different authors (VINUELA et al. 1984, KELTNER et al., 1987b, KUPERSMITH 1988). Interestingly enough, several authors have reported disappearance of the AV shunting following diagnostic angiography (GROVE 1984; KELTNER et al. 1987b; PHELPS et al. 1982; VOIGT et al. 1971). Thus, spontaneous cure seems possible and should be considered in therapeutic decision-making.

The classical Dandy's triad seen in Type A or traumatic CCFs (Fig. 6.1) – chemosis, exophthalmos and bruit – is rarely observed in patients with dural CSF. Because of the usually chronic, clinically milder and variform manifestation of symptoms, the diagnosis of a DCSF can be less straightforward and may not allow a standard procedural regimen.

If an individual patient presents with nonspecific symptoms, the clinical picture may provide initial

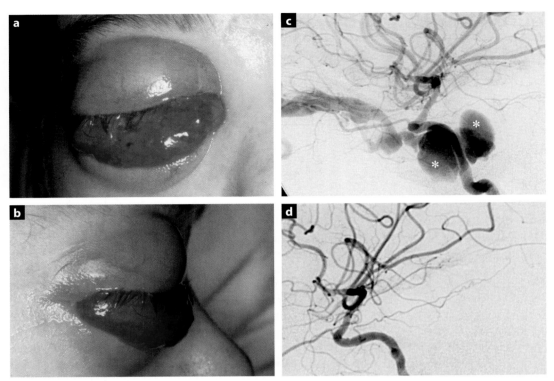

Fig. 6.1 a–d. Classic clinical presentation of a traumatic direct CCF that is often acute and fulminant, but can be delayed for several days or weeks, in some cases for several months. A 24-year-old man after a car accident seen in July 2002. **a–b** Severe exophthalmos and chemosis of the right eye, associated with audible bruit. **c** The arteriogram shows a massively enlarged CS (*asterisks*) with posterior bulging into the cranial cavity and dominant anterior drainage into a significantly enlarged SOV. No intracranial steal. Note that such severe chemosis is rare in DCSFs (see Fig. 6.4) **d** Fistula occlusion with one detachable balloon

signs pointing towards etiology, hemodynamics and prognosis. Therefore, knowledge and careful analysis of the neuroophthalmological symptoms are required for differential diagnosis, effective, individual, risk- and prognosis-oriented use of diagnostic and therapeutic measures in patients with DCSFs.

6.1
Extraorbital Ocular Symptoms

6.1.1
Orbital Pain

Persistent frontal or periorbital cephalgia of varying intensity, often starting acutely, is a frequent initial symptom in patients with DCSF. These headaches are usually caused by local thrombosis within the CS or the SOV.

Furthermore, hemodynamic turbulences in the fistula leading to painful irritation of the meninges can increase during physical exercise or elevated blood pressure. Extraocular or extraorbital symptoms beside headaches are rare. Anecdotal reports of life-threatening epistaxis or intracerebral hemorrhages in case of leptomeningeal venous drainage (KELTNER et al. 1987a) or ischemic brain stem infarcts after sinus venous thrombosis (UCHINO et al. 1997) and atypical trigeminal neuralgia (OTT et al. 1993) exist. Fistulous connections in the posterior CS may cause mechanical compression of the Gasserian ganglion or vascular steal phenomena affecting in particular the first or second division, resulting into neuralgia and dysesthesia (MADSEN 1970; PALESTINE et al. 1981). They can initially occur isolated and thus may easily be mistaken for idiopathic trigeminal neuralgia (OTT et al. 1993; RIZZO et al. 1982). Patients with periorbital cephalgia and accompany-

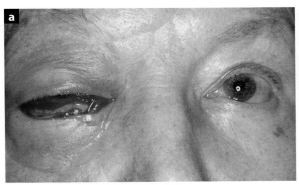

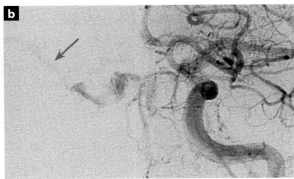

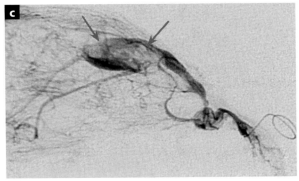

Fig. 6.2 a–c. Aggravated chemosis in a low-flow AV fistula. **a,** 88-year-old patient with diplopia due to 6th nerve palsy since 08/98. She presented with increasing proptosis and aggravated chemosis in 02/99. **b,** Left ICA injection AP view shows a low-flow fistula draining into the right SOV (*arrow*). **c,** This vessel turned out to be partially occluded by a large intraluminal thrombus as revealed by a superselective injection into the CS during the treatment session (*arrows*). Venous outflow obstruction associated with a low-flow AV shunt leads to venous hypertension and may cause dramatic symptoms (see also Chap. 10)

ing ophthalmoplegia, initially misdiagnosed as suffering from migraine, cluster headaches, Tolosa-Hunt syndrome or intracranial aneurysms, have been described as well (HAWKE et al. 1989; BRAZIS et al. 1994; KOMORSKY 1988).

6.1.2
Cranial Nerve Deficits and Ophthalmoplegia

Unilateral ophthalmoplegia can be seen in ca. 50% of the patients with DCSFs (MIYACHI et al. 1993) and often represents the first objective symptom. It usually becomes manifest after weeks or months following development of a fistula. The elevated intraorbital venous pressure leads to a progressive swelling of the ocular muscles and to a reduced contractility and limited motility of the eye bulb. On the other hand, dilated vessels and vascular steal phenomena result in mechanical and ischemic oculomotor nerve damage.

Due to their course through the CS, the sixth CN is most frequently (46%–85%), the third CN less frequently (36%) and usually in cases with posterior

drainage, and the fourth CN (11%) is rarely involved (KUPERSMITH et al. 1986, 1988).

In cases of anterior drainage, the ophthalmoplegia is often accompanied by other orbital symptoms such as exophthalmos and chemosis. In contrast, fistulas with posterior drainage via the IPS may be the cause for isolated ophthalmoplegia and should be included in the differential diagnoses of intracranial neoplasms, cavernous aneurysms and meningitis (ACIERNO et al. 1995). Although diplopia in these patients is usually reversible, it requires intensive neuro-ophthalmological care and early intervention. In some cases of longstanding AV shunting into the CS, diplopia may become permanent.

6.2
Orbital Symptoms

Several authors postulate anterior drainage or disturbance of the anterior venous outflow from the

Table 6.1. Incidence of frequent signs and symptoms in DCSFs in recent series (MEYERS et al. 2002; STIEBEL-KALISH et al. 2002; DE KEIZER 2003; THEAUDIN et al. 2006; SUH et al. 2005)

	MEYERS et al. (2002) % of 135	STIEBEL-KALISH et al. (2002) % of 85	DE KEIZER (2003)[a] % of 68	KIM (2006) % of 65	THEAUDIN et al. (2006) % of 27	SUH et al. (2005) 58
Conjunctival injection	93	76	66		41	*
Chemosis	87	21	-	32	37	*
Propotosis	81	76	65	21	37	*
Diplopia	68		45	34	45	*
Bruit	49	28[b]	27			*
Retroorbital pain	34		11	34		*
Elevated IOP	34	72				*
Decreased visual acuity	31		26	13	30	*
Retinal hemorrhage	-	18	18			*

[a]DE KEIZER (2003) differentiated in 68 spontaneous (dural, orbital and direct) and 33 traumatic (direct and dural) fistulas
[b]Subjective bruit in 24 and objective in 7 patients
*SUH et al. (2005): divided 58 patients into four main symptom pattern
- Orbital pattern (chemosis, exophthalmos,pain,eyelid swelling): 53%
- Cavernous pattern (ptosis,diplopia, anisocoria, ophthalmoplegia): 71%
- Ocular pattern (decreased vision, IOC > 20 mm Hg ocular pain, glaucoma, retinal hemorrhage): 64%
- Cerebral pattern (seizures, hemorrhage): 5%

CS as a precondition for the presence of orbital symptoms in patients with DCSFs, although its angiographic appearance may be mimicked by an anatomical variant or be caused by a thrombotic occlusion of the IPS (GROVE 1984; HOOPS et al. 1997).

6.2.1
Exophthalmos

As a result of the chronically elevated intraorbital venous pressure a prolapse of the orbital soft tissue may develop, which is commonly less prominent than in patients with direct CCFs. In most cases it is less than 5 mm and can initially be overlooked. The most precise method of measurement is to examine the patient in reclining head position using the Hertel Exophthalmometer.

A massive exophthalmos, rarely observed in cases of DCSF, can lead to chemosis, lid swelling, lagophthalmos and corneal damage. If an acute increasing exophthalmos, associated with pain and lid swelling occurs and is followed by a spontaneous improvement, a thrombosis of the SOV or the CS should be considered.

6.2.2
Conjunctival Engorgement and Chemosis

Typically, arterialization of conjunctival veins is associated with other ophthalmologic manifestations, particularly with exophthalmos, and can be found in 82%–100% of patients (PHELPS et al. 1982; PALESTINE et al. 1981; KUPERSMITH et al. 1988) with intraorbital symptoms. It may lead to dilatations and tortuosities of conjunctival veins, which are often the cause for misdiagnosis such as inflammatory conjunctivitis. However, the conjunctival injection in patients with CSF is, different from allergic, viral or bacterial conjunctivitis, characterized by bright-red, corkscrew veins. Except for cases of secondary infections, it usually occurs without inflammatory secretion.

These veins are called specific epibulbar loops by DE KEIZER (2003) and represent the most superficial layer, developing due to opening of small capillary connections at the outside of the orbit (Fig. 6.3). Enlarged connections on the eyeball develop between the recurrent conjunctival ciliary veins and posterior conjunctival veins (specific limbal loops) (DE KEIZER 1979, 2003).

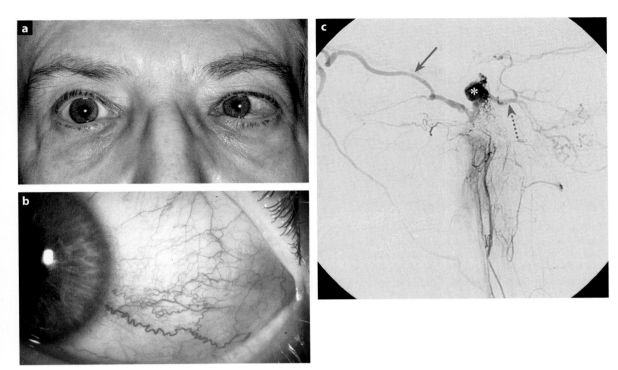

Fig. 6.3 a–c. Conjunctival injection (eye redness) in a DCSF. Symptoms in DCSFs can be similiar to that of direct CCF patients, but are usually milder and develop less dramatically. A bruit is infrequently reported. This 86-year-old woman presented in March 2002 with mild exophthalmos, eye redness and 6th cranial nerve palsy (**a**). The close-up shows the typical "corkscrew" dilation of epibulbar veins, which can be considered pathognomonic for DCSFs (**b**). The type of venous drainage (anterior or posterior) may determine the clinical presentation. This fistula's drainage involves anteriorly the SOV (*arrow*), and posteriorly the SPS (*dotted arrow*), the anterior pontomesencephalic vein, basal vein of Rosenthal and leptomeningeal veins of the posterior fossa (**c**). Only some of the patients with retrograde cortical or leptomeningeal venous drainage present with venous ischemia or hemorrhage. In most cases, the clinical symptoms are purely opththalmological. Treatment was performed using TVO (see Chap. 8, Fig. 8.4)

Conjunctival chemosis is defined as an edema of the sclera and occurs in 25%–90% (PALESTINE et al. 1981; KUPERSMITH et al. 1988; VINUELA et al. 1984) of the cases, accompanying conjunctival injection in patients with DCSFs. In particular, when exophthalmos occurs, it may cause significant prolapse of the conjunctiva with lagophthalmos and trophic damages of the cornea (Figs. 6.4, 6.4). Chemosis may occur before proptosis and is invariably limited to the inferior palpebral conjunctiva (MILLER 1998).

6.2.2.1
Retinal Hemorrhage

In severe cases of venous dilation and elevated intravenous pressure, optic disc swelling and retinal hemorrhages, caused by venous stasis and impaired retinal blood flow, with secondary ischemia or hypoxia, can occur (Fig. 6.5) (see Case Report I). These intraretinal hemorrhages can be both, flame-shaped (located in the nerve fiber layer) and punctuate (located in the outer retinal layers) (MILLER 1998) and can be associated with central retinal vein occlusion (KUPERSMITH et al. 1996). DE KEIZER (2003) as well as STIEBEL-KALISH et al. (2002) found them in up 18% of their patients.

6.2.3
Corneal Damage

Dehydration of the cornea, usually painful, caused by lagophthalmos, is the main cause for cornea irritations in patients with DCSFs. Therapeutic management of this exposure; a keratopathy may be complicated by dysfunction of the facial nerve with

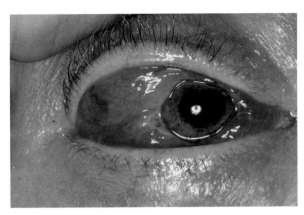

Fig. 6.4. Severe chemosis in a misdiagnosed DCSF. Despite repeated imaging studies including MRI and CT, the correct diagnosis in this 73-year-old woman was delayed for more than 4 months. During this period, her differential diagnoses included conjunctivitis, maxillo-facial tumor and orbital phlegmone. She underwent extractions of nine (!) teeth, held responsible for her "infectious process". The patient presented with retroorbital pain, exophthalmos, swelling and redness of her right eye with significant chemosis and visual loss (IOP 23 mmHg) when she was admitted in July 2000. Such chemosis with arterialized conjunctival and episcleral veins may be indistinguishable from that of a direct CCF (see also Case Report III).

paresis of the "orbicular oculi muscle" and reduced lacrimation. Progressive damages of the corneal epithelium can be initially painless but may lead to local infections, corneal ablations – and ulcerations and beside local hydration and antibiosis often a temporary tarsorrhaphy (eyelids partially sewn together) becomes necessary. Due to variform clinical manifestations, considering differential diagnoses is essential for optimizing therapy of patients with a prolapsed reddish eye bulb. In general, bulb-compressing methods should be avoided to minimize the risk of subconjunctival bleedings in case of an underlying arteriovenous fistula. Differential diagnoses include mainly thyroid related orbitopathy (most common cause of unilateral and bilateral proptosis in adults), neoplastic diseases (lymphoma, primary and secondary CNS tumors, in children particularly rhabdoid tumors and sarcomas), allergic reactions, inflammations (viral/bacterial conjunctivitis, myositis), vascular and pseudotumors of the orbit as well as intraorbital bleedings (post-traumatic, paraneoplastic).

6.2.4
Orbital Bruit

The bruit (French word for noise) over the temporal bone or the orbit can be subjective and/or objective (auscultatory) and is usually synchronous with the heartbeat. It may appear as a buzzing, swishing or roaring and represents one classical symptom of high-flow CCFs. It is found in only 25% of patients with DCSFs, mainly in cases with posterior drainage (HALBACH et al. 1987). The bruit develops due to arteriovenous turbulences within the CS, which may reach the inner ear organ via sound transmission through the skull. It may increase due to spontaneous occlusion of fistula feeder or during physical exercise or increase of blood pressure. Otherwise, the bruit may decrease or completely disappear following thrombosis, spontaneous occlusion of fistula feeder or during manual compression of the carotid artery in the neck. Bruit, commonly considered a benign symptom, can become a great source of annoyance preventing some patients from sleeping (MADSEN 1970). I have observed a patient with a DAVF of the sigmoid sinus who was unable to carry on his profession due to the distress. However, such severe discomfort caused by bruit is rare in DCSFs. A bruit may also not be reported because it is not very intense, the patient has got used to

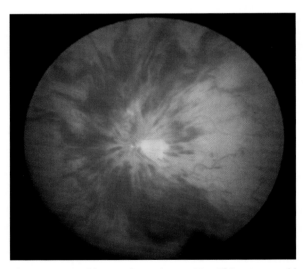

Fig. 6.5. Retinal hemorrhages in a DCSF. This 56-year-old woman presented in October 2000 with bilateral proptosis and eye-redness after not being correctly diagnosed for more than 22 months. The fundoscopy shows venous dilation and significant optical nerve swelling. Extensive flame-shaped (superficial) and some punctuate (deep) intraretinal hemorrhages, probably caused by central retinal vein occlusion. (see also Case Report I)

it or may not associate it with ocular symptoms (MILLER 2007).

Comparable (audible) bruits in the craniofacial region can be found in patients with arteriosclerotic stenoses of the carotid siphon, subclavian artery or vascular tumors. A congenital or posttraumatic hypo- or aplasia of the sphenoid bone may simulate the bruit of a CCF through transmission of brain pulsations to the orbit. A bruit may also be heard in rare cases of raised ICP or meningeomas (MILLER 1998).

6.2.5
Pulse-synchronous Pulsation of the Eyelid and Bulb

BIRCH-HIRSCHFELD (1930) was the first to describe pulse-synchronous movements of the eye lid and bulb in patients with CCFs. They develop due to the arterializations of intraorbital veins, also involve the bulb, and are visible or can be found by palpation in about 5%–20% of patients with DCSF. Bilateral assessment of ocular pulse amplitudes (OPA) using the pneumotonometer or Goldmann tonometer differs in 93% of patients with CCF by >1.6 mm, and is a reliable non-invasive method for identifying a CCF (GOLNIK and KULWIN 1997; GOLNIK and MILLER 1992).

6.2.6
Secondary Glaucoma and Visual Loss

After manifestation of orbital symptoms, the chronic elevated intraorbital venous pressure may lead in 20% of patients with DCSF to a blockage of Schlemm's canal. This may subsequently lead to gonioscopically detectable elevated intraocular pressure (secondary glaucoma), retinal ischemia and usually reversible loss of visual acuity. Many authors postulate that the elevated episcleral venous pressure is responsible for secondary glaucoma, rarely for papilla edema, retinal ablations, central vein thrombosis and hemorrhagic retinopathy (2%) (PHELPS et al. 1982; BARKE et al. 1991; JORGENSEN and GUTTHOFF 1985). In 11% of the patients bilateral symptoms are found. In general, the clinical severity of visual loss correlates more with the venous drainage pattern than with the volume and flow velocity of AV shunt. MEYERS et al. (2002) found diminished visual acuity is found in up to 31%.

In patients with rapid visual loss, neuropathy of the optic nerve and occlusion of the superior ophthalmic vein are found, respectively, while distal stenosis merely contributes to clinical improvement (HALBACH et al. 1992). Patients with a DCSF and fulminant glaucomatous loss of vision need, beside endovascular therapy, temporary local β-blocker or Diamox (Acetazolamide) application, or even more invasive ophthalmologic intervention (canthotomy, gonioplasty) (FIORE et al. 1990). It cannot be emphasized enough that in patients with unilateral glaucoma, a DCSF must always be included in the differential diagnosis.

STIEBEL-KALISH et al. (2002) have provided the most detailed description of frequency of signs and symptoms in a larger group (85) of patients so far. The authors differentiated cranial neuropathy accordingly into sixth (34%), third (19%), fourth (5%) nerve palsies, fifth nerve dysfunction (2%) and facial nerve paresis (1%). They found relatively frequent optic neuropathy (31%), vertigo in 5%, intracerebral hemorrhage in 2%, and cortical venous infarct in 1% of their patients.

6.3
Other and Neurological Symptoms

Intracranial hemorrhage caused by CSFs has already been reported to occur by SATTLER (1930), DE SCHWEINITZ and HOLLOWAY (1908) and others in about 3% of cases, most of which, however being caused by CSFs of traumatic origin. HARDING et al. (1984) reported on two patients with a DCSF, who experienced a spontaneous intracerebral hemorrhage within 18 months after onset of their symptoms. SAKUMA et al. (2006) reported recently a case where the hemorrhage developed contralateral to the fistula side, mimicking a hypertensive putaminal bleeding. KUWAYAMA et al. (1998) described a patient who presented with frontal subcortical hemorrhage and NAKAHARA et al. (1996) reported another who developed a temporo-parietal hematoma due to a ipsilateral fistula. Although cortical or leptomeningeal drainage can be found in 31% of the patients, intracerebral hemorrhage seem to occur less frequently than in DAVF, in only 1.5% (MEYERS et al. 2002). In general, central nervous system symptoms or dysfunction are less frequent and have been observed in larger patient groups in only 7/85 cases with vertigo

(5%), intracerebral hemorrhage (2%) and cortical venous infarct (1%) (STIEBEL et al. 2002).

Cerebral or cerebellar symptoms can be caused by a venous outflow restriction or venous hypertension. They are rare events and occur less frequently than in DAVFs and are only observed, if a cortical venous drainage is present. IWASAKI et al. (2006) have recently reported a DCSF complicated by pontine venous congestion. The authors observed isolated sixth nerve palsy in a 71-year-old woman that was caused by brain stem edema due to an AV shunt with exclusive venous posterior drainage into SPS, cerebellar cortical veins and inferior vermian vein. Only a few more of such cases have been reported so far (UCHINO et al. 1997; KURATA et al. 1999; KAI et al. 2004; TAKAHASHI et al. 1999), showing that in fact a "cortical" venous drainage is not always the cause, but often a leptomeningeal retrograde venous drainage of the AV shunt instead (DAVIES et al. 1997).

An unusual clinical presentation is posterior ischemic optic neuropathy (PION) as recently suggested by HASHIMOTO et al. (2005), who observed a patient with sudden unilateral vision loss after an ocular motor disturbance and pulsatile tinnitus. The arteriogram revealed a fistula which was in part supplied by a recurrent meningeal branch arising from the ophthalmic artery possibly causing arterial steal.

Other rare complications of DCSF include macular exudative retinal detachment (GARG et al. 2006), abnormal choroidal circulation (KLEIN et al. 1978), myelopathy (OHNISHI et al. 2003), and facial nerve paresis (MOSTER et al. 1988).

6.4
Differential Diagnosis

Dural CSFs presenting with mild and slowly progressing symptoms are often misdiagnosed in their early stage (MILLER 2007). Considering a DCSF in the differential diagnoses of inflammatory and other orbital diseases can be crucial. In a recent study, STIEBEL-KALISH et al. (2002) were able to demonstrate a good correlation between venous drainage pattern and clinical signs. Drainage into the anterior CS and SOV was well correlated with orbital congestion, elevated IOP and optic neuropathy. Drainage into the IPS was well correlated with third nerve palsy, drainage into the SPS allowed prediction for CNS symptoms. In series only 10 patients with bilateral signs had true bilateral AV shunts. While four patients had bilateral eye signs without evidence of drainage into the SOVs, three had unilateral congestion with bilateral shunts draining into both SOV.

IKEDA et al. (2005) reported recently on a patient with prominent anterior drainage who presented with absent orbito-ocular signs. By contrast, cases with dominant posterior drainage may present not with the typical "white-eyed cavernous shunt" as described by ACIERNO et al. (1995). I have seen patients that, despite exclusive posterior drainage, presented with eye-redness (Fig. 6.3). The angiographic demonstration of either anterior or posterior drainage alone will not always or not completely explain the symptoms (Fig. 6.6). Equally or even more important is probably the associated venous pressure. This pressure may, especially in low-flow fistulas, not be significantly elevated and only increases if venous outflow restriction starts to occur.

Various pathologies should be considered differential diagnoses in clinical practice, including conjunctivitis, thyroid orbitopathy, orbital pseudotumor, myositis, orbital cellulites, episcleritis, meningeoma or Tolosa-Hunt syndrome and allergic reactions. (Brazis 1994; Grove 1984; Miller 2007; Newton 1970; Oestreicher 1995; Phelps 1982; Procope 1994). Pulsating exophthalmos can also be caused by sphenoid dysplasia in neurofibromatosis (Recklinghausen) or after neurosurgical removal of the orbital roof. Dilated episcleral and conjunctival loops can be observed in CS thrombosis, venous malformations, brain AVMs or DAVFs (see Figs. 7.48, 7.49). Other causes include Graves' disease (LORE et al. 2003), idiopathic elevated episcleral pressure, orbital vein variation, superior vena cava syndrome, pulmonary hypertension (AKDUMAN et al. 1996), scleritis with vortex vein blockage and malignant endocrine exophthalmos (DE KEIZER 2003). If the fistula is small and thus not detectable by CT or MRI, a patient can be misdiagnosed, leading not only to distress but also to inadequate therapeutic measures and false treatment effects (Figs. 6.4 and 6.7). THEAUDIN et al. (2006) reported just recently a delay in diagnosis of up to 22 months; similar to my own experience (Fig. 6.5., Case Report I), underlining the diagnostic dilemma in patients with small AV-shunts, not detectable by CT or MRI. Selective catheter angiography is indispensable in these cases and can be performed by an experienced neuroradiologist with very low morbidity (WILLINSKY et al. 2003).

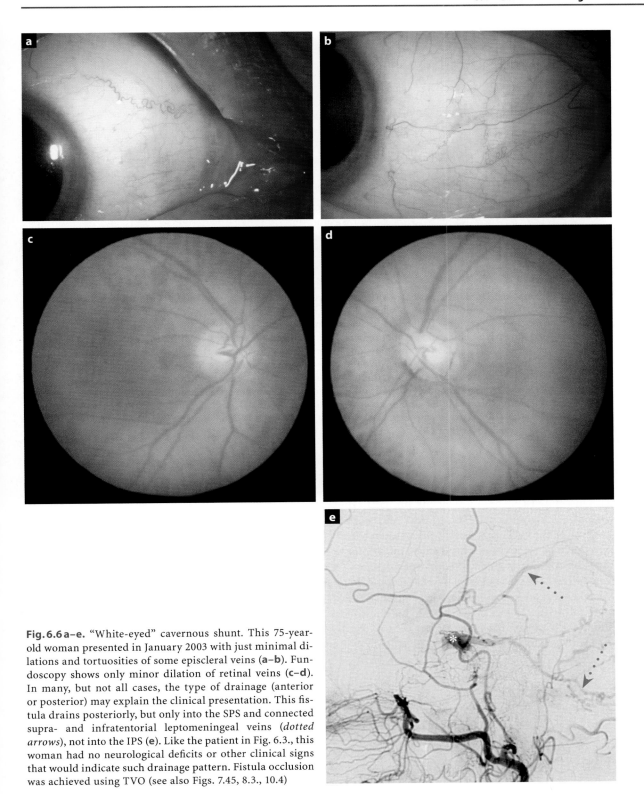

Fig. 6.6 a–e. "White-eyed" cavernous shunt. This 75-year-old woman presented in January 2003 with just minimal dilations and tortuosities of some episcleral veins (**a–b**). Fundoscopy shows only minor dilation of retinal veins (**c–d**). In many, but not all cases, the type of drainage (anterior or posterior) may explain the clinical presentation. This fistula drains posteriorly, but only into the SPS and connected supra- and infratentorial leptomeningeal veins (*dotted arrows*), not into the IPS (**e**). Like the patient in Fig. 6.3., this woman had no neurological deficits or other clinical signs that would indicate such drainage pattern. Fistula occlusion was achieved using TVO (see also Figs. 7.45, 8.3., 10.4)

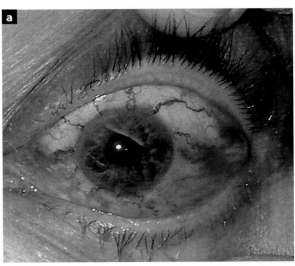
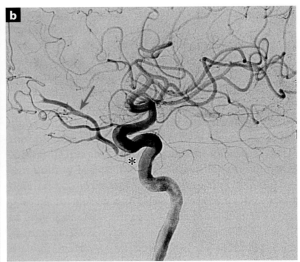

Fig. 6.7 a, b. Overlooked DCSF in a patient with eye-redness. a Eye-redness and chemosis with dilation, tortuosity and characteristic "corksrew" appearance of episcleral veins in a 54-year-old patient who presented after being incorrectly diagnosed for more than 3 months. Differential diagnoses included endocrine ophthalmopathy, inflammation, immunopathy and orbital tumor/lymphoma and pseudotumor cerebri, for which she was treated with corticosteroids and eventually even underwent a biopsy. The patient was seen by four different specialists: Endocrinologist, rheumatologist, neurologist and an ophthalmologist. She underwent a negative CT scan and MRI exam before the definite diagnosis could be made using a cerebral angiogram. **b** shows a tiny AV shunt (*asterisk*), supplied by the ILT with sluggish flow in the SOV that is not notably enlarged (*arrow*) and appears partially occluded, and thus may not appear prominent on CT or MRI (Courtesy: R. Klucznik, Houston). This and other similar cases (Case Reports I and III), with significant delays in correct diagnosis and proper treatment, still occur, emphasizing the key role of intraarterial DSA for timely diagnosis in patients with small AV shunts, not detectable by MRI or CT

In summary, the signs and symptoms in patients with low-flow DCSF are in principle similar to those with direct high-flow CCF, but milder and less progressive. In the initial stage of the disease, nonspecific signs such as retro orbital headaches, mild conjunctival injection or isolated diplopia may occur. Consequently, the disease may be overlooked and can be mistaken as endocrine orbitopathy, conjunctivitis or ocular myositis. Neglecting a DCSF in the clinical differential diagnoses may cause progression of the disease with serious deterioration of the patient's symptoms including the risk of complete vision loss.

References

Acierno MD, Trobe JD, Cornblath WT, Gebarski SS (1995) Painful oculomotor palsy caused by posterior-draining dural carotid cavernous fistulas. Arch Ophthalmol 113:1045–1049

Akduman L, Del Priore LV, Kaplan HJ, Meredith T (1996) Uveal effusion syndrome associated with primary pulmonary hypertension and vomiting. Am J Ophthalmol 121:578–580

Barke RM, Yoshizumi MO, Hepler RS, Krauss HR, Jabour BA (1991) Spontaneous dural carotid-cavernous fistula with central retinal vein occlusion and iris neovascularization. Ann Ophthalmol 23:11–17

Benndorf, G, et al. (1999) Occlusion of the inferior petrosal sinus (IPS) for endovascular treatment of a longstanding traumatic carotid cavernous sinus fistula (CCF). In Annual Meeting, European Society of Neuroradiology. Vienna.

Birch-Hirschfeld A (1930) Kurzes Handbuch der Ophthalmologie, vol 1. Springer, Berlin Heidelberg New York

Brazis PW, et al. (1994) Low flow dural arteriovenous shunt: another cause of „sinister" Tolosa-Hunt syndrome. Headache 34:523–525

Davies M, Saleh J, Ter Brugge K, Willinsky R, Wallace MC (1997) The natural history and management of intracranial dural arteriovenous fistulae. Intervent Neuroradiol 3

de Keizer RJ (1979) Spontaneous carotico-cavernous fistulas. The importance of the typical limbal vascular loops for the diagnosis, the recognition of glaucoma and the uses of conservative therapy in this condition. Doc Ophthalmol 46:403–412

de Keizer R (2003) Carotid-cavernous and orbital arteriovenous fistulas: ocular features, diagnostic and hemodynamic considerations in relation to visual impairment and morbidity. Orbit 22:121–142

De Schweinitz G, Holloway T (1908) Pulsating exophthalmos: its etiology, symptomatology, pathogenesis and treatment. Saunders, Philadelphia

Eggenberger, E, et al. (200) A bruital headache and double vision. Surv Ophthalmol. 45(2):147–153.

Fiore PM, Latina MA, Shingleton BJ, Rizzo JF, Ebert E, Bellows AR (1990) The dural shunt syndrome. I. Management of glaucoma [see comments]. Ophthalmology 97:56–62

Garg SJ, Regillo CD, Aggarwal S, Bilyk JR, Savino PJ (2006) Macular exudative retinal detachment in a patient with a dural cavernous sinus fistula. Arch Ophthalmol 124:1201–1202

Golnik C, Kulwin D (1997) CCF: neuro-ophthalmolgic findings. In: Tomsick TA (ed) Carotid cavernous fistula. Digital Educational Publishing, Philadelphia, pp 75–82

Golnik KC, Miller NR (1992) Diagnosis of cavernous sinus arteriovenous fistula by measurement of ocular pulse amplitude [see comments]. Ophthalmology 99:1146–1152

Grove AS Jr (1984) The dural shunt syndrome. Pathophysiology and clinical course. Ophthalmology 91:31–44

Halbach VV, Higashida RT, Hieshima GB, Reicher M, Norman D, Newton TH (1987) Dural fistulas involving the cavernous sinus: results of treatment in 30 patients. Radiology 163:437–442

Halbach VV, Hiogashida RT, Hieshima GB, Dowd CF (1992) Endovascular therapy of dural fistulas. In: Vinuela F, Halbach VV, Dion J (eds) Interventional neuroradiology. Raven Press, New York, p 32

Harding AE, Kendall B, Leonard TJ, Johnson MH (1984) Intracerebral haemorrhage complicating dural arteriovenous fistula: a report of two cases. J Neurol Neurosurg Psychiatry 47:905–911

Hashimoto M, Ohtsuka K, Suzuki Y, Hoyt WF (2005) A case of posterior ischemic optic neuropathy in a posterior-draining dural cavernous sinus fistula. J Neuroophthalmol 25:176–179

Hawke SH, Mullie MA, Hoyt WF, Hallinan JM, Halmagyi GM (1989) Painful oculomotor nerve palsy due to dural-cavernous sinus shunt. Arch Neurol 46:1252–1255

Hoops JP, Rudolph G, Schriever S, Nasemann JE, Bien S, Kuffer G, Schworm HD, Kampik A (1997) Dural carotid-cavernous sinus fistulas: clinical aspects, diagnosis and therapeutic intervention. Klin Monatsbl Augenheilkd 210:392–397

Ikeda K, Deguchi K, Tsukaguchi M, Sasaki I, Shimamura M, Urai Y, Touge T, Kawanishi M, Takeuchi H, Kuriyama S (2005) Absence of orbito-ocular signs in dural carotid-cavernous sinus fistula with a prominent anterior venous drainage. J Neurol Sci 236:81–84

Iwasaki M, Murakami K, Tomita T, Numagami Y, Nishijima M (2006) Cavernous sinus dural arteriovenous fistula complicated by pontine venous congestion. A case report. Surg Neurol 65:516–518; discussion 519

Jorgensen JS, Gutthoff RF (1985) 24 cases of carotid cavernosus fistulas: frequency, symptoms, diagnosis and treatment. Acta Ophthalmol Suppl 173:67–71

Kai Y, Hamada JI, Morioka M, Yano S, Ushio Y (2004) Brain stem venous congestion due to dural arteriovenous fistulas of the cavernous sinus. Acta Neurochir (Wien) 146:1107–1111; discussion 1111–1102

Keltner JL, Gittinger JW Jr, Miller NR, Burder RM (1987a)

A red eye and high intraocular pressure [clinical conference]. Surv Ophthalmol 31:328–336

Keltner JL, Satterfield D, Dublin AB, Lee BC (1987b) Dural and carotid cavernous sinus fistulas. Diagnosis, management, and complications. Ophthalmology 94:1585–1600

Kim, DJ, et al. (2006) Results of transvenous embolization of cavernous dural arteriovenous fistula: a single-center experience with emphasis on complications and management. AJNR Am J Neuroradiol. 27(10):2078–2082.

Klein R, Meyers SM, Smith JL, Myers FL, Roth H, Becker B (1978) Abnormal chloroidal circulation: association with arteriovenous fistula in the cavernous sinus area. Arch Ophthalmol 96:1370–1373

Komorsky GB (1988) Carotid cavernous sinus fistulas presenting as painful ophthalmoplegia without external ocular signs. J Clin Neuro Ophthalmol 8:131–135

Kupersmith MJ, Berenstein A, Flamm E, Ransohoff J (1986) Neuroophthalmologic abnormalities and intravascular therapy of traumatic carotid cavernous fistulas. Ophthalmology 93:906–912

Kupersmith MJ, et al. (1988) Management of nontraumatic vascular shunts involving the cavernous sinus. Ophthalmology 95:121–130

Kupersmith MJ, Vargas EM, Warren F, Berenstein A (1996) Venous obstruction as the cause of retinal/choroidal dysfunction associated with arteriovenous shunts in the cavernous sinus. J Neuroophthalmol 16:1–6

Kurata A, Miyasaka Y, Oka H, Irikura K, Tanaka R, Ohmomo T, Nagai S, Fujii K (1999) Spontaneous carotid cavernous fistulas with special reference to the influence of estradiol decrease. Neurol Res 21:631–639

Kuwayama N, Endo S, Kitabayashi M, Nishijima M, Takaku A (1998) Surgical transvenous embolization of a cortically draining carotid cavernous fistula via a vein of the sylvian fissure. AJNR Am J Neuroradiol 19:1329–1332

Lore F, Polito E, Cerase A, Bracco S, Loffredo A, Pichierri P, Talidis F (2003) Carotid cavernous fistula in a patient with Graves' ophthalmopathy. J Clin Endocrinol Metab 88:3487–3490

Madsen PH (1970) Carotid-cavernous fistulae. A study of 18 cases. Acta Ophthalmol (Copenh) 48:731–751

Meyers PM, Halbach VV, Dowd CF, Lempert TE, Malek AM, Phatouros CC, Lefler JE, Higashida RT (2002) Dural carotid cavernous fistula: definitive endovascular management and long-term follow-up. Am J Ophthalmol 134:85–92

Miller N (1998) Carotid-cavernous sinus fistulas. In: Miller N, Newmann N (eds) Walsh and Hoyt's clinical neuro-ophthalmology. Williams and Wilkins, Baltimore, pp 1524–1526

Miller, NR (2007) Diagnosis and management of dural carotid-cavernous sinus fistulas. Neurosurg Focus. 23(5): p. E13

Miyachi S, Negoro M, Handa T, Sugita K (1993) Dural carotid cavernous sinus fistula presenting as isolated oculomotor nerve palsy. Surg Neurol 39:105–109

Moster ML, Sergott RC, Grossman RI (1988) Dural carotid-cavernous sinus vascular malformation with facial nerve paresis. Can J Ophthalmol 23:27–29

Nakahara I, Taki W, Murao K, Ohkata N, Matsumoto K, Isaka F, Kikuchi H (1996) Endovascular treatment of cavernous dural AVFs (spontaneous CCFs): results in 50 patients. In: Taki W, Picard L, Kikuchi H (eds) Advances in interventional neuroradiology. Elsevier Science, Amsterdam, pp 251–256

Newton TH, Hoyt WF (1970) Dural arteriovenous shunts in the region of the cavernous sinus. Neuroradiology, 1970. 1:71–81

Oestreicher, JH, Frueh BR (1995) Carotid-cavernous fistula mimicking Graves' eye disease. Ophthal Plast Reconstr Surg,. 11(4):238–244

Ohnishi H, Deguchi J, Yamada M, Kuroiwa T (2003) Cavernous arteriovenous fistula presenting myelopathy: a case report. No Shinkei Geka 31:1119–1123

Ott D, Bien S, Krasznai L (1993) Embolization of a tentorial dural arterio-venous fistula presenting as atypical trigeminal neuralgia. Headache 33:503–508

Palestine AG, Younge BR, Piepgras DG (1981) Visual prognosis in carotid-cavernous fistula. Arch Ophthalmol 99:1600–1603

Phelps CD, Thompson HS, Ossoinig KC (1982) The diagnosis and prognosis of atypical carotid-cavernous fistula (red-eyed shunt syndrome). Am J Ophthalmol 93:423–436

Procope, JA, et al. (1994) Dural cavernous sinus fistula: an unusual presentation. J Natl Med Assoc, 1994. 86(5):363–364.

Rizzo M, Bosch EP, Gross CE (1982) Trigeminal sensory neuropathy due to dural external carotid cavernous sinus fistula. Neurology 32:89–91

Sakuma I, Takahashi S, Tomura N, Kinouchi H (2006) Dural arteriovenous fistulas of the cavernous sinus with onset of intracerebral haemorrhage mimicking hypertensive putaminal hemorrhage. Acta Neurochir (Wien) 148:915–918

Sattler H (1930) Pulsierender Exophthalmus. In: Graefe A, Saemisch T (eds) Handbuch der Gesamten Augenheilkunde. Springer, Berlin Heidelberg New York, pp 745–948

Stiebel-Kalish H, Setton A, Nimii Y, Kalish Y, Hartman J, Huna Bar-On R, Berenstein A, Kupersmith MJ (2002) Cavernous sinus dural arteriovenous malformations: patterns of venous drainage are related to clinical signs and symptoms. Ophthalmology 109:1685–1691

Suh DC, et al. (2005) New concept in cavernous sinus dural arteriovenous fistula: correlation with presenting symptom and venous drainage patterns. Stroke 36:1134–1139

Takahashi S, Tomura N, Watarai J, Mizoi K, Manabe H (1999) Dural arteriovenous fistula of the cavernous sinus with venous congestion of the brain stem: report of two cases. AJNR Am J Neuroradiol 20:886–888

Theaudin M, Saint-Maurice JP, Chapot R, Vahedi K, Mazighi M, Vignal C, Saliou G, Stapf C, Bousser MG, Houdart E (2006) Diagnosis and treatment of dural carotid-cavernous fistulae: a consecutive series of 27 patients. J Neurol Neurosurg Psychiatry

Uchino A, Kato A, Kuroda Y, Shimokawa S, Kudo S (1997) Pontine venous congestion caused by dural carotid-cavernous fistula: report of two cases. Eur Radiol 7:405–408

Vinuela F, Fox AJ, Debrun GM, Peerless SJ, Drake CG (1984) Spontaneous carotid-cavernous fistulas: clinical, radiological, and therapeutic considerations. Experience with 20 cases. J Neurosurg 60:976–984

Voigt K, Sauer M, Dichgans J (1971) Spontaneous occlusion of a bilateral caroticocavernous fistula studied by serial angiography. Neuroradiology 2:207–211

CONTENTS

7.1
Non-invasive Imaging Techniques

7.1.1
CT and MRI (Figs. 7.1–7.10)

The clinical presentation of patients with characteristic neuroophthalmic symptoms does not usually require invasive imaging techniques, and a correct diagnosis can be made with certainty using CT or MRI techniques. As outlined in the previous chapter, non-invasive imaging may fail in patients with low-flow AV shunts, and a patient with atypical symptoms may be misdiagnosed over time. If there is a clinical suspicion of an inflammatory or tumorous process in the orbital or peri-orbital region, computed tomography (CT) or magnetic resonance imaging (MRI) is commonly performed. In the case of a DCSF, the image may show a dilated or thrombosed vein, indicating an underlying vascular pathology. An exophthalmos or a proptosis can often be diagnosed using a routine CT scan (Figs. 7.1 and 7.2). However, only when the AV shunting volume is large enough will the CS become visible as an enhancing space occupying lesion.

OHTSUKA and HASHIMOTO (1999) performed serial enhanced computed tomography (DE-CT) scanning of the cavernous sinus and provided direct evidence of pathological shunting from the carotid artery to the cavernous sinus. By scanning serial axial images around the sella turcica at intervals of 3 s the authors were able to obtain an early filling of the CS in direct (two) as well as in indirect (five) fistulas. This technique was also found to be useful in revealing a CS thrombosis by non-filling even in late venous phases. A differentiation between Types A–B and C fistulas was possible, based on the delayed staining of the CS when only ECA branches supplied the fistula.

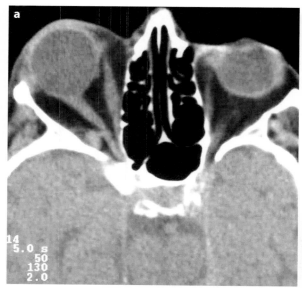

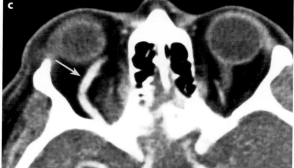

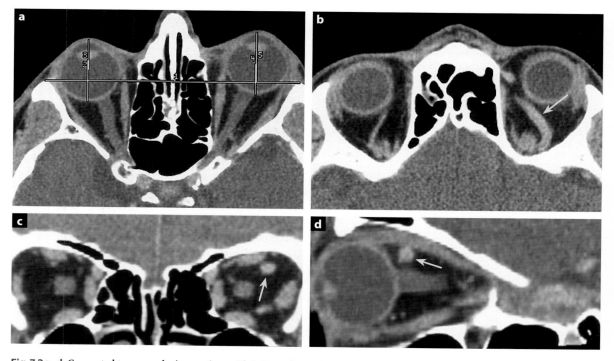

Fig. 7.1 a–c. Computed tomography findings in two patients with DCSFs. **a** Significant exophthalmos and enlarged SOV (**b**) on the right side. **c** Enhancement of the right (not notably enlarged) SOV after contrast administration, indicating an AV shunt at the CS in another patient. Note: In cases with posterior drainage, a CT of the orbit may appear normal

Fig. 7.2 a–d. Computed tomography in a patient with DCSF. **a,b** Axial views shows mild exophthalmos and an enlarged SOV on the left side. **c,d** Coronal and sagittal reformatted views show the enlarged SOV behind the eyeball. (Courtesy: A. Biondi, Paris)

A focal bulging or diffuse distension of the CS on contrast enhanced CTs has been detected in 50%–64% of the cases (AHMADI et al. 1983; UCHINO et al. 1992). The SOV can be enlarged on the fistula site in 86%–100% on post-contrast CTs and in 75%–100% on spin echo MR images (AHMADI et al. 1983; UCHINO et al. 1992; HIRABUKI et al. 1992; KOMIYAMA et al. 1990; ELSTER et al. 1991).

If a cortical venous drainage is present, those enlarged veins may become visible on axial CT. WATANABE et al. (1990) described a case of a Type D fistula with considerably enlarged veins visualized on contrast enhanced CT. In addition, a SPECT was performed showing reduced regional cerebral perfusion in this area, caused by elevated transvenous pressure. D'ANGELO et al. (1988) described a case with a Type A fistula and dilated veins in the temporal region, which were identified as Sylvian veins. TENG et al. (1991) reported a brain stem edema in two patients with Type D fistulas that became visible on CT after occlusion of the normal venous drainage, probably triggering the development of cortical venous drainage. In both cases complete disappearance of the edema was documented. UCHINI et al. (1997) reported two patients with pontine venous congestion due to DCSFs. Brain stem edema due to DCSFs has also been described by TAKAHASHI et al. (1999) in two patients, in which after occlusion of the fistula, reversal of the edema on MRI became evident. Edematous changes due to venous hypertension can also be seen in both hemispheres being mainly limited to the white matter, like a vasogenic edema (CORNELIUS 1997).

When an intracranial hemorrhage occurs as a complication of a CCF, CT is the preferred diagnostic tool (D'ANGELO et al. 1988). This type of complication is mainly seen in Type A fistulas, but only rarely observed in DCSFs (SATOH et al. 2001), even though cortical venous drainage is relatively frequently present (see Table 5.3).

In most cases the bleeding occurs adjacent to the dilated veins. MRI is superior to CT in showing discrete changes due to AV shunts of the CS, because it may demonstrate not only the enlarged SOV but also a minimal proptosis and extraocular thickening of the muscles. SATO et al. (1997) recently reported on flow voids shown in eight of 10 patients with Type D fistulas using spin echo sequences. In particular MRA can be helpful in low-flow conditions, as often present in DCSFs. MRI findings can be discrete on MIPs and raw data (source images) can be useful for analysis (CORNELIUS 1997; ACIERNO et al. 1995;

CHEN JC et al. 1992; DIETZ et al. 1994) (Figs. 7.3, 7.6 and 7.8).

MRA, as well as conventional spin echo sequences, can demonstrate abnormal cortical drainage (CHEN JC et al. 1992), as seen in Figure 7.5b and 7.8a. Under certain circumstances MRA is particularly helpful for early detection of CCF with posterior drainage (Fig. 7.8), also called "white eyed shunt syndrome" (ACIERNO et al. 1995). These patients present with headaches and painful oculoparesis but without orbito-ocular congestion, which may easily lead to a wrong diagnosis of, e.g. Tolosa Hunt syndrome or painful ophthalmoplegia. Conventional spin echo sequences can be normal in these patients; however, MRA would be diagnostic in showing abnormal vessels arising from the posterior CS (Figs. 7.5 and 7.6). The CS itself can become visible even due to normal venous flow causing flow voids in TOF-MRAs as has been observed by CORNELIUS (1997) in eight of 50 patients. Several authors have described flow voids within the CS on spin echo MR images in patients with CSFs (UCHINO et al. 1992; HIRABUKI et al. 1992; KOMIYAMA et al. 1990). HIRAI et al. (1998) saw flow voids in the CS less frequently in their patients and found in 3% false positive results, emphasizing the difficulty to differentiate normal venous flow in the CS from abnormal flow voids caused by an AV shunt based on spin echo MR images.

Another MR finding is the "flow-void" of the inter-cavernous sinus in contrast enhanced T1-weighted images (Figs. 7.3a, 7.4a, 7.6a, 7.7a). SERGOTT et al. (1987) recommended MRI as the initial exam in patients with known arteriovenous shunts and clinical deterioration. The authors observed three patients with paradoxical worsening of clinical symptoms due to thrombosis of the SOV, which was revealed by increased signal intensity in T1-weighted images. According to CORNELIUS (1997), intra-arterial DSA is not required in patients with clinical worsening if MRI shows a thrombosed SOV and an improvement under conservative management. On the contrary, GOLDBERG et al. (1996) observed that MRI led to a diagnosis in only 5 of 10 patients (50%). SCHUKNECHT et al. (1998) were able to show that high-resolution contrast enhanced CT and MRI exam can demonstrate not only thrombi within the CS, but also in its tributaries such as the SOV, the SPPS and even the IPS.

MRI may help to differentiate a CSF from malignant tumors, vasculitic processes and intracranial AV malformations. If thrombosis occurs, the signal appears as a white hyperdense spot on the T1-

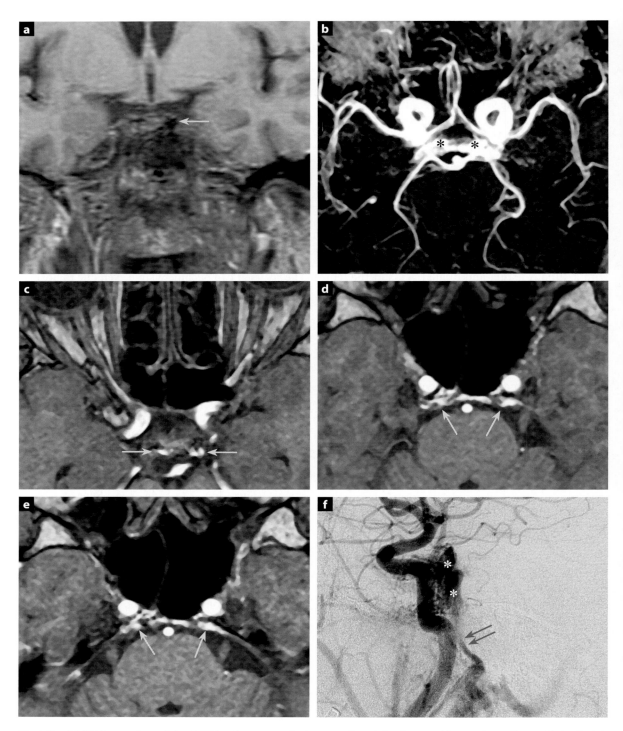

Fig. 7.3 a–f. MRI in a patient with a DCSF and posterior drainage. a T1-weighted coronal image shows flow voids in the left CS. **b** TOF MRA shows both CSs and the posterior ICS in MIP views; no anterior drainage towards SOV is apparent. **c–e** MRA source images reveal bright signal spots within the posterior CS on both sides and within the ICS (*arrows*). **f** DSA, right ICA shows intense opacification of the posterior CS (*asterisk*) and a dominant posterior drainage via the IPS (*double arrow*). (Courtesy: G. Gal, Odense)

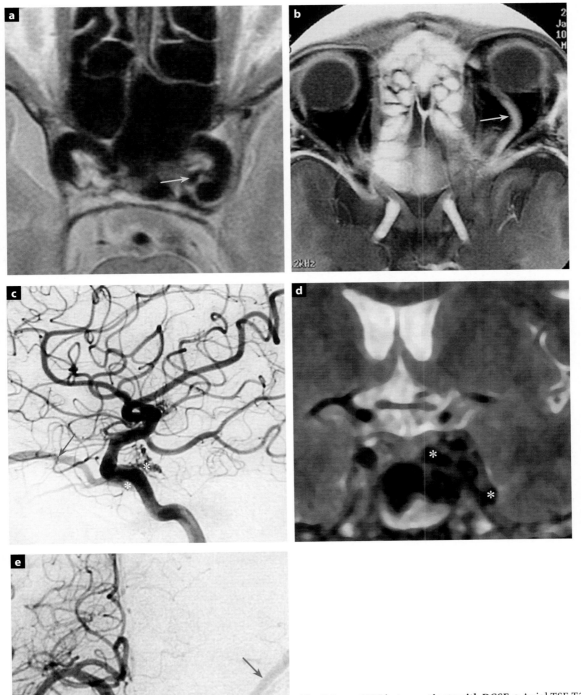

Fig. 7.4 a–e. MRI in two patients with DCSF. a Axial TSE T2-weighted image showing a flow void in the left CS (*arrow*). **b** Axial IR T1-image showing the enlarged SOV (*arrow*). **c** ICA injection lateral shows the AV shunt at the posterior CS draining anteriorly in the SOV (*arrow*). **d** T2-weighted coronal image shows numerous flow voids in the left CS. **e** DSA, right ICA injection fills the ICS and the left CS (*asterisks*) with drainage into cortical veins (*arrow*) and the IPS/IJV. (Courtesy: A. Biondi, Paris)

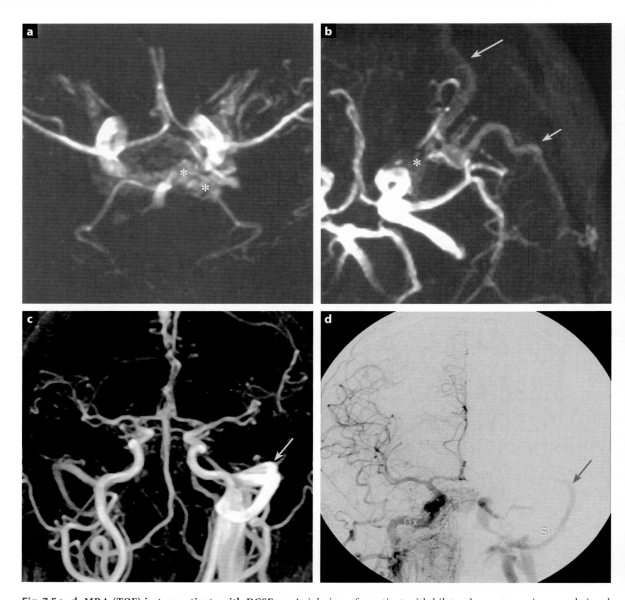

Fig. 7.5 a–d. MRA (TOF) in two patients with DCSFs. a Axial view of a patient with bilateral symptoms: increased signal intensity in the left posterior CS (*asterisk*) indicating a small low-flow fistula without clear demonstration of a draining vein (Courtesy: R. Parsche, Neuruppin). **b** Axial view of a patient with left-sided symptoms: Large AV shunt causing increased signal intensity (due to higher flow) in the anterior CS (*asterisk*), the SOV (*arrow*) and the superficial middle cerebral vein (cortical drainage, *short arrow*) (Courtesy: B. Sander, Berlin). **c** If the AV shunt itself is not evident, MRA may show indirect signs, such as retrograde filling of the left sigmoid sinus, as in this patient caused by a stenosis at the level of the JB. **d** DSA shows filling of left CS, SOV, IPS and sigmoid sinus (*arrows*) (Courtesy: Dr. G. Gal, Odense)

weighted image (DE KEIZER 2003). The visualization of draining veins may require using both phase contrast techniques (3D PC MRA) for demonstrating the dilated SOV and associated reflux, and 3D TOF MRA for demonstrating the IPS (IKAWA et al. 1996). If the SOV is not the draining vein it may not be demonstrated with 3D PC MRA. The IPS is usually shown better on TOF MRA, because it runs in a superior inferior direction causing stronger time of flight effects.

HIRAI et al. (1998) have compared the value of fast imaging with steady state precession (FISP) to

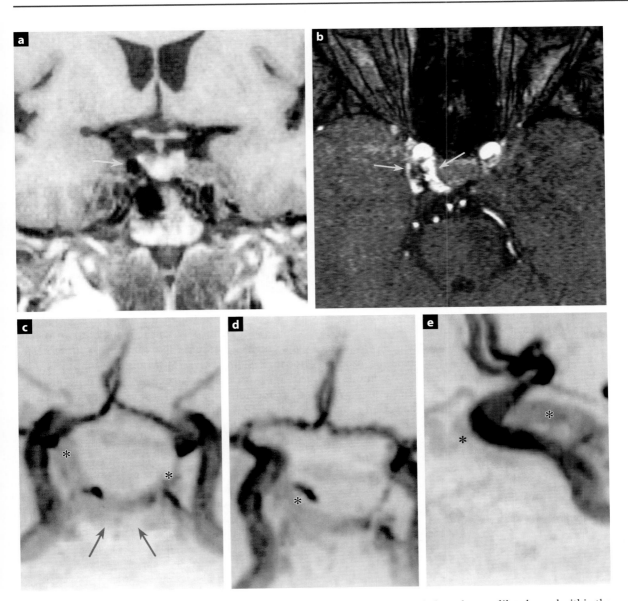

Fig. 7.6 a–e. MRI and MRA in two patients with DCSFs. a T1-weighted image, coronal plane shows a dilated vessel within the right CS (*arrow*) with flow voids, indicating AV-shunting. **b** Source image of the MRA (TOF) shows higher signal intensity (*arrows*) adjacent to the right ICA. **c–e** MRA in various projections reveals the cavernous sinus AV shunt, involving both CSs (*asterisks*) as well as the intercavernous sinus (*arrows*). **Note:** The exact type of the fistula (Type A–D), details of the arterial angioarchitecture or venous drainge pattern can often not be evaluated. (Courtesy: A. Campi, Milan)

contrast enhanced CT and spin echo MR imaging and found it superior in the diagnosis of CCF. Their group of 17 patients included 14 DCSFs in which a hyperintensity of the CS was noted in most cases (11/14). In DCSFs with very slow flow this hyperintensity can be missed, leading to false negative results and necessitating a careful search for other findings related to the venous drainage. In highly vascularized DCSFs, multiple hyperintensive curvilinear structures or spots adjacent to or within the CS were seen, likely corresponding to dural feeders. Because these findings were not observed in direct

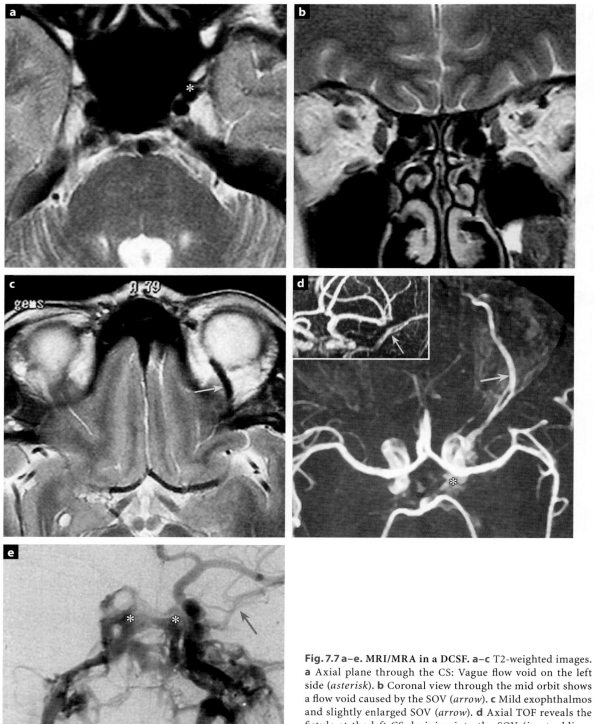

Fig. 7.7 a–e. MRI/MRA in a DCSF. a–c T2-weighted images. **a** Axial plane through the CS: Vague flow void on the left side (*asterisk*). **b** Coronal view through the mid orbit shows a flow void caused by the SOV (*arrow*). **c** Mild exophthalmos and slightly enlarged SOV (*arrow*). **d** Axial TOF reveals the fistula at the left CS draining into the SOV (*inset*: oblique view). **e** DSA with simultaneous arterial and venous injection for better understanding of the anatomy confirms a DCSF (*asterisks*), draining into the SOV (*arrow*). Note, there is no posterior drainage (*inset*), even though both IPSs are widely open as demonstrated by the jugular phlebogram. (Courtesy: A. Biondi, Paris)

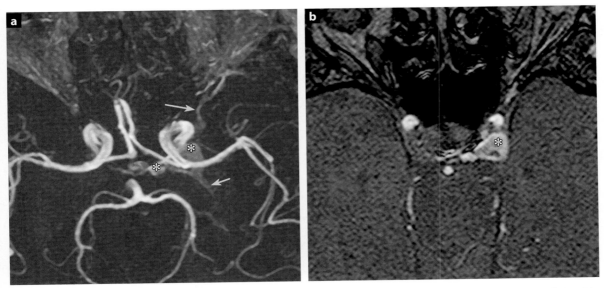

Fig. 7.8 a,b. MRI/MRA in a DCSF with anterior and posterior (leptomeningeal) drainage. a MRA TOF A, abnormal signal in the left CS (*asterisk*) and scarcely in the left SOV (*arrow*) as well as posterior to the CS, indicating possible leptomeningeal venous drainage (*short arrow*), which was confirmed by DSA. **b** MRA source image reveals the abnormal signal in the left CS (*asterisks*). (Courtesy: U. Schweiger, Berlin)

CCFs, they may help to differentiate direct from indirect fistulas. 3D FISP images showed posterior venous drainage, but were not helpful in detecting cortical drainage, which is an important detail not to be missed.

Because relying on MRI and 3D TOF MIP images alone may lead to underdiagnosis of indirect CSFs, MRA source images become quite valuable (Figs. 7.3, 7.6, 7.8 and 7.9). Tsai YF et al. (2004) recently encountered dilemmas in reviewing MRI flow voids and identified them in only five of eight patients with DCSFs. The authors detected an engorged CS only in four cases and swollen extraocular muscles in none. Flow artifacts resulting from pulsation of the cavernous ICA may corrupt CS details and CSF pulsation may result in flow voids in the prepontine cistern mimicking enlarged abnormal vessels. Air in the sphenoid sinus may cause susceptibility artifacts or partial volume effects. Because MIP reconstruction may cause vascular distortion they need to be reviewed carefully. Reliance on MIPs alone may lead to misdiagnosis in 50% of the cases. On the other hand, reading of the source images of 3D-TOF MRA allowed the correct diagnosis in all eight cases. Therefore, in order not to overlook small AV shunts, careful evaluating of MRA source images should be included in all

doubtful cases. Nevertheless, even with improved technology, MRI and MRA cannot replace high quality DSA for differentiating direct Type A and indirect Type D fistulas with certainty (Tsai YF et al. 2004).

Diagnostic sensitivity of MRI can be enhanced with contrast and magnetization prepared rapid gradient echo sequences (MP-RAGE), allowing for better assessment of retrograde venous drainage than T1-weighted SE imaging (Kitajima et al. 2005). Kwon et al. (2005b) found direct fistula visualization in 75%–86% of the 27 DAVF (11 DCSFs), although the reviewers were not blinded to angiography in this study. The authors suggest looking for any suspicious flow void cluster around a dural sinus.

Chen CC et al. (2005) have recently compared the utility of CTA and MRA source images in the diagnostic of 53 direct CCFs. They found CTA as useful as DSA and superior to MRA in accurately localizing the fistulous connection, in particular when it was located in segment four according to Debruns classification (Debrun et al. 1981).

Finally, CT and MRI can be used to rule out complications of EVT, for documentation of coil masses or liquid embolic agents within the CS, or to detect residual/recurrent AV shunting (Figs. 7.9 and 7.10).

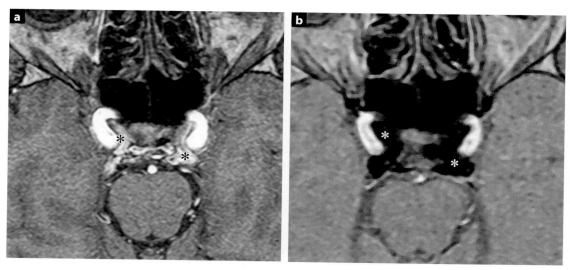

Fig. 7.9 a,b. MRA source images in a DCSF pre and post embolization. Contrast enhanced T1-weighted images pre- and post transvenous occlusion of a bilateral DCSF. The *dark areas* in **b** correspond to the *bright areas* in both CSs in **a** (*asterisks*), confirming that platinum coils have been packed in the previously AV shunting compartments. There is no signal abnormality that would indicate a residual shunt, suggesting that MRA could be used for non-invasive FU. Note, however, that a minimal AV shunt can be missed; to rule out a small residual fistula with certainty, intra-arterial DSA remains indispensable. (Courtesy: G. Gal, Odense)

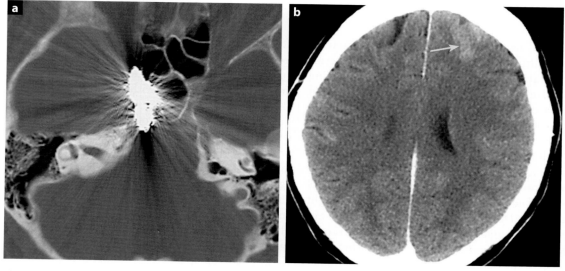

Fig. 7.10 a,b. Computed tomography in two DCSF patients post embolization. a Post-embolization CT reveals the positioning of the coils within the right CS. **b** Follow-up CT after a patient presented with transient deficit after TVO. The small hyperdense area in the left frontal lobe (*arrow*) is likely due to repeated contrast injections during endovascular treatment. Both indications for cross-sectional imaging have become clinical applications for DynaCT (see below)

7.1.2
Doppler and Carotid Duplex Sonography
(Fig. 7.11)

Ultra-sonography represents a cost-effective, non-invasive method for the study of intraorbital hemo-

dynamic parameters in patients with CSFs. However, ultra-sonography is not suitable to visualize the complex venous anatomy of the cavernous sinus, or to rule out cortical or leptomeningeal venous drainage (BELDEN et al. 1995; FLAHARTY et al. 1991); therefore, its value for treatment planning is limited.

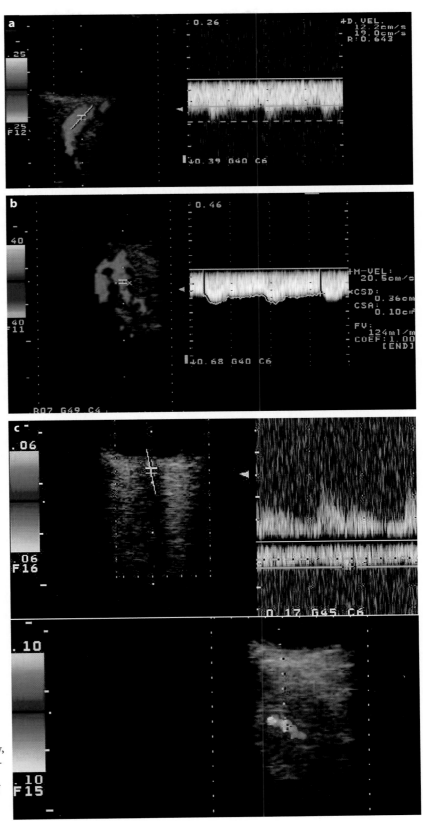

Fig. 7.11a–c. Color-Doppler ultrasound in a DCSF: Flow reversal in the superior ophthalmic vein.
a A 39 year-old man with dural AV shunt at the posterior CS causing orbital signs on the right side before embolization. Arteriovenous flow directed towards the probe, depth 4.5 cm. Total flow: 234 ml/min. **b** Measurement of the inferior ophthalmic vein also shows arterio-venous shunting flow, directed towards the probe. **c** Superior ophthalmic vein after successful embolization: Normalization of blood flow direction (Courtesy: R. de Keizer, Leiden)

In some studies, Doppler sonography has shown value for diagnosis and follow-up in patients with CSF (BELDEN et al. 1995; FLAHARTY et al. 1991; ERICKSON et al. 1989; MUNK et al. 1992). It allows for the assessment of direction and velocity of blood flow, as well as the differentiation of a typical venous flow pattern from an arterialized vein with characteristic bi-phasic flow (ERICKSON et al. 1989).

DE KEIZER (1986) performed Doppler flow velocity measurements in 35 patients with direct and indirect fistulas (14 traumatic, 21 spontaneous) and found a specific flow pattern in 100% of direct and in 80% of the indirect communications. He recorded his measurements as hematotachograms (HTGs) and found normalization of flow pattern in patients with direct fistulas after embolization. In a more recent article (DE KEIZER 2003) he points to the difficulty of separating the arterial flow in the supratrochlear artery from the abnormal arterialized flow velocities and pattern in the ophthalmic veins. When the flow velocity in the ICA was additionally found to be abnormal, a direct fistula could be identified in all cases. Color Doppler methods are helpful in differentiating arterial from venous flow. De Keizer also recommends the use of Doppler measurements for monitoring conservative treatment using manual compression.

LIN et al. (1994) suggested the application of duplex carotid sonography (DCS) for hemodynamic classification of CSFs (see Chap. 4) with special emphasis on the resistance index (RI) and the flow volume, based on 14 cases. The authors suggest the use of sonography for screening and follow-up because DCS cannot accurately identify Type B fistulas and is limited in its differentiation between Types C and D fistulas for which angiography remains indispensable. CHIOU et al. (1998) were able to verify the complete obliteration of carotid cavernous fistulas in 13 patients (10 posttraumatic and three spontaneous) with color Doppler ultrasonography. The authors found a spiculated waveform with turbulent flow pattern in most of their direct (Type A) fistulas, while patients with indirect fistulas showed a low-resistive arterial pulsatile pattern. In these six patients with DCSFs, radiosurgery was performed and a cure was documented by sonography, a reasonable approach when repeated angiography can be spared. Nevertheless, for final documentation of anatomical cure, angiography was performed. ARNING et al. (2006) studied 17 patients with DAVFs and were able to detect AV shunting lesions in 100% if the ECA was examined. In contrast to brain AVMs

that are detectable only in cases with large shunt volume, most DAVFs can be diagnosed because of their supply by ECA branches that lose their characteristic flow pattern as resistance vessels. Assessment of venous drainage pattern, however, is difficult if not impossible and DSA as an initial diagnostic tool remains necessary. TSAI LK et al. (2005) studied a similar series of patients with DAVFs, one group undergoing endovascular treatment and another undergoing only clinical and sonographic follow-up. The authors found a good correlation between the increase of the RI and the effectiveness of the treatment in DAVF located at major sinuses, but not at the CS. This finding was in agreement with a previous study of the same group (TSAI LK et al. 2004) in which the sensitivity of using the ECA-RI was only 54% for cavernous sinus fistulas while it was 86% for non-cavernous sinus AVFs. This discrepancy is likely explained by the relatively small AV shunting volume in most DCSFs thus having rather little impact on the flow in the ECA. Therefore, it appears advisable to combine DCS with Doppler flow imaging of the superior ophthalmic veins (CHEN YW et al. 2000). In patients with solely posterior drainage, it might be impossible to depict an abnormal Doppler flow pattern in the SOV, thus leaving angiography as a last resort for a correct diagnosis.

In summary, modern cross-sectional imaging such as CT and MRI provide a correct diagnosis in many cases or can at least raise the suspicion of a CSF. The combination of transcranial and transorbital Doppler sonography and carotid duplex sonography further increases the sensitivity of non-invasive imaging. Sonography provides information on blood flow, while CTA and MRI help to delineate the angiomorphology of the arteriovenous communication.

The venous drainage pattern, representing the main morphological feature of a DCSF, causing mainly the clinical symptoms and being often the potential endovascular approach, can often not be imaged to a satisfactory degree. Low-flow fistulas with small or partially thrombosed SOVs may be completely missed. Therefore, not only patients with unclear symptoms, but all patients with DCSFs should eventually undergo an i.a. (intra-arterial) DSA at least once during the course of the disease, regardless of the planned therapeutic management.

Intra-arterial Digital Subtraction Angiography (DSA)

7.2.1
Introduction

It was Egas Moniz, a Portuguese neurologist, who on July 7, 1927, presented a revolutionary diagnostic method to the Societé de Neurologie de Paris (MONIZ 1927). His *"L' Encephalographie arterielle: son importance dans la localization des tumeurs cerebrales"* was the birth of a novel way to detect intracranial tumors by injecting contrast into the surgically exposed cervical carotid artery. By 1931, Moniz was able to perform 180 arteriograms in this way and described arterial, capillary and venous angiographic phases 3 years later.. Cerebral angiography was further developed by numerous investigators among which Loehr, Lima, Bergstrand, Olivecrano, Toennis, Takahashi, Wolff and Krayenbuehl (LOEHR 1933; LIMA 1935; BERGSTRAND et al. 1936; WOLFF and SCHALTENBRAND 1939; KRAYENBUEHL 1941) provided significant contributions. DYES (1938) suggested bi-plane radiography. In 1944 Holm emphasized the advantages of cineradiography and sequential imaging became possible thanks to Erik Lysholm (LYSHOLM 1931). The surgical exposure of the carotid artery initially used was soon followed by percutaneous techniques in 1936 and 1940 (TAKAHASHI 1940). To replace Thorotrast, iodide contrast media were introduced in 1939 and were continuously improved over the following years. Interestingly enough, although arteriography was rapidly accepted in Europe, it was not until the studies by LIST et al. (1945) and ECKER (1951) appeared that this diagnostic technique gained a similar acceptance in the United States (KRAYENBÜHL and YASARGIL 1979). The introduction of Seldinger's technique (SELDINGER 1953) simplified and facilitated further the use of percutaneous needle placement and catheterization techniques.

Development of subtraction techniques (ZIESDSES DES PLANTES 1934, 1935, 1961a) and angiographic magnification (LEEDS et al. 1968; WENDE and SCHINDLER 1970) were technical milestones in the history of modern cerebral angiography. These were complemented by a new computerized technology, digital subtraction angiography (DSA) that was employed in the late 1970s to re-explore intravenous (i.v.) angiography. At the RSNA in 1980, three companies introduced DSA equipment and by 1983 more than 30 manufacturers sold X-ray systems capable of digital subtraction. Because of its limitations, i.v. DSA was soon replaced by intra-arterial (i.a.) DSA that permitted the use of smaller catheters and smaller amounts of iodine contrast and has persisted until today.

The introduction of computerized tomography (CT) in 1973 represented the beginning of a new era in diagnostic neuroradiology – cross-sectional imaging of soft tissue structures such as the brain parenchyma and the ventricular system (so-called low-contrast imaging). Numerous early predictions stated that, because of its invasiveness and the associated complication rate, cerebral angiography was soon going to disappear from the spectrum of diagnostic tools. However, due to remarkable technological improvements and reduced risks, it not only persisted over the last 20 years, it even went through a renaissance in the 1990s when manufacturers started investing in its further development. No longer just as a diagnostic modality, but more a minimal invasive means to gain access for endovascular techniques, it became one of the key tools for modern image-guided therapy in interventional cardiology and radiology. High-resolution intra-arterial DSA currently plays a major role in the management of patients with vascular diseases of the CNS and other areas of the human body.

7.2.2
Technique

Due to the large amount of anatomic, pathologic and functional information provided, i.a. DSA has remained the gold standard for diagnostic and treatment planning of intracranial AV-shunting lesions. As emphasized in the previous section, the use of i.a. DSA is essential for the timely diagnosis of small, low-flow AV shunts.

Modern angiographic systems reliably provide high quality visualization of the smallest vasculature in the CS region, facilitated by the use of bi-plane acquisitions, and not affected by artifacts. Frame rates up to 15 frames are currently possible, allowing a temporal resolution not obtainable with CT or MRI. This resolution is of particular importance in high-flow dural or direct AV shunts when identifying the dominant supply or the exact site of the fistula (Figs. 7.48 and 7.49) is crucial.

High-resolution monitors in the control room as well as in the angiosuite are required. Intra-arterial angiograms are obtained using 4-(author's preference) or 5-F diagnostic catheters, usually with HH1 configuration, allowing for easy and fast access to the ICA and ECA branches. Simultaneous acquisitions in AP and lateral projections are standard requirements for state-of-the-art cerebral angiography. Selective catheterizations of all supplying territories are mandatory; "overview" injections from the CCA are not acceptable. In order to obtain complete information on the cerebral vasculature and not only in the region of interest, large fields of view, in addition to magnified projections, are advisable. Attention should be paid as to whether proximal supraaortic vessels are tortuous or diseased. To exclude an AV shunt, a diagnostic angiogram can be performed without anesthesia in outpatients. Furthermore, angiography is helpful to rule out other causes of tinnitus such as fibromuscular dyplasia (ARNING and GRZYSKA 2004), dissections (PELKONEN et al. 2004), or carotid siphon stenoses (HARTUNG et al. 2004).

The risks of stroke associated with cerebral angiography are not trivial but have decreased with time and experience, with improvement of equipment and advancement of endovascular tools (HANKEY et al. 1990; DION et al. 1987; FISHER et al. 1985; KERBER et al. 1978; ANONYMOUS 1995). Recent studies reveal a rate of 1.3%–2.3% for all neurological complications and 0.4%–0.5% for permanent neurological deficits (LEFFERS and WAGNER 2000; WILLINSKY et al. 2003). WILLINSKY et al. (2003) reported on 2899 consecutive cerebral DSAs prospectively studied. Among 39 complications (1.3%), 20 were transient (0.7%), 5 (0.2%) were reversible and 14 (0.5%) were permanent. The authors also found that neurological complications were significantly more frequent in patients over 55 years of age, in patients with cerebrovascular disease and when the fluoroscopic time was longer than 10 min.

The latter fact reflects an important aspect, which is experience. The influence of catheter technique, operator experience and procedure time has been reported (McIVOR et al. 1987) and is, in my opinion, a key factor in reducing complications. The choice of catheter size for placement in cerebral vessels plays another important role. During my clinical INR practice at Charité, I used 4-F diagnostic catheters almost exclusively between 1993 and 2003 (Cordis SUPER TORQUE®, 0.035″). In approximately 6000 patients (ca. 25,000–30,000 selective injections) diagnostic cerebral angiograms a permanent neurological deficit was observed in three patients. More than 90% of these diagnostic

cerebral angiograms were performed without the aid of a guidewire, even in older patients. This became possible only after the introduction of braided catheter material in 1992–1993. It is my strong belief that reducing guidewire manipulations in general helps to lower the complication rate. Patients with DCSFs are often elderly, and may present with advanced arteriosclerotic disease. Because no large guiding catheter is being placed in the internal carotid artery, the length of an endovascular treatment session, as a risk factor in this age group, plays a minor role when performing transvenous occlusions. Usually only a 4-F diagnostic catheter needs to be placed in the ECA for road mapping or control injections throughout the procedure. Overall, in experienced hands, the complication rate of cerebral angiography, local and neurological, is below the numbers reported in the 1980s and justifies its use whenever clinically necessary.

7.2.3
Angiographic Protocol for DCSFs

As for brain AVMs, complete visualization of the intracranial vasculature is important, including the ipsi- and contralateral ECA territories (Figs. 7.12–7.23).

The arteriogram should provide the following angiomorphological information:

- Localization of the fistula site (Figs. 7.38–7.49)
- Differentiation between indirect and direct fistula (Figs. 7.12–7.23)
- Demonstration of the entire arterial supply, in particular in cases with DCSF with visualization of so-called "dangerous anastomoses"
- Visualization of the CS and its tributaries with possible stenosis, thrombosis, ectasias, draining veins such as IPS, SOV, ICS etc.
- Identification of fresh thrombus in the CS or IPS
- Identification of risk factors such as CS varices, intercavernous pseudoaneurysms or cortical drainage
- Identification of trauma signs such as dissection or transsection
- Identification of diseased, stenosed or tortuous supraaortic arteries
- Preexisting disease such as FMD or Ehlers-Danlos
- Visualization of collateral circulation with adjacent territories such as carotid bifurcation

DEBRUN (1995) suggested the following protocol for a diagnostic work-up in CCFs:

- Selective bilateral injection of the ICA
- Selective injection of the ascending pharyngeal artery, bilateral (if necessary through microcatheter)
- Selective injection of the internal maxillary artery

PICARD et al. (1987) also emphasized the need for an exhaustive angiographic work-up for visualization of all potential feeders: the cavernous branches of ILT and MHT, the jugular, hypoglossal and carotid rami arising from the APA, IMA branches (cavernous branch of MMA and AMA as well as artery of the foramen rotundum) and recurrent deep ophthalmic artery.

A dural arteriovenous fistula of the CS can be uni- or bilateral and often involves multiple feeders of both ICA and ECA territories, also in cases where the shunt is unilateral (DEBRUN 1995). Because current treatment is performed in most centers using transvenous routes, precise analysis of the venous anatomy has become crucial for a successful procedure. The aim of angiography in patients with Type B–D fistulas is to determine the exact location of the arteriovenous communication, and to decide which compartment of the CS is involved: anterior or posterior (or both), left or right (Figs. 7.38 and 7.49). To identify precisely the site of the fistula, selective injection of ICA and ECA branches is necessary. The differentiation between uni- and bilateral fistulas should be done in magnified AP projections (Fig. 7.38). Enlarged dural branches of the cavernous ICA should not be mistaken for an opacified CS. This differentiation is sometimes difficult and probably the reason why the incidence of bilateral fistulas appears overestimated in clinical practice as well as in the literature (ERNST and TOMSICK 1997). Dural arteries can cross the midline to supply an AV shunt at the contralateral CS, occasionally even when there is no significant ipsilateral supply. In fact, in some cases, the shunt is neither right nor left, but may involve the ICS (Fig. 7.40). For identification of ECA feeders, lateral and AP projections should be used, and sometimes AP views at various angulations are helpful. When performing the diagnostic work-up, one should be aware of the fact that a dural fistula involving the IPS is usually supplied by APA branches and drains often times first into the CS, then into the SOV and thus can cause a very similar clinical picture (Fig. 7.46). LASJAUNIAS et al. (1987) have recommended performing selective catheterizations using even a microcatheter if

necessary, to visualize the smallest pedicles and to identify the so-called "dangerous anastomoses" (LASJAUNIAS 1984). These anastomoses are not per se "dangerous" and consist mainly of the AFR, AMA and MMA with connections to ILT, and the APA connected to ICA and TMH. They are practically always present, but can be obscured on angiograms due to their small size, poor image quality and individual hemodynamics (see Sect. 3.3.1). Being aware of their existence is indispensable for avoiding ischemic complications during transarterial embolizations in ECA branches, the only "danger" being ignoring or neglecting normal vascular anatomy in the CS region.

7.2.4
Angiographic Anatomy of the Cavernous Sinus

- Arterial Anatomy: Figs. 7.12–7.23
- Venous Anatomy: Figs. 7.24–7.37
- CSF Anatomy: Figs. 7.38–7.49

In some cases of high-flow dural AV shunts, an extensive network of small dural arteries can be found, of which only some can be identified and most are not large enough to be catheterized with currently available devices. The angiographic anatomy of the venous system in the region is influenced by hemodynamics of the cerebral circulation and of the AV shunt, selectivity of injections (arterial or venous), and thrombotic processes in the CS, SOV or IPS.

In my own practice the following work-up has usually been performed:
- Selective bilateral ICA injections, AP and lateral
- Selective bilateral ECA injections, AP and lateral (including APA)
- Selective VA injections, AP and lateral
- Selective phlebography, AP and lateral (at different levels below the jugular bulb)

"Selective" injection into the ECA herein means that overflow of contrast into the ICA territory is avoided. The pressure during manual injection should be appropriate to the difference in vascular resistance between both vascular beds and distal catheter placement into the IMA is usually helpful.

It is important that ICA injections are obtained in magnified views and caudal angulations (Waters' view). These projections allow for easier differentiation between uni- and bilateral fistulas, as well as

(Text continues on p. 122)

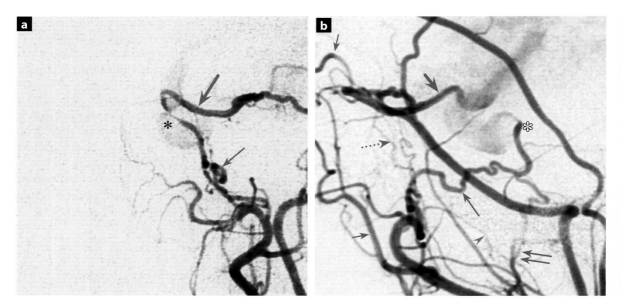

Fig. 7.12 a,b. A 30-year-old patient with a left temporal AVM. Selective left ECA injection, AP (a) and lateral (b) view. The arteriovenous shunt leads to increased flow in the ICA and to enlarged external-internal carotid anastomoses. From the MMA arises a recurrent meningeal branch, which fills the OA (*thick arrow*). The AFR (*arrow*) arises from the pterygopalatine artery and runs in AP projection cranially and medially through the foramen rotundum (*canalis rotundus*) to connect with the ILT (*asterisk*). The AMA (*double arrow*) reaches the ILT with a meningeal branch through the foramen ovale. Other anastomoses/branches: Anterior deep temporal artery (*short arrows*), SPA branches to the ethmoidal arteries of the OA, (*dotted arrow*), pterygovaginal artery (*arrowhead*). (Modified from Benndorf, 2002)

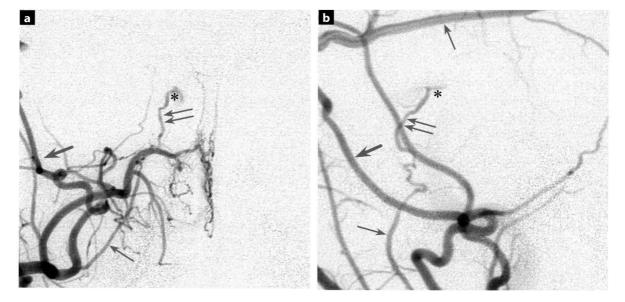

Fig. 7.13 a,b. A 5-year-old boy with a right temporal DAVF (*double arrowheads*). Selective ECA injection, AP (a) and lateral (b) view. The main supply of the arteriovenous shunt is provided by an enlarged MMA (*thick arrow*). Clearly visible is the AMA (*arrow*), passing with a branch through the foramen ovale and filling the ILT (*asterisk*) via its posteromedial ramus (*double arrow*). This vessel may run in AP projection in a medially convex turn

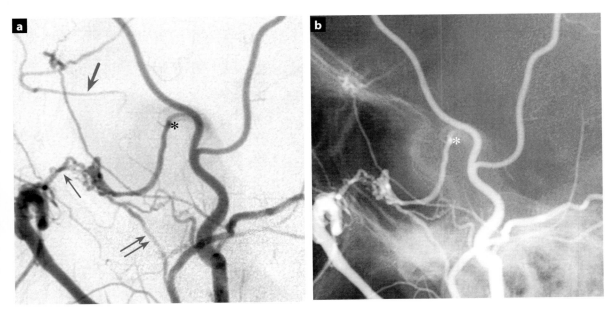

Fig. 7.14 a,b. A 33-year-old patient with a direct CSF (Type A), 2 years after car accident. Selective left ECA injection, lateral projection. **a** The ILT (*asterisk*) is enlarged due to the high-flow AV shunt and displaced posteriorly. It fills via the AFR (*arrow*), which has developed a network of multiple small dural vessels at the level of the foramen rotundum, and via a meningeal branch of the AMA (*double arrow*) that directly originates from the IMA. The frontal branch of the MMA is hypoplastic, however fills the ophthalmic artery (*thick arrow*) retrogradely. The non-subtracted image (**b**) shows the typical projection of the ILT origin onto the center of the sella

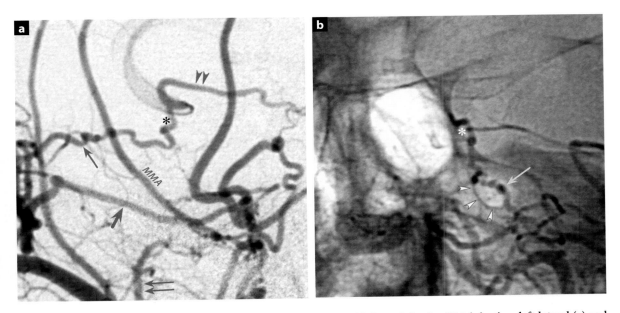

Fig. 7.15 a,b. A 65-year-old patient with bilateral DAVFs of the sigmoid sinus. Selective ECA injection, left lateral (**a**) and AP (**b**) projection. **a** The enlarged AFR (*arrow*) fills via the ILT (*asterisk*), the ramus superior (marginal tentorial artery, Bernasconi), which courses posteriorly and laterally towards the AV-shunt. In AP projection, the foramen rotundum (*arrowheads*) and the artery (*arrow*) coursing through, can be identified on a non-subtracted image (**b**). The enlarged artery of the pterygoid canal (vidian artery, *thick short arrow*), courses posteriorly and communicates with branches of the MMA and the APA and ICA. The AMA (*double arrow*) gives rise to a small branch that seems also to connect with the ILT

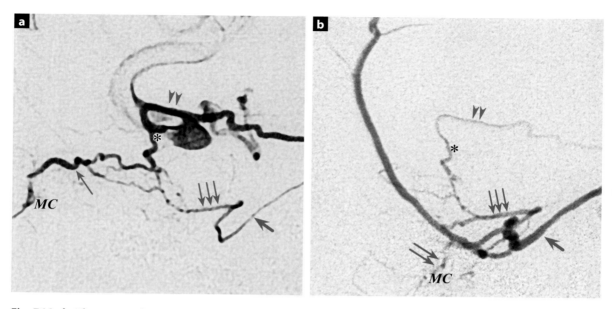

Fig. 7.16a,b. The same patient as in Fig. 7.15. Superselective injections in the artery of the foramen rotundum (**a**) and in the accessory meningeal artery (**b**) through a microcatheter (*MC*), lateral projections. **a** The AFR (*arrow*) passes through the foramen rotundum and is connected with the anterolateral ramus of the ILT (*asterisk*). From the connection with the ILT courses a small branch (*triple arrow*) to the MMA and reaches its petrous branch (*thick arrow*) distal to the foramen spinosum. **b** The AMA (*double arrow*) arises in this case directly from the internal maxillary artery giving off a branch to the foramen ovale, which connects to the ILT as well as to the the petrous branch of the MMA (*thick arrow*). (*Double arrowheads*, marginal tentorial, or medial tentorial artery with a typical undulating course (may also arise from the MHT or in rare cases from the AMA and MMA (BENNDORF 2008)

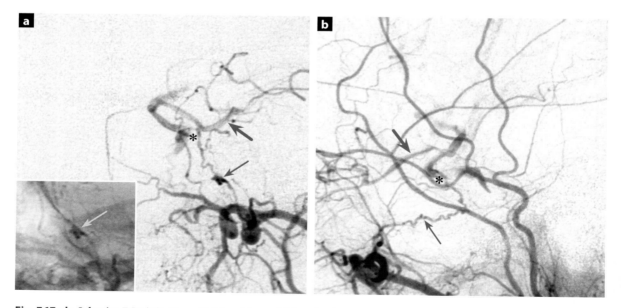

Fig. 7.17a,b. Selective ECA injection, AP (**a**) and lateral (**b**) projections. In this case, the carotid siphon fills not only via the retrogradely opacified ophthalmic artery (*thick arrow*), but also via the ILT (*asterisk*) which receives blood from the AFR (*arrow*) that often shows a typical irregular "zig-zag" course in lateral view. In AP view, this segment of the vessel usually projects as a dot with irregular contours (*arrow*), which is always centered in the foramen rotundum (*see inset*)

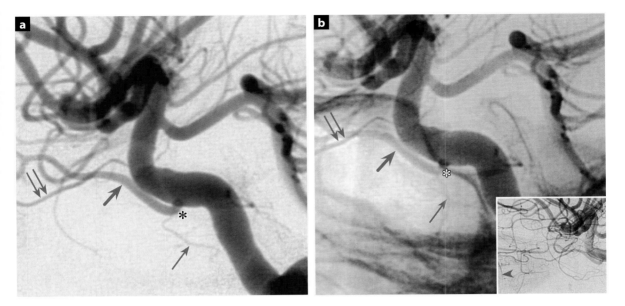

Fig. 7.18a,b. Selective ICA injection, lateral view subtracted (a) and non-subtracted (b) views. Anatomic variant of the ophthalmic artery. A large dorsal ophthalmic artery (*thick arrow*), from the C4 segment (**intracavernous OA, or recurrent OA**) and a very small ventral ophthalmic artery (*double arrow*) are visible. The former runs as the anteromedial branch of the ILT (*asterisk*) through the supraorbital fissure. The latter is, despite its smaller size, quite important because it usually supplies the central retinal artery. Note the choroidal blush from adjacent ciliary arteries in the late phase (*arrowhead, inset*). **Note:** The tiny branch (*arrow*) coursing posteriorly to reach the foramen spinosum is the posterolateral branch of the ILT)

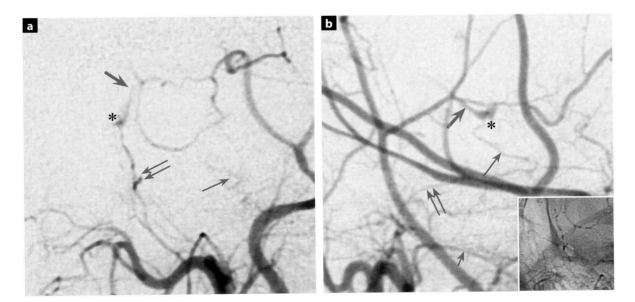

Fig. 7.19a,b. Same patient, selective left ECA injection, AP (a) and lateral (b) views. The MMA has a large ophthalmic branch, which retrogradely supplies also the dorsal ophthalmic artery (*thick arrow*). In the early arterial phase this vessel, however, is initially filled by the ILT (*asterisk*), which on the other hand is supplied by a very small AFR (*double arrow*) that connects with the very same, above-mentioned posterolateral branch (*arrow*). This example demonstrates the usefulness to look for the AFR in AP (*inset*), when the lateral view shows only a faint opacification. *Short arrow*: pterygovaginal artery well visible with its typical downward turn

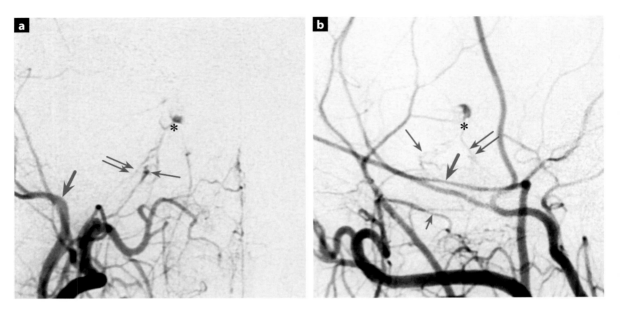

Fig. 7.20 a,b. Selective right ECA injection, AP (a) and lateral (b) views. The AFR (*arrow*) arises from distal internal maxillary artery in the pterygopalatine fossa, coursing cranially, medially and posteriorly to reach the ILT (*asterisk*), which in this case is only faintly opacified and appears additionally supplied by the posterolateral branch (*double arrows*) of the MMA (*thick arrow*). **Note:** Beside the fact that these branches are not enlarged due to an AV shunt, the spatial resolution of the II system used here, reaches its limits to display the minute arterial communications (see also Fig. 7.55). *Short arrow:* pteryvaginal artery with its characteristic downward turn

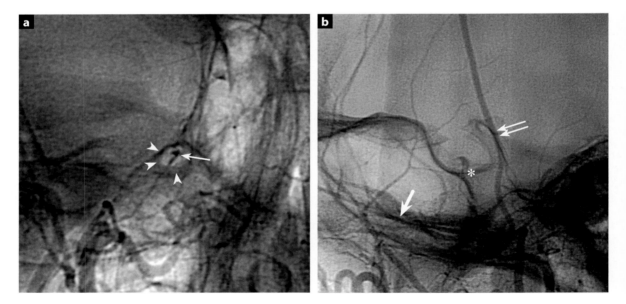

Fig. 7.21. Same projections as in Fig. 7.20, non-subtracted views. The AFR passes through the foramen rotundum and creates the typical above-mentioned irregular dot (*arrow*), projecting exactly onto this foramen (*arrowheads*). In some cases, the AFR is easier identifiable in AP than in the classic lateral view, where other anastomotic channels may take a similar course. In lateral view, the ILT reaches the C4 segment of the ICA approximately at the middle of the sella (*asterisk*), usually located between the superficial temporal artery (*double arrow*) and the MMA (*thick arrow*)

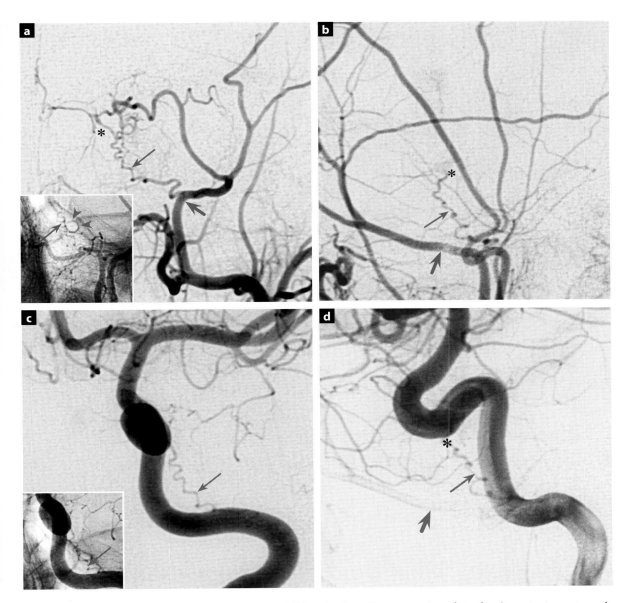

Fig. 7.22 a–d. Left ECA injection in AP (a) and lateral (b) projections. Demonstration of another important anastomosis between ECA and ICA: After passing the foramen spinosum, the MMA (*thick arrow*) gives off a small branch (*arrow*) that travels medially and cranially to connect with the posterolateral ramus of the ILT (*asterisk*). In non-subtracted AP view (*inset*) this vessel does not project onto the foramen rotundum. The corresponding ICA injections in AP and lateral projection in **c** and **d** show the same ramus that runs from the ILT (*asterisk*) caudally and laterally, leading to a faint opacification of the MMA (*thick arrow*) via its connection at the level of the foramen spinosum

118

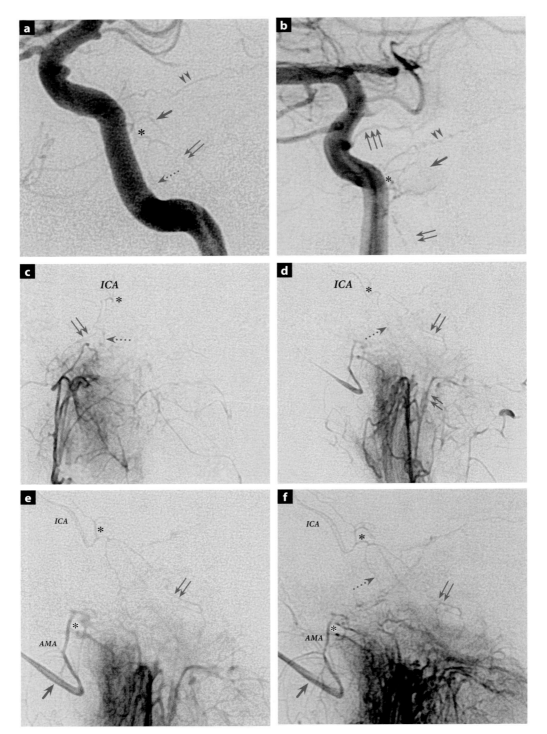

**Fig. 7.23 a–f. Communication between C5-segment of the ICA and ascending pharyngeal artery (APA). a,b ICA injection,
lateral and oblique projections:** Demonstration of the branches of the MHT (*asterisk*): The marginal tentorial artery (Bernasconi) with its characteristic undulating course ascends posteriorly (*double arrowheads*). Additional branches: Inferior
hypophyseal artery contributing to the blush of the posterior lobe of the pituitary gland (*thick arrow*), arteries to the clivus
(*double arrow*) from the dorsal meningeal artery, anastomosing with branches of the neuromeningeal ramus of the APA.
Dotted arrow: Recurrent artery of the foramen lacerum, *triple arrow*: Capsular artery after Mc Connell. **c–f Superselective
filling of the APA, AP and lateral view early arterial phase (c,d), lateral view mid and late arterial phase (e,f). d–f are identical projections to a:** Anastomosing branches between neuromeningeal ramus (*double short arrow*) and ICA: Lateral clival
artery (*double arrow*) from the jugular ramus. Further identifiable is the carotid branch (*dotted arrow*), arising from the
superior pharyngeal artery (*arrow*) and connecting with the recurrent artery of the foramen lacerum that arises from the C5
portion. These anastomoses provide a retrograde filling of the MHT (*asterisk*), which explains why a hypophyseal blush may
be seen in some selective APA injections. *Thick arrow:* Proximal internal maxillary artery opacified via an anterior branch
of the superior pharyngeal artery to the Eustachian tube (*white asterisk*) and AMA. (Modified from BENNDORF 2002)

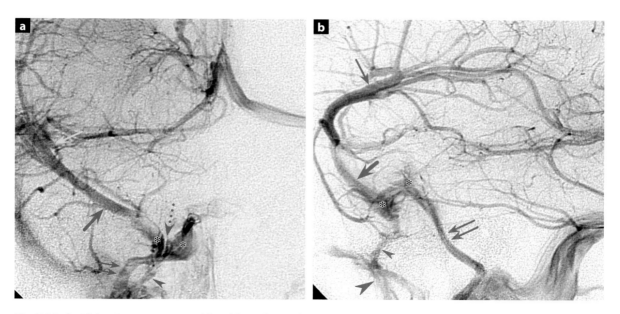

Fig. 7.24a,b. Right ICA venogram AP (a) and lateral view (b). A large SMCV (*arrow*) drains via the SPPS (*thick arrow*) into the anterior CS (*asterisk*). The CS drains into the inferior petrosal sinus of normal caliber (*double arrows*) and the pterygoid plexus (*large arrowhead*). The latter connects with the CS via a venous plexus in the foramen ovale (*arrowhead*), which lies in AP projection medial to the IPS. Note the white line (*dotted arrow*), separating the CS from a lateral structure that may correspond to a laterocavernous sinus (LCS)

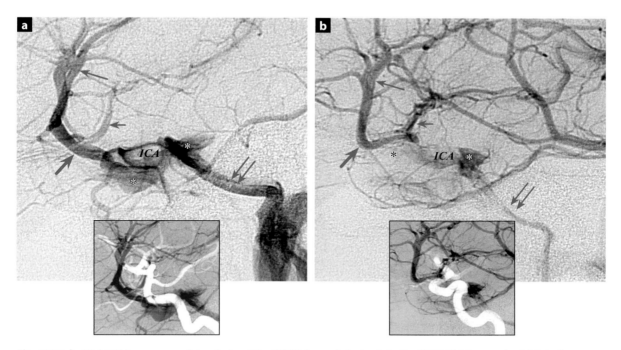

Fig. 7.25a,b. Right ICA venogram, lateral view. The SMCV (*arrow*) drains into the SPPS (*thick arrow*), which before opening into the CS (*asterisks*) is joined by the uncal vein (*short arrow*), a small CS tributary, often neglected in textbooks. No filling of the pterygoid plexus is seen. The CS may (angiographically) vary in shape and size (see also Fig. 7.34). In (**a**) there is a large anterior CS, and a smaller posterior CS, as opposed to (**b**), where the posterior CS appears the main compartment. The variform shape of the CS depends to some degree on the size and course of the ICA within the CS, as can be appreciated when using sequential subtraction technique (*insets*). Good visualization of the IPS in both cases (*double arrows*)

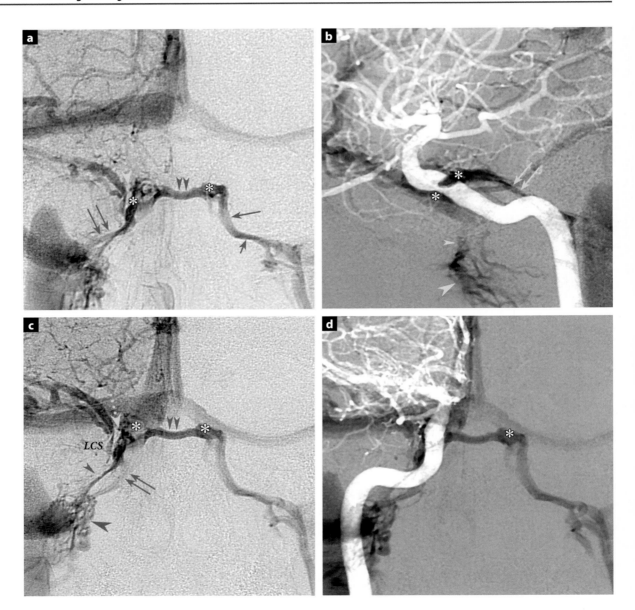

Fig. 7.26a–d. Right ICA venograms, AP (a) and lateral view (b). The right cavernous sinus (*asterisk*) fills via the SMCV and SPPS. It also drains via the intercavernous sinus (*double arrowheads*) to the contralateral side and via the left IPS (*short arrow* = pars horizontalis, *long arrow* = pars verticalis). Because of a superposition with the venous plexus of the foramen ovale (FO-plexus *arrowhead*) and the PP (*large arrowhead*) in AP projection, the ipsilateral IPS (*double arrow*) is difficult to identify. Both venous structures can be better distinguished – when a more caudal angulation, creating less foreshortening and projecting the FO-plexus cranial and lateral to the IPS, is used. These anatomical relationships also become clearer when sequential subtractions are used (**b,d**). *Dotted arrow*: Separating CS and laterocavernous sinus (LCS).

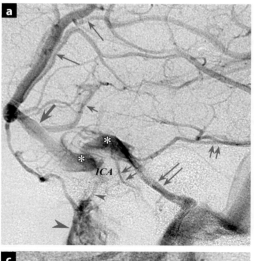

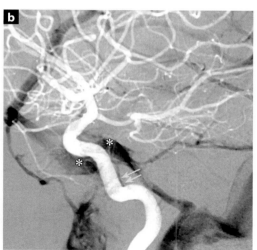

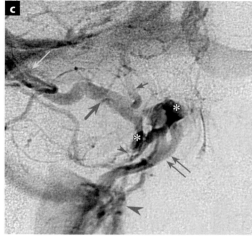

Fig. 7.27 a–c. Right ICA venogram, lateral (a, b) and AP (c) projection. The SMCV (*arrow*) runs as a large vein, draining several smaller vessels, towards the SPPS (*thick arrow*), which is joined by the uncal vein (*short arrow*), before reaching the CS (*asterisks*). From here, the blood drains via the IPS (*double arrows*) into the IJV, via the SPS (*short double arrows*) into the transverse sinus, and via a small emissary vein (*small arrowhead*) into the pterygoid plexus (*large arrowhead*). In the subtraction, the ICA marks a filling defect separating the anteroinferior and posterosuperior CS, as seen in the sequential subtraction (b). Note that in (a) the contours, outlining the non-opacified ICA lumen (*ICA*), belong to the internal carotid artery venous plexus (ICAVP) of Rektorzik (*double short arrows*). (See also Figs. 7.85–7.89)

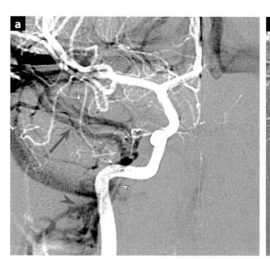

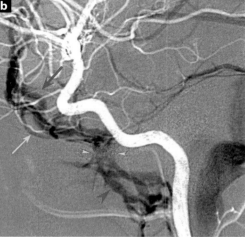

Fig. 7.28a,b. Right ICA venogram AP (a) and lateral (b) view with shifted mask (sequential subtraction). The Sylvian veins and the SPPS (*thick arrow*) do not reach the CS, but drain more laterally into a paracavernous sinus (PCS, *arrow*), that empties via a large emissary vein (*arrowheads*) into the pterygoid plexus (*large arrowhead*)

for better identification of the IPS, which may be opacified faintly during the late venous phase when filled via the normal venous drainage of the brain (Fig. 7.26). It is a widespread misconception that an IPS that is filled during the early arterial phase, or not angiographically involved in the fistula's drainage, must be considered either thrombosed or otherwise completely blocked (Fig. 7.29). In actual fact, a fistula that hemodynamically (or visibly) does not communicate with the IPS may be very well connected anatomically and could be approached by endovascular means (Fig. 7.42). Thus, careful analysis of the late venous phase in carotid and vertebral angiograms in both planes is advisable (Case report III, Figs. 7.41 and 7.42).

In my experience, the IPS is more frequently patent than assumed and, in contrast to the early statement from THERON (1972), may also well opacify in angiograms of the posterior fossa (Figs. 7.29 and 7.30).

As discussed in Sect. 4.1, arterial angioarchitecture has been the main basis for classifying spontaneous CS fistulas from a surgeon's point of view (BARROW et al. 1985). The arterial angiographic features are nonetheless of minor importance for planning transvenous embolizations. The differentiation between Types B–D and Type A fistulas, or between direct and indirect (dural) fistulas, is of little or no relevance for occlusion of fistulous CS compartments. More importantly, the radiologic work-up of CSFs must include detailed analysis of the venous angiomorphology. Such analysis requires knowledge and good understanding of the normal anatomy of the CS, its tributaries and its draining veins (Figs. 7.24–7.37).

The main tributaries of the anterior CS are the superior ophthalmic veins and the inferior ophthalmic veins, usually not visualized following ICA injections. Because the SOV usually drains the nasal mucosa, this vein is frequently seen on normal ECA arteriograms. In cases of hyperemic nasal mucosa, as seen under certain physiological conditions (e.g. in young girls during menstruation, this vein can appear surprisingly early and be intensely opacified, so that the inexperienced operator may suspect an AV shunt. The connection of the vein with the CS and its drainage via the IPS becomes visible in lateral views, while in AP view the typical omega configuration (Figs. 7.31–7.33) can be seen.

Other important tributaries are the superficial middle cerebral vein (SMCV Figs. 7.24–7.27) and the sphenoparietal sinus (SPPS, Fig. 7.27). The SMCV drains either directly or via the SPPS into the CS. Fre-

quently this vein may also bypass the CS and drain into a laterocavernous sinus (SAN MILLAN RUIZ et al. 1999) or directly into the foramen ovale plexus and the extracranial PP, a fact that has found little attention in the older literature. A minor tributary of the CS is the uncal vein. This small vein, best seen in lateral views coursing from postero-superior to antero-inferior, drains either directly or together with the SPPS into the CS (Figs. 7.25, 7.27, 7.32). Each tributary may change its function and turn into a draining vein when the venous pressure increases due to an AV shunt. Such changes gain particular importance in cases of high-flow lesions, but are less often seen in Type B–D fistulas as compared to direct CCF. However, when performing transvenous embolization, cortical or leptomeningeal drainage must not be missed. If coils are incorrectly placed, pressure increase with subsequent intracranial hemorrhage may result.

The SOV is most frequently opacified in a retrograde fashion and fills the angular vein, the facial vein and eventually the IJV. In case of a large AV shunt volume, the angular vein may also opacify the contralateral facial vein and the frontal vein. The caliber of these veins can be crucial for treatment planning, as are elongations, thrombi or stenoses, and other factors that could possibly compromise catheter navigation. In some cases, the supraorbital vein fills the medial temporal vein (Figs. 7.31, 7.32 and 7.91), which can be mistaken in lateral views as SOV, but can also serve as an approach to the CS (AGID et al. 2004; KAZEKAWA et al. 2003).

Increased blood volume may be directed to the contralateral CS and from there to the contralateral SOV and IPS. The AV shunt may also drain via the PP. Often the venous drainage will use the IPS, which may be opacified on both sides. The visualization of this sinus is of importance, because of its anatomical proximity and relatively straight course, making it the venous access route of choice.

The opacification of the CS as well as its draining veins in a DSA may vary significantly, depending on anatomical and hemodynamic factors (Fig. 7.35). Thrombotic processes within the CS or the IPS further influence their appearance in an angiogram obtained by arterial contrast injection. That is also why some of the most accurate descriptions of the CS and the SOV anatomy can be found in reports on orbital phlebography from the 1960s–1970s, where contrast medium was directly injected into a frontal vein and forced into the orbital venous system by the use of a tourniquet (LOMBARDI and PASSERINI 1967; CLAY et al. 1972; BRISMAR and BRISMAR 1976; BRISMAR et al. 1976).

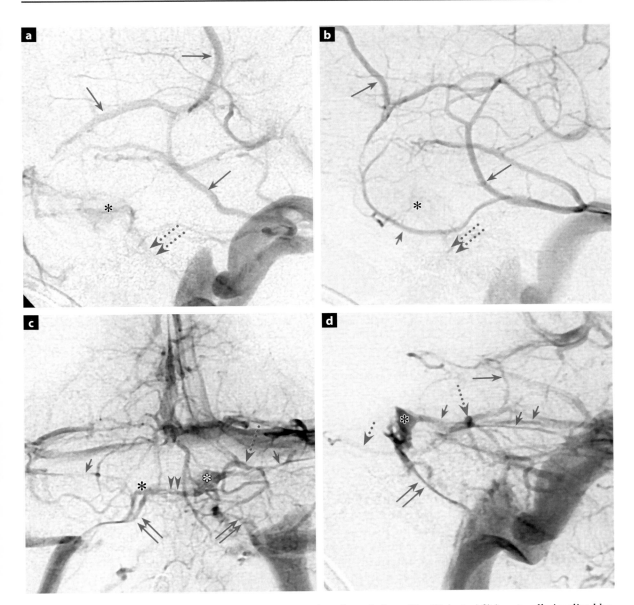

Fig. 7.29 a–d. Right (a) and left (b) ICA venogram, same patient, lateral views. The CS (*asterisk*) is not well visualized because most of the venous blood from the Sylvian fissure drains via superior and inferior anastomotic veins (*arrows*), and through a paracavernous sinus (*short arrow*). Accordingly, the IPS is just faintly opacified (*double arrows*), which does not necessarily mean that this sinus is thrombosed or occluded. **c, d Venogram of the posterior circulation of the same patient in AP (c) and lateral (d) projection.** The right, and less clearly the left IPS are opacified (*double arrows*). Their contrast filling is provided by both superior petrosal sinuses (*short arrows*), that reach the posterior CS (*asterisk*) and drain blood from the posterior fossa. The right and left cavernous sinus are joined by the posterior intercavernous sinus (*arrowheads*). Note that the paracavernous sinus, filled in **b,** is also faintly opacified (*short dotted arrow*). This example demonstrates that the assumption that a non-opacified IPS must be occluded and thus cannot be passed with a microcatheter is erroneous. Hemodynamic factors, type of injection and possible thrombus formation influence the angiographic appearance of a venous collector that receives blood from different tributaries of both hemispheres, the posterior circulation and the ECA territory. *Arrow*: Lateral mesencephalic vein; *dotted arrow*: Stem of petrosal vein

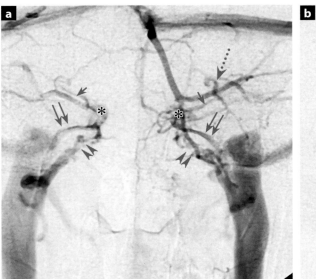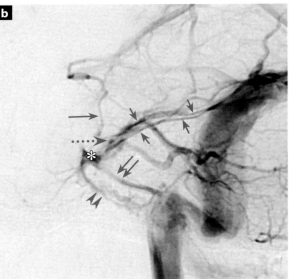

Fig. 7.30 a,b. CS visualization in a venogram of the posterior circulation AP (a) and lateral (b) projection. The right and left (*double arrows*) IPS are opacified via the posterior CS (*asterisk*) that receives blood from both SPSs (*short arrows*) and from draining veins of the posterior fossa (**a**). Note that the "mirror vessel" running parallel to the IPS in (**b**) is the inferior petroclival vein (IPCV, *arrowheads*) that lies at the inferior surface of the petroclival fissure (see Figs. 7.83–7.90). *Arrow*: Anterior pontomesencephalic vein, *dotted arrow*: Stem of petrosal vein

If the SOV is scarcely opacified or not visible at all due to thrombosis of the vein or of the CS, a selective phlebogram of the CS may help to clarify the situation and explain dramatic clinical symptoms in some small AV shunts. If an IPS does not fill at all during an angiogram early or late, it may indeed be thrombosed. It is believed that a recent thrombosis of the IPS is the cause for their clinical deterioration by increasing the venous pressure and rerouting the venous drainage anteriorly. This condition is otherwise not necessarily a reason to use an alternative approach, because a recently thrombosed IPS is usually not very difficult to pass with a microcatheter.

Transvenous phlebograms of the IJV/IJB region play a major role in the diagnostic work-up of DCSFs, more so when a transvenous approach is planned. Because the IPS is the most common approach, its precise anatomical relationship to the IJV is of key interest. Intravenous injections of contrast often provide more reliable information on the anatomy in this region than intra-arterial DSAs and are valuable when decide whether or not the IPS approach would be feasible (Fig. 7.41). In some cases simultaneous arterial and venous injections can further facilitate anatomic understanding (Fig. 7.7)

Such a situation is demonstrated in a case where the IPS was missed on intra-arterial injections due to local thrombosis (Case report III). Yet, the phlebogram showed a widely open IPS through which a microcatheter could easily be navigated. Even in cases of complete thrombosis of the IPS, often a tiny residual structure is seen as a sort of "stump" (Case report I, III). Because this venous stump or notch can be made more or less visible, the phlebogram should be repeated using different catheter positions, including injections below the jugular bulb. These will help to opacify the IPS in cases of a "deep termination" or aberrant IPS (Fig. 7.37). Section 3.3.2 discusses the variants of entry of the IPS into the IJV in more detail, of which I have observed five cases. When such an extracranially located connection between IPS and IJV is present, it may be used for transvenous catheterizations of the CS as well (BENNDORF and CAMPI 2001).

In cases where angiographic anatomy remains difficult to read, sequential subtraction (mask shifting into the arterial phase) is a simple and useful technique. Placing the mask within the early arterial phase provides white (ICA) and black (CS) contrast images displaying the anatomical relationship between portions of the CS, its afferent and efferent veins and the cavernous ICA (Figs. 7.34–7.36).

(Text continues on p. 139)

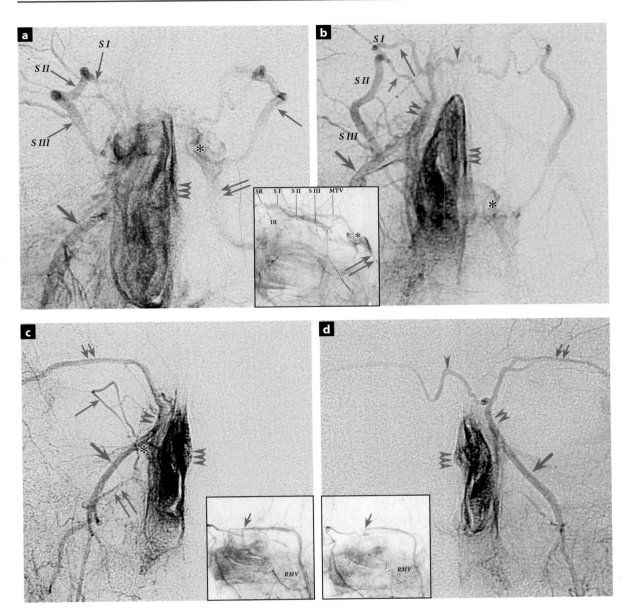

Fig. 7.31 a–d. Drainage of ECA territories in two patients. a,b Right and left ECA venogram, AP and lateral views (*inset*): Intense mucosal blush (*double arrowheads*) opacifying both SOVs (*arrows*) and the right facial vein (*thick arrow*). On the left side there is opacification of the CS (*asterisk*), which receives blood from the right CS (superimposed by nasal mucosa) and drains via the IPS (*double arrows*) into the internal jugular vein, as seen in lateral view (*inset*). The various segments of the SOV (typical Omega shape) are better demonstrated in Waters' view (**b**) that also demonstrates the nasal arcade (*arrowhead*) and the angular vein (*double arrowhead*), joining the facial vein (*thick arrow*). The latter can be differentiated from the posteriorly located junction of SOV and CS. Note the three segments of the SOV (I–III), and its superior (SR, *long arrow*) and inferior (IR, *short arrow*) root. Recognizing this anatomic disposition may become helpful for planning TVO through the facial vein and SOV. The superior root is more commonly used (BIONDI et al. 2003). **c, d Right and left ECA-venogram in AP and lateral projection (*insets*):** Intense blush of the nasal mucosa (*double arrowhead*), which in this case drains only partially via the right SOV (*arrow*), but mainly via angular veins into the facial veins (*double arrowheads* and *thick arrow* respectively), and via supraorbital veins (*short double arrows*) into the middle temporal veins (MTVs, *insets, short arrows,* The MTVs run in lateral projections parallel to the SOVs posteriorly and then turn caudally to join the retromandibular veins (RMVs). The CS (*asterisk*) and the IPS (*double arrows*) are faintly opacified on the right, but not on the left side. *Insets*: The MTV often has a distinctive sharp turn when coursing around the zygoma (*arrows*)

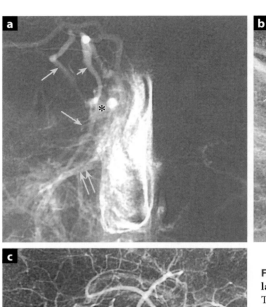

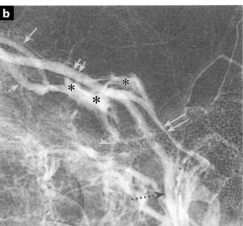

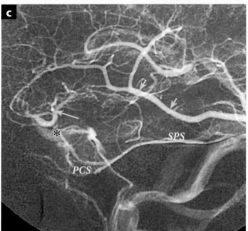

Fig. 7.32 a–c. Right ECA venogram AP (a) and lateral view (b). Right ICA venogram lateral (c). The intensely opacified nasal mucosa drains via the SOV (*arrow*) and the IOV (*thin short arrow*) into the CS (*asterisk*), which connects with the IPS (*double arrows*), as well as with the pterygoid plexus (*large arrowhead*) via a small emissary vein (*small arrowhead*). There is a significant component draining via the middle temporal vein (*short double arrow*) into the retromandibular vein (*dotted arrow*). The right cortical veins (**c**) drain mostly via a large vein of Labbé (*short arrows*), while the CS mainly drains a large uncal vein (*arrow*). *PCS*: Paracavernous sinus, *SPS*: Superior petrosal sinus. Note the typical Omega shape of the SOV in AP projection (**a**)

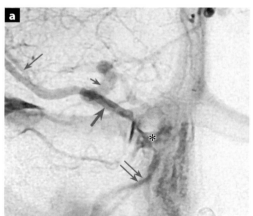

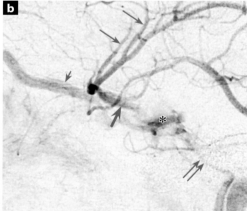

Fig. 7.33a,b. ICA and ECA drainage of the cavernous sinus. Right common carotid venogram AP (a) and lateral view (b). The late venous phase shows the drainage from the cavum nasi and the right cerebrum, both opacifying the CS. SOV: (*short arrow*) and its entry into the CS (*asterisk*). The sphenoparietal sinus (*thick arrow*), which brings blood from the Sylvian veins (*arrow*), is also visible. The cavernous sinus drains mainly into the IPS (*double arrows*) and the internal jugular vein

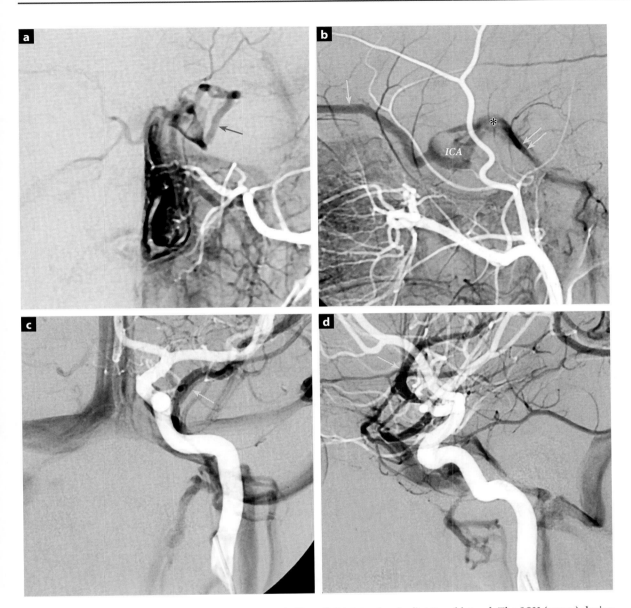

Fig. 7.34a–d. Cavernous sinus opacification via ECA (a,b) and ICA injection (c,d) AP and lateral. The SOV (*arrow*) drains into the CS (*asterisk*) and IPS (*double arrow*), while the SMCV drains (*arrow*), in addition, into the pterygoid plexus. Angiographic appearance of the CS and its draining veins depends on the injected territory and on local hemodynamics. A single territory angiogram may only partially visualize the venous anatomy and should not be used as the only diagnostic exam to assess the venous anatomy. The filling defect in **b** is not a thrombus in the CS, but caused by the ICA lumen (**d**)

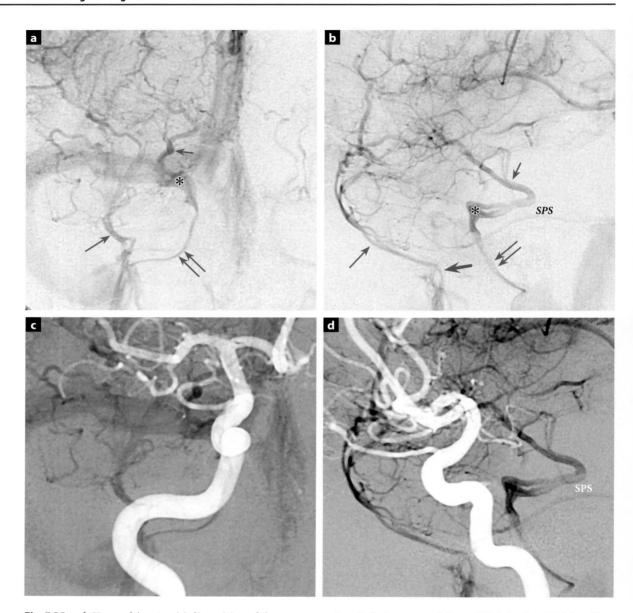

Fig. 7.35 a–d. Unusual (anatomic) disposition of the cavernous sinus/inferior petrosal sinus. ICA injection AP (a) and lateral (b). Sequential subtractions (c,d). The posterior CS (*asterisk*) is filled exclusively via a large uncal vein that takes an unusual posterior turn (*short arrow*) and drains into the IPS (*double arrow*). The anterior CS is not opacified. Cortical drainage from the Sylvian territory is directed towards a paracavernous sinus (*arrow*) that empties into the emissary vein of the foramen ovale (*thick arrow*) and reaches the pterygoid plexus. This angiographic appearance of an isolated posterior CS may in fact not represent the true anatomy

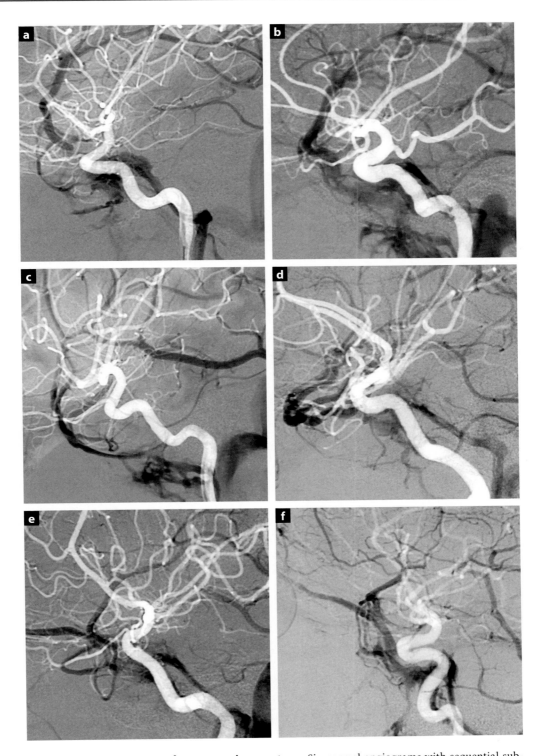

Fig. 7.36a–f. Variant angiographic appearance of cavernous sinus anatomy. Six normal angiograms with sequential sub-tractions allow for relating arterial (*white*) and venous (*black*) structures to each other. **a,b** Common configurations, drain-age via PCS into PP (**c**), Unusual anterior loop of SMCV and SSPS (**d**). **e,f** Interestingly, the SOV may serve not as tributary, but as a draining vein of the CS. This can be a normal finding, seen in some ICA injections under physiological condition. It does not always indicate a pathological condition, such as an AV shunt or elevated intracranial pressure as assumed in the past. In clinical practice, cerebral angiograms show numerous variations and no angiogram will look like another. Important is to understand the basic anatomic dispositions

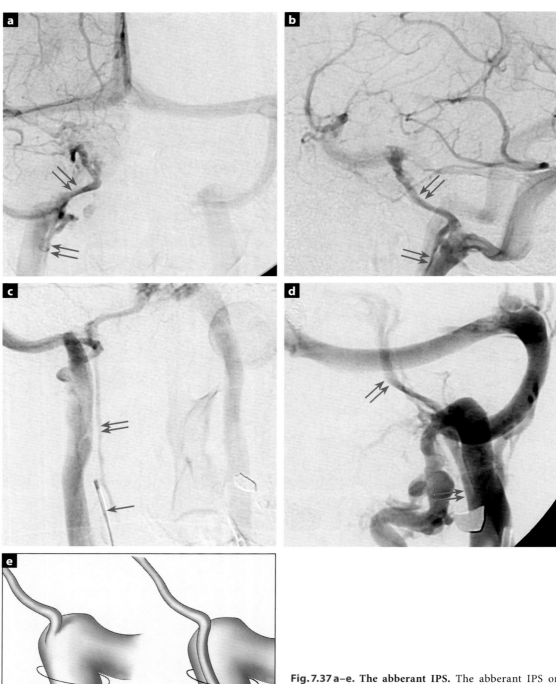

Fig. 7.37 a–e. The abberant IPS. The abberant IPS or "deep termination" can easily be overlooked on standard projections (**a, b**). The oblique projection in **c** facilitates understanding of this anatomic disposition and reveales that the IPS (*double arrows*) courses parallel to the IJV for several centimeters, before actually joining it. Recognizing this anatomic disposition may save valuable time during EVT. This anatomic variant has been successfully used as an approach for transvenous access to the CS in two cases (**d**, Benndorf et al. 2001). *Arrow* in **c**, catheter in ICA. **e** Illustration of normal and deep termination of the IPS

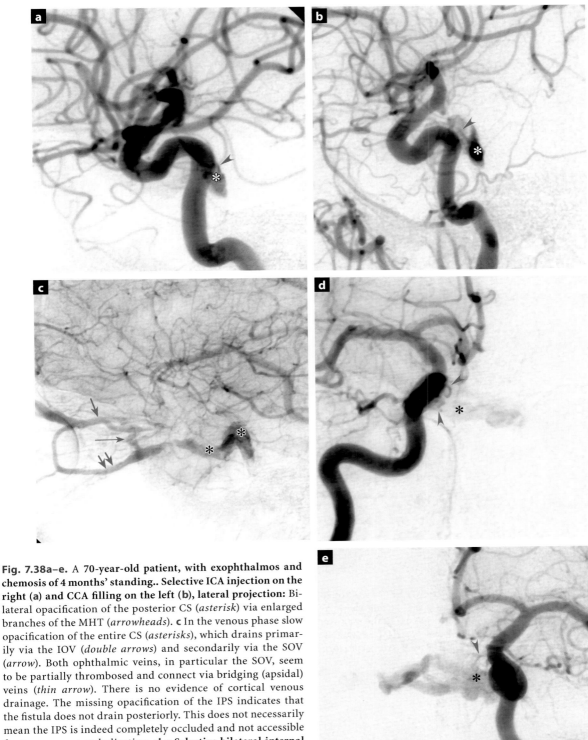

Fig. 7.38a–e. A 70-year-old patient, with exophthalmos and chemosis of 4 months' standing.. Selective ICA injection on the right (**a**) and CCA filling on the left (**b**), lateral projection: Bilateral opacification of the posterior CS (*asterisk*) via enlarged branches of the MHT (*arrowheads*). **c** In the venous phase slow opacification of the entire CS (*asterisks*), which drains primarily via the IOV (*double arrows*) and secondarily via the SOV (*arrow*). Both ophthalmic veins, in particular the SOV, seem to be partially thrombosed and connect via bridging (apsidal) veins (*thin arrow*). There is no evidence of cortical venous drainage. The missing opacification of the IPS indicates that the fistula does not drain posteriorly. This does not necessarily mean the IPS is indeed completely occluded and not accessible for transvenous embolization. **d,e** Selective bilateral internal carotid arteriograms, AP projection (same patient): The filling of the CS (*asterisk*) in the early arterial phase on the right (**a**), as well as on left (**b**) becomes more evident indicating a true bilateral fistula (*arrowheads*: tiny feeder arising from both, the right and left MHT)

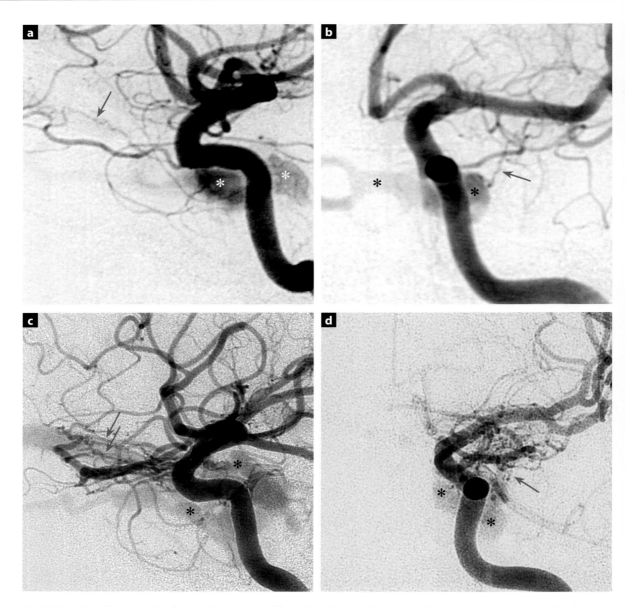

Fig. 7.39 a–d. Indirect supply of DCSFs by ICA-OA collaterals. a, b Not only TMH and ILT participate in the supply of DCSFs. Minute branches, such as this single recurrent meningeal branch arising from the ophthalmic artery, may contribute. **c, d** In this relatively high-flow dural AV shunt, the main supply from the ICA is not provided by ILT or TMH, but comes from multiple recurrent meningeal and posterior ethmoidal arteries (*arrows*) of the enlarged ophthalmic artery. This type of arterial supply is not fully covered by Barrows classification

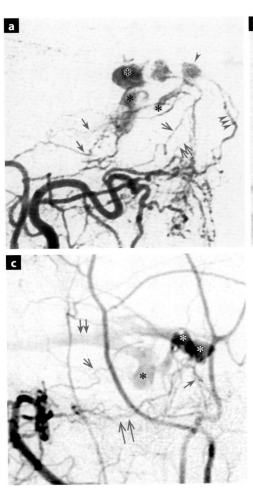

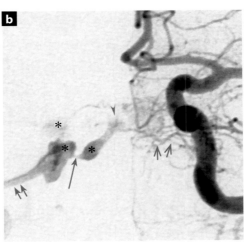

Fig. 7.40 a–c. Type-D fistula. A 77-year-old patient with diplopia and chemosis on the right side. Selective injection of the right ECA (**a**) and the left ICA (**b**) in AP view: Opacification of the intercavernous sinus (*arrowhead*) and the right CS (*asterisks*) by tiny dural arteries of the IMA: the AFR (*thin arrow*), the vidian artery (*thin double arrow*), and petrosal branches of the MMA (*short arrows*). Furthermore, supply by branches of the MHT (*thin arrows*) of the contralateral ICA. Note that some of the AV shunting is actually located in the midline (*arrowhead*) and that different fistulous compartments of the CS are opacified in **a** and **b**, communicating via a stenotic segment (*long arrow* in **b**). **c** Right ECA lateral view: The right CS (*asterisks*) drains the AV shunt initially into the IOV (*double arrows*) and secondarily in the SOV (not shown). Posterior drainage into the IPS is not visible. The AFR (*singular thin arrow*) and the vidian artery (*double thin arrows*) are shown. The branches supplied by midline anastomoses in **a** (*triple arrowhead*), are difficult to identify: Limitation of 2D-DSA.

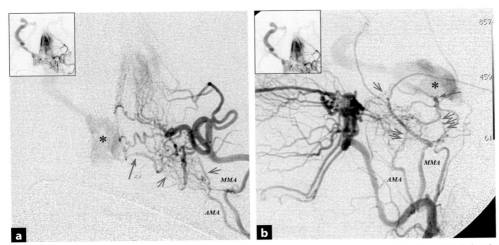

Fig. 7.41 a,b. A 78-year-old patient with exophthalmos, chemosis and diplopia. Selective ECA injection from the left side in Waters' (**a**) and lateral (**b**) views. **a** Opacification of the right CS (*asterisk*) by multiple feeding pedicles from the contralateral ECA, forming a network (*thin arrows*) and converging to a small channel (*arrow*) that connects with the right side. **b** The AFR (*singular thin arrow*), branches from the AMA (*thin double arrow*) and the MMA (*thin triple arrows*) can be identified better in lateral view. *Insets*: later phases. (Modified from BENNDORF 2002)

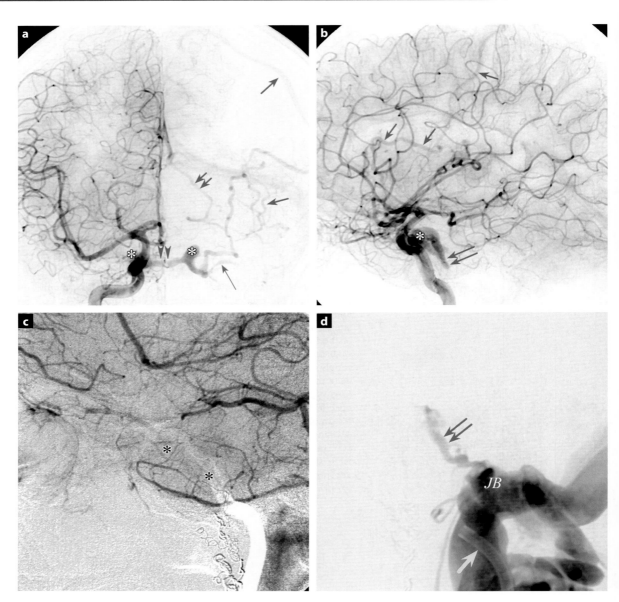

Fig. 7.42 a–d. A 71-year-old patient with left-sided conjunctival injection caused by a right CS AV shunt. **Right ICA injection AP (a) and lateral (b) views**: Opacification of the right CS from branches of the right MHT. Drainage to the contralateral side via the intercavernous sinus to the left CS. From here, only minimal filling of the presumably partially occcluded left SOV (*thin arrow*) is seen. Significant drainage via leptomeningeal and deep veins (*short double arrow*: basal vein of Rosenthal), as well as cortical veins (*arrow*) of the left hemisphere is evident. The tapered IPS appearance usually indicates a recent thrombosis, and thus does often not prevent catheterization. **c, d** Same patient. **Right ICA venogram, lateral (c)**: In the late venous phase, neither the CS (*asterisks*) nor the IPS is opacified. **Phlebogram of the right IJV, lateral (d)**: The 6-F guiding catheter (*thick arrow*) should be positioned below the jugular bulb (*JB*) so that vessels entering the IJV at a lower level are less likely missed. Often only then, the irregular lumen of the thrombosed IPS (*double arrow*) becomes more or less visible as a short stump. Changing position of the catheter and repeated injections may help to identify an aberrant IPS (Fig. 7.37). This patient was successfully treated using this IPS as a venous route (Benndorf et al. 2000)

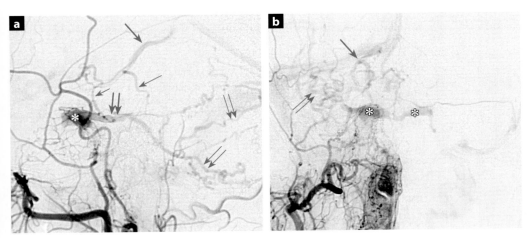

Fig. 7.43 a,b. Posterior leptomeningeal and deep venous drainage in a DCSF. a,b When a fistula involves mainly the posterior CS (*asterisks*), the drainage may not use anterior tributaries. In such a case, the IPS is most likely thrombosed and the only reamaining exit is the SPS (*double arrow*) subsequently emptying into the anterior pontomesencephalic vein (*short thin arrow*), the lateral mesencephalic vein (*thin arrow*), the basal vein of Rosenthal (*arrow*) and cerebellar veins (*thin double arrows*). This patient presented without neurological deficit, as do the majority of patients with DCSFs and cortcial drainage. The term "leptomeningeal venous drainge" may be a more suitable description for this drainage pattern than just "cortical venous drainage"

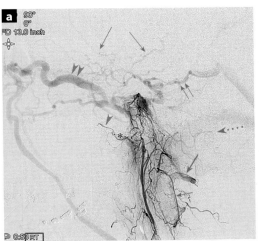

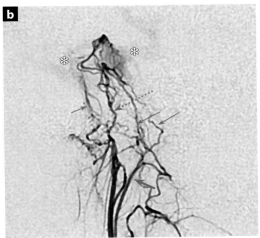

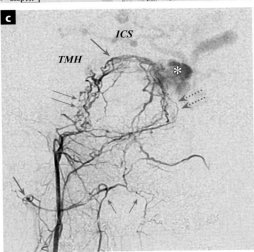

Fig. 7.44a–c. Complex DCSF. Selective injections into the APA are very useful for pre-treatment evaluation. They often reveal better the angioarchitecture than global ECA/ICA injections as there is little superimposition by normal vascular territories. **a** Right APA injections, lateral view, revealing the different types of venous drainage: anterior (SOV), cortical (Sylvian veins, *arrow*), deep (basal vein of Rosenthal, *double arrow*) and posterior (cerebellar veins, *dotted arrow*). Cortical venous drainage into Sylvian arises ususally from the lateral CS, while posterior leptomeningeal and deep venous drainage commonly arises from the posterior CS and SPS. Such a disposition may become important when selective coil packing is performed. Blocking the flow into the SOV will increase the flow and pressure in the other venous exits. Coil packing should ideally be performed so that blockage of the cortical and deep venous drainage is assured during the procedure (see Chap. 8). *Large arrow*: Vertebral artery, *short arrow*: Odontoid arch, *arrowhead*: Pterygovaginal artery, anastomosis with the internal maxillary territory via branches to the Eustachian tube (*asterisk*). **b** Magnified view shows the arterial supply from clival branches (*arrows*) of the neuromeningeal trunk (*thick arrow*), carotid branch from the superior pharyngeal artery (*long dotted arrow*) and an additional anterior anastomosis (*short arrow*). **c** Filling of clival branches of the right (*arrows*) and left (*dotted arrows*) side through midline anastomoses. There is some early filling of the right CS (*large arrow*), before draining via the ICS towards to the left side, indicating a small AV fistula on this side, while the main AV shunting involves the left CS (same patient as in Fig. 7.44c,d)

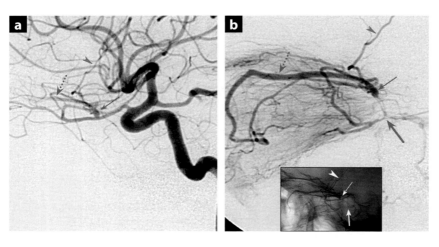

Fig. 7.45 a,b. Intraorbital, paracavernous DAVF. a ICA injection, lateral view. The AV shunt (*arrow*) is actually located at the level of the superior orbital fissure (SOF), supplied by the same recurrent meningeal branch as in Fig. 7.44, but shunting directly into the proximal SOV. **b** Superselective injection after navigation of a microcatheter into the CS and IOV (*thick arrow*, inset). The SOV is thrombosed in its distal portion and fills retrogradely from the IOV via a bridging (apsidal) vein. No angiographic evidence for a communication between SOV and CS. Not a true DCSF, although angiographic appearance is alike, and causing similiar symptoms (see Figs. 4.5. and 7.72). *Arrowheads:* Frontal MMA branch.

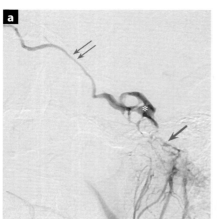
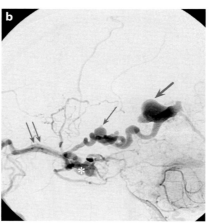

Fig. 7.46 a,b. Two non-cavernous DAVFs causing symptoms that mimic a DCSF. a APA injection, lateral view: DAVF of the IPS (*thick arrow*), supplied by clival branches of the neuromeningeal division and draining into the CS (*asterisk*) and SOV (*double arrow*), causing diplopia due to 4th and 6th nerve palsy. **b VA injection, lateral view:** Tentorial DAVF at the vein of Galen (*thick arrow*) with anterior drainage via the basal vein of Rosenthal (*arrow*) and CS (*asterisk*) into both SOVs (*double arrow*) causing exophthalmos and visual deficit (BENNDORF et al. 2003)

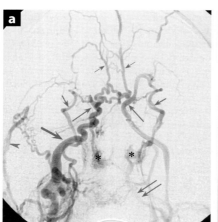
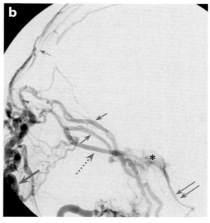

Fig. 7.47a,b. Maxillo-facial AVF draining into the SOV, CS and IPS. The main drainage of this AVF is directly via the enlarged and tortuous right facial vein (*thick arrow*), angular veins (*arrows*) filling both SOVs (*short arrows*) and the CSs (*asterisks*) and from here into the left IPS (*double arrow*). Note the filling of supraorbital and frontal veins (*short thin arrows*) and the middle temporal vein (*dotted arrow*)

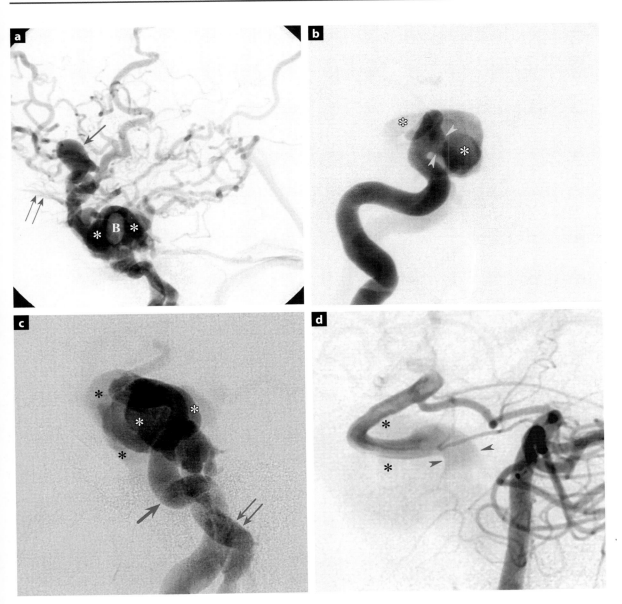

Fig. 7.48 a–d. True high-flow CSF. A 28-year-old patient, presented after car accident 2 years previously, Type-A fistula. **a ICA arteriogram, lateral:** In contrast to DCSFs, in direct fistulas, frequently multiple ectatic cortical veins develop due to a complete arterial steal that is caused by the high flow: No opacification of intracranial arteries in the ipsilateral hemisphere. Note, the venous aneurysm (*arrow*) is, according to current angiomorphologic criteria, a risk factor for bleeding. *Thin double arrows*: Superior ophthalmic vein, which is only to a minor extent involved in the drainage. Even in so-called "high-flow" DCSFs, such extensive cortical venous drainage is not observed. **ICA arteriogram (6 frames/second) early arterial phase, AP (b) and lateral (c):** The large defect in the carotid wall (*arrowheads*) is only recognizable in AP projection and despite the higher frame rate (6 frames/second) not clearly visible in lateral view, due to the very rapid filling of the enlarged CS (*asterisks*). Significant enlargement of the IPS (*double arrow*), which has gained a caliber, equal to the that of the ICA (*I*). **d Huber's maneuver:** Vertebral arteriogram, lateral view. Under manual compression of the carotid artery and simultaneous contrast injection into the vertebral artery, the location of the wall defect between C4- and C5-segment (*arrowheads*) can readily be identified. Its exact size and orientation (medial or lateral) remains difficult to evaluate: Limitation of 2D-DSA. (During EVT of a direct CSF, a detachable balloon can be navigated through the carotid tear and is inflated until occlusion of the fistula is documented. In some cases, such balloons may deflate after detachment and the fistula reopens (oval filling defect "*B*" in **a**)

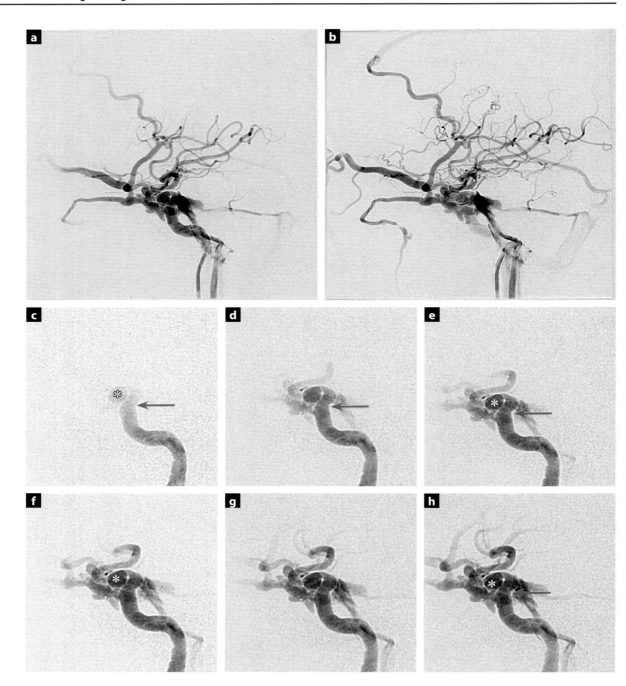

Fig. 7.49 a–h. Value of high frame rates for high-flow AV fistulas (here a direct CCF). a,b Standard 2D-DSA (3 frames/second) shows a high-flow CSF with an unclear fistula site. **c–h** Higher temporal resolution with 15 frames/second shows the fistula site better. Note that the earliest filled structure (*asterisk*) has a saccular, "aneurysm-like" appearance, which is most likely caused by a venous outpouching of the CS. This CCF was caused by a motorboat accident, not by a ruptured cavernous carotid aneurysm

7.2.5
Flat Detector Technology in Neuroangiography
(Figs. 7.50–7.57)

Flat detector (FD) technology was introduced in the early 1990s, almost 100 years after the discovery of X-rays by Conrad Roentgen. Initial medical applications were for thorax and skeletal X-rays, followed by digital mammography. Although it has only recently become possible to implement FDs in angiographic systems, image intensifier systems are rapidly being replaced in cardiac, general and neuroangiography. The main reason for this development is a clearly improved image quality of 2D DSA imaging combined with other technological advantages.

The currently dominating FD technology is based on an indirect X-ray conversion process, using a cesium iodide (CsI) scintillator and an amorphous silicon active pixel matrix (Figs. 7.52–7.54). Cesium iodide can be grown as needle-shaped crystals measuring 5–10 μm in diameter, and ensuring that light reaches the photodiode with only little scatter, while limiting its lateral diffusion. This scintillator also has very good X-ray absorption properties (SPAHN 2005). The detector used in the system described here is 30 cm×43 cm (A-plane) and 20 cm×20 cm (B-plane) with a pixel size of 154×154 and 184×184 μm respectively. This pixel size is optimized for high resolution required in diagnostic radiology and provides a square matrix of about 9 million pixels on the large detector.

FDs are smaller and add less weight to the C-arm allowing for faster rotations, providing more stability and fewer distortions. While image intensifier systems (II systems) used a multi-step conversion from X-ray beams into a digital image signal that causes increase of noise, this conversion is only a two-step process in FD technology (Figs. 7.50 and 7.52). Resulting advantages over II systems are more image formats, less geometric distortion, more homogenous exposure, excellent coarse contrast and high X-ray sensitivity. One of the most important features of FDs is their wide dynamic range (14 bit vs 12 bit in II systems). It allows one to cover a wider dose range without risking wrong exposure, which is particularly advantageous in angiography where broader dose ranges need to be covered from low levels of about 10 nGy to much higher system dose levels of about 5 μGy (SPAHN 2005).

The high dynamic range provides a better contrast resolution (16,384 different grey scale values available per pixel as opposed to 4096) allowing for soft tissue imaging using DynaCT (see below). In addition, an increase in image matrix from 1024×1024 (1 k) to 2480×1920 (2 k), allows for better identification of small arteries such as dural branches of the cavernous portion of the ICA. Figure 7.55 shows an example that demonstrates the improved image quality of 2D-DSA.

7.2.6
Rotational Angiography and 3D-DSA
(Figs. 7.58, 7.68 and 7.71–7.74)

Early experimental work on rotational angiography was performed in the 1970s and was quickly followed by clinical applications (CORNELIS et al. 1972; VOIGT et al. 1975). THRON and VOIGT (1983) were able to demonstrate that cerebral rotational angiography added value to the existing angiotomography or magnification angiography (WENDE and SCHINDLER 1970), techniques used at that time to improve visualization of cerebral aneurysms and AVMs. The authors used a 70-mm camera, mounted onto a C-arm that acquired one image every 5° during a 5–6 s sweep. Although digital subtraction was not possible at that time, the set up provided relatively good visualization of size, shape and orientation of cerebral aneurysms.

The next step was the development of the so-called 3D-morphometer by French investigators (HEAUTOT et al. 1998). The morphometer consisted of a CT gantry in which two X-ray tubes plus the image intensifier systems were integrated. This rather complex technology provided angiographic 3D images of aneurysms and AVMs of satisfactory quality.

Three-dimensional images of intracranial vasculature acquired with a rotating C-arm were presented for the first time by PICARD et al. (1997). Since then, a continuous improvement of 3D imaging using rotating C-arms has resulted in widely accepted clinical use of 3D angiography in neuroendovascular treatment.

Because the main focus in 3D angiography was initially on diagnosis of cerebral aneurysms and AVMs, bony structures adjacent to this vasculature compromised its visualization and were commonly removed during the image post processing (Siemens systems).

Advantages of simultaneous reconstructions of osseous and vascular structures have been demonstrated only to a limited degree (GAILLOUD et al. 2004), but are obvious in areas with a complex ar-

(Text continues on p. 142)

Image Intensifier

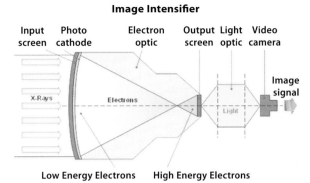

Fig. 7.50. Conversion process in an traditional image intensifier (II) uses multiple steps to convert an X-ray beam into a digital image signal (X-rays-light-electrons-light-electrons). This can cause increased background noise, while the spatial resolution is determined by the camera's resolution, which is usally 1K (1024×1024)

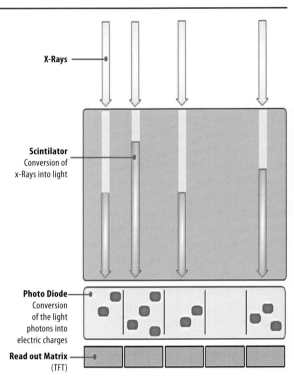

Fig. 7.52. As opposed to image intensifiers, the FD uses only a two-step (indirect conversion) conversion process (X-rays-light-electric signal)

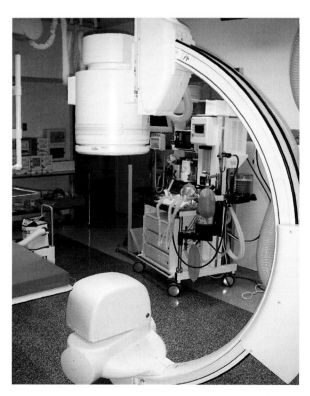

Fig. 7.51. C-arm mounted image intensifier of its last generation. This system has been used for rotational angiography and 3D-DSA since its introduction in the late 1990s (see examples in Figs. 7.70–7.73, 7.81, 7.83, 7.85)

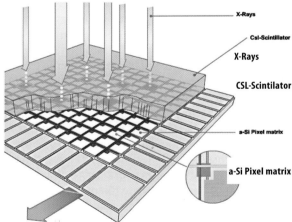

Fig. 7.53. New technologies employ flat detector (FD) with fast-imaging capability. The FD used in Siemens and Philips systems is based on Cesium Iodide (CsI), combined with an amorphous silicon active matrix array. This provides excellent quantum efficiency and a good resolution due to the needle-shaped or pillar-like crystal structure, limiting the lateral light diffusion. The matrix can be increased to 2K (2480×1920), although monitor systems for full 2K resolution are not commercially availabe yet. As an alternative, new medical grade displays (56 inch, 3840×2160 pixel) are recently available

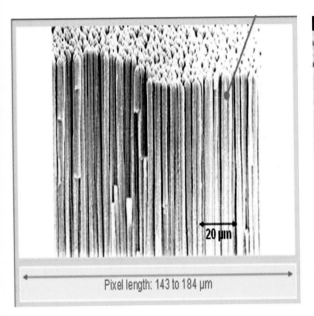

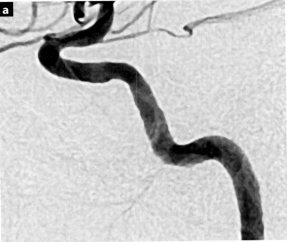

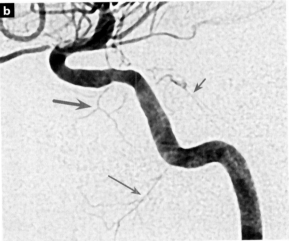

Fig. 7.54. The CsI crystals can be grown in needle-shaped form, measuring 5–10 μm. The size of one detector element (154 μm) defines (among other factors) the spatial resolution in an acquisition mode without binning (pixel binning). In order to reduce the size of data sets to be reconstructed, programs with various binning modes (1×1, 2×2 detector elements), faster rotations and fewer projections are used

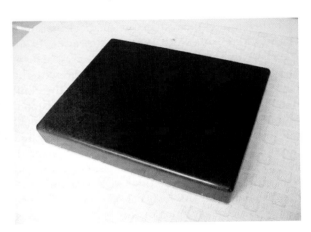

Fig. 7.55a,b. 2D-DSA demonstrating the improved image quality of cerebral angiograms using recent FD technology. Two arteriograms of the left ICA, same views in the same patient. **a** June 2004, **b** August 2006. Although the overall filling of the ICA in **a** appears better, opacification of the cavernous carotid branches, MHT (*short arrow*) and ILT (*arrow*), as well as of the mandibular artery (*thin arrow*) is clearly superior (not only sharper, but also reveals more branches). Note that in theory, the spatial resolution of an II system using the maximum zoom format is 6 LP/mm, while the FD reaches approximately 3 LP/mm. Various other factors including size of focal spot (0.3 mm), dynamic range (14 vs. 12 bit) and improved image post processing also play a role.

Fig. 7.56. Flat detector used in the current biplane systems Axiom Artis dBA.
  Area: 30×40 cm
  Pixel size: 154×154 μm (detector element size)
  Frame rates: Up to 30 fps (monoplane), 15 fps biplane. No binning: 7.5 fps
  Binning: 10 nGy–3.5 μGy
  Analog to digital conversion: 14 bit.

rangement of these components such as the skull base. For quite some time, investigators have been focusing on improving anatomic understanding using colored plastic casting of vessels in cadaver specimens as the main tool to investigate the minute and vascular anatomy imbedded in bony canals and foramina, especially in the middle cranial fossa and parasellar region (LASJAUNIAS 1984; SAN MILLAN RUIZ 1999; PARKINSON 1963, 1984; RHOTON et al. 1979, 1984). The use of 3D vascular imaging of the cavernous sinus and its related structures employing 3D angiography and modern reconstruction techniques, documented in the literature only scarcely (NISHIO et al. 2004; LASJAUNIAS et al. 2001, MITSUHASHI et al. 2007; HIU et al. 2009), has been of major interest for the author (BENNDORF 2002). Initial results of such 3D reconstructions (Figs. 7.70–7.73, 7.81 and 7.83–7.85), using non-subtracted rotational angiography, obtained with an II system (Neurostar, Siemens), which already encouraging. Using simultaneous reconstructions of the osseous and vascular structures, it has been possible to visualize small dural arteries and their course through skull base foramina. One can follow the artery of the foramen rotundum through its foramen and canal, the course of the AMA through the foramen ovale or anastomotic vessels through the foramen lacerum. Using this type of angiographic 3D imaging, identification of arteries feeding a DCSF becomes easier and is possible without using traditional 2D landmarks (BENNDORF 2002, 2008; HIU et al. 2009). Commonly, high-contrast tissue like bone causes reconstruction artifacts. Due to isotropic resolution of cone-beam reconstructions, as used in 3D-DSA, these artifacts become of minor importance (FAHRIG et al. 1997). Each voxel has the same size in the X, Y and Z directions, leading to a reduction of the non-linear partial volume effect. Visualization of vessels and bone in maximum intensity projections (MIPs) is possible because vascular density is increased up to 8000 HU, compared to 2000–2500 HU, typical for bone. The combination of high contrast and spatial resolution provides higher accuracy in displaying anatomic details, not obtainable using other imaging technology, including modern multi-slice CT scanners. Using an II system (C-arm mounted image intensifier), EL SHEIK et al. (2001) showed that high-resolution multiplanar reconstructions of osseous spongiosa can be obtained (rotational osteography). The usefulness of 3D reconstructions after cervical myelograms, revealing the relationship between contrast-filled thecal sac and osteophytes of the cer-

vical spine has also been demonstrated (KUFELD et al. 2003).

Image quality of angiographic 3D reconstructions has been significantly improved by the recent introduction of FD technology, as demonstrated in examples displaying small vessel reconstruction using the older II system (Neurostar, Siemens Medical) and the latest FD system (Axiom Artis, dBA, Siemens Medical) in Fig. 7.55. The current spatial resolution of the FD is defined by the size of its detector elements: 154 µm providing 0.13 mm which correspond to 4.1 Lp/mm (Nyquist frequency) in the unbinnend mode, while the maximum resolution of a Somatom 64 is 0.36 mm, corresponding to 1.4 LP/mm.

The available computing power can use a 20-s rotation with 543 projections only when two detector elements are combined (binned), which doubles the pixel size from 154 to 308 µm. Special programs, capable of using the full detector resolution, providing so-called 2 k datasets, are currently under evaluation.

Nonetheless, visibility of vascular and bony details is superior to conventional (II based) 3D-DSA or CT/CTA. This high spatial resolution is of importance for imaging small arteries such as the dural branches of the cavernous ICA and its communications with the ECA. The artery of foramen rotundum for example has a normal diameter of approximately 135 µm (LANG 1979).

Different from the arterial network within and around the CS, the venous anatomy appeared to be of rather minor interest in the medical literature (BRAUN and TOURNADE 1977; BRAUN et al. 1976). Hence, veins and sinuses in the middle cranial fossa and the CS region and its communications with the extracranial veins and venous plexus of the skull base are neither well studied nor fully understood. More recently, several investigators have pointed out the importance of these veins for anatomy and physiology (GAILLOUD et al. 2000; SCHREIBER et al. 2003; DOEPP et al. 2004; TAKAHASHI et al. 2005) of the cerebral blood circulation. Angiographic computed tomography (ACT, see below)-based MIPs, obtained using intravenous or intra-arterial contrast injections, can reveal even the smallest veins and sinuses in this area (BENNDORF 2002; NISHIO 2004; MITSUHASHI 2007).

Because of its superior spatial and temporal resolution, intra-arterial DSA is the imaging tool of choice for cerebral vascular lesions, primarily for arteriovenous shunting diseases. Analysis of radiology data is mostly done by reading 2D images. Interventional neuroradiologists and other endovascular neurosurgeons are forced to mentally combine multiple views to create a 3D model, adding further complexity to what is already a difficult task. This complex mental process constitutes a universal problem to be solved not only for surgeons using 2D information when operating vascular lesions in a 3D space, but also for the endovascular operator forced to use similar mental processing to translate 2D images. In order to monitor and control the catheter positions and the delivery of embolic devices and agents in a complex vascular structure such as the CS, complete understanding of 3D anatomy can become crucial.

Four main steps compose 3D angiography (Siemens system):

- Data acquisition:
  (Fig. 7.59) C-arm rotations between 5 and 20 s acquiring images in a projection matrix of 960×1240 (1 k) or 2480×1920 (2 k)
- Data transfer:
  The data are transferred using a fast 1:1 connection (100 Mb/s)
- Data reconstruction:
  Using the modified cone beam method of Feldkamp, axial slice images are calculated in a matrix of 256×256 or 512×512
- Data processing:
  Image post processing is performed using a dedicated software package (Syngo DynaCT, Leonardo, Siemens) in VRTs (In Space) or as MPRs or MIPs for cross-sectional imaging

The acquisition is obtained using a rotating C-arm with various program settings, depending on the clinical and diagnostic question. A standard 3D-DSA is performed using 5- or 10-s rotations, obtaining opacified 130 or 273 projections. After positioning the patient's head in both planes into the iso-center, the C-arm moves to two predetermined positions before starting the actual rotation. A 3D-DSA consists of an initial mask run and a second filling run. Projections are acquired in identical positions of the C-arm and angle triggered, allowing for a precise projection-angle determination for the reconstruction.

The total angle per rotation is typically 200° or 220°. During the filling run, contrast medium is injected either manually or using a power injector according to the length of rotation. A typical injection protocol for a 10-s rotation is 2.5 cc/s, a total of 28 cc. Images are then transferred to a workstation for post processing and automatically reconstructed using either a 256×256 or a 512×512 matrix, either as a subtracted or non-subtracted dataset. Second-

ary reconstructions can be performed using various matrix sizes, kernels and volumes of interest (VOIs). The steps necessary to obtain a 3D reconstruction may slightly differ among various manufacturers. The Allura system from Philips for example acquires usually a filling run only. For a subtracted reconstruction, the mask run has to be performed separately as a second step which causes delay and possible additional motion artifacts.

7.2.6.1
Dual Volume Technique (DVT) (Fig. 7.60)

Current software for angiographic systems (Axiom Artis dBA, Siemens Medical Solutions) allows for separately reconstructing the two components of a DSA rotational angiogram. The mask run is reconstructed to provide information on radiopaque objects within the projection field like bony structures, coils, clips or stents. Then, a second reconstruction is performed using the subtracted filling run, which contains only information on vascular structures filled during the rotation. In a 5-s rotation mainly arteries will be filleds, but during a 10-s rotation cerebral veins will also be filled. Both volumes can be loaded and interactively displayed on the Leonardo (Siemens Medical Solution) workstation. The user can freely choose the extent to which each volume is shown. This tool, initially developed to better separate coils or clips from residual or recanalized aneurysms, allows excellent imaging of the vascular-osseous relationships in complex anatomical regions.

DVT permits visualization of vascular and osseous anatomy simultaneously and allows for identifying their precise anatomical relationship without interfering with each other. DVT is further helpful for demonstrating a coil mass, clip or stent in relation to an aneurysm neck. Consequently, aneurysm regrowth, misclipping and stent malapposition can be detected more easily than on 2D-DSA images.

7.2.6.2
Angiographic Computed Tomography (ACT), DynaCT (Siemens), C-arm Flat Detector CT (FD-CT), Flat Panel CT (FP-CT) or Cone Beam CT (Figs. 7.58, 7.59, 7.61–7.69)

The integration of flat detectors into rotating C-arms in combination with a higher number of projections per rotation has led to another new modality that allows cross-sectional "CT-like" images to be obtained. The use of multiplanar reconstructions, based on rotational angiograms or radiograms, is per se not new

(Text continues on p. 146)

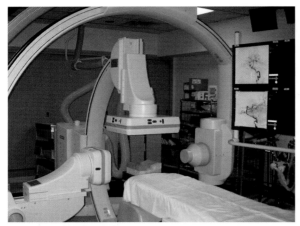

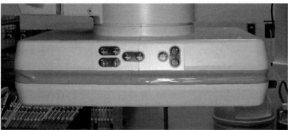

Fig. 7.57. Biplane FD system with a large FD (30×40 cm) for the A-plane and a small FD (20×20) for the B-plane (or two large FDs are currently also available). Reconstructions based on rotational angiograms (radiograms) allow cross-sectional (CT-like) imaging that provides soft tissue visualization (DynaCT) superior to that obtainable with image intensifier systems (The Methodist Hospital Houston)

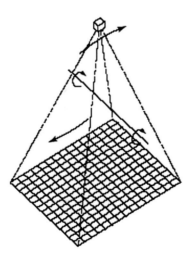

Fig. 7.58. Cone beam CT is based on the measurement of an entire volume (cone) in one single orbit, obtained with either image intensifier or flat panel detector systems (from SUETENS 2002)

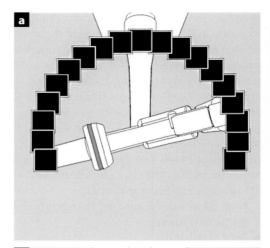

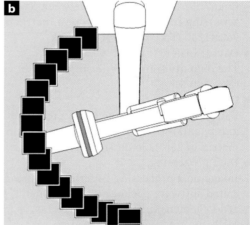

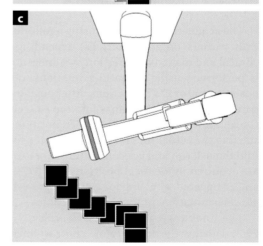

Fig. 7.59a–c. The rotating C-arm is capable of aquiring up to 543 projections (20 s, increment 0.4) that are mostly used to reconstruct a 3D dataset within less than a minute. This 3D volume can be viewed in a cross sectional imaging mode either as multiplanar reconstructions (MPRs), maximum intensity projections (MIPs) or in volume rendering technique (VRT)

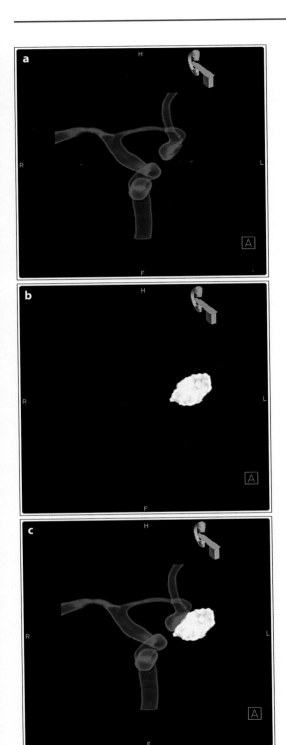

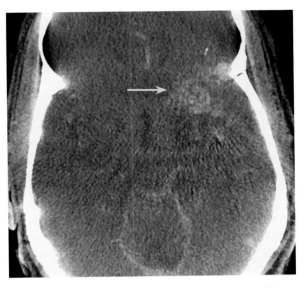

Fig. 7.61. DynaCT (543 projections in 20 s, 512×512 "bone normal"), 1 mm MPR. Intraprocedural bleeding that occurred during AVM embolization. Note, although the contrast resolution is lower than in conventional CT, hyperdensities caused by intraparenchymal blood (here mixed with some contrast after vessel perforation) become visible. In this case, no significant mass effect and no hydrocephalus was noted so that the procedure could be continued

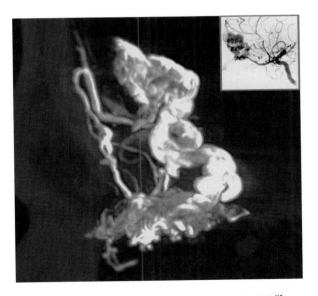

Fig. 7.62. DynaCT (543 projections in 20 sec, 512×512 "bone sharp") 20 mm MIP, shows postembolization cast of Onyx® after endovascular occlusion of a DAVF of the cribiforme plate (*inset*). The resolution of high-contrast objects, such as a cast of liquid embolic material is more detailed than achievable by digital radiography or conventional CT. This data set was obtained immediately postembolization, while the patient was still under general anesthesia on the angio table

Fig. 7.60. Dual volume technique (DVT). Both rotational sweeps are used for reconstructing two separate data sets. The filling run provides the vascular anatomy, while the mask contains the relevant background information, usually consisting of high-contrast objects, in this case the platinum coils. Both volumes are simultaneously viewed, while the amount of information being displayed can be freely chosen

and has been reported in a number of clinical applications. Its clinical use, however, has been limited to multiplanar reformatted images for visualization of high-contrast objects, such as contrast filled vessels or bony structures (3D myelogram, etc.).

In the past, cross-sectional imaging in neuroradiology has been mainly performed using conventional CT and MRI. The use of rotating C-arms in the angiographic suite was initially focused on 3D imaging of intracranial vascular lesions such as aneurysms and AVMs, employing mainly volume-rendering techniques.

Conventional CT or X-ray computed tomography produces cross-sectional images, based on X-ray attenuation. The word tomography stems from the Greek words tomos (slice) and graphe (write). Angiographic computed tomography (ACT, when contrast is used to opacify vascular structures) or DynaCT (Siemens) is a similar cross-sectional imaging modality based on the cone beam algorithm from Feldkamp, while in conventional CT parallel beam geometry, or in recent CT generations fan beam geometry, is usually employed. The terms flat detector CT, flat panel CT or C-arm CT are meanwhile synonymously used for what is technically cone beam CT.

The cone beam CT technology using C-arms was pioneered by Siemens but is meanwhile implemented by other vendors too (X-perCT by Philips). The description of technological details in the following chapter is based on the use of the first installed angiographic bi-plane FD system at the Methodist Hospital Houston, Texas. This system has been improved and continuously upgraded since September 2004.

The cone beam reconstruction algorithm is the basis for rotational 3D angiography, where the 3D datasets are reconstructed from a series of 2D projections. The method is derived from the standard fan beam formula. The density in one voxel is obtained as the sum of contributions from all projections through the voxel while the angle between two projections (increment) and the distance between the X-ray tube and the detector are taken into account (Suetens 2002).

With the introduction of FD technology into modern angiographic systems, cross sectional imaging in the angiographic suite has gained importance providing so-called low-contrast imaging. In particular, the improved contrast resolution due to the wider dynamic range (see above) currently allows for "soft tissue imaging" in the angiographic room. Using a 20-s single rotation acquiring 543 non-subtracted projections (Axiom Artis, Siemens), a contrast resolution of < 10 HU can be achieved, allowing for visualizing low contrast structures such as grey and white matter and the delineation of brain tissue from the intracranial ventricular system. In other words, this cross-sectional imaging allows for visualization of hyperdense intracranial lesions such as subarachnoid hemorrhage (SAH), hematoma caused by vessel perforation during an endovascular treatment or a developing hydrocephalus. Early recognition and monitoring of intraprocedural complications during neuroendovascular treatment has become possible and is of great value for interventional neuroradiologists and endovascular neurosurgeons (Heran et al. 2006). DynaCT contributes to the overall safety of EVT (Figs. 7.61 and 7.62), which is of particular importance for the often time-consuming transvenous embolizations of DAVFs or DCSFs.

7.2.6.3
Image Post-Processing (Figs. 7.63–7.65)

Various software tools for post-processing and analyzing angiographic volume data sets are in use today. Similar to CTA, they employ dedicated display modes, such as MPRs, MIPs or VRTs. Because not every interventional neuroradiologist or endovascular neurosurgeon may be familiar with 3D imaging some of the basic principles are explained in the following.

- 1. MPR: Multiplanar Reformatting – technique to display up to three orthogonal cut planes using the averaged voxel values along one beam, which can be correlated with a true 3D image.
- 2. MIP: Maximum Intensity Projection – technique to display up to three orthogonal cut planes using the maximum voxel values along one beam.
- 3. VRT: Volume-Rendering Technique – technique to visualize the structure of volume datasets.
- 4. SSD: Surface Shaded Display – technique to visualize a surface that corresponds to an iso-value in the dataset.

1. Multiplanar Reformatting (MPR) is one of the oldest visualization techniques used for viewing 3D medical images, providing the possibility for an arbitrarily positioned and oriented 2D plane to be placed in a 3D data set so that the projection of the data on that plane may be viewed. In modern software packages there are usually three planes simultaneously shown, each of them corresponding to one of the major axes, sagittal, coronal and axial (Fig. 7.63). This allows for precise orientation and localization of any object in the 3D data set. The

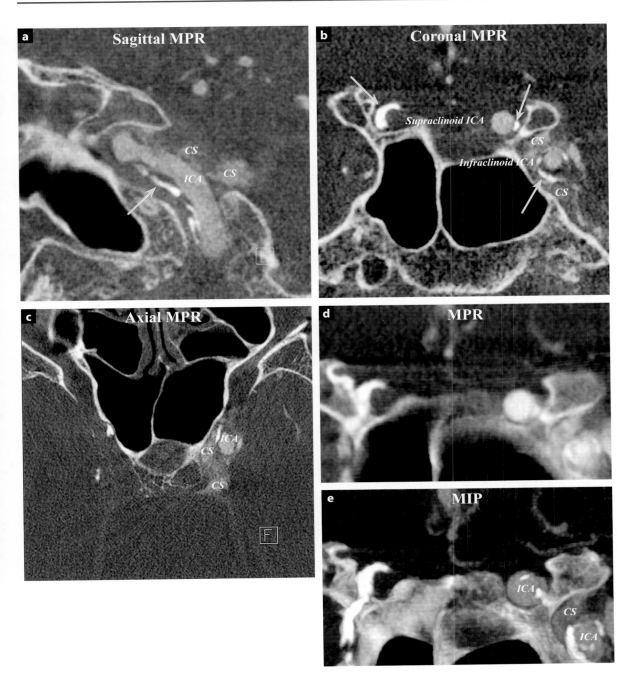

Fig. 7.63 a–e. Cross-sectional imaging in the angiographic room. a–c 1-mm Multiplanar reformatted images (MPRs) of a DynaCT (20 s, 543 projections, 20% of 300 mg Iodine, 2 cc/s, 40 cc) showing the CS region. Views are available in three orthogonal planes (sagittal, frontal and axial) that can be tilted and rotated into any desired angle. Curved reformatted images are also possible. Note the calcifications of the carotid wall on both sides (*arrows*). **d–e** 5-mm MPR and 5-mm MIP: Increasing thickness of the MPR causes blurring of the object contours while the MIP remains relatively sharp, allowing for delineation of the ICA, surrounding bone and calcifications

thickness of the planes can be adjusted to the size of the object (e.g. vessel diameter) and they can be moved along a relevant axis to provide the desired view. Curved reformations in any direction are possible and extremely useful to provide views inside the lumen of a curved anatomic structure (vessels, osseous canals etc.).

2. Maximum Intensity Projection (MIP) is a volumetric imaging technique that uses only the brightest voxel (hence maximum intensity) along one beam to be projected into a picture (Fig. 7.64). Objects with high density, such as contrast filled vessels, calcifications and metal structures such as clips, stents and coils, appear brighter while the surrounding tissue remains dark grey. MIPs can visualize very small structures with high density; however, they do not provide a depth perception. Thus, the viewer cannot decide if a bright structure is in front or in the background of the volume he is looking at. To improve the visualization, background structures suppressed by appropriate windowing, whereby an effect of semi-transparency can be obtained. The volumes can be interactively rotated and three orthogonal planes can be simultaneously visualized. The lack of depth information has to be considered when viewing thick MIP images (10–40 mm), because it may exaggerate certain findings and more importantly, obscure others (RYBICKI et al. 2006).

MIPs are visually appealing and provide superior detection of details in high contrast objects such as very small vessels or stents. For diagnostic purposes or measurements, MIPs are of limited value and should be used prudently.

3. Volume Rendering Technique (VRT), probably the most widely applied method for display of three-dimensional structures, uses a mean value corresponding to a value of absorption as seen in an X-ray image (Figs. 7.65 and 7.66). A volume rendered image represents the complete dataset and does not rely on surface information. All voxels are rendered with a specifically assigned opacity (VAN OOIJEN and IRWAN 2006). In contrast, in an MIP obtained out of 256 slices of a 256×256 matrix, less than 1% of the original information is used. In other words, the original information is reduced to about 1%. Today, VRT has replaced SSD in most software packages on graphic workstations. In VRT, the identification of different tissue types is based on grey or color-grey value rendering, in which the visible part can be modified using a so-called histogram (transfer function). Since all information is stored, the range of visible objects can be interactively modified by changing this window and only structures relevant to the viewer, e.g. blood vessels, coils and clips, are made visible.

This transfer function is advantageous as compared to SSD, where after each change of the threshold a new calculation is required. The additional use of colors allows for a better separation of certain structures such as vessels and coils or clips.

A volume rendered image is intrinsically not a 3D image, but opacity and brightness can be modified so that the surface of a dataset becomes a more-dimensional appearance. Using a specific cutting tool and six variable clip planes, further editing is possible. Bones or overlying vessel loops can be eliminated so that only relevant structures in the volume of interest (VOI) are left. Semitransparent images may be of particular value when visualizing AVMs or cerebral aneurysms.

For vascular lesions at the skull base or parasellar region, it is generally of interest to visualize adjacent osseous structures as well. For this purpose, both non-subtracted projections and appropriate windowing allows for the display of bony structures in a more or less "radiolucent" (X-ray like) or transparent fashion. This facilitates identifying not only the vasculature of the skull base, but also its actual relationship with imbedding osseous structures.

7.2.6.4
3D Studies of the Cavernous Sinus Region
(Figs. 7.68–7.91)

In the past, both radiologists and manufacturers have given little attention to the imaging of normal vascular anatomy using 3D angiography. Angiographic visualization of small arteries, such as dural branches of the cavernous ICA, has been limited by the spatial resolution and the traditional 2D display of a standard DSA. Thus, 3D imaging of small arteries and veins in complex anatomical regions would have significant value as it contributes to our understanding of both normal vascular anatomy as well as pathological lesions. The following section focuses particularly on 3D imaging of the cavernous sinus region using rotational angiography and radiography. Of major interest for the author was: (1) the visualization of small anastomosing branches between ECA and ICA territories when coursing through the skull base, middle cranial fossa and the cavernous sinus and (2) the detailed venous ar-

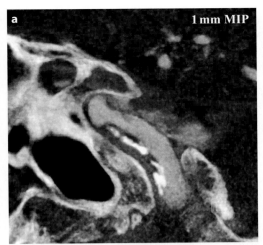

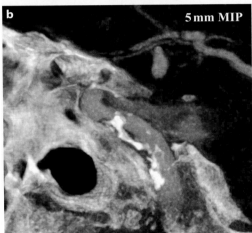

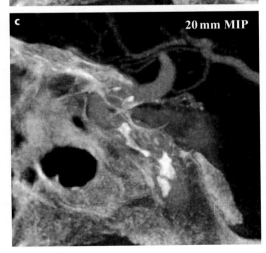

Fig. 7.64 a–c. Maximum intensity projections (MIPs) of a carotid syphon in different thicknesses. With increasing thickness of the MIP, more objects, or an entire vessel segment become visibile, while other information, such as the non-calcified lumen may become obscured by overlay with adjacent osseuous structures. There is no depth perception (**c**)

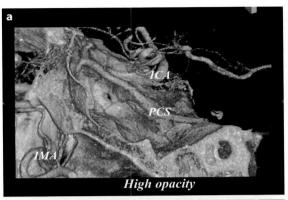

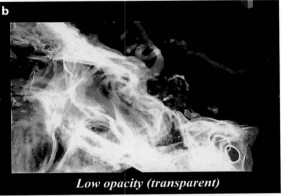

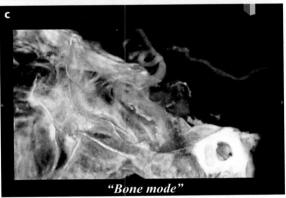

Fig. 7.65a–c. Volume rendering techniques (VRTs) of the same dataset in three different viewing modes using sagittal clip planes. Manipulations of the transfer function, opacity and brightness permit choosing a display setting that provides the most relevant information. Increasing opacity (**a**) allows visualization of vessels closer to the viewer, such as the paracavernous sinus (PCS) and the internal maxillary artery (IMA). **b** The transparent mode is useful for identifying vascular loops. Calcifications of the ICA wall may be obscured and are better seen in **c**. Note also the difference in depth perception between the VRTs and the MIPs in Fig. 7.64c

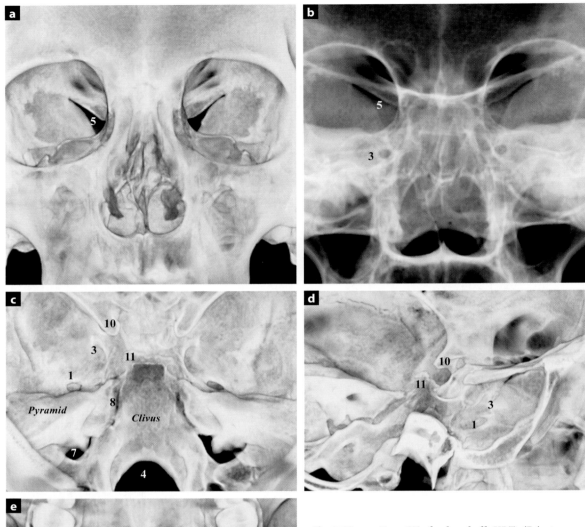

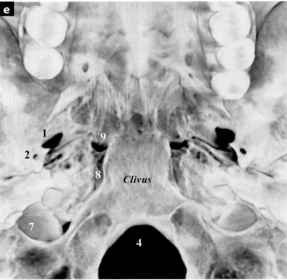

Fig. 7.66 a–e. DynaCT of a dry skull, VRTs (B in transparent mode resembling a skull X-ray): **20 s rotation, 543 projections, 1024×1024.** Excellent visualization of the skull in opaque (**a**), and transparent (**b** resembling a skull X-ray) mode. Bony landmarks and foramina of the middle cranial fossa can be readily identified at the inner surface (**c, d**). **e** View onto the outer surface of the central skull base. Compare to Fig. 3.1

  1 Foramen ovale
  2 Foramen spinosum
  3 Foramen rotundum (canalis rotundis)
  4 Foramen magnum
  5 Superior orbital fissure
  6 Carotid canal
  7 Jugular foramen
  8 Petroclival fissure
  9 Foramen lacerum
10 Anterior clinoid process
11 Posterior clinoid process

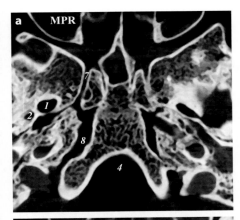

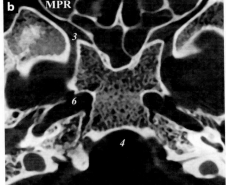

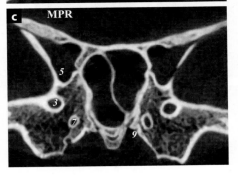

Fig. 7.67a–c. DynaCT of a dry skull: 0.2 mm multiplanar reconstructions (MPRs) (20 s rotation, 543 projections, 1024×1024).

Visualization of the osseus skull base in orthogonal planes, usually sagittal, coronal and axial (oblique and curved MPRs are possible). Osseous foramina, canals and fissures can be simultaneously visualized in three orthogonal planes, here showing two axial (**a, b**) and one coronal plane(s) (**c**). Note in coronal plane, the most common alignment of the three posterior foramen of the pterygopalatine fossa carrying each an artery that may serve as anastomosis between ECA and ICA territory: The foramen rotundum most lateral and superior, the vidian canal in the middle, and the pterygovaginal canal most medial and inferior (Rumboldt et al. 2002). In this example the pterygovaginal canal is incomplete (semicanal). Also visible is the SOF that is not directly connected to the PPF, but indirectly via the orbit and IOF.

1 Foramen ovale
2 Foramen spinosum
3 Foramen rotundum (canalis rotundis)
4 Foramen magnum
5 Superior orbital fissure
6 Carotid canal
7 Vidian canal
8 Petroclival fissure
9 Pterygovaginal canal (semicanal)

chitecture of the CS and its connections with the IPS/IJV junction.

The majority of small dural arteries that arise from the ECA enter the intracranium through skull base foramina, and are often not sufficiently visualized on standard 2D-DSA. Although their topography has been studied extensively by various investigators (Parkinson 1984; Rhoton et al. 1984; Lasjaunias et al. 2001; Lang 1979; Hacein-Bey et al. 2002), these vessels are not always easy to identify due to their small size and overlying bony structures. Likewise, the venous anatomy in this region is to date not fully understood due to limited capacity

of 2D-DSA to visualize peculiar and complex venous structures.

The origin and course of dural branches involved in the complex angioarchitecture of the cavernous sinus has been the topic of numerous anatomical-radiological studies. Superselective arteriography of ECA branches has been introduced by Castaigne et al. (1966), Newton and Hoyt (1968) and others (Djindjian and Merland 1978). The extensive work of Djindjian and Merland (1978) has invaluably contributed to our understanding of cranio-facial vascular anatomy and still remains unmatched to this date. Lasjaunias and Berenstein (1987) and

(Text continues on p. 156)

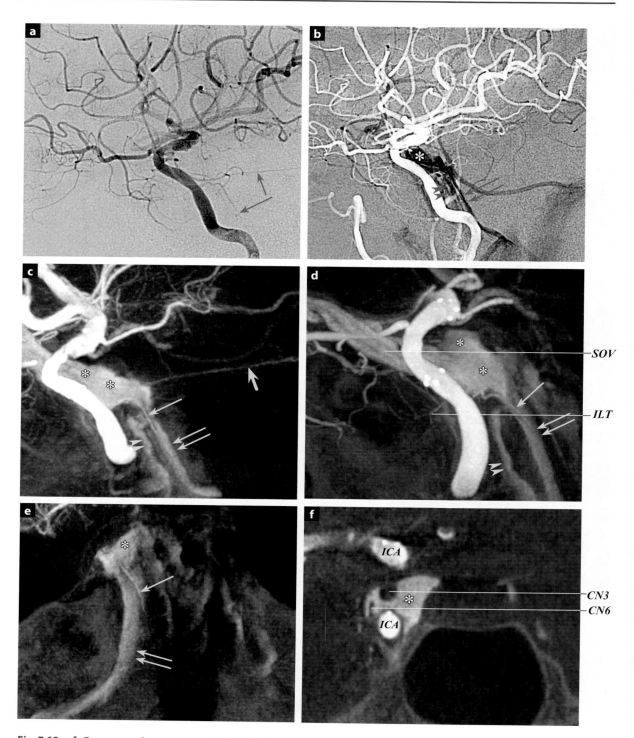

Fig. 7.68 a–f. Cavernous sinus anatomy. DSA (prior) and ACT (after) in a patient undergoing intracranial stenting. **a** Note the opacification of the marginal tentorial artery (*short arrow*) and the clival branch arising from the MHT (*long arrow*). **b** Early filling of the CS (sequential subtraction). **c–f** Simultaneous opacification of the ICA (bright) and the CS that drains into the IPS (*double arrow*) and IPCV (*arrowheads*). **c** Lateral, **d** oblique view. **e** Posterior view that shows the course of the clival artery (*arrow*) crossing the IPS (*double arrow*). **f** Delineation of the oculomotor and the abducens nerves within the opacified CS. CN3 is the most cephaled nerve, while CN6 is considered the only nerve lying in fact within the CS. ACT has very low temporal resolution as compared with DSA, but provides valuable three dimensional anatomic information

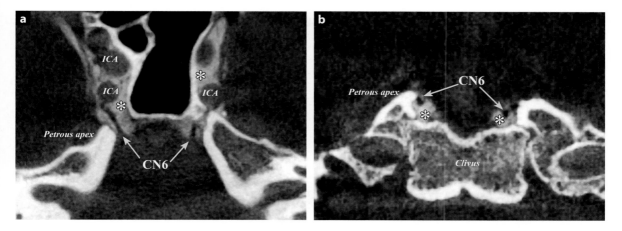

Fig. 7.69a,b. Visualization of cranial nerves in the CS using ACT (10 s 3D-DSA, Axiom Artis). The axial (**a**) and coronal (**b**) MIPs (0.2 mm) show an indirect opacification of the CS (*asterisks*), delineating its vascular and neural contents. The course of the abducens nerve (*CN6*) through Dorellos canal between the petrous apex and the clivus becomes well visible. The bow-shaped Dorello's canal, through which the abducens nerve courses before reaching the cavernous sinus, is located inside a venous confluence, which occupies the space between the dural leaves of the petroclival area. The abducens nerve perforates the dura, courses below the petrosphenoidal ligament of Gruber and reaches the lateral wall of the intracavernous *ICA*

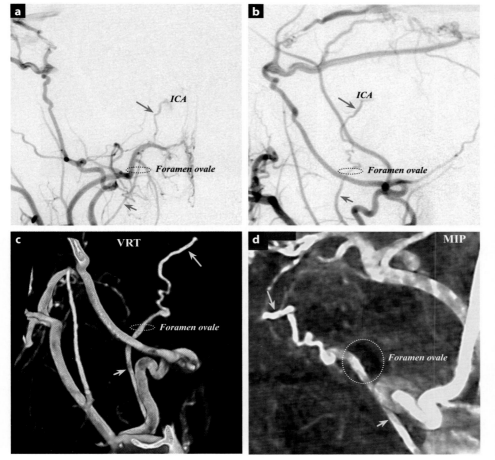

Fig. 7.70a–d. Angio-architecture of ECA/ ICA anastomoses using 3D-DSA. Right ECA arteriogram in AP (a) and lateral (b) views. Arteriovenous shunt, supplied by the MMA with an additionally enlarged AMA (*short arrow*) giving rise to a branch that courses cranially to reach the ILT (*arrow*). 3D Rotational angiography with Neurostar (non-subtracted, 8 s rotation, 80 projections), lateral view. **c** The VRT shows the AMA (*short arrow*) and its connection to the posteromedial branch of the ILT (*arrow*). In axial view (MIP), the related osseous structure (**d**) is visualized and the course of the anastomosing branch (*arrow*) through the foramen ovale (*dotted circle*) can be seen. (Modified from BENNDORF 2002)

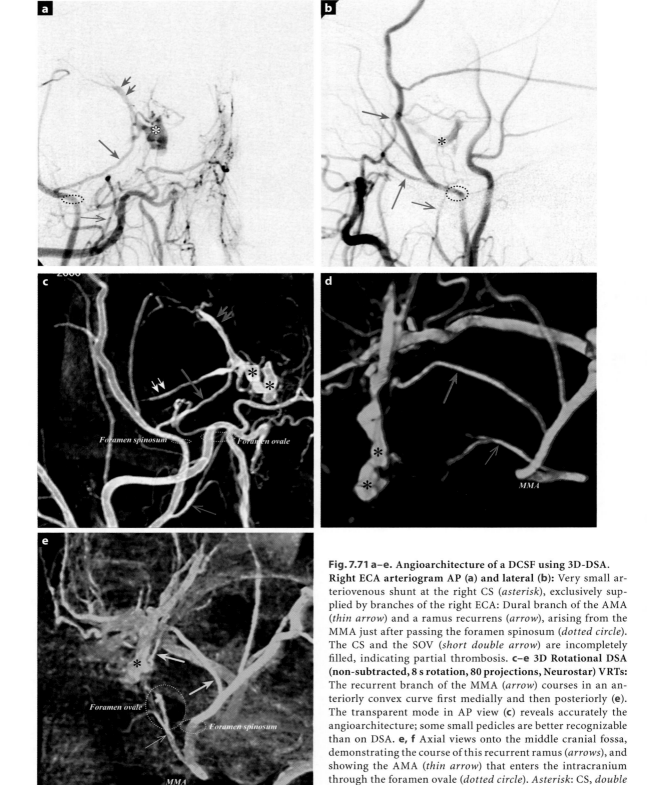

Fig. 7.71 a–e. Angioarchitecture of a DCSF using 3D-DSA.
Right ECA arteriogram AP (a) and lateral (b): Very small arteriovenous shunt at the right CS (*asterisk*), exclusively supplied by branches of the right ECA: Dural branch of the AMA (*thin arrow*) and a ramus recurrens (*arrow*), arising from the MMA just after passing the foramen spinosum (*dotted circle*). The CS and the SOV (*short double arrow*) are incompletely filled, indicating partial thrombosis. **c–e 3D Rotational DSA (non-subtracted, 8 s rotation, 80 projections, Neurostar) VRTs:** The recurrent branch of the MMA (*arrow*) courses in an anteriorly convex curve first medially and then posteriorly (**e**). The transparent mode in AP view (**c**) reveals accurately the angioarchitecture; some small pedicles are better recognizable than on DSA. **e, f** Axial views onto the middle cranial fossa, demonstrating the course of this recurrent ramus (*arrows*), and showing the AMA (*thin arrow*) that enters the intracranium through the foramen ovale (*dotted circle*). *Asterisk*: CS, *double white arrow*: IOV. (Modified from BENNDORF 2002).

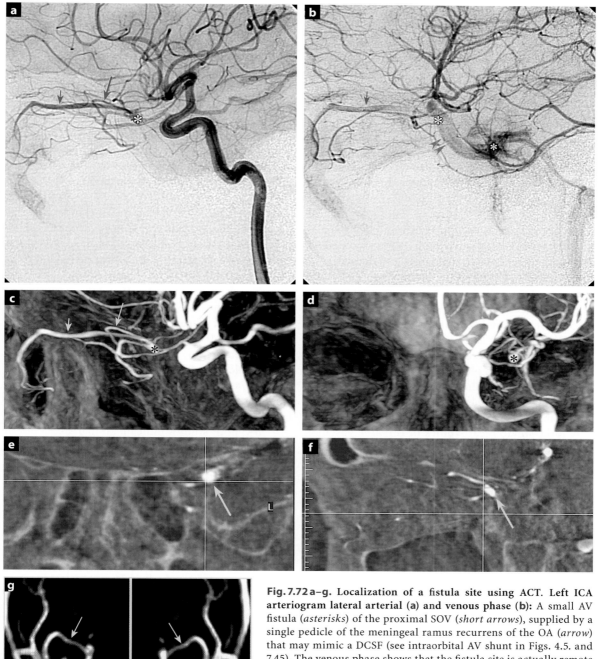

Fig. 7.72 a–g. Localization of a fistula site using ACT. Left ICA arteriogram lateral arterial (**a**) and venous phase (**b**): A small AV fistula (*asterisks*) of the proximal SOV (*short arrows*), supplied by a single pedicle of the meningeal ramus recurrens of the OA (*arrow*) that may mimic a DCSF (see intraorbital AV shunt in Figs. 4.5. and 7.45). The venous phase shows that the fistula site is actually remote from the CS (BW *asterisk*) and superimposed onto the SPPS (*arrowheads*). 3-Rotational Angiography (ACT with Neurostar, 14 s rotation, 132 projections). Thick MIPs, AP lateral (**c**) and AP (**d**) views: Visualization of the AV fistula with a feeding pedicle arising from the OA and draining vein in good quality, providing anatomical information equal to the DSA. **e–f** Coronal and sagittal, thin MPRs allow for localization of the fistula site (*arrow*) at the level of the superior orbital fissure (SOF). **g** In the VRTs, the course of the supplying feeder (*arrow*) arising from the OA and traveling lateral to the fistula point (*arrowheads*) is seen either from cranial (*left*) or from caudal (*right*). (Modified from BENNDORF 2002)

Lasjaunias (1984) followed this tradition in the late 1980s, using meticulously superselective arteriographs, obtained by manual subtraction techniques and providing an image quality superior to that of DSA at that time.

Digital subtraction angiography, developed in the late 1970s, but remarkably improved in the 1980s and 1990s, meanwhile allows for visualizing in greater detail arterial and venous anatomy in one of the most complex anatomic regions of the human body. But even this high-resolution DSA, the current gold standard for vascular imaging, is limited in its capacity to demonstrate reliably and understandably peculiar vascular anatomy. Thus, not only in the past but to date, angiographic studies have frequently been verified and complemented by detailed anatomic dissections (Lasjaunias and Berenstein 1987; Lasjaunias 1984; Parkinson 1963, 1984; Rhoton et al. 1979). Colored casts of cadaver vessels, obtained by injecting liquid plastics, were used to study detailed arterial and venous anatomy (Rhoton et al. 1984; San Millan Ruiz et al. 2002; Martins et al. 2005; Rhoton 2000). On the other hand, improved modern X-ray technology, using high resolution 3D DSA and contrast enhanced DynaCT, is capable of displaying 3D vascular and osseous anatomy in the CS region in surprising quality, facilitating remarkably radio-anatomical studies of this fine vascular network in vivo (Benndorf et al. 2000; Hiu et al. 2009).

The usefulness of 3D angiography for endovascular treatment of direct carotid cavernous fistulas has been recently reported by Kwon et al. (2005a) who found 2D-DSA less reliable in detecting a remaining pseudoaneurysm after balloon detachment. 2D-DSA indicated the possibility of traction-induced instability or intra-arterial balloon position, but 3D volume rendered images were superior in terms of diagnostic information. Cut planes, perpendicular to the vessel axis, provided orthogonal views, which permitted better identification of a residual fistula. Because a detachable balloon is contrast filled, as is the parent vessel, both structures can be made visible in their precise relationship. This type of imaging can become very helpful, after incomplete or subtotal balloon occlusion The exact site of a CCF can angiographically be identified performing Huber's or Mehringer's maneuver (Huber 1976; Mehringer et al. 1982); however, its exact orientation and size within the carotid wall can remain difficult to evaluate due to unopacified blood and large AV shunt volume, even when using higher frame rates such as 15 f/s (Fig. 7.43). VRTs may facilitate the identification of such a fistula site; however, its measured size depends on the threshold that is subjectively chosen by the viewer, a problem that is not solved by most current 3D software. Ishida et al. (2003) described a CCF, identified by 3D-DSA using VRT and virtual endoscopic view. The anatomical orientation of the fistula was easily understood. Yet its dimensions were not found measurable in a precise manner and the balloon size could not be selected based on the 3D-DSA. Both studies indicate an increasing use of 3D-DSA for evaluation of carotid cavernous fistulas.

MPRs or MIPs obtained by either DSA or ACT (contrast enhanced DynaCT) are in this regard superior to VRT as they allow a more precise analysis of the vessel morphology. Less dependant on subjective thresholding, the site of the carotid tear can

Fig. 7.73 a–h. Angioarchitecture of DCSF at the right CS using ACT. Right ECA injection AP and lateral view (**a, b**). The AV shunt is located at the right CS and supplied by several dural branches arising from the AMA (*thin arrow*), MMA (*long thick arrow*) and distal IMA (*short thick arrow*). **c–h** 3D-DSA (non-subtracted, 14 s rotation, 132 projections, manual injection, Neurostar). This example shows the course of dural branches supplying the AV shunt at the CS (*asterisk*); MIPs in coronal (*left*) and sagittal (*right*) plane. The AMA (*long arrow*) courses vertically and passes the foramen ovale to reach the intracranial dural network supplying CS AV shunt (**c,d**). The AFR (*short thick arrows*) courses posteriorly and vertically through the canalis rotundis and connects to the same network (**e,f**). The ACT further allows for identifying precisely the fistula site (*asterisk*, see also Figs. 7.72, 7.78). It is interesting to observe that an additional branch appears to arise from the sphenopalatine portion of the IMA, and courses similarly, but actually superior to the AFR, posteriorly to reach the AV shunt (*arrowheads*). This small artery passes apparently through both the inferior and superior orbital fissures and is also demonstrated in Figs. 7.77–7.79. *Insets*: showing the passage of corresponding branches through the foramen ovale (axial view in **e**), and through the foramen rotundum (coronal view in **f**). Additionally seen in **g** is the contribution from petrosal branches of the MMA (*long thick arrows*), as well as from clival branches of the APA (*dotted arrows*). *Asterisk*: CS AV shunt, *PPF*: Pterygopalatine fossa

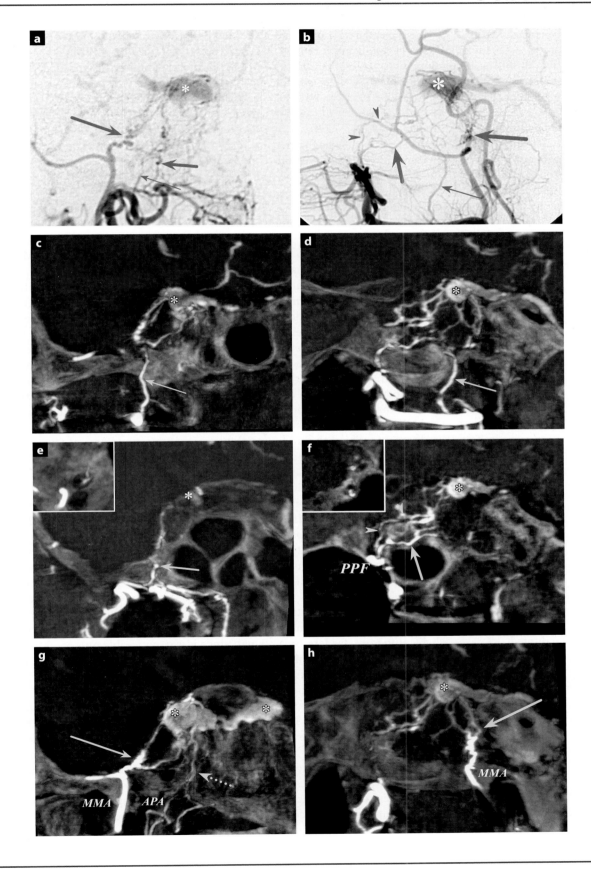

be easier identified; size measurements for potential use of detachable balloons becomes more reliable. In addition, accompanying osseous lesions, such as fractures of the temporal bone, can be detected. For precise localization of a dural CSF, ACT can be helpful too, as shown in an earlier study by the author using previous II technology (Figs. 7.71, 7.72).

Recently, the value of 3D-DSA has beens further enhanced by DVT, which specifically improves the understanding of anatomical arrangements between arteries or veins and their surrounding osseous structures. As shown in Figures 7.75 and 7.77, DVT allows for correlating the course of any vessel within its osseous neighborhood, along bony sutures and canals as well as through foramina in the skull base. The reconstruction matrix is usually 512×512, providing a voxel size of approximately 0.1 mm. Contrast application is performed using a 4- or 5-F diagnostic catheter, placed for standard angiography in the ECA or ICA. In some cases, a superselective injection using a microcatheter, placed within an ECA branch, the IPS or the CS itself, is useful and makes obtaining opacification of a selectively chosen territory possible. The advantage of DVT compared to anatomic dissections is that tissue can be virtually cut in slices without destroying it. The 3D volume remains entirely intact and such computerized graphic dissection can be repeated and reproduced as often as necessary. Also, the vessels have their physiologic dimensions as they are filled with blood under a certain pressure. MPRs simultaneously display three different cut planes, facilitating the orientation in space for the operator enormously. Curved reformatting mode allows for reconstruction along irregular and curved anatomic structures such as canals or vessel courses.

Figures 7.70–7.80 show how the identification of small arteries feeding an arteriovenous shunt is facilitated. In cases where numerous feeders or a network of arteries supplies a DCSF, 2D-DSA may not always provide sufficient information to fully understand the vascular topography. Despite extensive descriptions in textbooks using dissections and complex illustrations, mental translation of 2D images into 3D anatomy remains a difficult task, even for the experienced angiographer.

Figures 7.74–7.76 show that in some cases of dominant ECA supply of a cavernous AV shunt, the vessel referred to as artery of the foramen rotundum represents in fact not a single vessel but may instead consist of two or more small branches, passing through the canalis rotundis. This observation has not been reported in the literature.

Furthermore, in many arteriograms, the AP projection shows a bundle of vessels coursing posteriorly that are difficult or impossible to distinguish from each other, even when using lateral views. Figure 7.76 is an example of a DAVF at the sigmoid sinus with this type of complex arterial supply from the internal maxillary artery. By using 0.1–0.2 mm MPRs, 3D imaging of the osseous skull base in excellent quality is possible and allows depiction of fine details such as foramina and canals that provide the passage for nerves and vessels, as well as for spread of infectious or tumorous diseases. Every single branch of the arterial network, e.g. the MMA, AMA, the vidian artery, and the artery (-ies) of the foramen rotundum, can be related to their surrounding osseous structure, allowing for precise identification.

These thin slice MPRs are simultaneously displayed in three perpendicular planes, so that each vessel can be followed along its anatomical course in every possible projection, not obtainable on 2D-DSA. For example, orthogonal views of foramina and canals, and the simultaneous display of corresponding sagittal and axial projections, are particularly helpful in image analysis. Due to their traditionally analogous use in most anatomical textbooks, axial planes for display of vascular anatomy are didactically useful. In cases where an artery takes an irregular or oblique course, curved reformatted images can be used accordingly.

This technique, facilitating understanding of normal vascular anatomy, may also be used to detect arteries and veins (see below) that have been widely ignored in textbooks. For example, Figs. 7.73 and 7.76–7.78. show an artery that appears quite similar to the artery of the foramen rotundum, arising from the distal internal maxillary artery and coursing posteriorly and cranially. This artery is apparently very small since it was noticeable only in cases with AV shunts at the CS. It lies superior to the AFR on lateral DSA views and courses through the IOF and then through the SOF to reach the CS. DynaCT and DVT show more clearly the topography of this distal IMA branch that represents possibly an additional ECA/ICA anastomosis. The distal portion of the IMA, the pterygopalatine artery, as described in the current literature, divides into three posterior branches from lateral to medial (in AP views): the AFR, the vidian artery and the pterygovaginal artery (LASJAUNIAS et al. 2001; HARNSBERGER et al. 2006; OSBORN 1980). An additional branch coursing above the AFR crani-

(Text continues on p. 163)

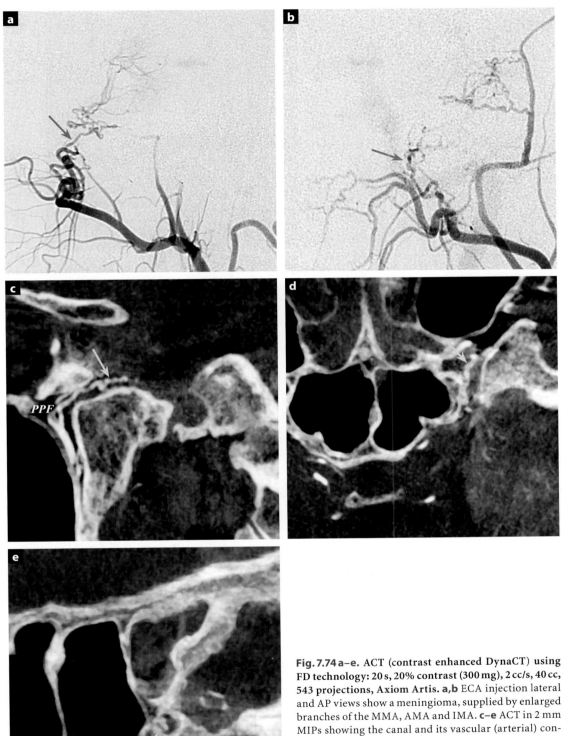

Fig. 7.74 a–e. ACT (contrast enhanced DynaCT) using FD technology: 20 s, 20% contrast (300 mg), 2 cc/s, 40 cc, 543 projections, Axiom Artis. a,b ECA injection lateral and AP views show a meningioma, supplied by enlarged branches of the MMA, AMA and IMA. **c–e** ACT in 2 mm MIPs showing the canal and its vascular (arterial) contents, **c** in sagittal, **d** in axial and **e** in coronal planes. It reveals the course of the artery of the foramen rotundum through the canalis rotundis. This artery is often not just a single vessel, but may consist of 2–3 branches that follow this route and may resemble a small network (see also Figs 7.75, 7.76)

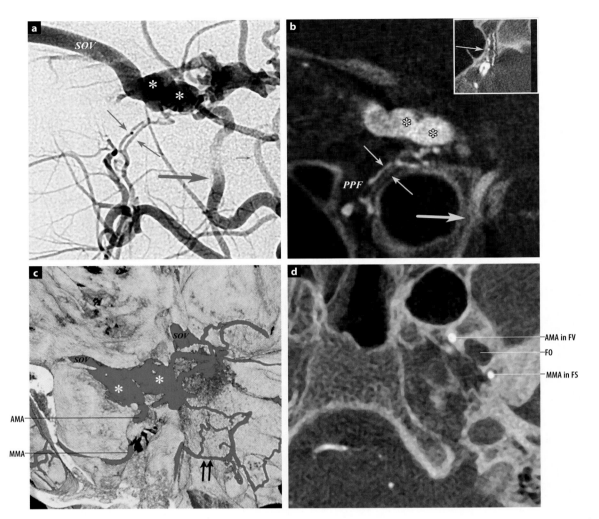

Fig. 7.75 a–d. Traumatic "(D)CSF". DSA, ACT and DVT (10 s 3D-DSA, Axiom Artis). **a** External carotid arteriogram, lateral view, shows a fistulous communication between the AMA (*thick arrow*) and the CS. The AV shunt has also recruited two distal branches of the sphenopalatine artery, taking the course of the artery of the foramen rotundum (*small arrow*: MMA). **b** 0.4 mm MPR, sagittal view through the pterygopalatine fossa reveals both branches passing through the canalis rotundus (*inset*: Axial view), thus could be called "arteries of the foramen rotundum". **c** (DVT) and **d** (0.2 mm MIPs) reveal that the AMA (*arrow*) does not actually course through the foramen ovale as observed in the majority of the cases (78%), but through the sphenoidal emissary foramen (foramen of Vesalius) that lies directly medial and anterior. *PPF*: Pterygopalatine fossa, *asterisk*: CS, *SOV*: Superior ophthalmic vein, *FO*: foramen ovale, *FS*: Foramen spinosum, *FV*: Foramen venosum. *Double arrow*: Drainage into pontomedullary and spinal veins.

Fig. 7.76 a–h. 3D angioarchitecture of a DAVF of the transverse sinus, supplied by multiple feeders, arising from the IMA, AMA and MMA. a, b Left ECA injection AP and lateral. The network of enlarged feeding pedicles is hard to evaluate in AP projection, while in lateral view this seems at least partially possible. Three major feeding pedicles appear to arise from the sphenopalatine artery. 1) Superior: Artery traveling through the IOF and SOF (*thin arrows*); 2) Middle: Artery(ies) of the foramen rotundum (2 vessels, *short thick arrows*). 3) Inferior: Vidian artery (*double arrows*). The branch coursing through the IOF and SOF appears to arise distal from the AFR and courses in lateral view almost parallel, but above the AFR. The vidian artery is the most medial and most distal branch of all involved feeders. **c–h** ACT (**c,d**) based on a non-subtracted reconstruction of a 10 s 3D-DSA (273 projections, Axiom Artis). 20 mm MIPs show the origin and course of the vessels in their relation to the osseous structures: through the canalis rotundis (**e**); Through the vidian canal reaching the carotid (**f**); Through the IOF and SOF (**g**). *Insets*: Corresponding axial views. Coronal view (**h**) showing the three main feeding vessels, while coursing through the corresponding bony foramina in orthogonal projection. The pterygovaginal artery that usually lies medial to the vidian artery and passes through the pterygovaginal canal is not shown here (see Fig. 7.80j) SPA: Spheno-palatine artery in the pterygopalatine fossa

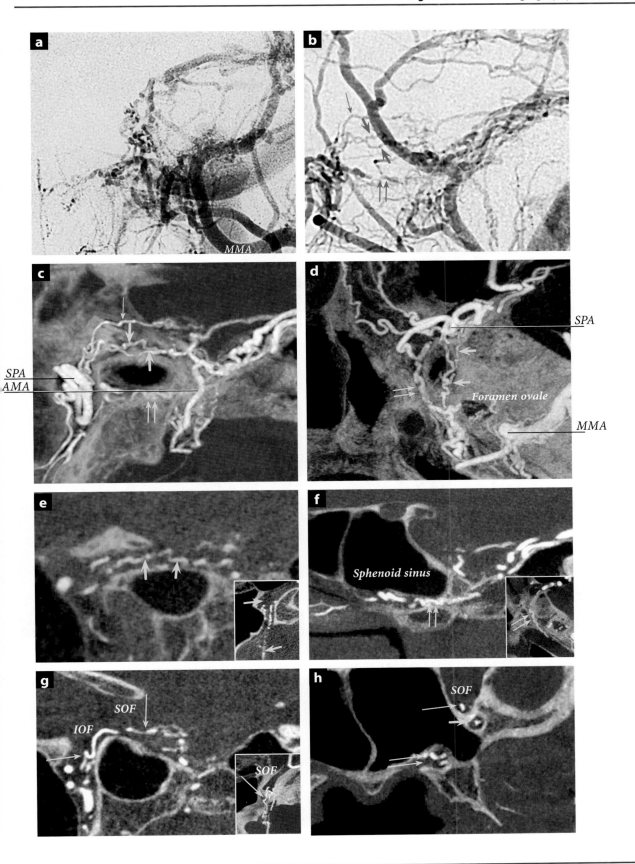

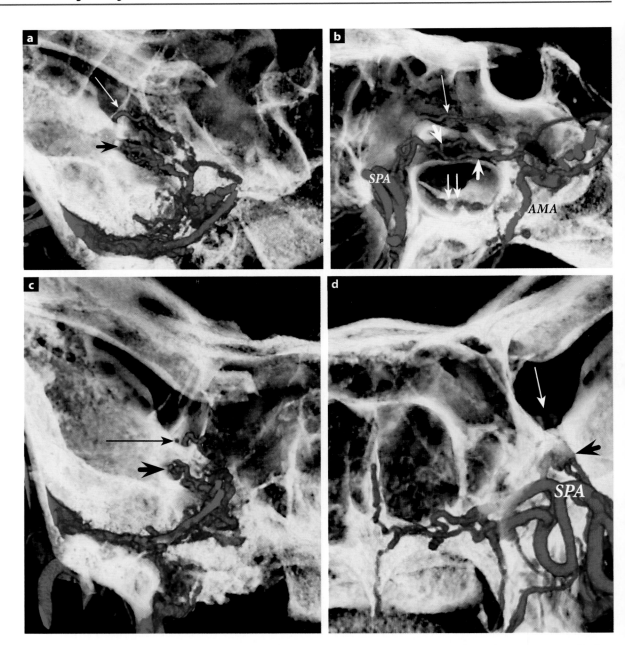

Fig. 7.77 a–d. DAVF of the transverse sinus, supplied by multiple feeding vessels, arising from the IMA, AMA and MMA (same case as in Fig. 7.76). DVT based on a 10 s 3D-DSA. **a** Oblique view from posterior. **b** Lateral view using sagittal clip planes. **c,d** PA and AP view using coronal clip planes. Although providing lower spatial resolution, DVTs enable one to appreciate better the three-dimensional osseous-vascular relationships shown in Fig. 7.76. *Thin arrow:* The branch passing first through the IOF and then through the SOF, arising more distally than the AFR and courses in lateral view almost parallel to the AFR. *Short thick arrows:* Artery(ies) of the foramen rotundum. *Double arrow:* Vidian artery as the most inferior artery in lateral view (pterygovaginal artery not shown). SPA: Sphenopalatine artery

ally through the supraorbital fissure, as seen by the author in several cases, has not been reported so far (see Fig. 7.79a). Referring to the osseous structures, which this vessel courses, the name "artery of the orbital fissures" could be suggested (Fig. 7.79b). It is not clear whether this branch anastomoses with a ramus from the ILT or another (dural) artery from the ICA. Because it was only seen in AV shunting lesions of the CS region, more detailed studies are necessary to further validate this anatomic disposition. Such an observation confirms the enormous value of high-resolution cross-sectional and 3D imaging of neurovascular anatomy.

Figure 7.80 shows the indirect supply of long standing CCF after ineffective ligation. In this case the fistula's supply on the right side comes directly from the supraclinoid ICA. On the left side, however, the ECA appears to be a significant contributor as well. While the DSA does not give certainty regarding the topography of the dominant feeder, the MIPs readily show the location of this specific vascular segment: in axial views, this artery projects exactly onto the course of the carotid canal in the petrous bone, identifying this vessel as a revascularized segment of the petrous ICA. This information is difficult to obtain using 2D-DSA only and, if possible, is likely to require meticulous knowledge of this specific anatomic area. Relating arteries to their corresponding osseous structures in the skull base provides a new level of accuracy in imaging minute arterial angioarchitecture. Hiu et al. (2009) recently described the efficacy of DynaCT digital angiography in detecting the fistula sites in dural AV shunts.

Thus, currently obtainable angiographic 3D datasets not only contain more relevant anatomic information. Another major benefit is that this information is made available in a more didactive manner as it facilitates understanding of spatial relationships between complex structures of different origin. Knowledge of neuroradiological and surgical anatomy remains essential for learning endovascular (and surgical) procedures. The major drawback of 3D-DSA and DynaCT, when compared to anatomic dissections, is their limitation to display non-radiopaque structures. Soft and fat tissue, and thus neural structures in the CS region, cannot be directly visualized using X-rays, but are well delineated when the CS is opacified.

Similar to the advanced 3D imaging of arterial network involving the CS, venous anatomy of the skull base and the middle cranial fossa can be studied using modern 3D-DSA and ACT. Three dimensional visualization of venous anatomy can in principle be obtained using two different approaches.

The first approach is 3D venography: as part of a reconstruction obtained on the basis of an arterial injection as is usually performed for a standard 3D-DSA. During a 10-s rotational angiogram, part of the venous circulation is opacified and reconstructed. Because of contrast dilution and fewer projections containing contrast-filled veins per rotation, venous structures are usually not sufficiently opacified and frequently superimposed by arteries dominating the dataset. To reverse this "arterial dominance" in the data set, the arterial injection is started during the last seconds of the back sweep, before the filling run begins. Thus, fewer projections with arterial than with venous filling are reconstructed and veins will consequently dominate in the reconstructed 3D volume. This technique, called "3D rotational venography", has been successfully used by the author (BENNDORF 2002) using a conventional (II) C-arm system and is shown in Fig. 7.81.

NISHIO et al. (2004) have reported on the value of 3D rotational venography using a C-arm mounted flat detector system. The authors obtained venograms, based on rotational DSA, using a delayed third rotation (filling run) with intervals between 5.5 and 9 s. The amount of contrast injected was 13.9 ml (2.2 ml/s) in the CCA and 12 ml (2.3 ml) in the ICA. It is concluded that neurosurgeons will benefit from a better understanding of venous anatomy in the posterior fossa and the skull base when choosing surgical approaches to vascular or neoplastic lesions in this region. Figure 7.82 shows a rotational venography using the currently available FD modality that illustrates the improved visualization of venous anatomy by isolating the venous part of the circulation from the rotational angiogram. The following setting was used in the case shown: 5-s rotation, 5-s delay of contrast injection, 2 cc/s injection rate, 10 cc total volume. Employing a 960×1240 projection matrix, exclusive visualization of the venous circulation in the injected cerebral territory is possible with a spatial resolution superior to CTA and MRA. Other advantages are that overlays with arterial structures or vessels from territories other than the injected ones do not compromise the diagnostic information. MITSUHASHI et al. (2007) recently reported the successful application of this technique for evaluation of inferior petrosal sinus anatomy and developed a new classification based on their results.

The second approach is "3D phlebography". Another way of obtaining high quality 3D datasets of

(Text continues on p. 167)

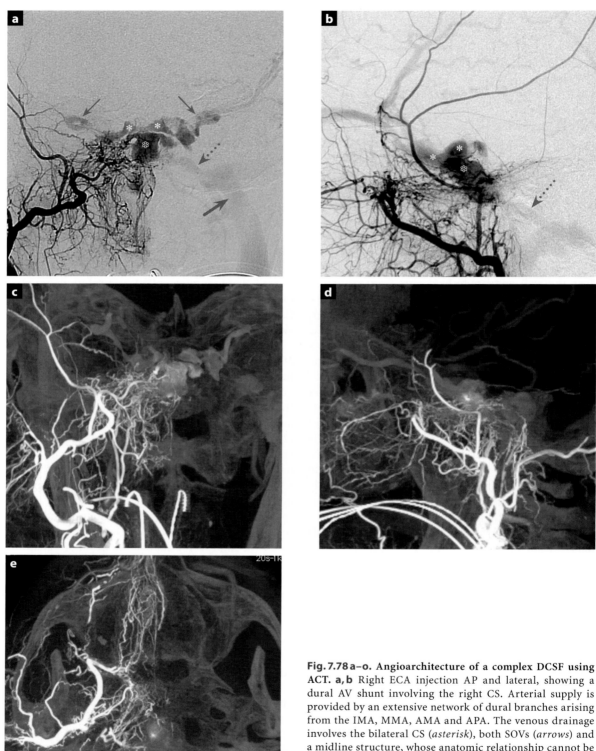

Fig. 7.78 a–o. Angioarchitecture of a complex DCSF using ACT. **a, b** Right ECA injection AP and lateral, showing a dural AV shunt involving the right CS. Arterial supply is provided by an extensive network of dural branches arising from the IMA, MMA, AMA and APA. The venous drainage involves the bilateral CS (*asterisk*), both SOVs (*arrows*) and a midline structure, whose anatomic relationship cannot be readily determined (*B/W asterisk*). There is also a faint communication (*dotted arrow*) with the left IJV (*thick arrow*). **c–e** ECA-ACT (20 s, 2% contrast, 40 cc, 543 projections, Axiom Artis) of the left ECA territory shows the extensive arterial network, providing the arterial supply arising also

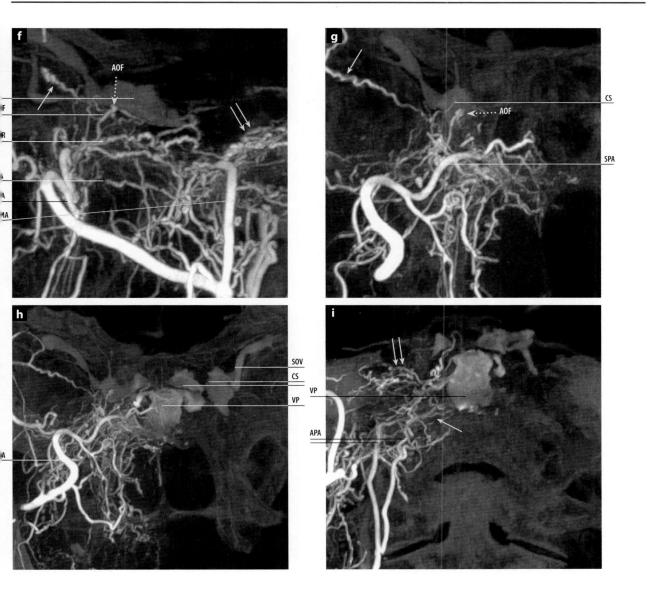

from the APA (clival branches). Three orthogonal MIPs provide a good overview showing the feeding arteries in bright contrast and the venous drainage in dark grey. The window level is chosen to display the osseous background as well. In particular, axial views like in **e** can become very helpful in understanding complex vascular anatomy. (The case was treated successfully by the author and Dr. A. Biondi in 2008 at Pitié-Salpêtrière Hospital, Paris). **f–k** Higher resolution secondary reconstruction based on the same rotation reveals more details. Main feeding pedicles can be better separated, especially when the thickness of the MIPs is changed. *Arrow*: Recurrent meningeal MMA branch. *Double arrow*: Petrosal

MMA branches. **h** demonstrates the more anterior supply from the sphenopalatine artery (SPA) with the artery of the foramen rotundum (AFR), vidian artery (ViA) and arteries coursing through the orbital fissures (AOF). Choosing a more posterior plane, the coronal view in **i** reveals enlarged clival branches (*arrow*) of the APA and petrosal MMA branches (*double arrow*) that seem to supply mainly the venous pouch in the midline (VP).

Continued on next page

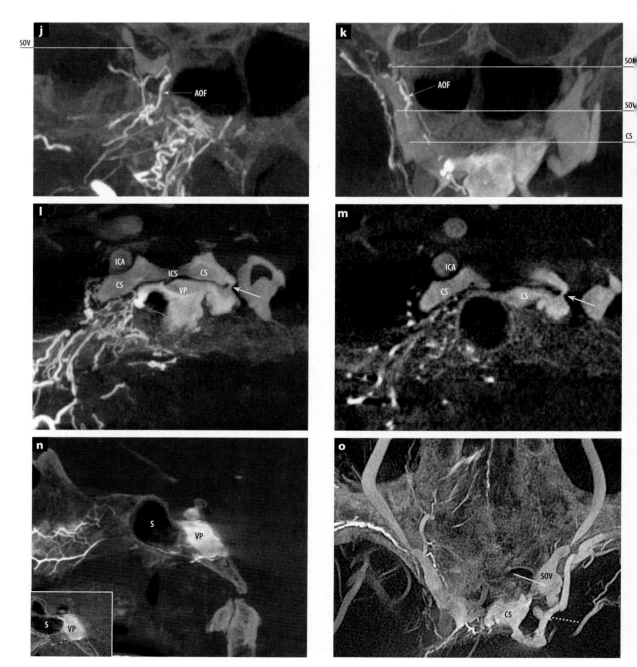

Fig. 7.78 a–o continued. j–k This case is the third observation of the aforementioned additional posterior communication between the SPA and the CS area (see Figs. 7.73, 7.76-7.77). The branch initially takes a vertical course through the inferior orbital fissure and courses then horizontally through the superior orbital fissure (SOF). Accordingly, "Artery of the orbital fissures" (AOF, *dotted arrow*) may be suggested (see also Fig. 7.79). This vessel, also visible in **f** and **g**, is not mentioned in textbooks, and was observed by the author in cases with AV shunts, causing enlargment of ECA-ICA anastomotic branches. **l–m** The CS appears to be clearly separated from the venous pouch and communicates only via a small channel on the far left side (*yellow arrow*). The main fistulous connection is also visible (*red arrow*). **n** This sagittal (midline) plane demonstrates that the venous pouch (VP) is not located on the superior surface of the clivus and thus, less likely represents the basilar plexus, as initially assumed. It appears to be located inside the bone, delineating the sphenoid sinus (S, *inset*). **o** shows further details on the venous angioarchitecture that are impossible to gain from 2D-DSA. The SOV carries an aneurysm like pouch (*arrow*); before passing the SOF, a second, smaller venous aneurysm (*dotted arrow*) is seen at the cortical vein that leaves the posterior CS and courses in parallel to the SOV before turning lateral to reach the temporal cortex

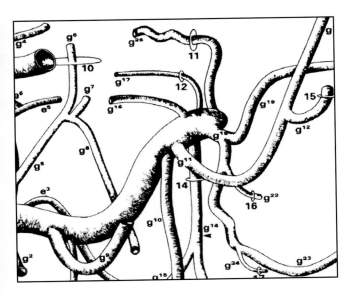

Fig. 7.79. Traditional description of terminal posterior branches of the internal maxillary artery: The artery of the foramen rotundum (superior "g^{26}"), the vidian artery (middle, "g^{17}") and the pterygo-vaginal artery (inferior, "g^{16}"). (From LASJAUNIAS et al. 2001)

the intracranial venous circulation is to directly inject contrast into veins or sinuses during a rotational DSA. By eliminating arteries completely from the data set, this technique allows for a retrograde (against the physiological blood flow) opacification of venous structures including veins and sinuses, obscured during a regular contrast passage after arterial injection. The result may, depending on the selectivity of catheter placement and the communications between adjacent veins, show extensive visualization of veins and sinuses not obtainable through arterial injections. Employing DVT, a direct comparison of venous structures to the imbedding osseous anatomy in multiplanar cross-sectional images is possible. This reveals 3D information on venous anatomy in much greater detail than that available by other clinical imaging modalities, including DSA, so far. In practice, for the CS region a 5-F catheter is placed at the level of the jugular bulb or into the IPS (during sampling) to perform either unilateral or even bilateral injections during a 10-s DSA or even a 20-s ACT (contrast enhanced DynaCT). Reconstructions are performed in a non-subtracted mode, or are obtained as DVT (DSA).

Figures 7.86–7.91 demonstrate how this method remarkably facilitates the perception of the complex venous anatomy in the CS region. The connections between CS, the ICS and draining veins such as the IPS and emissary veins, passing through the foramina, are displayed. Simultaneous bilateral injections of contrast provide extensive opacification of venous structures, commonly not visualized on a standard 2D-DSA. Three dimensional phlebography using

ACT and DVT allows for the most accurate identification of veins and sinuses embedded in their adjacent osseous structures.

Venous structures usually obscured on 2D-DSAs by dense bony structures, such as the internal carotid artery venous plexus (Rektorzik), or

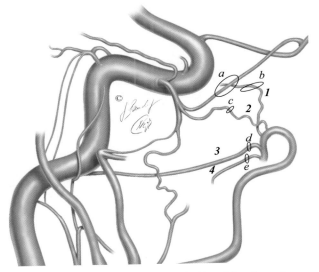

Fig. 7.80. Additional posterior branch (*1*), arising from the distal sphenopalatine artery and coursing through the inferior and superior orbital fissures to reach the CS. This course was identified using ACTs and DVT in three cases. While the AFR (*2*) often has a posteriorly ascending oblique course, this "artery of the orbital fissures" (AOF) courses more vertically first, and then turns horizontally to reach the CS region. *3*: Vidian artery, *4*: Pterygovaginal artery. *a*: SOF, *b*: IOF, *c*: Foramen rotundum, *d*: Vidian canal, *e*: Pterygovaginal canal

(Text continues on p. 171)

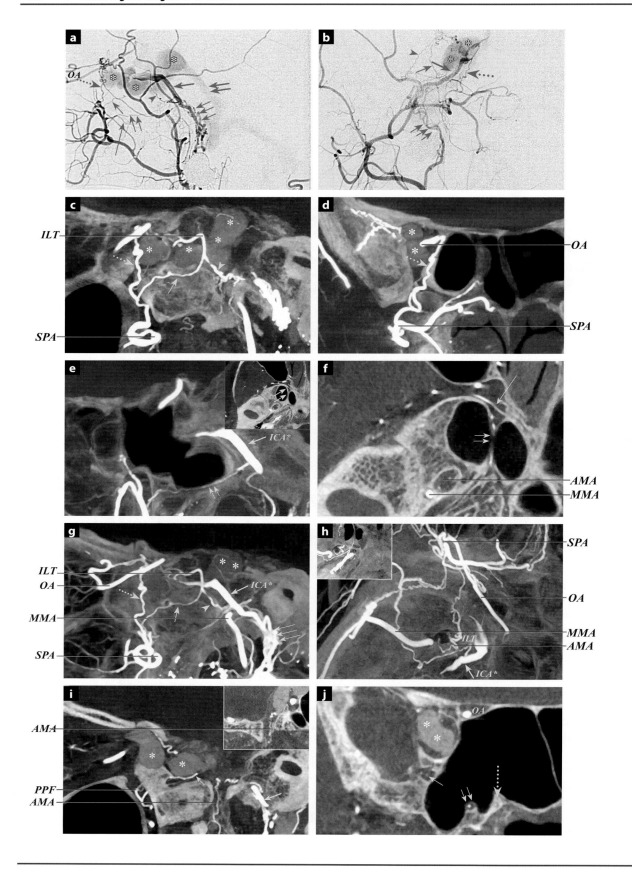

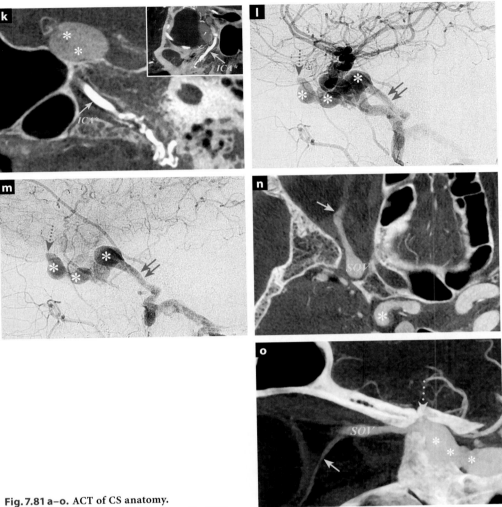

Fig. 7.81 a–o. ACT of CS anatomy.

Long-standing (20 years) right traumatic CCF, ineffectively treated by carotid ligation. **a, b Right ECA lateral and RAO projections:** Recruitment of various ipsilateral ECA collaterals: Artery of the foramen rotundum (*small arrow*), vidian artery (*double arrow*), and collateral branches by the ascending pharyngeal artery (APA, *triple arrows*). Note the retrograde filling of the ophthalmic artery (OA) via an anastomosing branch passing through the inferior orbital fissure (IOF, *dotted arrow*). **c–k ECA-ACT** (20 s rotation, 50% contrast, 2 cc/s, 40 cc, 543 projections): MIPs reveal filling of the residual ICA lumen (*arrow*) via branches of the APA (vasa vasorum), as well as the vidian artery. The ILT does not directly contribute, but fills the OA via its anteromedial branch. **c** The AFR connecting with the anterolateral branch of the ILT, and the anastomosis with the OA (*dotted arrow* in **c–d**). **e–f** The vidian artery sagittal and axial (*double arrows*), while **f** also depicts the pterygovaginal artery (*long arrow*, also in **a**), as a tiny vessel in the pteryovaginal canal. **c** The postero-lateral branch (*arrowhead*) of the ILT, filled by the MMA. **g–h** 30 mm MIPs lateral and axial, provide overviews of the complex network. **i** Sagittal 2 mm MIP shows the AMA and its contributing pedicle through the foramen ovale, not clearly visible on DSA (*inset*: Frontal view, *short arrow*: AFR). Regular arrows in **e–h**: Pointing to the residual ICA lumen (*ICA**). Triple arrow in **g** APA branches reconstituting the ICA lumen. **J** is a 0.2 mm frontal view (*MPR*), slightly posterior to the pterygopalatine fossa showing three posterior branches of the sphenopalatine artery (*SPA*) from medial to lateral: Pterygovaginal artery (*long arrow*), vidian artery (*double arrow*) and artery of the foramen rotundum (*short arrow*). The vidian canal and the smaller pterygovaginal canal may lie very closely together with only a subtle demarcation in between (in this cases the AOF was not visualized). **k** Oblique 2 mm sagittal MIP along the course of the carotid canal (inset axial view) showing the residual/reconstituted ICA lumen (*ICA**, *arrow*) that may involve some vasa vasorum. *Asterisk*: Cavernous sinus, *PPF*: Pteryopalatine fossa, *OA*: Ophthalmic artery, *SPA*: Sphenopalatine artery. **l, m** Right ICA early and late phase: Rapid retrograde filling of the AV shunt I (*asterisks*), mainly draining posteriorly into the IPS (*double arrows*). **n, o** Interestingly, the ACT reveals that the SOV is actually not completely occluded in its proximal segment, as could be assumed from the DSA (*dotted arrows*). It clearly fills also a segment inside the orbit, and even a small vein coursing behind the eyeball (*yellow arrows*)

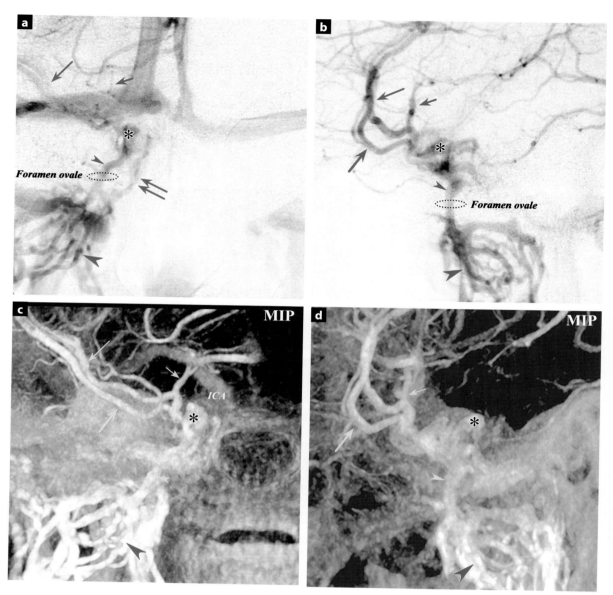

Fig. 7.82 a–d. 3D angioarchitecture of normal CS drainage. **Right ICA venogram AP (a), lateral (b).** Normal drainage via the Sylvian vein (*arrows*) that courses parallel to the sphenoparietal sinus (*thick arrow*) and receives the uncal vein (*short arrow*), just before entering the CS (*asterisk*). From here, the drainage uses a venous emissarium (*arrowhead*), which courses through the foramen ovale to reach a large pterygoid plexus (*large arrowhead*). The IPS (*double arrow*) is only in AP projection visible. **c,d Venous 3D Rotational venography.** MIPs, obtained by manual contrast injection during the mask run (non-subtracted, 14 s rotation, 132 projections, Neurostar). Intense opacification of the Sylvian veins and SPPS. Particularly well visible is the uncal vein (**c**, *shorter arrow*). ICA: The remaining contrast in the ICA superimposes partially onto the venous structures. (Modified from BENNDORF 2002)

the inferior petroclival vein (IPCV) become visible and can be followed along their course through the petrous pyramid and along the petroclival suture, respectively. Rektorzik's plexus, for example, is poorly described in the radiological literature and scarcely mentioned in older textbooks. This internal carotid artery venous plexus (ICAVP) was originally described by Rektorzik in 1858 and was observed by KNOTT (1882) and some other authors (SAN MILLAN RUIZ et al. 2002; HAIKE 1902; KNECHT 1937; PAULLUS et al. 1977; AUBIN et al. 1974; LANG and WEIGEL 1983). In many recent textbooks on venous anatomy of the skull base, as well as in numerous angiographic studies of the CS anatomy, the ICAVP is more or less neglected (THERON 1972; BRAUN et al. 1976; TAKAHASHI et al. 2005; SHIU et al. 1968; MILLER et al. 1993). This may in part be due to the fact that more recent imaging studies on the venous anatomy in this area were focused on structures that represent potential transvenous approaches to the CS for endovascular occlusion of CSFs. The ICAVP is certainly too small in caliber for such endeavor; however, its appearance on angiograms and cross-sectional imaging modalities should be known to everybody involved in diagnosis or treatment of arteriovenous shunting lesions in this area.

DVT imaging precisely reveals the origin, the course of the ICAVP through the carotid canal as well as its connection with the IPS/IJV junction. The plexus leaves the CS between the emissary vein (plexus) of the foramen ovale and the IPCV that arises from the CS just anterior to the IPS (Figs. 7.83–7.91). This creates an apparently consistent configuration of four major veins leaving the lateral and latero-posterior CS:

1. Foramen ovale plexus
2. Internal carotid artery plexus (Rektorzik's, ICAVP)
3. Inferior petroclival vein (IPCV)
4. Inferior petrosal sinus (IPS)

(1) The emissary vein coursing through the foramen ovale (foramen ovale plexus) often appears relatively small when it leaves the CS but may increase in size on its ways through the foramen and usually connects to a large pterygoid plexus. This vein was used as a transvenous approach for occlusion of a DCSF by JAHAN et al. (1998).

(2) After emerging from the CS, Rektorzik's plexus initially appears more like a continuous venous lining within the osseous petrous canal, covering the wall of the carotid artery with a very thin inner lu-

men. Following the course of the ICA, it travels more laterally than the other efferent veins and appears to transform into a plexiform arrangement of small veins. In this study material, this plexus-like structure ended somewhere in the carotid canal and was not directly connected with the IPS, but gave rise to a small vein that curved medially to reach the IPS/IJV junction (Figs. 7.86, 7.89 and 7.91).

The course and architecture of the ICAVP cannot be appreciated on a DSA, where in AP views it is often times superimposed or mistaken as the emissary vein to the foramen ovale. In lateral projections only the portion covering the anterior and posterior wall of the ICA, where the X-ray beam passes tangentially through its contrast filled lumen, the plexus is somehow recognizable (Figs. 7.27, 7.83–7.84, 7.86, 7.89). In orthogonal views obtainable only using high resolution 3D data sets, the fact that the plexus does not cover the entire carotid artery circumference, becomes evident by a figure "C" appearance.

(3) The IPCV arose between Rektorzik's plexus and coursed almost in parallel to the IPS, postero-laterally and caudally towards the IPS/IJV junction. This vein indeed creates a "mirror image" of the IPS as described by RHOTON (2000) and lies so close to the IPS that it can easily be mistaken on a 2D-DSA for a "doubled IPS" or a "plexus type of IPS". As revealed by DVT, this vein lies on the external surface of the lower skull base, is connected to the foramen lacerum plexus (FLP), which was not always identifiable, and travels along the petroclival suture to reach the IPS/IJV junction, where it may drain directly or via the ACC into the IJV. It is interesting to note that the partially extracranial course of the IPCV is mentioned by several authors, but it is to my knowledge not reported through which osseous opening this vein courses. Based on the material studied it can be assumed that the foramen lacerum serves as an exit for the IPCV, but more detailed studies are required to confirm this topography. No report on the use of this vein as transvenous access to the CS exists in the literature, but based on anatomical course and size of this vein, such an approach could be feasible in selected cases. Due to difficulties distinguishing between IPCV and IPS based on DSA only, an accidental use of the former instead of the latter is possible, especially in case of poor angiographic image quality.

(4) The IPS is the best known efferent vein of the CS and its anatomy has been studied extensively mainly because of its frequent use for petrosal sinus sampling. This sinus has also been increasingly

(Text continues on p. 179)

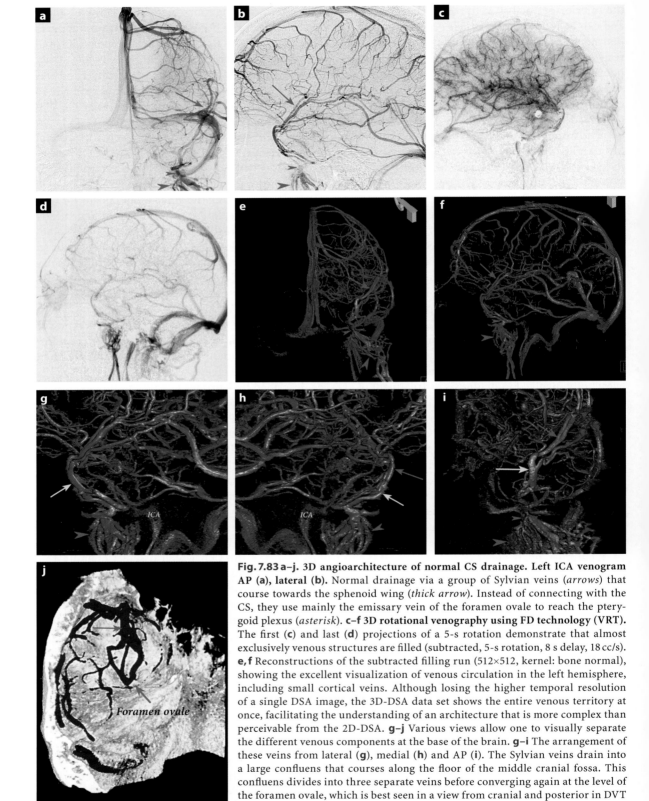

Fig. 7.83 a–j. 3D angioarchitecture of normal CS drainage. Left ICA venogram AP (**a**), lateral (**b**). Normal drainage via a group of Sylvian veins (*arrows*) that course towards the sphenoid wing (*thick arrow*). Instead of connecting with the CS, they use mainly the emissary vein of the foramen ovale to reach the pterygoid plexus (*asterisk*). **c–f 3D rotational venography using FD technology (VRT).** The first (**c**) and last (**d**) projections of a 5-s rotation demonstrate that almost exclusively venous structures are filled (subtracted, 5-s rotation, 8 s delay, 18 cc/s). **e,f** Reconstructions of the subtracted filling run (512×512, kernel: bone normal), showing the excellent visualization of venous circulation in the left hemisphere, including small cortical veins. Although losing the higher temporal resolution of a single DSA image, the 3D-DSA data set shows the entire venous territory at once, facilitating the understanding of an architecture that is more complex than perceivable from the 2D-DSA. **g–j** Various views allow one to visually separate the different venous components at the base of the brain. **g–i** The arrangement of these veins from lateral (**g**), medial (**h**) and AP (**i**). The Sylvian veins drain into a large confluens that courses along the floor of the middle cranial fossa. This confluens divides into three separate veins before converging again at the level of the foramen ovale, which is best seen in a view from cranial and posterior in DVT (**j**). *ICA*: Some residual contrast opacifies the proximal ICA as well

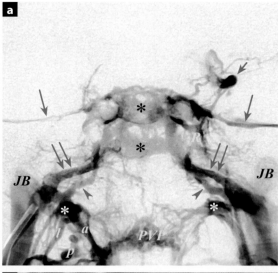

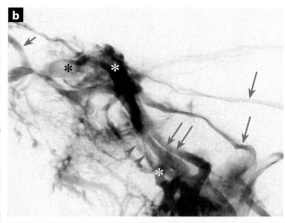

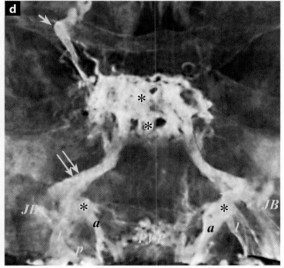

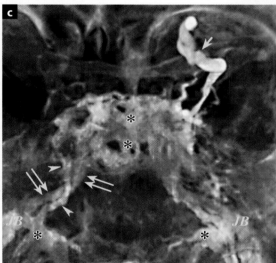

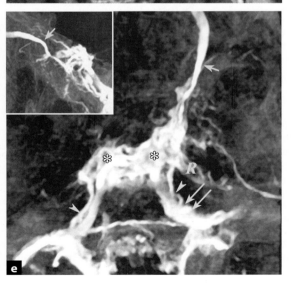

Fig. 7.84a–e. 3D angioarchitecture of the CS in a DCSF (Case report III). Phlebography via a 6-F guiding catheter in the left IJV, AP (**a**) and lateral views (**b**): Both CSs (*asterisks*) and IPSs (*double arrows*) are intensely opacified. Visualization of the SPS (*arrows*) as well as of the left SOV. No opacification of a fistulous connection on the right side. Additional visualization of the inferior petro-clival vein (IPCV) on each side (*arrowheads*) and of the internal carotid artery venous plexus (ICAVP, Rektorzik, *R*). The latter is difficult to identify on standard projections due to its thin, plexus-like structure, lining the wall of the carotid canal. **3D rotational phlebography with Neurostar** (**non-subtracted 14 s rotation, 132 projections**), VRT (**c,d**) and MIP (**e**), seen from anterior (**c**), posterior (**d**) and caudal (**e**): Opacification of both CSs with demonstration of its partial trabecular ("septated") structure. Visualization of both IPSs and the left SOV. The osseus background facilitates the anatomical orientation. The IPCV is best seen in **c** and **e** seemingly "crossing" the course of the IPS from medial to lateral. **e** The more lateral course of the internal carotid plexus (Rektorzik). **d** The anterior condylar confluens (ACC, *large asterisk*) medial to the jugular bulb (*JB*). Note the connections with anterior (*a*), lateral (*l*) and posterior (*p*) condylar veins. (Modified from BENNDORF 2002)

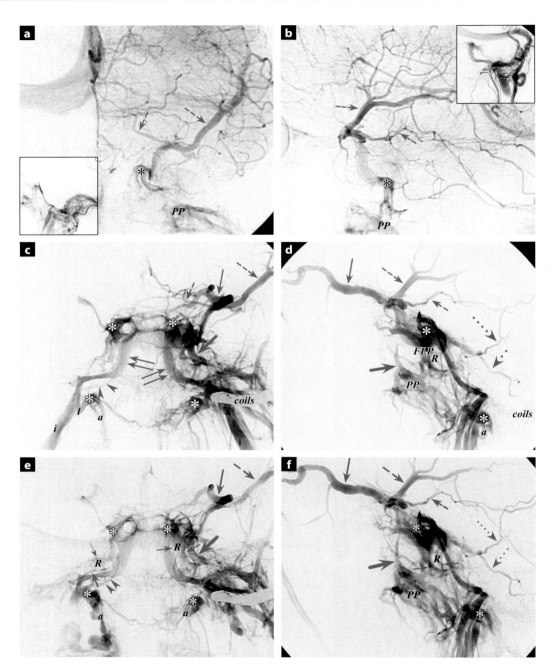

Fig. 7.85 a–f. Venogram (**a,b** obtained by arterial injection) and phlebogram (**c–f** obtained by venous injection) of a patient with a DAVF of the sigmoid sinus draining retrogradely into the IPS, CS and SOV due to a IJV stenosis. As seen in this example, the ICAVP (Rektorzik) is usually not visible in the venous phase of a carotid angiogram, although the filling defect (if present) caused by the intracavernous ICA, may indicate its location. Due to higher pressure when injecting contrast directly into the IPS or IJV, the phlebogram may reveal more architectural details of the cavernous sinus and its communications. It shows the pial veins, commonly involved in the drainage of a CSF: SMCV (*dashed arrow*), uncinate vein (*short dashed arrow*), lateral mesencephalic vein (*dotted arrow*), cerebellar vein (*short dotted arrow*). The IPCV (*arrowheads*) and the ICAVP (*short arrows* outlining its contours) are better visible in later phases (**e,f**). In this case, a more prominent vein, coursing through the foramen ovale (*thick arrow*), is seen in AP view lateral to the ICAVP. This example further underlines how unreliable a venogram for the visualization of the venous anatomy may be: No IPS is seen in **a,b** but is clearly filled bilaterally in **c–f**! *B/W asterisk*: CS, *white asterisk*: ACC, *a*: Anterior condylar vein, *l*: Lateral condylar vein, *i*: Internal jugular vein, *FLP*: Foramen lacerum plexus. *Insets*: DAVF of the sigmoid sinus

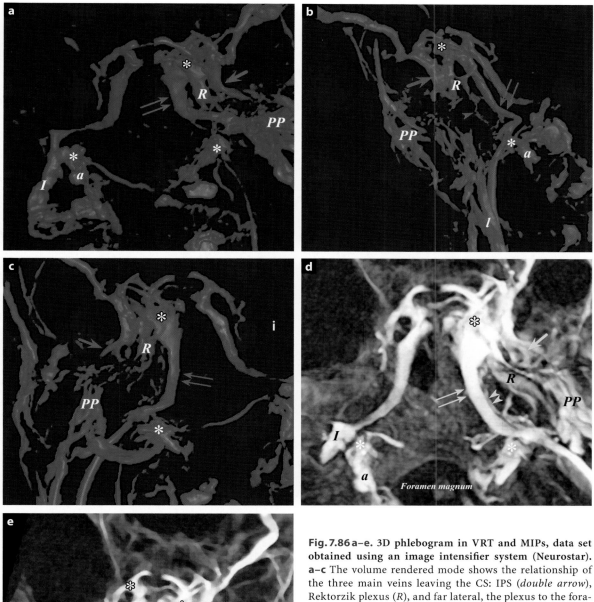

Fig. 7.86 a–e. 3D phlebogram in VRT and MIPs, data set obtained using an image intensifier system (Neurostar). **a–c** The volume rendered mode shows the relationship of the three main veins leaving the CS: IPS (*double arrow*), Rektorzik plexus (*R*), and far lateral, the plexus to the foramen ovale (*thick arrow*). The IPCV (*arrowheads*) is not well shown, but becomes apparent in the two MIPs (**d, e**). Note that the quality of the reconstruction using older technology is inferior to that of current FD systems, which provide higher spatial and better contrast resolution and allow for easier identification of visualized sinuses and veins (see examples below). **d, e** ACT, manual contrast injection (non-diluted), obtained using a 14 s rotation, 132 projections (Neurostar, post-processed with Leonardo). *B/W asterisk*: CS, *white asterisk*: ACC, *a*: Anterior condylar vein, *l*: Lateral condylar vein, *i*: Internal jugular vein, *PP*: Pterygoid plexus

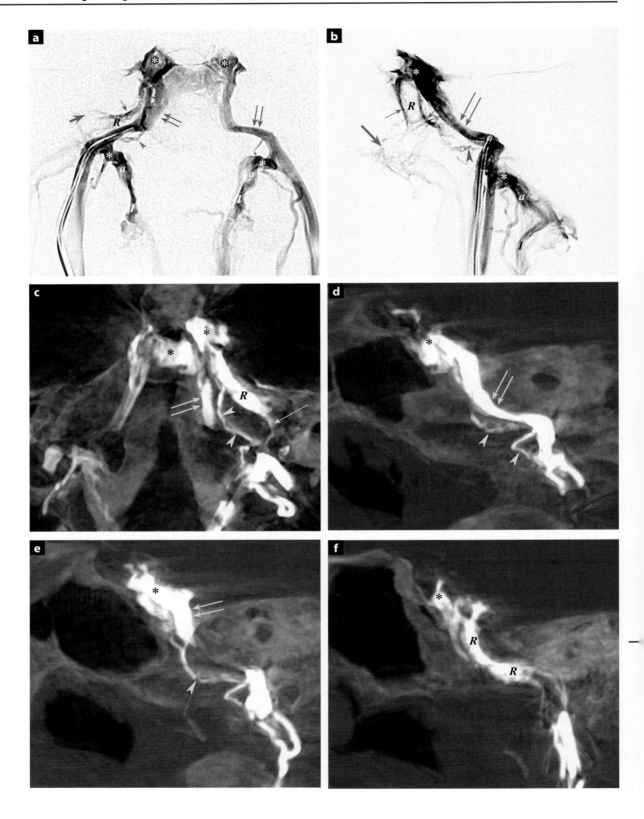

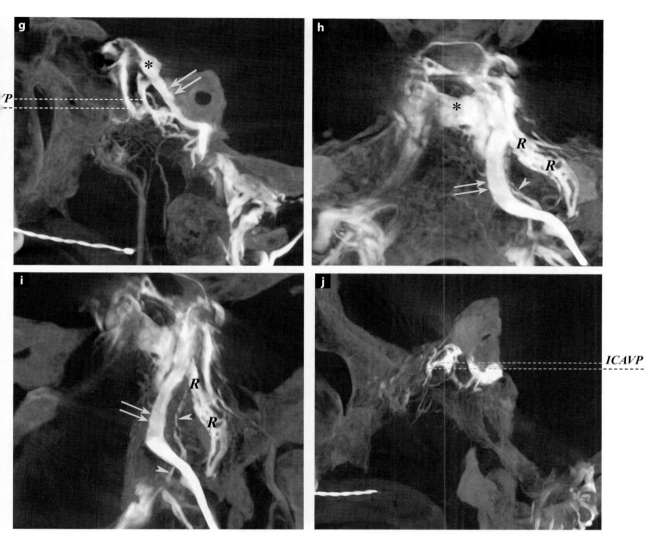

Fig. 7.87 a–f. Venous Anatomy of the CS/IPS/IJV. a,b IJ Phlebography, AP and lateral, obtained during IPS sampling. **c–f** 3D Phlebography using ACT (20 s, 2% contrast, 40 cc, 543 projections, Axiom Artis), MIPs. **c** View from posterior and above, **d–f** lateral views in 5 mm sections from medial to lateral. Note that on lateral DSA views, the ICAVP is visible only as anterior and posterior contours of the filling defect caused by the ICA lumen. On DSA the IPS can usually be identified, while IPCV and Rektorziks plexus are usually difficult to recognize. Viewing MIPs from posterior allows for a better understanding. The IPCV crosses the IPS from medial to lateral and has a similar course (mirror image according to KATSUTA et al. 1997). **c** shows a relatively consistent arrangement from medial to lateral: **IPS-IPCV-ICAVP** that can be applied to angiograms, although often not readily perceivable there. *B/W asterisk*: CS, *double arrows*: IPS, *arrowhead*: IPCV, *thick arrow*: Emissary vein to the PP (foramen ovale plexus), *white or black asterisk*: ACC, *a*: Anterior condylar vein, *l*: Lateral condylar vein, *R*: Internal carotid artery venous plexus (ICAVP, Rektorzik, outlined by the *short arrows* in **b**). **g–j. 3D-phlebography using ACT (20 s, 2% contrast, 40 cc, 543 projections, Axiom Artis).** Bilateral IPS injections provide a better filling of the veins, allowing for a more complete image analysis and a better separation between IPS, IPCV and ICAVP. **g** is a 5 mm MIP that shows the same "filling defect" as **b**. **h,i** reveal the rather plexiform structure of the ICAVP that is impossible to perceive using 2D-DSA. **j** is an oblique almost view orthogonal view, demonstrating the thin venous lining between the unopacified ICA and the osseous carotid canal that creates an incomplete circle or a "figure c". *B/W asterisk*: CS, *double arrows*: IPS, *arrowhead*: IPCV, *regular arrow*: Emissary vein to the PP (foramen ovale plexus), *thick short arrow*: PP, *white asterisk*: ACC, *a*: Anterior condylar vein, *l*: Lateral condylar vein, *R*: Internal carotid artery venous plexus (ICAVP, Rektorzik)

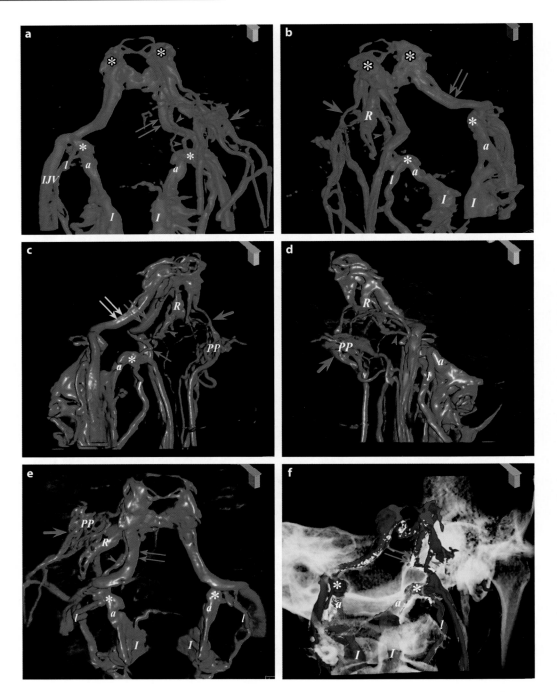

Fig. 7.88 a–f. Venous anatomy of the CS/IPS/IJV. 3D phlebography (10 s 3D-DSA, Axiom Artis) in different views from ante-rior (a), lateral (d), right posterior (b), right anterior (c) and cranio-caudal (e). f DVT from RAO (Same case as Fig. 7.87). The three-dimensional angioarchitecture can be better perceived using these VRTs in DVT. The IPCV and Rektorziks plexus can be readily differentiated. The IPCV makes a sharp zig-zag turn (*arrow*) to communicate with the IPS, before entering the ACC. The course of Rektorzik's plexus is best seen in **e**, where it passes more lateral than IPS and IPCV towards the carotid canal in the petrous bone. It appears to become thinner on its way and drains via a small curved vein that is only visible on MIPs (*long thin arrow* in **7.86c**) into the IJV. **f** shows the relationship of the venous architecture to the posterior skull base (oblique view from posterior. *Double yellow arrows* in **c**: Left IPS. *B/W asterisk*: CS, *double arrows*: IPS, *arrowheads*: IPCV, *thick short arrow*: Emissary vein to the PP (foramen ovale plexus), *white asterisk*: ACC, *a*: Anterior condylar vein, *l*: Lateral condylar vein, *R*: Internal carotid artery venous plexus (ICAVP, Rektorzik), *I*: Anterior internal vertebral venous plexus. *PP*: Pterygoid plexus

used as transvenous approach for endovascular occlusion of CSFs that will be covered in detail in the next chapter. One interesting aspect of my observations is the fact that the IPS and the IPCV may be connected through several small bridging veins (Figs. 7.89 and 7.90), which may play a role in cases of sinus thrombosis, and which could also resemble the plexiform type of the IPS/IJV junction that has been described in the literature (SHIU et al. 1968; MILLER et al. 1993). MITSUHASHI et al. (2007) have classified the IPS-IJV junction into six types based on 3D rotational venograms. They found that the IPS drains directly into the JB in only 1.2%, while most frequent was the drainage either into the upper IJV (34.9%), or into the lower IJV (37.3%). These results emphasize the value of 3D-DSA imaging for understanding venous anatomy.

The ACC was demonstrated in all 3D phlebograms. This venous collector, originally described by TROLARD (1868), was recently "rediscovered" by SAN MILLAN RUIZ et al. (2002). The authors performed high quality radiograms on cadaver casts and correlated their findings with MRA studies. It was found that the ACC connected with six main venous structures: inferior petrosal sinus (IPS), internal carotid venous plexus (ICAVP, Rektorzik), anterior condylar vein (ACV), lateral condylar vein (LCV), prevertebral venous plexus (PVP), and internal jugular vein (IJV).

This is to some extent different from my observations, where Rektorzik's plexus did not seem directly connected to the ACC, but rather through a small medially curved vein, reaching the IPS, which may correspond to the medial petrosal vein.

The IPCV was not included as tributary of the ACC by SAN MILLAN RUIZ et al. (2002), but as a connecting vein between ICAVP and ACC. In contrast the IPCV was found in our material to be connected to the ACC, independently from Rektorzik's sinus. The illustration of SAN MILLAN RUIZ et al. (2002) showed the IPCV (called there inferior petro-occipital vein) arising from Rektorzik's plexus which is not confirmed by this study where both veins appeared to arise separately from the CS: the IPCV coursing mainly extracranially to reach the ACC, while the ICAVP travels intracranially through the petrous pyramid.

TAKAHASHI et al. (2005) recently studied the anatomy of the craniocervical junction around the suboccipital sinus using MRI and also described six tributaries to the ACC, including the IPCV, but neglecting the ICAVP.

Figure 7.92 summarizes some of the observations in the IPS/ACC/IJV junction so far, adding the IPCV to the tributaries of the ACC. More detailed studies are on-going and will add knowledge of the topography of the venous anatomy in the parasellar and skull base region. For successful catheter navigation into the CS, knowledge of the possible anatomical arrangements and communications between IPS, IJV and ACC is essential, since variations from normal anatomy are not seldom and 2D angiograms may look confusing, especially when local thrombosis is present or the IPS has to be approached through the ACC.

Bilateral retrograde injections through diagnostic angiographic catheters within each IPS and 3D reconstructions using DynaCT and DVT provide an extensive three-dimensional visualization of the venous anatomy at the posterior skull base and of the CS, including its afferent and efferent veins. This technique provides anatomic information, not obtainable by 2D-DSA or other cross-sectional imaging modalities such as CTA or MRA, and is without doubt regarding its topographic accuracy and image quality comparable to colored plastic casts in cadaver vessels. Advanced three-dimensional imaging using modern rotational angiographic techniques based on high-resolution FD technology enhances not only our existing knowledge of venous anatomy in the parasellar region and the skull base. It also allows the study of small venous structures and their communications, traditionally obscured on angiograms and thus poorly described or even neglected in the literature.

In summary, modern bi-plane DSA based on FD-technology allows for precise and detailed visualization of all relevant arterial and venous structures. It remains the gold standard for timely and correct diagnosis as well as for optimizing treatment planning in patients with DCSFs. The combination of 2D-DSA with novel 3D imaging tools such as ACT and DV technique, as well as 3D venography and 3D phlebography provides anatomical information in a quality that sets a new standard for vascular imaging in this area, allowing for computerized graphic dissection of vascular structures within their osseous embedment. Beside high-quality angiographic equipment and sufficient training, profound knowledge of the vascular anatomy, including its angiographic appearance, remains the essential basis for successful and safe endovascular occlusion of CSFs.

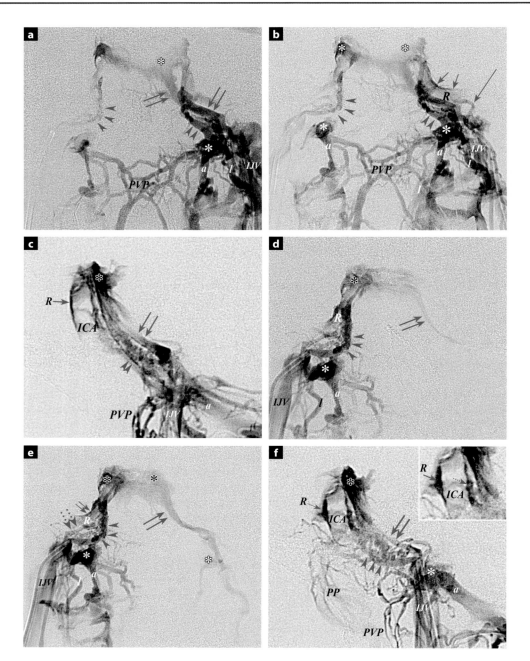

Fig. 7.89a–f. Venous anatomy CS/IPS/IJV. a–f IJ phlebography, left (**a–c**) and right (**d–f**) side AP and lateral, obtained during IPS sampling. On the left side, both the IPS (*double arrow*) and the IPCV (*double arrowhead*) can be identified, while on the right side, there is a dominant filling of the IPCV (*triple arrowhead*). Its course is very similiar and could be easily mistaken for that of the IPS. The right IPCV drains directly into the IJV, but is also connected to the ACC via several small veins (**d,e**). The left IPCV "crosses" in AP projection the IPS to reach the ACC (**a,b**). Cross-flow through the ICS fills the IPS on the left (*double arrow* in **d,e**) and the IPCV on the right (*triple arrow* in **a,b**). The right IPS is vaguely identifiable in **e** (*dotted double arrow*), but unclear in **f** due to superimposition with the left IPS (cross-flow filled). **c** and **f** show a longitudinal filling defect, corresponding to the ascending course of the C5 ICA segment that is outlined by Rektorziks venous plexus (*R, small arrows*). The very thin lumen of this plexus is clearly seen only in a tangential projections of its anterior and posterior part (see also inset in **f**). Note in **b** a small curved intrapetrosal vein, connecting the ICAVP and the ACC (*long thin arrow*). *B/W asterisk*: CS, *double arrows*: IPS, *arrowheads*: IPCV, *white asterisk*: ACC, *a*: Anterior condylar vein, *l*: Lateral condylar vein, *R*: Internal carotid artery venous plexus (ICAVP, Rektorzik), *I*: Anterior internal vertebral venous plexus. *PP*: Pterygoid plexus

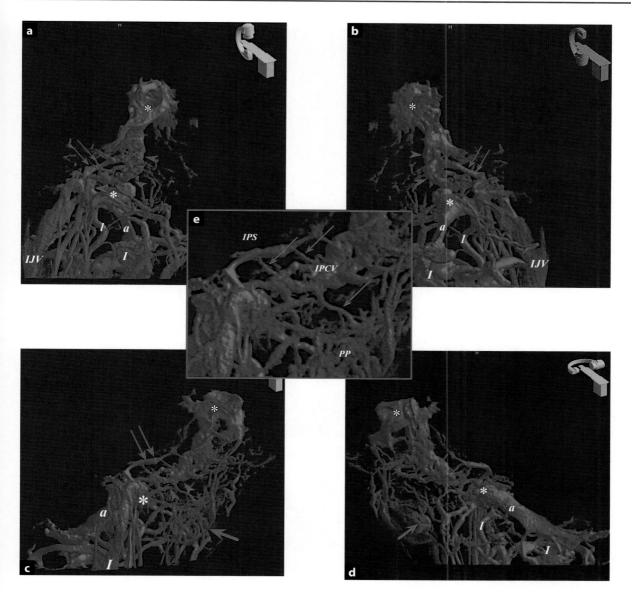

Fig. 7.90 a–k. Venous anatomy CS/IPS/IJV (compare to Fig. 7.89). 3D phlebography (10 s 3D-DSA, Axiom Artis), right side, AP (**a**) and PA (**b**) lateral (**c**) and medial (**d**) view, obtained during IPS sampling using bilateral injections (sagittal clip plane used to exclude the left side). The IPCV (*double arrowheads*), and especially the IPS (*double arrow*), although only in fragments possibly due due to thrombosis, are visualized. The IPCV, which appears enlarged and plexiform shows several bridging veins to the pterygoid plexus (*thick arrow*), as well as to the IPS (**c, d** *arrows* in **e**) and courses inferiorly, in parallel to the IPS (**c, d**). This detailed anatomy cannot be perceived from the 2D-DSA. The IPS appearance could easily be interpreted as plexiform Type III (**Fig. 7.89 d** and **e**) type after SHIU et al. (1968, see Fig. 3.11). *B/W asterisks:* CS, *double arrows:* IPS, *arrowhead:* IPCV, *thick short arrow:* Emissary vein to the PP (foramen ovale plexus), *white asterisks:* ACC, *a:* Anterior condylar vein, *l:* Lateral condylar vein, *I:* Anterior internal vertebral venous plexus, *PP:* Pterygoid plexus, *R:* Internal carotid artery venous plexus (ICAVP, Rektorzik)

Continued on next page →

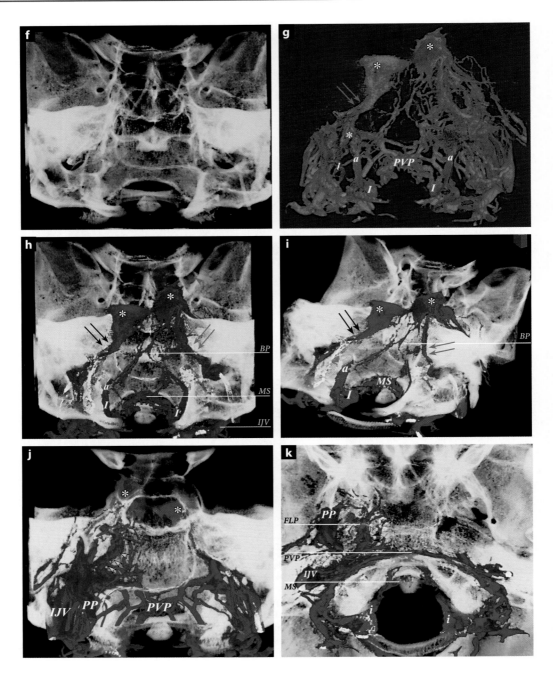

Fig. 7.90a–k. Continued. f–k Venous anatomy IPS/IJV in DVT obtained by bilateral 3D phlebography (10 s 3-D DSA, Axiom Artis). f,g DVT, two volumes separately reconstructed based on identical projections of mask (**f**) and filling run (**g**). **h,i** View at the posterior skull base from above and oblique. **j** View at the central skull base from below. **k** Cranio-caudal view onto the foramen magnum, clivus and sella. The venous structure seen in **h** and **i** represents the right IPS (*red double arrowhead*), as it courses along the inner (superior) surface of the petroclival fissure to reach the ACC and IJV, while the IPCV is not shown. The sinus is not readily identifiable on high-resolution DSA (compare with **7.89d,e**) that shows predominantly the IPCV. The rather plexiform structure of the vein can, on the other hand, readily be identified in **j**, where it courses along the outer (inferior) surface of the petroclival fissure (*triple arrowheads*). There are numerous small connections between the IPCV and the PP, the PVP as well as the FLP. *B/W asterisk: CS, double arrows:* IPS, *arrowhead:* IPCV, *white asterisk:* ACC, *a:* Anterior condylar vein, *l:* Lateral condylar vein, *R:* Internal carotid artery venous plexus (ICAVP, Rektorzik). *BP:* Basilar plexus, *MS:* Marginal sinus, *PVP:* Prevertebral plexus, *IJV:* Internal jugular vein, *PP:* Pterygoid plexus, *FLP:* Foramen lacerum plexus, *i:* Anterior internal vertebral venous plexus

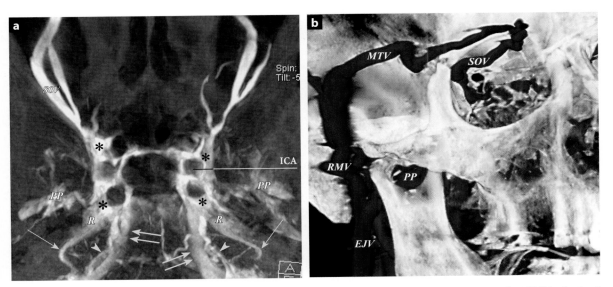

Fig. 7.91a,b. Venous anatomy of the IPS/IJV junction. ACT (a) using 20 s rotation, 20%, 2 cc/s, 40 cc, and DVT (b), obtained by 10 s 3D-DSA (simultaneous bilateral IPS injections).

a Thick MIP (20 mm) revealing the extensive opacification of both CSs, including some of its efferent and afferent veins. Note the bilateral ICAVP and the medially coursing intrapetrosal veins (*long arrows*). The arrangment of the four main draining veins leaving the lateral and posterolateral CS:

 - Emmissary vein to the foramen ovale (foramen ovale plexus, FOP)
 - Internal carotid artery venous plexus (ICAVP, Rektorzik)
 - Inferior petroclival vein (IPCV)
 - Inferior petrosal sinus (IPS)

was found consistently in six patients undergoing 3D phlebography during petrosal sinus sampling (see also Fig. 7.92).

b DVT showing the connection between superior ophthalmic vein and middle temporal vein that drains into the retromandibular vein and the external jugular vein (EJV). *Asterisk: CS, double arrows:* IPS, *arrowhead:* IPCV, *R:* Internal carotid artery venous plexus (ICAVP, Rektorzik). *MTV:* Middle temporal vein, *RMV:* Retromandibular vein, *EJV:* External jugular vein, *PP:* Pterygoid plexus, *SOV:* Superior ophthalmic vein.

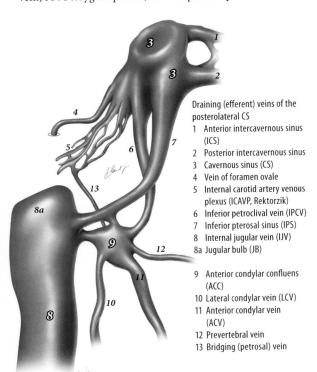

Draining (efferent) veins of the posterolateral CS
1 Anterior intercavernous sinus (ICS)
2 Posterior intercavernous sinus
3 Cavernous sinus (CS)
4 Vein of foramen ovale
5 Internal carotid artery venous plexus (ICAVP, Rektorzik)
6 Inferior petroclival vein (IPCV)
7 Inferior pterosal sinus (IPS)
8 Internal jugular vein (IJV)
8a Jugular bulb (JB)

9 Anterior condylar confluens (ACC)
10 Lateral condylar vein (LCV)
11 Anterior condylar vein (ACV)
12 Prevertebral vein
13 Bridging (petrosal) vein

Fig. 7.92. Artistic drawing of the posterolateral cavernous sinus and its main draining veins, based on observations using 2D-DSA, 3D phlebograms (view from posterior). The ICAVP (Rektorzik) and the inferior petroclival vein (IPCV), often not readily identifiable on angiograms, are illustrated. The IPCV courses almost in parallel to the IPS, yet slightly lateral and inferior along the outer (inferior) petroclival fissure (suture) and has no vertical and horizontal portion. This vein is not well described in textbooks; in some it is called "petrooccipital sinus" (relating to "petrooccipital suture") or "inferior petrooccipital vein" after Trolard. It makes in its distal portion a medial turn, while the IPS courses laterally. Rektorzik's sinus appears rather like a plexus, surrounding the carotid wall and may be difficult to identify on angiograms, and thus has been widely neglected in the angiographic literature. It is named here ICAVP and courses more lateral than the IPCV following the ICA into the carotid canal and may be connected to the IPS, ACC or IJV via small veins. The ICAVP may not serve as access route to the CS, but can be involved in the venous drainage of traumatic or dural CSFs. The ACC lies medial and slightly anterior to the jugular bulb and may communicate with the IPS, IPCV, Rektorzik's sinus, IJV, ACV, LCV and several small prevertebral veins. In one case several small veins, connecting the IPCV with the PP and the IPS, were found.

References

Acierno MD, et al. (1995) Painful oculomotor palsy caused by posterior-draining dural carotid cavernous fistulas. Arch Ophthalmol 113:1045–1049

Agid R, et al. (2004) Targeted compartmental embolization of cavernous sinus dural arteriovenous fistulae using transfemoral medial and lateral facial vein approaches. Neuroradiology 46:156–160

Ahmadi J, et al. (1983) Computed tomography of carotid-cavernous fistula. AJNR Am J Neuroradiol 4:131–136

Anonymous (1995) Endarterectomy for asymptomatic carotid artery stenosis. Executive Committee for the Asymptomatic Carotid Atherosclerosis Study. JAMA 273:1421–1428

Anxionnat R et al. (2001) Intracranial aneurysms: clinical value of 3D digital subtraction angiography in the therapeutic decision and endovascular treatment. Radiology 218(3):799–808

Anxionnat R, et al. (1998) 3D angiography. Clinical interest. First applications in interventional neuroradiology. J Neuroradiol 25(4):251–262

Arning C, Grzyska U (2004) Color Doppler imaging of cervicocephalic fibromuscular dysplasia. Cardiovasc Ultrasound 2:7

Arning C, Grzyska U, Lachenmayer L (1997) Lateral cranial dural fistula. Detection with Doppler and duplex ultrasound. Nervenarzt 68(2):139–146

Arning C, Grzyska U, Lachenmayer L (2005) Duplex ultrasound of external carotid artery branches for the detection of dural arteriovenous fistulae. ROFO 177:236–241

Ayanzen RH, et al. (2000) Cerebral MR venography: normal anatomy and potential diagnostic pitfalls. AJNR Am J Neuroradiol 21(1):74–78

Barrow DL, et al. (1985) Classification and treatment of spontaneous carotid-cavernous sinus fistulas. J Neurosurg 62:248–256

Belden CJ, Abbitt PL, Beadles KA (1995) Color Doppler US of the orbit. Radiographics 15:589–608

Bendszus M, et al. (1999) Silent embolism in diagnostic cerebral angiography and neurointerventional procedures: a prospective study. Lancet 354(9190):1594-1597.

Benndorf G (2002) Dural cavernous sinus fistulas. Diagnosis and endovascular treatment. Berlin: Charité. Humboldt University, pp 67–75

Benndorf G (2008) Anomalous Origin of the Marginal Tentorial Artery: Detection by Contrast-Enhanced Angiographic Computed Angiography (CE-ACT). Clinical Neuroradiology 18:261–264

Benndorf G, et al. (2000) Transvenous occlusion of dural cavernous sinus fistulas through the thrombosed inferior petrosal sinus: report of four cases and review of the literature [In Process Citation]. Surg Neurol 54(1):42–54

Benndorf G, Campi A (2001b) The abberrant inferior petrsoal sinus: an unusual approach to the cavernous sinus. Neuroradiology DOI 10.1007/s002340100659

Bergstrand H, Olivecrano H, Toennis W (1936) Gefaessmissbildungen und Gefaessgeschwuelste des Gehirns. Thieme, Leipzig

Braun JP, Tournade A (1977) Venous drainage in the craniocervical region. Neuroradiology 13:155–158

Braun JP, Tournade A (1978) The venous topography of the small circumference of the tentorium. J Neuroradiol 5(1): 13–15

Braun JP, Tournade A, Ammerich H (1976) Transverse anastomoses of the veins at the base of the brain. Neuroradiology 12:165–169

Braun JP, et al. (1978) Anatomical and neuroradiological study of the veins of the tentorium and the floor of the middle cranial fossa, and their drainage to dural sinuses. J Neuroradiol 5(2):113–132

Brink JA (1995) Technical aspects of helical (spiral) CT. Radiol Clin North Am 33(5):825–841

Brismar G, Brismar J (1976) Orbital phlebography. Technique and clinical applications. Acta Ophthalmol (Copenh) 54:233–249

Brismar G, Brismar J, Cronqvist S (1976) Orbital phlebography in evaluation of the cavernous sinus and adjacent basal veins of the skull. Acta Radiol Suppl 347:43–51

Cares HL, et al. (1978) A safe technique for the precise localization of carotid-cavernous fistula during balloon obliteration. Technical note. J Neurosurg 49(1):146–149

Castaigne P, et al. (1966) Spontaneous arteriovenous communication between the external carotid and the cavernous sinus. Rev Neurol (Paris) 114:5–14

Cellerini M, et al. (1999) Phase-contrast MR angiography of intracranial dural arteriovenous fistulae. Neuroradiology 41(7):487–492

Chaloupka JC, et al. (1993) True anatomical compartmentalization of the cavernous sinus in a patient with bilateral cavernous dural arteriovenous fistulae. Case report [see comments]. J Neurosurg 79(4):592–595.

Chen CC, et al. (2005) CT angiography and MR angiography in the evaluation of carotid cavernous sinus fistula prior to embolization: a comparison of techniques. AJNR Am J Neuroradiol 26:2349–2356

Chen JC, Tsuruda JS, Halbach VV (1992) Suspected dural arteriovenous fistula: results with screening MR angiography in seven patients. Radiology 183:265–271

Chen YW, et al. (2000) Carotid and transcranial color-coded duplex sonography in different types of carotid-cavernous fistula. Stroke 31:701–706

Chiou HJ, et al. (1998) Verifying complete obliteration of carotid artery-cavernous sinus fistula: role of color Doppler ultrasonography. J Ultrasound Med 17:289–295

Clay C, Theron J, Vignaud J (1972) Value of jugulography and orbital phlebography in pathology of the cavernous sinus. Arch Ophtalmol Rev Gen Ophtalmol 32:123–135

Cochran JW, et al. (1982) Transient global amnesia after cerebral angiography. Report of seven cases. Arch Neurol 39(9):593-4

Cornelis G, et al. (1972) Rotational multiple sequence roentgenography of intracranial aneurysms. Acta Radiol (Diagn) 13:74–76

Cornelius R (1997) CCF: Imaging evaluation In: Tomsick TA (ed) Carotid cavernous fistula. Digital Educational Publishing, Cinncinati, pp 23–31

Coskun O, et al. (2000) Carotid-cavernous fistulas: diagnosis with spiral CT angiography. AJNR Am J Neuroradiol, 21(4):712–716

Cromwell LD, Kerber CW, Vermeere WR (1977) A wedge filter for craniocervical angiography. AJR Am J Roentgenol 129(6):1125–1127.

D'Angelo VA, et al. (1988) Intracerebral venous hemorrhage in „high-risk" carotid-cavernous fistula. Surg Neurol 30:387–390

Davies KN, Humphrey PR (1993) Complications of cerebral angiography in patients with symptomatic carotid territory ischaemia screened by carotid ultrasound. J Neurol Neurosurg Psychiatry 56(9):967–972.

de Keizer R (1986) Carotid cavernous fistulas and Doppler flow velocity measurements. Neuro-ophthalmology 8:205–211

de Keizer R (2003) Carotid-cavernous and orbital arteriovenous fistulas: ocular features, diagnostic and hemodynamic considerations in relation to visual impairment and morbidity. Orbit 22:121–142

de Keizer RJ (1982) A Doppler haematotachographic investigation in patients with ocular and orbital symptoms due to a carotid-cavernous fistula. Doc Ophthalmol 52(3-4):297–307

de Keizer RJ (1983) Carotid cavernous fistulas. Fortschr Ophthalmol 79(5):391–392

Debrun GM (1995) Angiographic workup of carotid cavernous sinus fistulas (CCF). What information does the interventionalist need for treatment? Surg Neurol 44:75–79

Debrun G, et al. (1981) Treatment of 54 traumatic carotid-cavernous fistulas. J Neurosurg 77:678–692

Dichgans M, D. Petersen D (1997) Angiographic complications in CADASIL. Lancet 349(9054):776-777

Dietz RR, et al. (1994) MR imaging and MR angiography in the evaluation of pulsatile tinnitus [see comments]. AJNR Am J Neuroradiol 15:879–889

Dion JE, et al. (1987) Clinical events following neuroangiography: a prospective study. Stroke 18:997–1004

Djindjian R, et al. (1968) Neuro-radiologic polymorphism of carotido-cavernous fistulas. Neurochirurgie 14(8):881–890

Djindjian R, Merland J-J (1978) Super-selective arteriography of the external carotid artery. Springer, Berlin Heidelberg New York

Djindjian R, Manelfe C, L. Picard L (1973) External carotid-cavernous sinus, arteriovenous fistulae: angiographic study of 6 cases and review of the literature. Neurochirurgie 19(1):91-110

Djindjian R, Picard L, Manelfe C (1973) Internal carotid-cavernous sinus, arteriovenous fistulae: current radio-anatomic aspects and therapeutic perspectives. Neurochirurgie 19(1):75–90

Doepp F, et al. (2001) Venous collateral blood flow assessed by Doppler ultrasound after unilateral radical neck dissection. Ann Otol Rhinol Laryngol 110(11):1055–1058

Doepp F, et al. (2004) How does the blood leave the brain? A systematic ultrasound analysis of cerebral venous drainage patterns. Neuroradiology 46:565–570

Dohrmann PJ, et al. (1985) Recurrent subarachnoid hemorrhage complicating a traumatic carotid-cavernous fistula. Neurosurgery 17(3):480–483

Dyes (1938) Gleichzeitige Roentgenaufnahmen mit gekreuzten Strahlenkegeln. Roentgenpraxis 10:252–256

Earnest Ft, et al. (1984) Complications of cerebral angiography: prospective assessment of risk. AJR Am J Roentgenol 142(2):247–253

Ecker A (1951) The normal cerebral angiogram. Thomas, Springfield

el-Sheik M, et al. (2001) Multiplanar reconstructions and three-dimensional imaging (computed rotational osteography) of complex fractures by using a C-arm system: initial results. Radiology 221:843–849

Elster AD, et al. (1991) Dilated intercavernous sinuses: an MR sign of carotid-cavernous and carotid-dural fistulas. AJNR Am J Neuroradiol 12:641–645

Erickson SJ, et al. (1989) Color Doppler flow imaging of the normal and abnormal orbit. Radiology 173:511–516

Ernst RJ, Tomsick TA (1997) Classification and angiography of carotid cavernous fistulas. In: Tomsick TA (ed) Carotid cavernous fistula. Digital Educational Publishing, pp 13–21

Fahrig R, et al. (1997) Use of a C-arm system to generate true three-dimensional computed rotational angiograms: preliminary in vitro and in vivo results. AJNR Am J Neuroradiol 18(8):1507–1514

Fahrig R, Holdsworth DW (2000) Three-dimensional computed tomographic reconstruction using a C-arm mounted XRII: image-based correction of gantry motion nonidealities. Med Phys 27(1):30–38

Fahrig R, Moreau M, Holdsworth DW (1997) Three-dimensional computed tomographic reconstruction using a C-arm mounted XRII: correction of image intensifier distortion. Med Phys 24:1097–1106

Fahrig R, et al. (1999) A three-dimensional cerebrovascular flow phantom. Med Phys 26(8):1589–1599

Fischgold H (1962) The Ziedses des Plantes subtraction method.]. Presse Med 70:193.

Fisher M, Sandler R, Weiner JM (1985) Delayed cerebral ischemia following arteriography. Stroke 16:431–434

Flaharty PM, et al. (1991) Color Doppler imaging. A new noninvasive technique to diagnose and monitor carotid cavernous sinus fistulas. Arch Ophthalmol 109:522–526

Gailloud P, et al. (2000) Angiographic anatomy of the laterocavernous sinus [in process citation]. AJNR Am J Neuroradiol 21:1923–1929

Gailloud P, et al. (2004) Three-dimensional digital angiography: new tool for simultaneous three-dimensional rendering of vascular and osseous information during rotational angiography. AJNR Am J Neuroradiol 25:571–573

Glickman MG, Gletne JS, Mainzer F (1971) The basal projection in cerebral angiography. Radiology 98(3):611–618.

Goldberg RA, et al. (1996) Management of cavernous sinus-dural fistulas. Indications and techniques for primary embolization via the superior ophthalmic vein [see comments]. Arch Ophthalmol 114:707–714

Goncalves M, Reis J, Almeida R (1994) Carotid-cavernous fistulae. The diagnostic and therapeutic prospects. Acta Med Port 7(7-8):427–432

Grass M, Kohler T, Proksa R (2000) 3D cone-beam CT reconstruction for circular trajectories. Phys Med Biol 45(2):329-47

Grass M, Kohler T, Proksa R (2001) Angular weighted hybrid cone-beam CT reconstruction for circular trajectories. Phys Med Biol 46(6):1595–1610

Grass M, et al. 1999) Three-dimensional reconstruction of high contrast objects using C-arm image intensifier projection data. Comput Med Imaging Graph 23(6):311–321

Haike H (1902) Zur Anatomie des Sinus caroticus (Plexus venous caroticus) und seine Beziehungen zu Erkrankungen des Ohres. Archiv f. Ohrenheilkunde:17–22

Halbach VV, et al. (1989) Embolization of branches arising from the cavernous portion of the internal carotid artery. AJNR Am J Neuroradiol 10(1):143–150

Hankey GJ, Warlow CP, Sellar RJ (1990) Cerebral angiographic risk in mild cerebrovascular disease. Stroke 21:209–222

Harding AE, et al. (1984) Intracerebral haemorrhage complicating dural arteriovenous fistula: a report of two cases. J Neurol Neurosurg Psychiatry 47(9):905–911

Harnsberger H, Osborn A, Ross J (2006) Diagnostic and surgical imaging anatomy. Amirsys, Salt Lake City

Harrison MJ, et al. (1997) Preliminary results on the management of unruptured intracranial aneurysms with magnetic resonance angiography and computed tomographic angiography. Neurosurgery 40(5):947–955; discussion 955-7.

Hartung O, Alimi YS, Juhan C (2004) Tinnitus resulting from tandem lesions of the internal carotid artery: combined extracranial endarterectomy and intrapetrous primary stenting. J Vasc Surg 39:679–681

Hasuo K, et al. (1997) Dural non-cavernous sinus arteriovenous fistulas symptomatically simulating spontaneous carotid-cavernous fistulas: an analysis of angiographic findings. Radiat Med 15(4):203–208

Heautot JF, et al. (1998) Analysis of cerebrovascular diseases by a new 3-dimensional computerised X-ray angiography system. Neuroradiology 40:203–209

Heran NS, et al. (2006) The utility of DynaCT in neuroendovascular procedures. AJNR Am J Neuroradiol 27:330–332

Hirabuki N, et al. (1992) Follow-up MRI in dural arteriovenous malformations involving the cavernous sinus: emphasis on detection of venous thrombosis. Neuroradiology 34:423–427

Hirai T, et al. (1998) Three-dimensional FISP imaging in the evaluation of carotid cavernous fistula: comparison with contrast-enhanced CT and spin-echo MR. AJNR Am J Neuroradiol 19:253–259

Hiramatsu K, et al. (1991) Intracerebral hemorrhage in carotid-cavernous fistula. Neuroradiology 33(1):67-69

Hoff DJ, et al. (1994) Rotational angiography assessment of cerebral aneurysms. AJNR Am J Neuroradiol 15(10):1945–1948

Holm O (1944) Cinematography in Cerebral Angiography. Acta Radiol 25:163–173

Hoops JP, et al. (1997) Dural carotid-cavernous sinus fistulas: clinical aspects, diagnosis and therapeutic intervention. Klin Monatsbl Augenheilkd 210(6):392–397

Huber P (1976) A technical contribution of the exact angiographic localization of carotid cavernous fistulas. Neuroradiology 10:239–241

Ikawa F, et al. (1996) Diagnosis of carotid-cavernous fistulas with magnetic resonance angiography-demonstrating the draining veins utilizing 3-D time-of-flight and 3-D phase-contrast techniques. Neurosurg Rev 19:7–12

Ishida F, et al. (2003) Traumatic carotid-cavernous fistula identified by three-dimensional digital subtraction angiography – technical note. Neurol Med Chir (Tokyo) 43:369–372; discussion 373

Jahan R, et al. (1998) Transvenous embolization of a dural arteriovenous fistula of the cavernous sinus through the contralateral pterygoid plexus. Neuroradiology 40:189–193

Jorgensen JS, Gutthoff RF (1985) 24 cases of carotid cavernosus fistulas: frequency, symptoms, diagnosis and treatment. Acta Ophthalmol Suppl 173:67–71

Katsuta T, Rhoton, AL Jr, Matsushima T (1997) The jugular foramen: microsurgical anatomy and operative approaches. Neurosurgery 41(1):149–201; discussion 201-2

Kerber CW, et al. (1978) Cerebral ischemia. I. Current angiographic techniques, complications, and safety. AJR Am J Roentgenol 130:1097–1103

Kilic T, et al. (2001) Value of transcranial Doppler ultrasonography in the diagnosis and follow-up of carotid-cavernous fistulae. Acta Neurochir (Wien) 143(12):1257–1264, discussion 1264–1265

Kim JK, et al. (1996) Traumatic bilateral carotid-cavernous fistulas treated with detachable balloon. A case report. Acta Radiol 37(1):46–48

Kitajima M, et al. (2005) Retrograde cortical and deep venous drainage in patients with intracranial dural arteriovenous fistulas: comparison of MR imaging and angiographic findings. AJNR Am J Neuroradiol 26:1532–1538

Knecht B (1937) Die Bedeutung der Arteria carotis interna in der hlas-Nasen-Ohrenheilkunde. Archiv f. Ohren-, Nasen-, u. Kehlkopfheilkunde 143:1–47

Knosp E, Mueller G, Perneczky A (1987) The blood supply of the cranial nerves in the lateral wall of the cavernous sinus, in The cavernous sinus, V.V. Dolenc, Editor. Springer: Wien-New York. p. 67–79

Knott JF (1882) On the cerebral sinuses and their variations. J Anat Physiol 16:27–42.

Koch RL, Bieber WP, Hill MC (1967) The hanging head position for detection of site of internal carotid artery occlusion. Am J Roentgenol Radium Ther Nucl Med 101(1):111–115

Komiyama M, et al. (1990) MR imaging of dural AV fistulas at the cavernous sinus. J Comput Assist Tomogr 14:397–401

Komiyama M, et al. (1989) Magnetic resonance imaging of intracavernous pathology. Neurol Med Chir (Tokyo), 29(7)573–578

Komiyama M, et al. (1990) Indirect carotid-cavernous sinus fistula: transvenous embolization from the external jugular vein using a superior ophthalmic vein approach. A case report. Surg Neurol 33(1):57–63

Krayenbuehl H (1941) Das Hirnaneurysma. Schweiz Arch Neurol Psychiatr 47:155–236

Krayenbühl H, Yasargil MG (1979) Zerebrale Angiographie in Klinik und Praxis. Thieme, Stuttgart

Kufeld M, et al. (2003) Three-dimensional rotational myelography. AJNR Am J Neuroradiol 24:1290–1293

Kumazaki T, (1998) Development of rotational digital angiography and new cone-beam 3D image: clinical value in vascular lesions. Comput Methods Programs Biomed 57(1-2):139–12

Kurata A, et al. (1998) The value of long-term clinical follow-up for cases of spontaneous carotid cavernous fistula. Acta Neurochir (Wien) 140(1):65-72.

Kurokawa Y, et al. (2000) The usefulness of 3D-CT angiography for the diagnosis of spontaneous vertebral artery dissection-report of two cases. Comput Med Imaging Graph 24(2):115–119

Kurokawa Y, et al. (2000) The use of three-dimensional computed tomographic angiography in the accurate diagnosis of internal carotid artery aneurysms: degree for expression of posterior communicating and anterior choroidal arteries. Comput Med Imaging Graph 24(4):231–241.

Kwon BJ, et al. (2005a) Endovascular occlusion of direct carotid cavernous fistula with detachable balloons: usefulness of 3D angiography. Neuroradiology 47:271–281

Kwon BJ, et al. (2005b) MR imaging findings of intracranial dural arteriovenous fistulas: relations with venous drainage patterns. AJNR Am J Neuroradiol 26:2500–2507

Lang J (1979) Kopf, Teil B, Gehirn und Augenschädel, vol 1. Springer, Berlin Heidelberg New York

Lang J, Weigel M (1983) Nerve-vessel relation in jugular foramen region. Anat Clin 5:1–16

Lasjaunias P (1984) Arteriography of the head and neck:normal functional anatomy of the external carotid artery. In: Bergeron T (ed) Head and neck imaging excluding the brain. Mosby, St Louis, pp 344–354

Lasjaunias P, Berenstein A (1987) Functional anatomy of craniofacial arteries in surgical neuroangiography. In: Surgical neuroangiography. Springer, Berlin Heidelberg New York, pp 239–244

Lasjaunias P, Berenstein A, terBrugge K (2001) Clinical vascular anatomy and variations. Springer, Berlin Heidelberg New York

Leeds NE, et al. (1968) Serial magnification erebral angiography. Radiology 90:1171–1175

Leffers AM, Wagner A (2000) Neurologic complications of cerebral angiography. A retrospective study of complication rate and patient risk factors. Acta Radiol 41:204–210

Liang EY, et al. (1995) Detection and assessment of intracranial aneurysms: value of CT angiography with shaded-surface display. AJR Am J Roentgenol, 1995. 165(6): p. 1497-502.

Lima PA (1935) La technique de l'angiographie cerebrale. Rev Neurol 64:623–624

Lin TK, Chang CN, Wai YY (1992) Spontaneous intracerebral hematoma from occult carotid-cavernous fistula during pregnancy and puerperium. Case report. J Neurosurg, 1992. 76(4):714–717

List CF, Burge C, Hodges F (1945) Intracranial angiography. Radiology 45:1–14

Lombardi G, Passerini A (1967), The orbital veins. Am J Ophthalmol 64(3):440-7.

Lysholm E (1931) Apparatus and technique for roentgen examination of the skull. Acta Radiol Suppl 12

Martins C, et al. (2005) Microsurgical anatomy of the dural arteries. Neurosurgery 56:211–251; discussion 211–251

Mascalchi M, et al. (1997) MRI and MR angiography of vertebral artery dissection. Neuroradiology, 1997. 39(5):329–340

McIvor J, et al. (1987) Neurological morbidity of arch and carotid arteriography in cerebrovascular disease. The influence of contrast medium and radiologist. Br J Radiol 60:117–122

Medina LS (2000) Three-dimensional CT maximum intensity projections of the calvaria: a new approach for diagnosis of craniosynostosis and fractures. AJNR Am J Neuroradiol 21(10): p. 1951-4.

Medina LS, et al. (2001) Children with macrocrania: clinical and imaging predictors of disorders requiring surgery. AJNR Am J Neuroradiol, 2001. 22(3):564-70.

Mehringer CM, et al. (1982) Improved localization of carotid cavernous fistula during angiography. AJNR Am J Neuroradiol 3:82–84

Metens T, et al. (2000) Intracranial aneurysms: detection with gadolinium-enhanced dynamic three-dimensional MR angiography-initial results. Radiology 216(1):39–46

Miller DL, Doppman JL, Chang R (1993) Anatomy of the junction of the inferior petrosal sinus and the internal jugular vein. AJNR Am J Neuroradiol 14:1075–1083

Missler U, et al. (2000) Three-dimensional reconstructed rotational digital subtraction angiography in planning treatment of intracranial aneurysms. Eur Radiol 10(4):564–56

Modic MT, Berlin AJ, Weinstein MA (1982) The use of digital subtraction angiography in the evaluation of carotid cavernous sinus fistulas. Ophthalmology 89(5):441–444

Modic MT, et al. (1982) Digital subtraction angiography of the intracranial vascular system: comparative study in 55 patients. AJR Am J Roentgenol 138(2):299-306.

Molnar LJ, et al. (2001) Doppler mapping of direct carotid-cavernous fistulae (DCCF). Ultrasound Med Biol 27(3):367–371

Moniz E (1927) Encéphalographie artérielle: son importance dans le diagnostic des tumeurs cérébrales. Rev Neurolog 1:48–72

Moniz, E., L'angiographie cerebrale. Ses applications et resultats en anatomie, physiologie et clinique. 1934, Paris: Masson. 327pp.

Moniz E, Lima A, Caldes P (1934) Angiographies en serie de la circulation de la tete. Rev. neurol 1: p. 489-510.

Montane D, Casado J (1997) Treatment of carotid cavernous fistulas. Rev Neurol 25(148):1963–1967

Morris L (1970) A lateral oblique view in cerebral angiography. Radiology 96(1):61–65

Motoyama Y, et al. (2000) A case of high flow CCF with congestive hemorrhage. No Shinkei Geka 28(7):647–651

Munk PL, et al. (1992) Colour-flow Doppler imaging of a carotid-cavernous fistula. Can Assoc Radiol J 43:227–229

Newton TH, Cronqvist S (1969) Involvement of dural arteries in intracranial arteriovenous malformations. Radiology, 1969. 93(5):1071–1078

Newton TH, Hoyt WF (1968) Spontaneous arteriovenous fistula between dural branches of the internal maxillary artery and the posterior cavernous sinus. Radiology 91:1147–1150

Newton TH, Hoyt WF (1970) Dural arteriovenous shunts in the region of the cavernous sinus. Neuroradiology 1:71–81

Ning R, Wang X (1996) Acad Radiol

Nishijima M, et al. (1985) Spontaneous occlusion of traumatic carotid cavernous fistula after orbital venography. Surg Neurol 23(5):489–492

Nishio A, et al. (2004) Three-dimensional rotation venography using the digital subtraction angiography unit with a flat-panel detector: usefulness for the transtemporal/transtentorial approaches. Neuroradiology 46:876–882

Ohshima S, et al. (2006) Venous infarction associated with carotid-cavernous fistula. Rinsho Shinkeigaku 46(4):261–265

Ohtsuka K, Hashimoto M (1999) The results of serial dynamic enhanced computed tomography in patients with carotid-cavernous sinus fistulas. Jpn J Ophthalmol 43:559–564

Ouanounou S, et al. (1999) Cavernous sinus and inferior petrosal sinus flow signal on three-dimensional time-of-flight MR angiography. AJNR Am J Neuroradiol 20(8):1476–1481

Parkinson D (1963) Normal anatomy of cavernous carotid and its surgical significance. Presented at the Annual Meeting of the Harvey Cushing Society, April 1963, Philadelphia

Parkinson D (1984) Arteries of the cavernous sinus. J Neurosurg 61:203

Parlea L, et al. (1999) An analysis of the geometry of saccular intracranial aneurysms. AJNR Am J Neuroradiol 20(6):1079–1089

Paullus WS, Pait TG, Rhoton AI (1977) Microsurgical exposure of the petrous portion of the carotid artery. J Neurosurg 47:713–726

Pelkonen O, et al. (2004) Pulsatile tinnitus as a symptom of cervicocephalic arterial dissection. J Laryngol Otol 118:193–198

Phatouros CC, et al. (2000) Carotid artery cavernous fistulas. Neurosurg Clin N Am 11(1):67–84, viii.

Picard L (1997) 3D-Angiography – techniques, results, interest for interventional neuroradiology. Presented at ASITN/WFITN Scientific Conference, September 13–16 1997, New York,

Rao VM, et al. (2001) Use trends and geographic variation in Neuroimaging: nationwide medicare data for 1993 and 1998. AJNR Am J Neuroradiol 22:1643–1649.

Rektorzik E (1858) Sitzungsber. Akad. Wiss. Wien. Math.-naturwiss. Kl. 32:466.

Rey A, et al. (1973) Treatment of carotid-cavernous fistulae. Neurochirurgie 19(1):111–122

Rhoton AL Jr (2000) Jugular foramen. Neurosurgery 47:S267–285

Rhoton AL Jr, Hardy DG, Chambers SM (1979) Microsurgical anatomy and dissection of the sphenoid bone, cavernous sinus and sellar region. Surg Neurol 12:63–104

Rhoton AL Jr, Fujii K, Fradd B (1979) Microsurgical anatomy of the anterior choroidal artery. Surg Neurol 12(2):171–187

Rhoton A, Harris F, Fujii K (1984) Anatomy of the cavernous sinus. In: Kapp J, Schmidek H (eds) The cerebral venous system and its disorders. Grune & Stratton, Orlando, pp 61–91

Rybicki FJ, et al. (2006) Utilization of thick (>3 mm) maximum intensity projection images in coronary CTA interpretation. Emerg Radiol 13:157–159

Saint-Felix DM, Trousset Y (1994) Phys Med Biol

San Millan Ruiz D, et al. (1999) Laterocavernous sinus. Anat Rec 254:7–12

San Millan Ruiz D, et al (2002) The craniocervical venous system in relation to cerebral venous drainage. AJNR Am J Neuroradiol 23:1500–1508

Sato N, et al. (1997) Pituitary gland enlargement secondary to dural arteriovenous fistula in the cavernous sinus: appearance at MR imaging. Radiology 203:263–267

Satoh K, et al. (2001) Cerebellar hemorrhage caused by dural arteriovenous fistula: a review of five cases. J Neurosurg 94:422–426

Schreiber SJ, et al. (2004) Doppler sonographic evaluation of shunts in patients with dural arteriovenous fistulas. AJNR Am J Neuroradiol 25(5):775-80.

Schreiber SJ, et al. (2005) Internal jugular vein valve incompetence and intracranial venous anatomy in transient global amnesia. J Neurol Neurosurg Psychiatry 76(4):509–513

Schreiber SJ, et al. (2003) Extrajugular pathways of human cerebral venous blood drainage assessed by duplex ultrasound. J Appl Physiol 94:1802–1805

Schuknecht B, et al. (1998) Tributary venosinus occlusion and septic cavernous sinus thrombosis: CT and MR findings. AJNR Am J Neuroradiol 19:617–626

Schumacher, M., K. Kutluk, and D. Ott, Digital rotational radiography in neuroradiology. AJNR Am J Neuroradiol, 1989. 10(3): p. 644-9.

Seldinger SJ (1953) Catheter replacement of the needle in percutaneous arteriography. Acta Radiol 39:368–376

Sergott RC, et al. (1987) The syndrome of paradoxical worsening of dural-cavernous sinus arteriovenous malformations. Ophthalmology 94:205–212

Seynaeve PC, Broos JI (1995) The history of tomography. J Belge Radiol 78(5):284–288

Shimizu T, et al. (1988) Transvenous balloon occlusion of the cavernous sinus: an alternative therapeutic choice for recurrent traumatic carotid-cavernous fistulas. Neurosurgery 22(3):550–553

Shiu PC, et al. (1968) Cavernous sinus venography. Am J Roentgenol Radium Therm Nucl Med 104:57–62

Slaba S, et al. (1998) Cavernous dural fistulas: Importance of trans-ocular Doppler ultrasound in evaluating venous patency and therapeutic choices. J Radiol 79(2):153–156

Soderman M, et al. (2006) Gamma knife surgery for dural arteriovenous shunts: 25 years of experience. J Neurosurg 104(6):867–875

Spahn M (2005) Flat detectors and their clinical applications. Eur Radiol 15:1934–1947

Spector RH (1991) Echographic diagnosis of dural carotid-cavernous sinus fistulas [see comments]. Am J Ophthalmol 111(1):77–83

Suetens P (2002) Fundamentals of medical imaging. Cambridge University Press, Cambridge, NY

Takahashi K (1940) Die perkutane Arteriographie der A. vertebralis und ihrer Versorgungsgebiete. Arch Psychiatr Nervenkr 111:373–379

Takahashi S, Tomura N, Watarai J, Mizoi K, Manabe H (1999) Dural arteriovenous fistula of the cavernous sinus with venous congestion of the brain stem: report of two cases. AJNR Am J Neuroradiol 20:886–888

Takahashi S, Sakuma I, Omachi K, Otani T, Tomura N, Watarai J, Mizoi K (2005) Craniocervical junction venous anatomy around the suboccipital cavernous sinus: evaluation by MR imaging. Eur Radiol 15:1694–1700

Tanoue S, et al. (2000) Three-dimensional reconstructed images after rotational angiography in the evaluation of intracranial aneurysms: surgical correlation [In Process Citation]. Neurosurgery 47(4):866–871

Teng MM, et al. (1991) Brainstem edema: an unusual complication of carotid cavernous fistula. AJNR Am J Neuroradiol 12:139–142

Thanapura C, (2004) Treatment of traumatic carotid-cavernous fistula at the Udon Thani Center Hospital. J Clin Neurosci, 2004. 11(5):498–500

Theron J (1972) Cavernous plexus affluents. Neurochirurgie 18:623–638

Theron J, Djindjian R (1973) Cervicovertebral phlebography using catheterization. A preliminary report. Radiology 108(2):325–331

Theron J, Djindjian R (1973) Comparison of the venous phase of carotid arteriography with direct intracranial venography in the evaluation of lesions at the base of the skull. Neuroradiology 5(1):43–48

Thron A, Voigt K (1983) Rotational cerebral angiography: procedure and value. AJNR Am J Neuroradiol 4:289–291

Toennis, Bergstrand, Olivecrona (1937) Gefaessmissbildungen und Gefaessgeschwuelste des Gehirns

Tomandl BF, et al. (2001) Local and remote visualization techniques for interactive direct volume rendering in neuroradiology. Radiographics 21(6):1561–1572

Trolard P (1868) Anatomie du systeme veineux de l'encephale et du crane. In: These de la Faculte de Medicine de Paris, Paris, pp 1–32

Tsai LK, et al. (2004) Diagnosis of intracranial dural arteriovenous fistulas by carotid duplex sonography. J Ultrasound Med 23(6):785–791

Tsai LK, et al. (2005) Carotid duplex sonography in the follow-up of intracranial dural arteriovenous fistulae. AJNR Am J Neuroradiol 26(3):625–629

Tsai YF, et al. (2004) Utility of source images of three-dimensional time-of-flight magnetic resonance angiography in the diagnosis of indirect carotid-cavernous sinus fistulas. J Neuroophthalmol 24(4):285–289

Turner DM, et al. (1983) Spontaneous intracerebral hematoma in carotid-cavernous fistula. Report of three cases. J Neurosurg 59(4): p. 680–686

Uchino A, et al. (1992) MRI of dural carotid-cavernous fistulas.

Comparisons with postcontrast CT. Clin Imaging 16:263–268

Uchino A, et al. (1997) Pontine venous congestion caused by dural carotid-cavernous fistula: report of two cases. Eur Radiol 7:405–408

Uehara T, et al. (1998) Spontaneous dural carotid cavernous sinus fistula presenting isolated ophthalmoplegia: evaluation with MR angiography. Neurology 50(3):814–816

Unger B, et al. (1999) Digital 3D rotational angiography for the preoperative and preinterventional clarification of cerebral arterial aneurysms. Rofo Fortschr Geb Rontgenstr Neuen Bildgeb Verfahr 170(5):482–491

Vaghi MA, Savoiardo M, Strada L (1983) Unusual computerized tomography appearance of a carotid-cavernous fistula. Case report. J Neurosurg 58(3):435–437

van Ooijen P, Irwan R (2006) Coronary 3D MRI, EBT, and MDCT. In: Baert AL, Sartor K (eds) Coronary radiology. Springer, Berlin Heidelberg New York, pp 245–273

Voigt K, Stoeter P, Petersen D (1975) Rotational cerebral roentgenography. I. Evaluation of the technical procedure and diagnostic application with model studies. Neuroradiology 10:95–100

Volk M, et al. (1997) Flat-panel x-ray detector using amorphous silicon technology. Reduced radiation dose for the detection of foreign bodies. Invest Radiol 32(7):373–377

Wang Y, Xiao LH, Imaging diagnosis of carotid cavernous fistula. Zhonghua Yan Ke Za Zhi 40(10):674–678

Watanabe A, et al. (1990) The cerebral circulation in cases of carotid cavernous fistula. Findings of single photon emission computed tomography. Neuroradiology 32:108–113

Waugh JR, Sacharias N (1992) Arteriographic complications in the DSA era. Radiology 182(1):243–246

Weisberg LA (1970) Computed tomographic findings in carotid-cavernous fistula. Comput Tomogr 5(1): 31–36

Wende S, Schindler K (1970) Technique and use of X-ray magnification in cerebral arteriography. Neuroradiology 1:117–120

Wetzel SG, et al. (2000) Cerebral dural arteriovenous fistulas: detection by dynamic MR projection angiography. AJR Am J Roentgenol 174(5):1293–1295

Wicky S, et al. (2000) Comparison between standard radiography and spiral CT with 3D reconstruction in the evaluation, classification and management of tibial plateau fractures. Eur Radiol, 10(8):1227–1232

Willinsky R, et al. (1994) Venous congestion: an MR finding in dural arteriovenous malformations with cortical venous drainage. AJNR Am J Neuroradiol 15(8):1501–1507

Willinsky RA, et al. (2003) Neurologic complications of cerebral angiography: prospective analysis of 2,899 procedures and review of the literature. Radiology 227:522–528

Wolff H, Schaltenbrand G (1939) Die perkutane Arteriographie der Hirngefaesse. Zbl Neurochir 4:233–239

Wolff H, Schmid B (1993) Das Arteriogramm des pulsierenden Exophthalmus. Zbl. Neurochir 4:241–250, 310–319.

Yasuda A, et al. (2005) Microsurgical anatomy and approaches to the cavernous sinus. Neurosurgery 56(1 Suppl):4–27; discussion 4–27.

Zeidman SM, et al. (1995) Reversibility of white matter changes and dementia after treatment of dural fistulas. AJNR Am J Neuroradiol 16(5):1080–1083

Ziedses des Plantes B (1934) Planigrafie en Subtractie. University of Utrecht, The Netherlands

Ziedses des Plantes BG (1935) Subtraktion. Fortschr Roentgenstr 52:69–79

Ziedses des Plantes BG (1961) Application de la soustraction a l'angiographie carotidienne. Ann Radiol 4:625–631

Ziedses des Plantes, BG (1961b) Subtraktion. Stuttgart: Thieme. 69–79.

Endovascular Treatment

(Case Reports I–VII, Case Illustrations I–XI)

8

C O N T E N T S

8.1

Techniques of Transvenous Catheterization
(Figs. 8.1–8.4)

Manual techniques of catheterization and embolization may differ from center to center and vary significantly between operators. The following descriptions are based on the author's personal experiences

gained over more than a decade performing EVT in cerebrovascular lesions. Although mainly based on subjective manual handlings and personal preferences, these accounts may be beneficial, especially for younger colleagues. As for most endovascular procedures in the treatment of cerebrovascular lesions, the embolization of DCSFs is performed under general anesthesia, preferably under supervision of an experienced neuroanesthesiologist. Transvenous

catheterizations and embolizations are often lengthy procedures (2–4 h), during which the typically elderly patients would have difficulties remaining still on an angiographic table. General anesthesia with endotracheal intubation is therefore widely used in most centers in the world, as it also allows for safer monitoring and easier management in cases of intraprocedural complications such as rupture and hemorrhage.

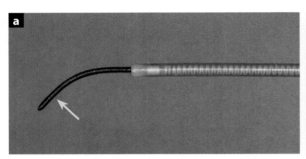 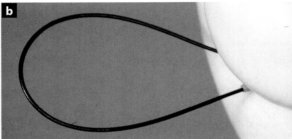

Fig. 8.1 a, b. Endovascular tools preferably used by the author for transvenous catheterizations of the cavernous sinus: a Microcatheter Tracker Excel®-14 (BSC, Fremont CA), braided and hydrophilic coated, outer diameter of the distal tip: 0.65 mm. *Arrow*: introduced hydrophilic micro guidewire Headliner® 0.012″ (Terumo®, Japan), very flexible with a 1:1 torquability, diameter of the 45° preshaped tip: 0.3 mm. It adapts well to very narrow and irregular venous structures and enables use of the "Loop Technique" (**b** Fig. 8.3) to pass thrombosed venous segments. This very supple guidewire has been used alternately with the hydrophilic coated Transend® 0.014″ (BSC, Fremont, CA) that has a stiffer tip, but also provides more support for the microcatheter

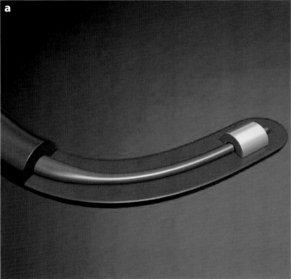 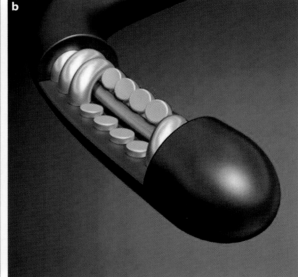

Fig. 8.2 a,b. Terumo® microguidewires with hydrophilic coating. a Glidewire® Gold Neuro with a 8 cm tapered distal end and a 2 mm Gold tip comes in 0.011″, 0.014″, 0.016″ and 0.018″. **b** Headliner (MicroVention, Terumo, Japan) has a superelastic kink-resistant Nitinol core with a 20 cm or 35 cm distal taper and a 20 mm gold tip for enhanced radiopacity. The wire is available in various pre-shaped tip configurations, such as 45° and 90°, or as 90°/150° double angle and comes in sizes of 0.012″, 0.014″ and 0.016″. Although available for more than 10 years, microguidewires from Terumo are still considered superior to their competitors, mainly because of their durability. The Headliner proved particularly useful for advancement in narrowed and thrombosed sinuses (Figs. 8.3, 8.15, 8.17, 8.20, 8.31, 8.38)

8.1.1
Inferior Petrosal Sinus Approach
(Case Reports I–III, Fig. 8.3)

After arterial and venous femoral punctures and placement of 6-F introducer sheaths, an intravenous bolus of 50 IU/kg of body weight heparin is administered. Monitoring is routinely performed in most centers to keep the activated clotting time (ACT) at a level of approximately 250–300 s or 2× above the normal level.

A 4-F Headhunter 1 catheter (H1, Cordis, Miami, FL) is advanced into the ECA or ICA on the side of the dominant fistula supply to allow for road mapping and control injections throughout the procedure. A 5-F or 6-F angled guiding catheter (e.g. Envoy, Cordis Endovascular, Miami Lakes, FL) is placed in the IJV on the side that shows dominant drainage, or that looks most promising on the diagnostic angiograms. The catheters are flushed with heparinized saline (1500 IU per liter). Arterial and venous femoral punctures may be performed uni- or bilaterally (Fig. 8.13).

Alternatively, a direct stick of the jugular vein may be used, especially in cases with a thrombosed jugular vein on the fistula side. Because the entire catheterization system becomes shorter and provides better support for a supple microcatheter, a direct jugular stick makes microcatheter navigation through the IPS easier. A microcatheter may even be navigated directly through a 4-F or 5-F sheath when the IPS is widely open. The less access tools and devices are used, the easier the technical part of the procedure is, including deployment of coils, glue or a catheter exchange. The guiding catheter should be advanced close to the jugular bulb for performing phlebograms using either manual injections (20-cc syringe), or a power injector. If the anatomy looks abnormal, or the IPS appears thrombosed or is absent, contrast injections should be repeated from different positions and combined with a 3D phlebogram. Changing the position of the guide may be helpful, because in some cases the IPS may terminate at a lower level or even outside the skull base, and thus will be missed on standard 2D angiograms as seen in Fig. 7.37 (BENNDORF and CAMPI 2001b; CALZOLARI 2002).

If the IPS is not identifiable on either side, even after repeated phlebograms, careful image analysis is crucial in order to identify the small "notch" or a stump that is often the only residual filling of a thrombosed sinus (Figs. 8.3, 8.4, 8.14). This should include diagnostic arterial injections, particularly in cases in which there is no posterior drainage, or the IPS is thrombosed. In those cases, the sinus may be wide open, utilized as an efferent vein by the normal cerebral venous drainage, and in fact representing a feasible transvenous approach (Case report III). If the IPS can be identified, retrograde catheterization is readily performed using a small hydrophilic-coated microcatheter, such as a 2.6-F FasTracker 10, (Boston Scientific, Fremont, CA).

Braided, reinforced microcatheters such as the 2.4-F Tracker Excel-14, 1.7-F Excelsior SL 10 (Boston Scientific, Fremont, CA) or the 3.0-F Rapid Transit 18 (Cordis, Endovascular, Miami Lakes), advanced over a 0.012″, 0.014″or 0.016″ guidewire, usually allow easier navigation through the IPS and the CS, especially in cases, where the contralateral CS (cross-over) needs to be reached. Reinforced microcatheters are more stable throughout the procedure, an important factor in achieving a dense coil packing in the fistulous compartment. They also show fewer tendencies to kink, which is advantageous when using larger coils. An experimental study showed that even some reinforced catheters, such as the Rapid Transit 18 (Cordis Endovascular, Miami Lakes, FL) may develop luminal irregularities in a curved model that may create high resistance for embolic agents (KIYOSUE et al. 2005). Significant friction may result when pushing fibered coils (Case Report IV).

In cases where the IPS cannot be identified with certainty, the residual "notch", if visible, should be catheterized very gently with a small, hydrophilic guidewire. For this purpose, the 0.012″ hydrophilic-coated wire (Headliner, Terumo Corporation, Tokyo, Japan) is considered the most suitable guidewire to be use. It is a highly flexible, kink-resistant wire with a super-elastic nitinol core providing a 1:1 torque ratio, and has a 20-mm gold coil at the tip for enhanced radiopacity (Fig. 8.2). The Headliner has a superior lubricity and is available in 200 cm length in various pre-shaped tip configurations such as 45°, 90°, 1.5-mm J-Tip angle and double angle.

Some operators may prefer the Synchro2 wire (BSC, Natick, MA) that is available as 0.014″ hydrophilic guidewire (external diameter 0.36 mm), or 0.010″ guidewire (external diameter 0.3 mm) with pre-shaped platinum-tungsten alloy tips. The proximal portion is coated with a polymer (Polytetrafluoroethylene, PTFE) to enhance tracking and manipulation. An alternate choice is the Mirage, a 0.008″ hydrophilic coated guidewire (0.20 mm) manufactured by MTI (Microtherapeutics, Irvine,

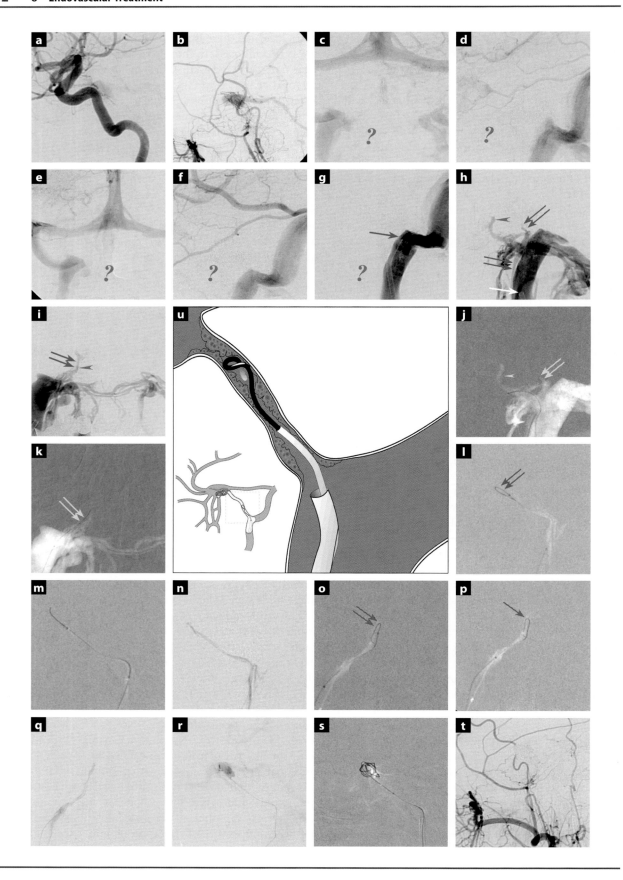

CA; Fig. 8.11). Another new development is the steerable guidewire Watusi (Micrus Endovascular Corporation, San Jose, CA) available in 0.014″ (0.36 mm), made of stainless steel with a hydrophilic coating of the distal 40 cm. The smallest guidewire currently available is the 0.007″ Sorcerer, (Balt Extrusion, Montmorency, France), a hydrophilic nitinol wire. The choice of microguidewires and microcatheters depends, to a large degree, on personal preferences, as well as on the type and level of acquired manual skills.

Using the microcatheter, the Headliner should be advanced only a few mm into the thrombosed IPS and then exchanged for a more stable hydrophilic coated guidewire such as the Transend 0.014″ (Boston Scientific, Fremont, CA). This guidewire provides more stability to advance the microcatheter, while its tip is less flexible than that of the Headliner. The technique, utilized by the author to pass a thrombosed IPS, is to alternately and slowly advance both guidewires with the help of the microcatheter towards the posterior CS. It requires patience and full concentration and should be performed by an experienced operator. Aggressive or forceful manipulations may cause rupture of the IPS. For advancing a catheter through an irregular, stenosed, or even occluded sinus, the following technique proved particularly useful:

The guidewire is advanced not with a straight end, but instead with a loop that is formed within the narrowed lumen by bending the tip. Such a distal shape can be navigated much more easily than one would expect as it adapts better to an irregular lumen than a straight guidewire. It gets less entangled in small septi or stenotic segments of the trabeculated cavernous sinus structure.

This method, also called the "Loop Technique" (Figs. 8.3, 8.15, 8.20, 8.17), published earlier, has been used since with great success (BENNDORF et al. 2000a), and has been adapted by others (CHENG et al. 2003). A Terumo guidewire such as the Headliner-12 with a pre-shaped 90° angle or double angle is particularly easy to form.

In order to avoid unintentional catheterization of bridging or pontine veins and to prevent perforation with subsequent intracranial hemorrhage, as reported by some authors (HALBACH et al. 1988; OISHI et al. 1999), the simultaneous use of bi-plane "blank road mapping" and fluoroscopy of the native background are helpful.

When the posterior CS is approached through the IPS, it is usually possible to navigate the microcatheter into the anterior compartment and its connection with the SOV without difficulties. It is advisable to bring the microcatheter as close as possible to the SOV, preferably in its first segment. Coil deployment should begin within the SOV approximately 2–3 mm before its entry into the CS. This initial coil positioning is crucial to avoid increased drainage of the AV shunting into the SOV and ophthalmological deterioration. On the other hand, coils deployed in the anterior SOV (2nd or 3rd segment) may cause thrombosis and occlusion of the entire vein with blockage of the central retinal venous drainage leading to serious clinical consequences. To achieve dense packing from the beginning, it is wise to start with a coil size that can be easily stabilized in an enlarged SOV (e.g. 5 mm/15 cm). Three-dimensional or complex coils may also be used to create a basket that, similar to aneurysms, is subsequently filled with smaller and softer coils (Fig. 8.5). The more stable this initial packing within the proximal SOV or at the CS-SOV junction is, the better it may be used as a scaffold for subsequent coils. It will allow a dense packing of the CS, without the risk of dislodging coils into the draining vein. Commonly, the coil placement is performed from anterior to posterior to keep the access through the IPS free until the end of the procedure. This is a useful strategy because there is always the chance that coils get inadvertently placed early dur-

Fig. 8.3 a–u. Loop Technique for catheter navigation through the thrombosed IPS. Type D fistula in an 80-year-old female with 6th nerve palsy and mild red eye. **a, b** Initial DSA demonstrating an AV shunt at the posterior CS draining into SPS and leptomeningeal veins, not into the IPS. **c–f** Bilateral late venous phase. Note there is no filling of the IPS here. **g–i** Jugular phlebogram showing the residual "notch" of the IPS. Note that in (**g**) due to the catheter position (too high, *white arrow*), the IPS is not opacified. **h, i** When the guiding catheter is positioned lower (*white arrow*), several communicating veins are visualized. In this case, it is mainly the inferior petroclival vein (IPCV, *arrowhead*), while the IPS (*double arrow*) is only faintly opacified. **j, k** Road Map and retrograde catherization of IPS using the loop techniqe (lateral view). **l–r** Stepwise, gentle advancement of the microcatheter with alternating guidewires (Transend and Headliner). Control sinograms (**n, q**) may not show any connection to the CS or to the fistula during navigation through the IPS. **r, s** Successful navigation into the posterior CS and subsequent coil packing with complete occlusion by the end of the procedure (**t**). **u** Artist's illustration of the loop technique using an angled (90°) Headliner that allows advancement of the microcatheter even through a narrowed and thrombosed IPS (BENNDORF et al., 2000a)

ing the procedure in the posterior CS, or even in the IPS. If this happens, before the actual AV shunt is occluded, complete packing of anteriorly located fistulas may become difficult, or the entire procedure may be jeopardized. Losing access to the CS or to a fistulous compartment in cases of an incomplete occlusion creates the risk of rerouting the drainage

towards cortical veins, causing cortical venous hypertension and possibly hemorrhages.

In cases with drainage towards the contralateral side of the fistula, the microcatheter should always be advanced there first. Such a "cross-over" approach via the intercavernous sinus allows blocking the drainage before withdrawing the catheter and pack-

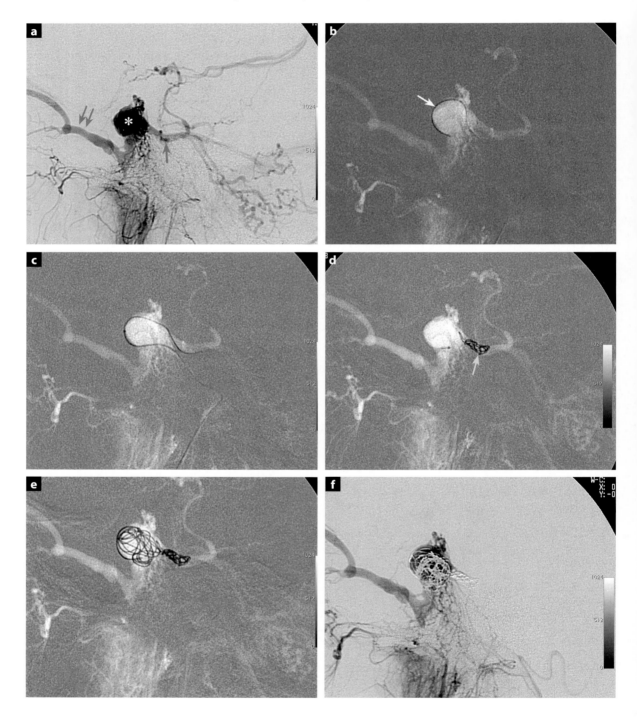

ing coils at the fistula's side (Fig. 8.15, 8.17, 8.22). This helps the operator to avoid leaving fistulous compartments behind that usually require more challenging catheterizations later on. Moreover, this is crucial in cases with bilateral fistulas, especially when the CS approach is possible from only one side (Fig. 8.22). Failing to occlude the contralateral fistula side first

may result compartmentalization, and second may complicate the management of the patient.

If cortical drainage is present, the most crucial part of the procedure is to block the connection between the CS and the cortical vein at the beginning of the occlusion, even before placing coils into the SOV (Fig. 8.4). Only such blocking will prevent per-

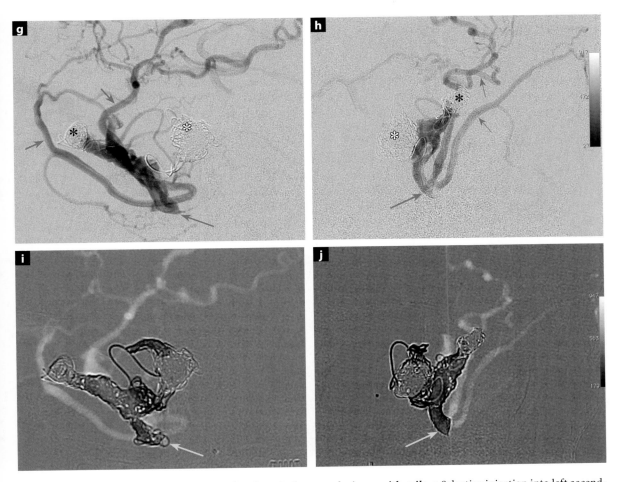

Fig. 8.4 a–j. Disconnection of leptomeningeal and cortical venous drainage with coils. a Selective injection into left ascending pharyngeal artery. AP view demonstrates AV shunt at the posterior CS (*asterisk*) draining into the SOV (*double arrow*) and the SPS (*arrow*) causing leptomeningeal and deep venous drainage. **b–e** Lateral road maps. An Excelsior® SL-10 was navigated around the venous pouch into the SPS first. Two GDC®-10 UltraSoft® coils (3/8) were used to block the drainage into the SPS before packing the CS itself. Then, the microcatheter was slightly withdrawn into the CS and a 3D-GDC® (8/20) was deployed into the venous pouch and subsequently filled with multiple GDC Soft and UltraSoft coils (total of 15 coils) until complete occlusion was documented. Note that during the coiling of the CS, the fistula continued to drain into the SOV, wheras it was disconnected from the SPS (**f**). *Note*: In this case, one coil could not be electrolytically detached and had to be manually separated from the pusher wire by clockwise rotation until it broke ("mechanically detached", LEE et al. 2008). No adverse clinical event occured. **g, h** Selective injection into the CS, lateral and "AP"* view shows the blocked venous drainage at the posterior CS (*b/w asterisk*) and the SOV (*black asterisk*) using two microcatheters (dual IPS approach, Fig. 8.31). There was significant cortical venous drainage left (*thin arrows*). **i, j** Lateral and AP* road maps show the selective packing of the lateral venous exit, blocking the cortical venous drainage. Note that due to superimposition with the SOV in standard lateral and "AP"* views, the venous exit to the cortical veins may be difficult to perceive. Cranio-caudal angulation of the B-plane (**g, i**) and a caudal-oblique* working-projection of the A-plane (**h, j**) demonstrated better this connection (*arrows*) and helped to navigate the catheter to the proper position for selective occlusion (*yellow arrows*). See also Case Illustration XI.

sistence, or even worsening by rerouting of the venous drainage that is associated with increased risk of intracranial hemorrhage. At the end of the procedure, occluding the IPS itself should be avoided as it may be needed as an access route in a subsequent session. Secondly, an occlusion of the IPS may, if it serves as drainage for the CS, compromise the normal cerebral circulation of the posterior fossa. Although a 4-F or 5-F guiding catheter can be advanced into the IPS, one should remember that, especially in cases with cortical venous drainage, such a maneuver may elevate venous pressure sufficent enough to cause intracerebral hemorrhage as recently reported (THEAUDIN et al. 2007).

The angiographic endpoint of the endovascular procedure is either subtotal or complete occlusion of the fistula. If there is a minimal residual AV shunt visible, the procedure can usually be stopped, because the postoperative normalization of the ACT will further promote ongoing thrombosis within the CS. Ongoing thrombosis in the CS may be impeded by the heparinization of the patient during the procedure. Subtotal occlusion is often sufficient and will lead to complete occlusion within a few days or even 24 h when the coagulation system is normalized (Case Reports II and IV). Whenever possible, it is advisable to avoid overpacking the CS.

Additional particulate embolization using PVA or Embospheres after TVO, although performed by some investigators, has rarely been necessary in the author's experience. After extubation, the patients are usually transferred to a post-anesthesia care unit, and then to a normal unit. Only if adverse effects or signs of visual deterioration are observed, will the patient be heparinized for 48 h. Some operators suggest reversal of systemic heparinization with protamine sulfate (10 mg per 1000 U) (VINUELA et al. 1997). In order to avoid post-procedural complications, the additional use of a closure device such as Angio-Seal™ (St. Jude Medical Inc.) is increasingly practiced by many operators.

Postoperative headaches due to mechanical pressure induced by the coils can usually be controlled with analgesics (300 mg ASA daily). If postoperative CN palsy occurs, additional corticosteroids can be administered (e.g. Decadron 4–8 mg every 6). Every patient should undergo an ophthalmological exam a few days after the procedure. Many times, symptoms improve during the first 24 h. The patient may be discharged either the next day or after 2–3 days, and is then seen for clinical follow-up after 3 months with at least one angiographic follow-up after 6–9 months.

8.1.2
Alternative Approaches to the Cavernous Sinus

8.1.2.1
Transfemoral Superior Ophthalmic Vein Approach (Case Report IV)

When the ipsi- or contralateral IPS approach clearly fails, a transfemoral SOV approach may be performed during the same or a subsequent session. This is done in the following way: A 4-F guiding catheter (0.038″ inner lumen) is introduced into the facial vein and navigated as distally as possible. The closer the tip of this catheter is placed to the angular vein, the easier the catheterization of the SOV will be with a microcatheter. A too proximally placed guide often requires more microcatheter manipulations in the facial and angular veins. These veins tend to become more mobile within the subcutaneous soft tissue, making advancing the microcatheter through a tortuous SOV difficult. A slightly stiffer microcatheter, such as the braided Rapid Transit 18, may be feasible. The use of a triaxial catheter systems (8 F-4 F-2 F), although never employed by the author, can also be helpful (SUZUKI et al. 2006).

8.1.2.2
Transcutaneous Superior Ophthalmic Vein Approach (Cannulation, Case Report V)

This approach is chosen if both the IPS and the transfemoral SOV approach fail to provide access. Under general anesthesia, the patient gets prepared in the surgical OR, or (under sterile conditions) in the angiography suite. An experienced ophthalmic surgeon, ophthalmologist or, as in the author's practice, a maxillo-facial surgeon should perform an upper-lid or sub-brow cut to mobilize the angular vein. The vessel is then gently held with a suture and cannulated with a 20- or 21-G thin or ultra-thin wall needle (e.g. Terumo UTW 21). A small microguidewire, preferably a 0.010″ wire, is carefully introduced and navigated into the distal SOV. The the blunt plastic cannula is stabilized with a suture until the end of the procedure. Then, the patient may be transferred to the OR (if not already prepared in the angiography suite). A small 0.010″ microcatheter (Tracker-10, Excelsior SL-10) is introduced and navigated into the proximal SOV or CS, which is usually possible without difficulties.

Some operators suggest a slightly different technique, where the microcatheter is directly introduced into the vein, which has been ligated proximally and distally with silicon vascular loops. These loops are passed through small pediatric feeding tubes to control the bleeding while advancing the catheter using a two-person technique (MILLER 2007).

For all SOV approaches, the packing of coils is performed in the reverse order compared to the IPS approach, starting at the most posterior aspect of the CS and finishing the coil packing at the SOV–CS junction. In this manner, the coil packing begins at the posterior or contralateral compartment of the CS; the disconnection between CS and SOV is done as the last step. At the end of the procedure, the vein is manually compressed for a few minutes before the skin is sutured.

8.1.2.3
Transorbital Puncture of the Superior or Inferior Ophthalmic Vein (Case Report VI)

Failure of all previously described approaches justifies a more aggressive technique, in the same or a subsequent session. A bi-plane road map is obtained using the 4-F diagnostic catheter demonstrating the course of the vein deep in the orbit. Under sterile conditions, a 21- or 22-gauge needle (e.g. Terumo UTW 21 or micropuncture set) is gently advanced along the medial wall of the orbit posterior to the globe, using bi-plane fluoroscopy. When the needle reaches the deep orbit, the SOV or the IOV is carefully cannulated and a small microcatheter (Tracker-10) is introduced. The IOV is punctured by advancing the needle along the inferior orbital rim (WHITE et al. 2007). After the microcatheter is advanced into the CS, coils are deployed, as described above. Puncturing an arterialized vein within the orbit is a delicate maneuver. Stabilizing the needle is crucial while manipulating a microcatheter or pushing coils into the CS. Losing this access can not only jeopardize the procedure, but may also cause intraorbital hemorrhage with potential vision loss. Avoiding excessive tension on the fragile venous wall by a lesser dense packing within the SOV may be advisable.

8.1.3
Other Techniques

For alternative transfemoral, transcutaneous and transorbital CS approaches, including the superior petrosal sinus (SPS), pterygoid plexus (PP), the facial vein (FV), the middle temporal vein (MTV), the frontal vein (FV), superficial middle cerebral vein (SMCV) and direct puncture of the CS, see discussion below.

Embolic Agents (Figs. 8.5–8.13)

To cover the wide range of various embolic materials and their handling is beyond the scope of this chapter. Embolic agents of particular interest for transarterial or transvenous occlusions of dural CSFs will be described below.

8.2.1
Polyvinyl Alcohol (PVA) and Embospheres

PVA particles (Contour PVA, Boston Scientific, Fremont; TruFill™ PVA, Cordis Endovascular, Miami Lakes, FL) have been employed for a long time in a wide range of applications and are used frequently in preoperative embolization of vascularized tumors such as meningiomas, glomus tumors or capillary hemangiomas (BENDSZUS et al. 2000; MANELFE et al. 1976; WRIGHT et al. 1982; BERENSTEIN and GRAEB 1982; KERBER et al. 1978). In the 1980s and early 1990s, PVA was also used for embolizing brain AVMs (SCIALFA and SCOTTI 1985). PVA particles can be injected wherever liquid embolic agents are considered unsafe, and coils are unsuitable for anatomic or hemodynamic reasons (WRIGHT et al. 1982; KERBER et al. 1978; JACK et al. 1985). The particles are manufactured by different vendors in a size between 45–150 μm and up to 700–2000 μm, and are selected based on the caliber of the vessel in the targeted territory. One long-standing disadvantage of PVA has been the fact that these particles not only varied in size (ranges), but also had an irregular surface causing aggregation, clumping and occlusion of catheters and proximal vessel segments. In addition, the particles showed a tendency to swell after being in a contrast suspension for some time and usually had to be replaced by a new mixture several times throughout the treatment session.

Newer PVA particle types come as hydrophilic microspheres in a calibrated size (Contour-SE, Boston Scientific). They are naturally opaque with a more uniform size distribution, a wider range of sizes and come pre-hydrated in saline in a prefilled syringe.

Alternatively, Trisacryl gelatin microspheres (Embospheres, Guerbet Biomedical, Louvres, France) can be used and may offer some advantages because they are precisely calibrated at 100–300 μm and have fewer tendencies to aggregate (LAURENT et al. 2005; BEAUJEUX et al. 1996; DERDEYN 1997). A recent comparison has shown that they produce less blood loss when used for embolization of meningiomas, presumably because of more distal penetration (BENDSZUS et al. 2000). In general, smaller particles are used for embolizing tumors (45–150 μm), because they will better penetrate small tumor capillaries. Because small PVA particles may migrate into the pulmonary circulation when embolizing AV shunts, larger particles up to 1000 μm have to be used for TAE of DCSFs.

Injection of PVA is performed under fluoroscopy after the particles are suspended in iodine contrast material (BERENSTEIN and GRAEB 1982; SZWARC et al. 1986), the concentration of which should be adjusted to the inner lumen of the microcatheter and to the flow in the targeted territory.

The use of particles and embospheres is different from injecting acrylic glue into an AVM nidus. In order to allow for particles and embospheres to reach the desired vascular target, sufficient flow must be maintained within the feeding pedicle. The concentration of PVA in the contrast suspension is chosen depending on the size of the vessels supplying the DCSF, but should be very dilute at first to avoid obstruction of the microcatheter. According to changes in the local hemodynamics that progressively occur during injection due to increasing blockage of the vascular bed, the concentration of particles and their size may be adjusted throughout the procedure. To start with smaller and continue with gradually increased particle sizes is usually most effective. For optimal visual monitoring of the embolic flux and early detection of reflux a magnified "blank road mapping" is strongly recommended. The more distal a catheter is placed, the smaller the particles that should be chosen. On the other hand, the injection of particles smaller than 150–300 μm into the MMA, IMA or AMA may lead to cranial nerve palsy. A more global injection into the IMA using larger particles (possible through a 4-F diagnostic catheter) may show an immediate angiographic change, but is usually ineffective to achieve a long-term occlusion of an AV shunt. As an adjunct for transvenous coil occlusion, or when the aim is mainly to induce flow reduction and to promote thrombosis, such a strategy may be appropriate. The angiographic endpoint should be slow antegrade or stagnant flow.

8.2.2
Stainless Steel Coils

Coils made of stainless steel, also named Gianturco coils after its inventor Cesare Gianturco

(ANDERSON et al. 1977, 1979; BRAUN et al. 1985; CHUANG et al. 1980), have a diameter between 0.035 and 0.038 inches and have been used for a long time for embolizations in peripheral vascular territories. Interwoven Dacron fibers increase the thrombogenicity of the coils, which require a larger diagnostic catheter, limiting their application in the neurovascular territory. They are the forerunners of the various detachable and non-detachable platinum coils available today.

8.2.2.1
Platinum (Non-detachable) Pushable Microcoils (Fig. 8.6)

These coils have also been called "free" or pushable coils and are available in different lengths, diameters and shapes (straight, helical, flower or spiral) (GRAVES et al. 1990; MORSE et al. 1990; YANG et al. 1988), provided by several companies. Some manufacturers have added Dacron fibers to increase the thrombogenicity while friction is minimized for the use in small microcatheters. Constant flushing of the microcatheter with heparinized saline is required to avoid friction within the microcatheter that may cause blockage and damage of the catheter lumen, necessitating exchange. Such catheter change often leads to loss of a distal position, lengthening of the procedure or even necessitates rescheduling for a subsequent session. Thus, for pushing coils, specifically fibered coils, it is recommended to have little or no friction at all, minimal wall tension and preferably no kinks in the catheter. Especially larger coils may produce friction when advanced through a sharp vessel turn and sometimes have to be deployed by forceful injection of a saline bolus using a 2- or 5-cc syringe. This will propel the coil through the catheter lumen, a technique that may save time and costs. Coil positioning can be slightly less accurate and some coils may be malpositioned by flow reversal. Thus, this technique should be applied only with some experience in endovascular techniques. In general, the use of pushable coils may in some cases be associated with coil migration or recoil of the microcatheter, leading to coil placement in unwanted and sometimes catastrophic positions (HALBACH et al. 1998). Pushable fibered coils have only been used by the author in addition to detachable coils, to increase the thrombogenicity of the bare platinum coil mesh. They are also available in complex configurations, such as VortX-coils (Boston Scientific). VortX-coils and other fibered coil configurations have become available with a detachment system as GDCs (HALBACH et al. 1998). Other manufacturers have developed similar devices such as the nylon fibered coils (NXT, EV3), in sizes ranging from 2×20 mm to 3×100 mm, combining the advantages of being highly thrombogenic and controllable by a similar detachment system (HENKES et al. 2004; HUNG et al. 2005; TAKAZAWA et al. 2005; ZINK et al. 2004). One main advantage of platinum as a material for coils is its high opacity compared to stainless steel and its MR compatibility.

Some operators have used this type of coil for transarterial embolization of ECA feeders (GIOULEKAS et al. 1997). However, while their placement leads to a proximal occlusion, resulting in a shunt reduction, it seldom produces a permanent obliteration. The major downside of transarterial coil embolization in AV shunting lesions is that future arterial approaches through the same pedicle are compromised and new treatment sessions may become jeopardized, unless TVO is used (Fig. 8.7). Thus, proximal arterial occlusion with coils should be avoided whenever possible. It has never been considered useful by the author, except when targeting a selective vessel blockage to avoid untoward migration of embolic agents via ECA-ICA anastomoses (e.g. MMA-OA anastomoses in preoperative embolization of meningiomas).

On the other hand, for transvenous occlusions of DAVFs in general, and for DCSFs in particular, even non-detachable fibered coils are quite useful and effective in accelerating the occlusion process due to their high thrombogenicity. However, if these coils are not properly positioned or densely enough packed, the chances of leaving a residual AV shunt in a compartmentalized CS is high.

8.2.2.2
Detachable Platinum Coils (Fig. 8.5)

The first detachable coil, the GDC system (Guglielmi detachable coil system), is a non-fibered, soft bare platinum coil mounted on a stainless steel wire that can be detached by electrolysis after placement in the desired location. This coil system was primarily developed for safer embolization of intracranial aneurysms, after it became evident in the 1980s that using pushable coils and detachable balloons was associated with too many serious complications due to their inherent limitations.

MULLAN (1974) was already able to induce an occlusion of a CSF using an electric current applied through copper wires surgically introduced into the CS. Guglielmi became interested in animal experiments on electrothrombosis in arteries and in 1979, accidentally observed, during attempts to induce electrothrombosis in an experimental aneurysm, a detachment of the electrode from the steel wire (STROTHER 2001). This incident was in principle the discovery of the electrolytic detachment of platinum coils that was implemented in the GDC system in 1991 and subsequent systems. GDC has meanwhile proved highly effective in the treatment of intracranial aneurysms and was FDA approved in 1995.

The use of a precise detachment mechanism is important not only for aneurysm treatment, but also for transarterial or transvenous occlusions of AV shunting lesions. Proper positioning of the coils in a distant location, while always having the possibility to retrieve the coil, is of key importance for safely and effectively performing TVOs. In fact, one of the first successful treatments using GDCs was a direct CCF, occluded by F. Vinuela in 1990 using only two coils (GUGLIELMI et al. 1992).

GDCs are made of a soft platinum alloy and are usually available in the configurations shown in Table 8.1.

GDC Soft coils are made of a thinner wire than standard coils and thus more pliable (e.g. GDC-10 Soft coils are 38% softer than GDC-10 standard coils). In order to minimize the mechanical stress applied to cranial nerves coursing through the CS, the use of softer coils for the CS packing is beneficial. At the same time a denser coil mesh can be achieved that is similar to aneurysm treatments – a major factor for achieving complete occlusion of the fistula.

The use of coils with a complex or spherical configuration at the beginning of the coil packing, when a basket in a certain compartment of the CS needs to be accurately built, is also advantageous. This is the case at the connection between the CS and the SOV or a cortical vein. Buckling and kick-back of

Table 8.1. Available lengths and diameters of GDCs

Coil	Platinum wire Ø (inch)	Outer Ø (inch)	Helix Ø (mm)	Length (cm)
GDC-18	0.0040	0.015	5–20	15–30
GDC-18 SOFT	0.0030	0.0135	2, 3, 4, 5, 6	4–15
GDC-10	0.0020	0.010	2–10	4–30
GDC-10 SOFT	0.00175	0.0095	2, 3, 4	2–10
GDC-10 U-SOFT	0.0015	0.010	2; 2,5; 3, 4	1–8

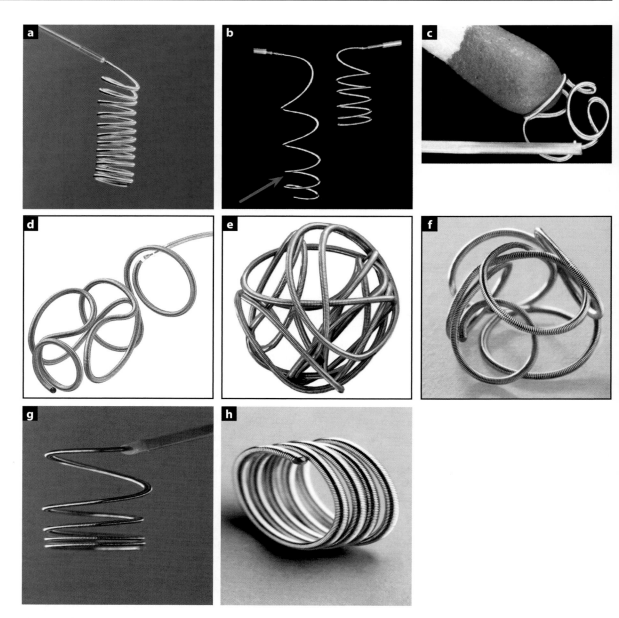

Fig. 8.5 a–h. Platinum detachable coils. a GDC-18 coil, used only in a few cases because of its stiffness. **b** GDC-10 Soft® and Ul-traSoft coil (*arrow*, ca. 50% softer than regular soft coils) with similar size (3 mm/4 cm). GDC-10 coils were the preferred type of coils used in the authors early experience, often combined with soft coils (Case Reports I–VI, Figs. 8.3, 8.4). Bare platinum coils are available in different lengths and diameters, provided today by various manufacturers. They are less thrombogenic than fibered coils, but usually more pliable and thus more suitable for dense packing. The major advantage of all detachable over pushable coils is the possibility of repositioning them until optimal deployment is achieved. Softer coils can be packed very densely, while minimizing mechanical pressure to the cranial nerves within the CS. **c** 3D coils (BSC) and other coils with a spherical configuration can be useful as starter coils to block the connection between the CS and the SOV or cortical veins as precisely as possible. This first 3D-coil generation was relatively stiff and could dislodge the microcatheter during detachment, leading to loss of position. **d** The newly developed 360° coil for the GDC system with an improved design (BSC). Several other manufacturers have developed coils with complex or spherical configurations that are superior to the original 3D coil (**e** Complex coil, MicroVention; **f** MicruSphere®, Micrus Endovascular). **g** MicroPlex® HyperSoft™ Coil (MicroVention). This new, highly compliant coil provides a remarkable packing density. Its extremely soft proximal end minimizes movement and deflection of the microcatheter tip and reduces buckling or kick-back. The coil allows for more precise coil placement or targeted venous compartments and facilitates repositioning (see Case Illustration VI). HyperSoft coils are available in 2–6 mm × 1–8 cm length. **h** Ultipaq™ Coil (Micrus Endovascular), partiallly used in Case Illustration III

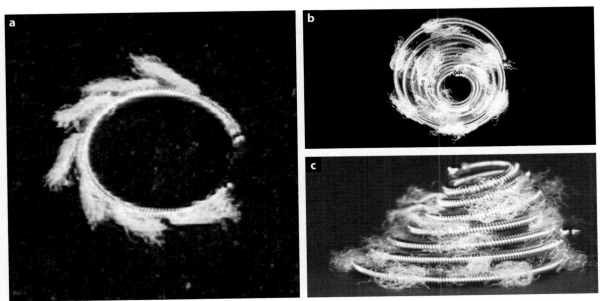

Fig. 8.6 a–c. Various fibered (pushable) coils (BSC). a Simple, fibered coil, here as a C-shaped spiral (3/7 mm) with attached Dacron fibers for increased thrombogenicity. These spiral coils are compatible with Tracker-10 and -18 and are introduced using a special pusher or injecting saline. The main drawback of all pushable coils is that they cannot be repositioned. Furthermore, the fibers may cause friction and damage to the microcatheter, requiring a catheter exchange that is undesirable during lengthy transvenous occlusions. **b, c** Fibered coils (2/6 mm) with complex configuration such as this VortX® coil can be added to accelerate thrombosis. However, because of their size and stiffness, they may not always adapt to the small spaces and interstices in the CS. Consequently, the catheter may dislodge, leading to a loose packing or loss of access. This may result in partial occlusion or compartmentalization of the CS. Fibered coils, also available as detachable versions, have been used by the author as adjunctive device in some cases

a microcatheter has occasionally been a problem, especially with the relatively stiff first 3D-GDC generation from BSC. This has been overcome with newer coils from other manufacturers (Fig. 8.5d–f). SR Coils (stretch resistant coils) have interwoven double strands of polypropylene or other material that prevent stretching and unraveling, which is advantageous when a long-used microcatheter develops friction or even kinks and cannot be replaced. Although coil unraveling or failure to detach during TVO are technical complications, their consequences are less dramatic than during aneurysm treatment. As a bail out, the coil may be "mechanically detached" (LEE and YIM et al. 2008) by 15–20 clockwise rotations until it breaks, which does not cause harm, even when the rest of the basket in the CS gets entangled (personal unpublished experience; see also Fig. 8.4).

So-called UltraSoft coils (BSC) provide a further stiffness reduction of about 50%, allowing for a packing density of up to 55% in experimental aneurysms (PIOTIN et al. 2004). These coils may be deployed in extremely small vascular pockets (BENNDORF et al. 2002). Recently, a new HyperSoft coil (MicroVention

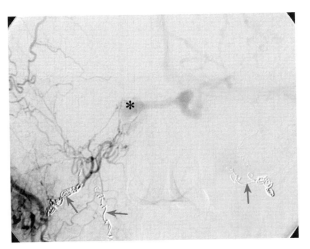

Fig. 8.7. Ineffective transarterial embolization of IMA branches with coils. Right ECA injection. AP view shows an AV shunt at the righ CS (*asterisk*) draining to the left side and causing cortical venous drainage. This patient was tranferred from another institution after undergoing TAE with coils (*arrows*). Proximal occlusion of ECA supply of an AVF with any type of coil (or glue) usually has little or no effect. It seriously compromises future attempts of catheterization instead and should be avoided. This patient was successfully managed by TVO and fully recovered (BENNDORF et al., 2000a)

Inc., Aliso Viejo, CA) with a remarkable compliance and a shorter, softer detachment zone has been introduced (Fig. 8.5g). This coil allows high packing density while minimizing microcatheter movement and proves very useful for treating DCSF (Case Illustrations V).

Platinum detachable coils have been used to a large degree in the group of patients studied by the author and only in some cases have been combined with fibered coils. Detachable coil systems from various other manufacturers are available today providing equal, if not better, mechanical properties compared to GDCs. Beside electrolysis, other detachment techniques have been developed using a mechanical mechanism such MDS (Balt Extrusion) or DCS (William Cook Europe), heat (Micrus Endovascular Corporation, San Jose, CA) or hydraulic pressure (MicroVention, Cordis Neurovascular) that allow deployment of a platinum coil in a quick, safe and reliable manner.

The additional coating of coils with bioactive materials such as polyglycolic-polyactic biopolymer (PGLA) to promote fibrocellular proliferation and increased endothelialization is of little relevance for occlusion of DCSFs. A fundamentally different approach to the problem of coil compaction and long-term occlusion of aneurysms has been the introduction of coils covered with a hydrogel (HydroCoils).

8.2.2.3
HydroCoils (Figs. 8.8–8.10)

Among the new coil generations with a "bioactive" surface coating, hydrogel, mounted on a detachable platinum coil (HydroCoil, HES,) has attracted attention for the treatment of DAVFs. The Hydro-Coil™ is a platinum-based coil with a Hhydrogel coating, a material that expands while in contact with water or blood. The water absorption leads to swelling of the material which results in an increase of the coil diameter after being deployed in the blood circulation. This rather unique property of the HES proved advantageous in treating cerebral aneurysms (KIRSCH et al. 2006; GOTO and GOTO 1997; NEMOTO et al. 1997; HANAOKA et al. 2006; SCHUKNECHT et al. 1998; MIRONOV 1994; HALBACH et al. 1992; SATOMI et al. 2005; TAPTAS 1982). It is currently believed that while the HES increase their diameter, they actually do not "over-swell", so that additional mechanical pressure will not occur. A HydroCoil 18 expands from 0.018″ to 0.034″, a HydroCoil 14 expands from 0.014″ to 0.027″ and the HydroCoil 10 expands from 0.013″ to 0.022″. The maximum reposition time of these coils is 5 min. in a 0.021″, 0.019″ or 0.015″ inner lumen microcatheter, respectively. A new detachment system (V-Trak) utilizes thermo-mechanical technology by sending a current to a heating coil at the end

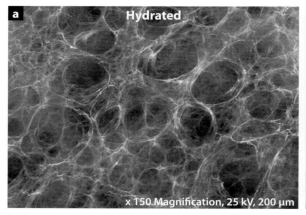 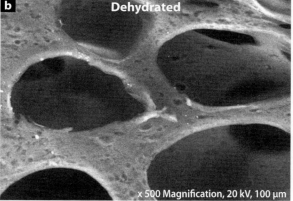

Fig. 8.8 a,b. Hydrogel after contact with water. **a, b** The porous hydrogel provides an excellent substrate for healing (neointima formation, smooth muscle cell migration) because blood components (proteins, etc.) are absorbed into the hydrogel during the swelling process. Hydrogel is a polymeric material that is capable of swelling in water (diffusion of water through the polymer causing disentanglement of polymer chains and swelling). Intelligel technology provides a pH-dependant, controlled expansion in response to changes in the environment. The hydrogel preparation is a liquid reaction mixture that contains: A monomer cross-linker, a polymerization initiator, and a porosigen. A controlled expansion rate is imparted through the incorporation of unsaturated monomers with ionizable functional groups

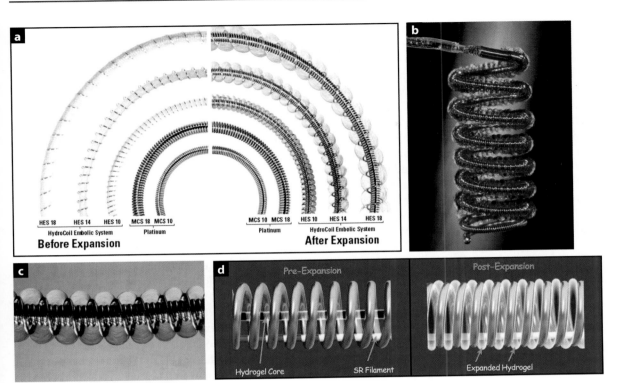

Fig. 8.9 a–d. HydroCoils. a HydroCoils-10, -14, and -18 before and after expansion. HydroCoils-18 are deliverable through a 0.021″ lumen microcatheter. The outer diameter is unexpanded 0.018″ and expanded 0.034″. The maximum repositioning time in a 0.021″ lumen microcatheter is 5 min. **b** The HydroCoil-10 is pushable through a 0.015″ lumen microcatheter, has a maximum repositioning time of 10 min (Excelsior® 10/18), 7 min (SL 10 & Prowler®-14) and 5 min (Prowler®-10). This coil is stretch-resistant and expands from 0.013″ to 0.022″. The stiffness is comparable to a MicroPlex-10 coil. HydroCoils® appear advantageous over standard platinum coils for occlusion of venous channels, such as the CS. They increase the overall volumetric packing, while causing less pressure to the cranial nerves. This reduces the total amount of coils as well as radiation exposure. **c** HydroCoil-14 Platinum coil core (0.008″) with gel covering and platinum "overcoil". The Hydrogel polymer expands 3× in the presence of blood to a diameter of 0.027″. The coil has a helical configuration and can be delivered through a 0.019″ lumen or larger microcatheter. **d** HydroSoft Coils. The Hydrogel expands beyond the platinum wind providing up to 70% more volume fill than a 10 system coil for better volumetric filling and mechanical stability. Swelling of the gel occurs to a lesser degree and reaches about 0.013″. Coils are available in 2–6 mm × 1–8 cm length

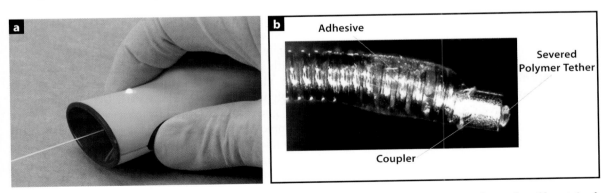

Fig. 8.10 a,b. V-Trak system. The newer detachment system consists of a more flexible delivery pusher and a self-contained, disposable integrated power supply. The coil is detached via a thermo-mechanical detachment mechanism. Heat acts as a catalyst to sever a polymer tether connecting the pusher to the implant. The tether is tied and adhesively bonded to the proximal end of the implant. Because of that only a very short tail (**a**) is left after detachment. No melted polymer or particles are released during the detachment and the end of the implant is a square, reducing risk of jamming with other coils inside the microcatheter. Coils are detached in 0.75 s

of the pusher. The coil is attached with a polymer tether under tension. The heat severs a polymer tether, detaching the coil in about 0.75 s.

The use of HES for AV shunting lesions is described only in a limited number of reports to date (MARDEN et al. 2005; MORSI et al. 2004). First, the swelling of the hydrogel is ideal for progressive mechanical occlusion of a venous AVF compartment, as it will adjust to the irregular surrounding anatomy better than bare metal coils. Such a progressive swelling and occlusion process can help to reduce the total number of coils needed for transvenous occlusion, as seen in cerebral aneurysms (DESHAIES et al. 2005). Second, the softness of the gel will allow a dense packing of the coils, while reducing mechanical pressure on intracavernous structures and the risk of CN deficits. It has been shown that the hydrogel expansion does not contribute to any change in the intraaneurysmal pressure (CANTON et al. 2005). Intervals of 5–10 min between control angiograms after each coil deployment (allowing for a full expansion of the gel) may already reveal a significant reduction of the AV shunting flow, indicating progressive occlusion and thrombosis. The swelling may increase the diameter of the coils up to five to 11 times of a standard platinum coil, which allows for achieving higher volumetric packing than possible with bare platinum coils while reducing the total amount of metal. The fact that the gel will swell after the coil has been deployed makes this coil very suitable for progressive occlusion of larger venous compartments such as dural sinuses.

Thus, the usefulness of HydroCoils for occluding DAVFs and DCSFs is rather obvious. In Case Illustration IV, effective transvenous occlusion using HydroCoils is demonstrated.

8.2.3
Liquid Embolic Agents: Cyanoacrylates (N-butyl-cyanoacrylate, Acrylic Glue, Histoacryl, Trufill™ n-BCA, Glubran™)

In the 1980s, NBCA (N-butyl-2-cyanoacrylate), initially known as Avacryl in the US and as Histoacryl in Europe (Braun-Melsungen, Germany) replaced IBCA (Isobutyl-2-cyanoacrylate), being the first acrylic glue for medical application (BROTHERS et al. 1989). Histoacryl is a tissue adhesive that polymerizes when in contact with ion solutions such as contrast, saline or blood, and was initially developed for use in dermatology. Cyanoacrylate was for a long

time considered the only agent capable of causing a permanent occlusion when injected intravascularly. Because of this property, it has been widely used in the treatment of brain AVMs and AVFs. The experience in using glue is extensively published (BROTHERS et al. 1989; DUFFNER et al. 2002; LIU et al. 2000a,b; HENKES et al. 1998; CROMWELL and KERBER 1979; KERBER et al. 1979; GOUNIS et al. 2002; LI et al. 2002; SADATO et al. 2000; RAFFI et al. 2007; TROFFKIN and GIVEN 2007; WAKHLOO et al. 2005). Its liquid form allows penetration into very small vessels and is particularly suitable for completely occluding an AVM nidus (BROTHERS et al. 1989).

The polymerization of NBCA starts after a few seconds of contact with blood and can be controlled only to some degree, depending on various factors such as blood flow velocity, speed of the injection, pH of the blood and temperature of the glue. In order to increase radiopacity for fluoroscopic control, Histoacryl is mixed by most investigators with Lipiodol (ethiodized oil), a cottonseed-oil-based contrast agent made by Laboratorie Guerbet (France). In addition, this mixture decelerates the polymerization depending on the concentration of lipiodol from 1–30 s (CROMWELL and KERBER 1979). Introducing the mixture with lipiodol significantly improved the handling of glue (STOESSLEIN et al. 1982). While concentrations of approximately 50% (60/40) were used in early years, glue has been increasingly diluted recently. For AVMs, dilutions of 20%–25% or less are meanwhile preferred. A concentration below 15%, although still usable, significantly impairs the polymerization; its adhesive properties are reduced, and the glue may easily migrate into the venous side of the AV shunt. Because of the potential hazardous complications, the handling of acrylics has to be studied and practiced extensively before it may be safely and effectively used. Prior to the embolization with glue, the microcatheter must be flushed with 5% glucose (dextrose in water) to avoid premature polymerization within the catheter. Each injection of glue must be carefully observed under fluoroscopic control in order to recognize early even the smallest reflux into the proximal feeder and to avoid gluing the catheter to the vessel wall. Additional use of tantalum powder in the mixture further enhances radiographic visibility. A small reflux (up to 5 mm) may be tolerated with modern hydrophilic catheters, depending on the concentration of the glue and the location of the microcatheter, prior to removal. When glue is injected directly into a sinus or a venous compartment such as the CS, gluing of the microcatheter is less of a problem. It has been found that polymerization of glue may be further prolonged by adding tantalum powder. A concentration as low as 10%–15% has been used by adding tungsten and lipiodol for TAE of five complex DCSFs (LIU et al. 2000b). GOUNIS et al. (2002) showed that predictability of the embolization process with NBCA can be improved by adding glacial acetic acid to the embolic mixture. Due to regulatory issues in North America in the 1990s, the use of acrylic glue was limited in the US compared to Europe. In 2000, a slightly modified version of Histoacryl, Trufill™ n-BCA (Cordis Neurovascular, Miami lakes, FL) received FDA approval for treatment of brain AVMs, and showed a good combination of penetration and permanence (JORDAN et al. 2005). It is also mixed with Ethiodol (Trufill™-NBCA Cordis Neurovascular) in various concentrations from 2:1, 3:1, etc. The intravenous injection of glue for occlusion of DCSFs has been reported only to a limited degree (WAKHLOO et al. 2005) and was used in a few cases in the studied group of patients (BENNDORF et al. 2004 , see also Fig. 8.35). A modified cyanoacrylate, Glubran™ (and Glubran 2™), was recently introduced in Europe (RAFFI et al. 2007).

8.2.4
Onyx™ (Ethylene-Vinyl Alcohol Copolymer) (Fig. 8.11)

Ethylene-vinyl alcohol copolymer (EVOH, Onyx, EV3, irvine CA) is a newer liquid embolic agent whose main characteristic is its non-adhesiveness. In contrast to adhesive acrylates, Onyx™ is a precipitating embolic agent that mainly causes a mechanical vessel occlusion. It prevents microcatheters from gluing to the vessel wall, and thus allows significantly prolonged injection times (up to 40 min or more). It is mixed with a solvent, dimethyl sulphoxide (DMSO) and tantalum powder (JAHAN et al. 2001) and comes in ready-to-use vials for AVMs and AVFs in three concentrations: 6% (Onyx 18), 6.5% (Onyx 20) and 8% (Onyx 34), dissolved in DMSO (SUZUKI et al. 2006).

Onyx is a pre-mixed, radiopaque, injectable embolic fluid that solidifies upon contact with aqueous solutions or physiologic fluids. In contrast to NBCA, this property allows for temporarily pausing the injection to prevent untoward leakage into a non-targeted territory (JORDAN et al. 2005). It forms a spongy polymeric cast and a "skin" – solidifying

from the outside while continuing to flow, "much like lava", in the liquid center. Thus, Onyx™ can be delivered in a relatively cohesive manner.

The initial description of its use for embolization of AV shunting lesions came from TAKI et al. (1990) and TERADA et al. (1991). The authors reported the successful embolization of cerebral AVMs with EVAL (ethylene vinyl alcohol copolymer) dissolved in DMSO. Safety concerns emerged after animal studies conducted by CHALOUPKA et al. (1994), who discovered significant angiotoxicity of the DSMO. A reexamination, however, showed no acute hemodynamic effects, and no infarction or SAH at slower injections rates of 30, 60 and 90 s (CHALOUPKA et al. 1999).

Subsequent studies revealed that the main factors influencing vascular toxicity are the contact time with the arterial wall and the total volume of DMSO. It was demonstrated that DMSO enters the bloodstream, is absorbed into tissue and metabolized to dimethyl sulfone ($DMSO_2$) and dimethyl sulfide (DMS) (CHALOUPKA et al. 1999). These metabolites are eliminated via the kidneys (within 1 week; 80%), and via the skin or lungs, causing a garlic odor to the breath until complete elimination: 13–18 days.

Onyx received FDA approval for the treatment of cerebral AVMs in 2005 and has been increasingly used since (NOGUEIRA et al. 2008; MOUNAYER et al. 2007; TOULGOAT et al. 2006; COGNARD et al. 2008; ARAT et al. 2004).

The use of Onyx has a number of technical advantages over cyanoacrylate, the most important of which is the possibility of prolonged injections in a slow and controlled fashion. If properly performed, it allows achieving deeper nidus penetrations in AV shunting lesions. Whether or not long-term occlusion rates are comparable or superior to the ones obtainable with NBCA remains to be answered by ongoing and future studies.

Among the disadvantages of Onyx is its limitation to DMSO compatible microcatheters such as the Rebar, a braided, relatively stiff microcatheter, the Ultraflow and the Marathon (Ev3, Irvine CA) both flow-guided microcatheters. The Echelon is a nitinol braided, over-the-wire catheter and is available as Echelon 10 (1.7F) and Echelon 14 (1.9F). It has a pre-shaped tip of 45 or 90 degrees and is particularly useful for transvenous occlusions, as it also allows placement of coils (see Figs. 8.31 and 8.34). Other compatible catheters are the flow-guided 1.2-F–1.8-F Baltacci and the braided Corail+ balloon catheter (Balt Extrusion, Montmorency, France). A novel

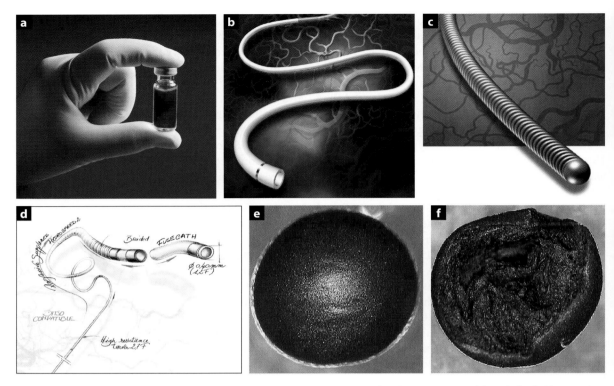

Fig. 8.11 a–f. Onyx and tools for its use. a Onyx (EV3, Irvine CA) is a pre-mixed, radiopaque, injectable embolic fluid. It consists of ethylene-vinyl alcohol copolymer (EVOH), dimethyl sulfoxide solvent (DMSO) and micronized tantalum powder. **b** Ultra-flow HPC™ (EV3, Irvine CA): Flow-guided DMSO compatible microcatheter. **c** Mirage™ (EV3, Irvine CA): 0.008″ hydrophilic coated tapered guidewire (0.2 mm) with proximal part of 0.012 mm for additional support. **d** Balt-Sonic® microcatheter (Balt Extrusion, Montmorency, France). This novel microcatheter with a detachable tip (Fusecath) makes the use of Onyx safer and more efficient. The detachable distal segment allows a longer reflux so that the cast can reach more of the vascular bed distal to the microcatheter. **e, f** Polymer precipitation occurs upon contact with ionic solutions. The solvent diffuses away and a spongy polymeric cast forms. This forms a "skin" - solidifying from the outside in. The liquid center continues to flow (like lava)

concept is the recent introduction of a microcatheter with a detachable tip (Detachable Fusecath, 1.5–2.5 cm) that allows removal of the microcatheter even when entrapment occurs (Balt-Sonic). This will improve safety and efficacy because it allows penetration of more vascular beds (Fig. 8.11d).

Some operators consider a second drawback the fact that the long injections, required in some cases for complete nidus casting, may be associated with an increased radiation dose.

Although unlike with NBCA gluing of microcatheters is not an issue, catheter entrapment by Onyx reflux may still occur and can in some cases lead to clinical complications, such as embolic infarction or cerebral hemorrhage. Finally, it must be mentioned that, even though appealing as a new material, the use of Onyx for transarterial embolization or transvenous occlusions is not without potential hazards. Transient or permanent CN deficits may occur (ELHAMMADY et al. 2009; Lv et al. 2008).

8.2.5
Stents

Stenting has been used in the recent past for occluding direct CCFs either in combination with coils or as single treatment (WEBER et al 2001; MEN et al. 2003; AHN et al. 2003; MORON et al. 2005). In order to primarily support coil placement or to secondarily keep coils within the CS, several intracranial stents are available, such as the Neuroform 3 (Boston Scientific, Fremont, CA), Enterprise (Cordis Neurovascular, Miami Lakes, Fl), LEO (Balt Extrusion, Montmorency, France) or Pharos (Biotronik, Micrus Corporation, Sunnyvale, CA) and others.

However, their use for occlusion of DCSFs is, if at all, of limited value, and thus a detailed description is beyond the scope of this chapter. A relevant reduction of arterial fistula supply by placing high-porosity intracranial stents cannot be expected.

The only stents with some application for dural AV shunts of the CS are covered stents. Covered stents have been used to some degree in the recent past to seal leaks in the carotid wall of direct CCFs (ARCHONDAKIS et al. 2007; NAESENS et al. 2006; REDEKOP et al. 2001; KOCER et al. 2002; FELBER et al. 2004). The device being mainly used is the Jostent (Abbott Vascular Devices, Illinois), a coronary stent graft that consists of a stainless steel 316L body, covered with a polytetrafluoroethylene (PTFE) layer. It is available in various sizes between 3 mm–5 mm diameter and 9 mm–26 mm length (Fig. 8.12). The Jostent has been primarily developed for treating coronary aneurysms and pseudoaneurysm (HEUSER et al. 1999; GERCKEN et al. 2002).

This stent has markers for accurate placement and a low-crimped profile, comparable to conventional coronary stent systems. The PTFE material is placed between two stainless steel struts allowing for stent expansion in one direction, while remaining rigid in the other. Ideally, the fully expanded stent retains its radial strength to resist vessel wall pressure. In order to achieve optimal apposition to the vessel wall, the stent is balloon-expanded with a minimum expansion pressure of 14 atm. Although the stent comes with a tapered tip design for increased crossability and enhanced trackability and is compatible with a

0.018″ guidewire, the device is relatively stiff to be used in the cerebral circulation and its placement requires dual antiplatelet therapy and ASA for an indefinite period of time.

Therefore, the use of such a device in patients with a DCSF needs to be carefully balanced against the potential risk of arterial dissection and stent thrombosis. The development of devices dedicated for neurovascular applications is under way and will hopefully find its introduction into clinical practice soon.

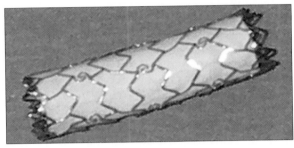

Fig. 8.12. Covered stent. Jostent Coronary Stent Graft (Abbot Vascular, IL), balloon expandable, stainless steel (316L) with an ultra thin, expandable PTFE layer. The stent requires a 7-F or 8-F guiding catheter and is a relatively stiff device. Expansion range is between 3.0–5.0 mm, 9–26 mm lengths are available. Advancement through the tortuous intracranial anatomy, like the petrous or cavernous ICA, may become difficult and is in some cases impossible

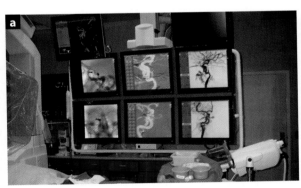 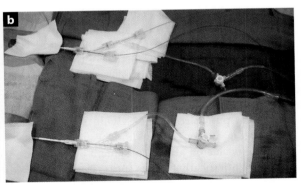

Fig. 8.13 a, b. Bi-plane angiographic suite for neuroendovascular treatment (Interventional Neuroradiology Suite, Ben Taub General Hospital, Houston, Tx). Although personal preferences, habits and choices of tools and devices may vary from center to center, general rules to be followed are quite similar. **a** Modern systems should have at least six monitors for simultaneous radiographic control in two projections (*Left*: Live fluoro, *middle:* Road map, *right:* Reference). Additional monitors may be used for displaying 3D data or physiological monitoring. Latest developments feature a full-color, 56-inch large screen display that enables users to select their preferred screen layout for the planned procedure step at tableside. **b** Bilateral femoral access for EVT of a CSF. Arterial access on the *right*, venous access on the *left side*. For control angiograms, placement of a 4F diagnostic catheter in the ICA or ECA is sufficient. In this case, a 6-F guiding catheter was used to navigate a HyperGlide™ balloon (EV3) into the ICA for temporary inflation during transvenous coilpacking of a direct CCF. The venous side was accessed with a 6-F guiding catheter and two rotating hemostatic valves (Y-connectors) that allow dual placement of microcatheters into the CS (above). Both systems are connected to a three-way stopcock with an extension that allows contrast injections for road mapping or angiographic controls. Continuous pressure flushings for guiding and microcatheters are mandatory to avoid contamination with air or clots. A clean and organized work environment in the angio suite (which should preferably be maintained throughout the procedure) is key to avoiding thrombembolic and other technical complications. Well trained, dedicated nurses and technicians play an important role for a successful team

Results of Transvenous Embolizations (Figs. 8.14–8.40, Tables 8.2–8.8)

8.3.1
Approaches (BENNDORF et al. 2004)

The inferior petrosal sinus (IPS) most frequently served as a venous route in a total of 37 cases (82%), among which 25 procedures (67.5%) resulted in successful occlusion without employing an additional route. In ten of these cases (27%), the IPS was successfully catheterized despite an apparent partial or complete thrombosis. In three cases (8.1%), the IPS was accessed using a direct stick of the internal jugular vein. The facial vein (FV)/superior ophthalmic vein (SOV) approach was used in 13 cases (29%). The SOV was surgically cannulated in eight, while the remaining five patients underwent transfemoral catheterization or direct puncture. In all 13 cases, an IPS approach was attempted first and either did not allow complete occlusion or failed entirely. In one patient, transfemoral approach and percutaneous cannulation failed and the patient underwent needle puncture of the deep (intraconal) SOV. In four cases (8.8%), the superior petrosal sinus (SPS) approach was chosen, in three as single approach, and in one patient with bilateral fistula, it was combined with an IPS approach. One patient (2.2%) with primary drainage via the frontal vein underwent percutaneous puncture of the vein using an 18-G needle with subsequent complete occlusion of the fistula. Another patient, in whom all transfemoral techniques failed, underwent open surgery and direct puncture of the Sylvian vein using an 18-G needle and a Tracker-18. The fistula showed complete occlusion after deployment of two fibered coils. The microcatheter was successfully navigated to the contralateral side in 13 patients (29%), in 11 cases (24%) using the IPS and in two (4%) using the SOV approach.

8.3.2
Angiographic and Clinical Outcome

In the group of patients studied (BENNDORF et al. 2004), complete occlusion of the fistula was achieved in 42/45 patients (93%). Final angiographic follow-up was still pending in three. This result was accomplished in 35 cases, using a single treatment session, while in ten cases two or three sessions were re-

Table 8.2. Summary of results achieved in the group studied (BENNDORF et al. 2004)*

Demographics:
- 45 Patients
- Female/male: 32/13
- Age: 32–90
- Symptoms: red eye (20), chemosis (22), exophthalmos (29), diplopia (25), retroorbital pain (7), visual loss (9), bruit (4), vertigo (1)
- Fistula type: D (41), B (3), C (1)
- Bilateral fistula site: 8
- Cortical drainage: 9 (20%) no neurological deficit, no ICH

Transvenous approaches:
- IPS: 37, thrombosed IPS: 10
- FV/SOV: 13, transfemoral (4), surgical exposure (8), direct (transorbital) puncture (1)
- Superior petrosal sinus: 4
- Frontal vein: 1
- Sylvian vein: 1
- Combined: 10
- Cross-over: 8
- Direct puncture of IJV: 3

Results:
- *Anatomic cure:* 42/45 (93%), (3 final follow-up pending)
    Single/multiple sessions – 35/10
    Initial result – complete occlusion: 28 (12 subtotal)
- *Clinical cure:*   41/45 (91%) – four improved
    (final follow-up pending)
- *Complications:*
    Death: 0
      Major permanent: 0
      Minor permanent: 0
      Minor transient: 1/45 (2.2%, 6th CN-palsy)
      Minor extravasation (IPS): 1/45 (2.2%, clinically silent)
- Transient increased IOP: 2/45 (4.4%)

*Awarded with Magna Cum Laude, ASNR 2004 Seattle

quired to achieve complete occlusion. Complete occlusion as immediate post-embolization result was documented in 30 (66%) cases, while in 12 (26.6%) subtotal or incomplete occlusion was documented. Follow-up at 3 months confirmed complete occlusion of the AV shunt. These numbers refer to the total number of patients ($n = 45$), while the ones seen for angiographic follow-up ($n = 42$) showed 100% angiographic occlusion. Clinical cure was achieved in 41/45 (91%); four patients reported improved symptoms by telephone interview, final follow-up was still pending.

There were no procedure-related permanent ophthalmological or neurological deficits. One patient (2.2%) developed a minor transient 6th CN palsy after coiling of the right and left CS using IPS approach through a thrombosed sinus. She was treated with corticosteroids for 1 week and was symptom free when seen for her clinical follow-up. In one patient (2.2 %), venous extravasation was observed during catheterization of the IPS. The patient woke up without any clinical sequelae. In two patients (4.4%), a transient aggravation of their ophthalmologic symptoms was seen after a transfemoral SOV approach failed to provide access to the fistula site. Both patients underwent more aggressive procedures (one had surgical SOV cannulation, the other deep SOV puncture). Both recovered fully after complete occlusion of the fistula.

Out of this group of patients (BENNDORF et al. 2004), seven typical venous approaches to the CS will be described in the following as Case Reports (Figs. 8.14–8.28) illustrating technical possibilities for gaining endovascular access and associated problems. These cases were treated by the author at the Charité, Humboldt University Berlin between 1992 and 2003. They are complemented by Case Illustrations (Figs. 8.29–8.40) showing valuable alternative approaches or techniques provided by other experienced operators from international centers.

8.3.3
Cases Reports (Figs. 8.14–8.28)

8.3.3.1
Case Report I: Approach via the Thrombosed IPS (Figs. 8.14–8.16).

A 56-year-old patient presented in October 2000 with an 18-month history of a swollen eye, conjunctival engorgement and retroorbital pain. Since February 1999, the patient noticed occasional occipital pain combined with dizziness and nausea for 2–3 days as well as bilateral diplopia. After several hospital stays and treatment with corticosteroids because of suspected endocrine orbitopathy, ocular myositis and pseudo tumor cerebri in July 1999, a DCSF was diagnosed using intraarterial DSA. By that time, the patient had undergone several CT and MRI exam that remained inconclusive. After an unsuccessful attempt to embolize the fistula in another institution, and clinical worsening, the patient was referred 14 months later to our institution. At that time, she had a moderate bilateral exophthalmos and a noticeable conjunctival injection with intraocular pressures of 18 mm Hg in the right eye and 20 mm Hg in the left eye. The patient further complained about horizontal diplopia. Her funduscopy showed significantly elongated veins and massive

retinal hemorrhages. Intraarterial DSA revealed a small AVF at the left posterior CS. The fistula was exclusively supplied by ipsilateral branches of the TMH (Type B after Barrows) and drained into the left SOV and via the ICS into the right CS and SOV. Because there was no posterior drainage identifiable, a phlebography was performed prior to the endovascular procedure. Repeated intravenous injections from different catheter positions in the IJV revealed a tiny "notch" in the vicinity of the jugular bulb. Here, a 0.014″ hydrophilic microguidewire (Transend-14) was introduced a few mm and used to navigate a small microcatheter, the Tracker Excel (0.014″). Then, a more flexible guidewire, the Terumo Headliner™ (0.012″, 90°), whose tip was formed into a small loop, was advanced. This loop was gently advanced within the presumably thrombosed IPS lumen. Control angiograms were performed using minimal manual injection pressure that showed a narrowed, irregular lumen without any recognizable communication to the CS or to the fistula. A bi-plane "blank road map" allowed control of the catheter navigation, while avoiding inadvertent entry into small pontine veins. After reaching the left posterior CS, a superselective contrast injection demonstrated the fistula's drainage into both partially thrombosed SOVs. In this manner, the microcatheter was advanced through the ICS into the right CS. The occlusion of the fistula started with placement of detachable platinum coils, at first with 3/8 mm (GDC-10), and was continued from right to left through the ICS initially with 2–3 mm coils and some GDC Soft coils (13 coils total). After a relatively dense packing of the posterior venous (CS) pouch on the left side was accomplished, the control series indicated an occlusion of the fistula. The patient partially recovered from her symptoms within the following week and noticed a complete disappearance of her diplopia 8 weeks later. The venous congestion resolved as well and a control angiogram after 5 months confirmed complete and permanent occlusion of the fistula.

8.3.3.2
Case Report II: Cross-Over Approach via the IPS (Figs. 8.17, 8.18)

In February 1999, a 77-year-old woman reported flickering in front of her right eye of 4 years' standing. She also presented with proptosis of her right eye, increasing diplopia due to 3rd, 4th and 6th CN palsy as well as chemosis and decreased vision for

(Text continues on p. 215)

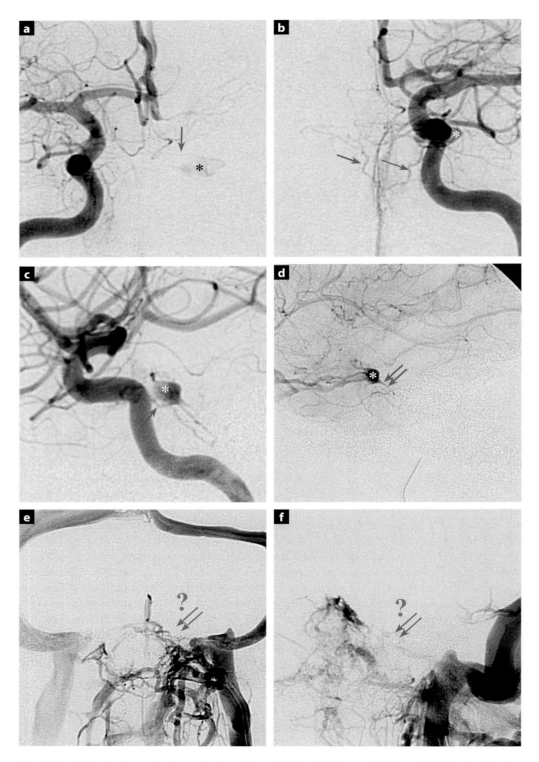

Fig. 8.14 a–f. Case I: Approach through a thrombosed IPS, initial DSA. Right (**a**) and left (**b**) ICA injections, AP views: Small arteriovenous shunt at the left CS (*asterisk*), supplied by branches from the ipsi- and contralateral MHT (*arrows*). Left ICA injection lateral view, early (**c**) and late (**d**) phase: Opacification of the posterior CS (*asterisk*). No drainage via the IPS, which is narrowed and does not opacify in the late venous phase, except for a short tapered segment (*double arrows*). Such residual tapering may indicate a more recent thrombosis that often facilitates catheter navigation. **e, f** Phlebogram of the left IJV, AP (**e**) and lateral (**f**): No clear (*?*) visualization of the IPS (*double arrows*)

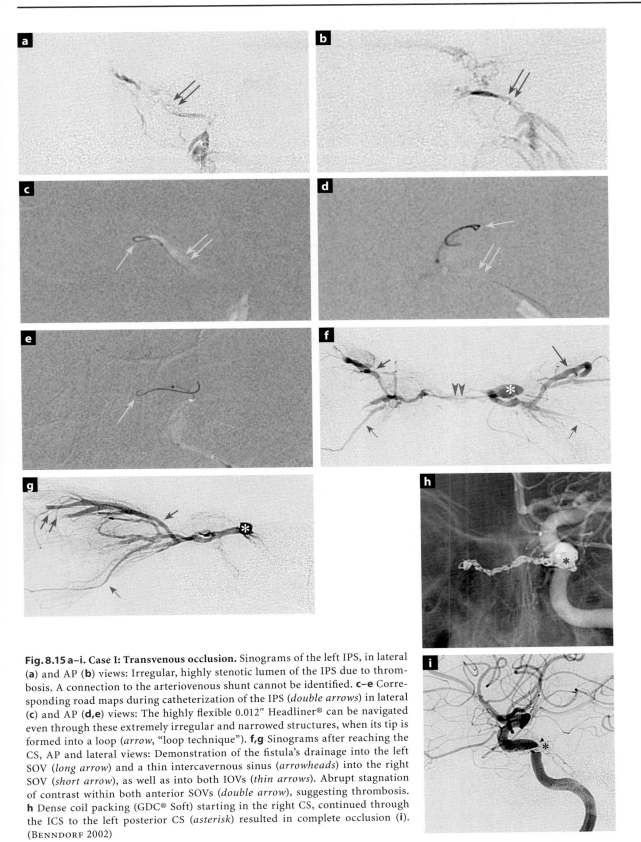

Fig. 8.15 a–i. Case I: Transvenous occlusion. Sinograms of the left IPS, in lateral (**a**) and AP (**b**) views: Irregular, highly stenotic lumen of the IPS due to thrombosis. A connection to the arteriovenous shunt cannot be identified. **c–e** Corresponding road maps during catheterization of the IPS (*double arrows*) in lateral (**c**) and AP (**d,e**) views: The highly flexible 0.012″ Headliner® can be navigated even through these extremely irregular and narrowed structures, when its tip is formed into a loop (*arrow*, "loop technique"). **f,g** Sinograms after reaching the CS, AP and lateral views: Demonstration of the fistula's drainage into the left SOV (*long arrow*) and a thin intercavernous sinus (*arrowheads*) into the right SOV (*short arrow*), as well as into both IOVs (*thin arrows*). Abrupt stagnation of contrast within both anterior SOVs (*double arrow*), suggesting thrombosis. **h** Dense coil packing (GDC® Soft) starting in the right CS, continued through the ICS to the left posterior CS (*asterisk*) resulted in complete occlusion (**i**). (BENNDORF 2002)

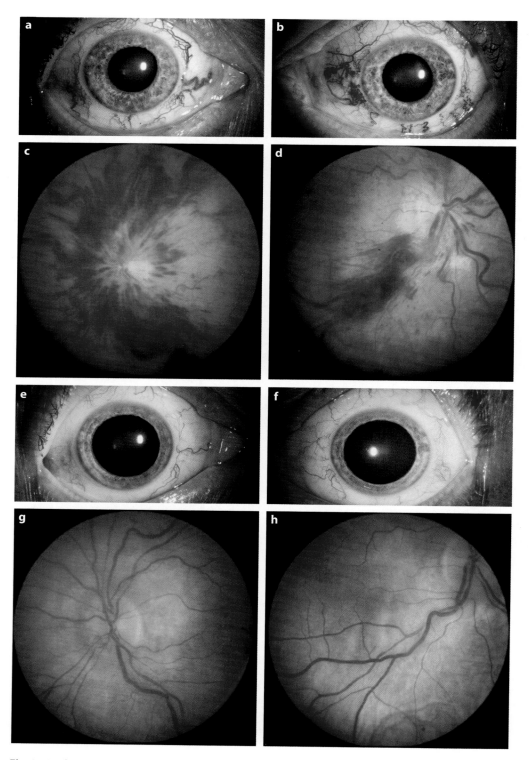

Fig. 8.16 a–h. Case I: A 56-year-old woman with an at least 18-month history of bilateral eye redness and diplopia. Proptosis, irritation of the conjunctiva and the fundus. **a–d** Before embolization: Bilateral episcleral congestion and hyperemia of the iris. Fundoscopy shows significant tortuousities and congestion of retinal veins as well as extensive retinal hemorrhages and papillary edema in both eyes. **e–h** At 3 months after embolization: Nearly complete resolution of the conjunctival signs and normalization of the fundus (BENNDORF 2002)

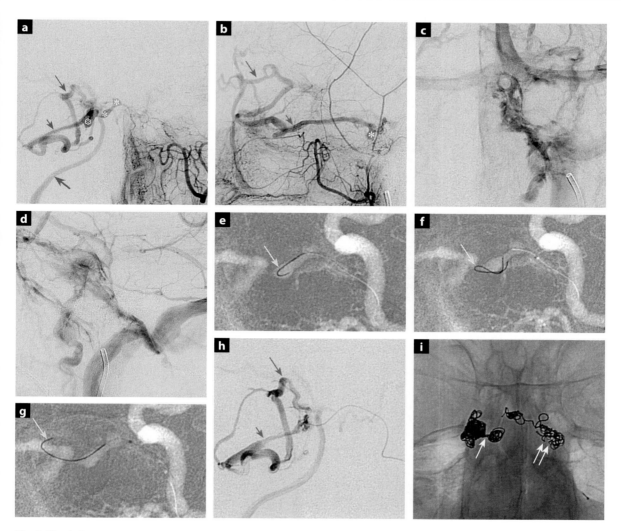

Fig. 8.17a–i. Case II: Cross-over IPS approach, initial DSA and transvenous occlusion. a,b Left ECA injection, AP and lateral views: Arteriovenous shunt involving the ICS (*white asterisks*) and right CS (*b/w asterisk*), which exclusively drains into the IOV (*short arrow*) while the SOV (*arrow*) is filled secondarily. Arterial feeders also arise from the ipsilateral ECA and ICA (Type D). *Thick arrow*: Facial vein. Both IPSs are not opacified. **c,d** ICA injection, late venous phase, AP view: Opacification of the irregular left IPS, suggesting ongoing thrombosis. **e–g** Road maps, LAO views: Successful navigation of the microcatheter from the contralateral IPS into the right CS. Note: The partially thrombosed intercavernous sinus with a highly stenotic segment can be passed using the Headliner and loop technique (*arrows*). **h** Sinogram after reaching the right CS, AP view: Opacification of the fistula's drainage via the IOV (*short arrow*), and secondarily via the SOV (*arrow*), that appears occluded in its posterior segment. **i** Non-subtracted AP view: Coil occlusion starting in the right CS and continued to the left side. Dense packing on the right side, where GDC Soft coils could be deployed even in the narrowed segment between CS and ICS (*white arrow*). On the left side, VortX coils caused disadvantageous friction in the microcatheter preventing a denser packing (*white double arrow*).

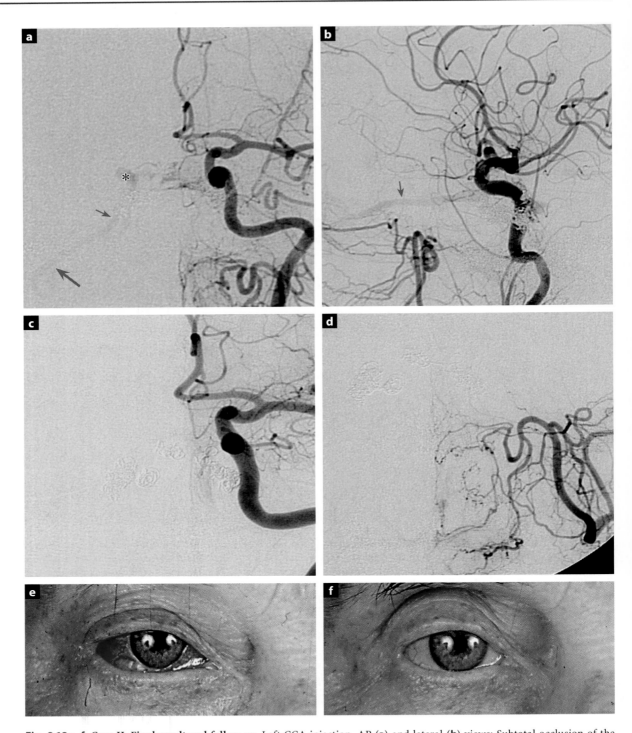

Fig. 8.18 a–f. Case II: Final result and follow-up. Left CCA injection, AP (**a**) and lateral (**b**) views: Subtotal occlusion of the fistula at the end of the procedure. Minimal residual AV shunt at the right CS (*asterisk*), opacifying the IOV (*short arrow*) and the facial vein (*thick arrow*). **c,d** Follow-up: Left ICA and ECA injections AP views: The follow-up exam after 9 months shows complete occlusion. The coils in the right CS are placed medially and laterally to the internal carotid artery. (BENNDORF et al. 2000). Note: A subtotal occlusion of the AV shunt can often be sufficient as long as the coil packing is dense enough. Reversal of Heparin contributes to the induced thrombosis and follow-up exams usually show complete occlusion of the fistula (see also Fig. 8.22c). **e** A 77-year-old patient suffering from proptosis for 4 years presented with eye redness and chemosis, diplopia due to 3rd, 4th and 6th nerve palsy as well as decreased vision for 2 months. **f** At 6 months after endovascular therapy, complete recovery

2 months. DSA showed a small AVF on the right CS (Barrows Type B) with primary drainage via the right inferior ophthalmic vein and secondarily into the right superior ophthalmic vein in the anterior orbit. Posterior drainage via the IPS was not recognizable on either side. The late venous phase of the left ICA injection showed a faintly opacified IPS on the left side that was chosen for transvenous approach. After placement of a 6-F guiding catheter a Transend-14 (0.014″) and a Terumo-12 (Headliner-0.012″) were used to navigate a microcatheter (Tracker Excel) through the left IPS into the ipsilateral CS. Advancing a Headliner's tip, formed to a loop, allowed for passage through a high-grade stenosis within the intercavernous sinus and for entry into the right CS. Occlusion of the sinus was started within the right CS using GDC-10 (5 mm/15 cm) and continued with smaller and more pliable GDC Soft coils. Coil packing was carried out from contra- to ipsilateral and within the highly stenotic segment. On the left side, the packing was completed by two VortX-18 coils, which caused suddenly increased friction within the microcatheter, thus dense packing was not achievable in this compartment (total number of coils=21). The procedure was terminated when the angiogram showed a subtotal occlusion with minimal residual flow in the IOV. The patient's ophthalmoplegia improved within the a few days. Her visual acuity had increased at the time of discharge, 1 week later. She was completely symptom free after 6 months; a control angiogram after 9 months confirmed complete occlusion.

8.3.3.3
Case Report III: Approach via the
Thrombosed Cavernous Sinus (Figs. 8.19, 8.20)

A 73-year-old former nurse presented in July 2000 with persistent visual problems. In her history, eye redness, retroorbital pain and minor exophthalmos on the right side were found over the previous 3 months. A CSF was assumed but "ruled out" by an initial MRI exam. Various differential diagnoses including inflammatory (conjunctivitis, myositis, phlegmon) and tumorous diseases of the orbit and the adjacent sinuses, were considered. In this context, the patient underwent extractions of nine teeth and an orbital biopsy. Because her symptoms did not improve, the patient was eventually transferred to perform a DSA at our institution. On admission, she showed exophthalmos and a con-

siderable vision loss, as well as an increase of the intraocular pressure to 32 mm Hg. The angiogram showed a very small low-flow fistula of the right CS that was exclusively supplied by the ipsilateral AMA (Barrows Type C). The venous drainage was provided by the ipsilateral partially thrombosed SOV and IOV, while the IPS did not seem involved, but showed faint opacification in the late venous phase. After placement of a 6-F guide in the IJV, a phlebogram showed a widely open IPS of normal caliber on both sides and a filling of the left SOV. The AV shunt in the right CS, however, was not identifiable. A microcatheter (Tracker Excel) could be advanced without difficulty into the posterior CS. Repeated control injections through the microcatheter showed a filling of the posterior portion of the sinus, but no communication with the fistula site in the anterior CS. Attempts to navigate the microcatheter into the anterior compartment remained initially unsuccessful. After several exchanges of guidewires, advancing a Headliner 0.012‴, 90° in loop technique was eventually successful and the microcatheter could be pushed into the previously not visualized fistulous anterior CS compartment. Here, the connection between anterior CS and SOV was blocked with one GDC-10 (4 mm/10 cm) first, then the anterior CS compartment was packed until complete occlusion of the fistula was documented (total of four GDCs).

Postoperatively, the patient was heparinized for 48 h during which her symptoms slightly improved. She reported the next day subjectively improved vision. After 1 week, she was discharged and recovered completely within 4 weeks. Her intraocular pressure decreased to 10 mm Hg. In a clinical follow-up 4 months later, the patient's symptoms were completely resolved and she still reported further improved vision. The patient suffered from an unrelated minor stroke a couple of months later, and was reluctant to undergo another control angiogram.

8.3.3.4
Case Report IV: Transfemoral Cross-Over Approach
via the Facial Vein and SOV (Figs. 8.21, 8.22)

A 74-year-old woman presented at the hospital (July 1999) with persistent retro-orbital pain. In addition, she suffered from diplopia and ptosis, underwent acupuncture without any significant improvement and was transferred by her neurologist for invasive vascular diagnostics. Intra-arterial

(Text continues on p. 220)

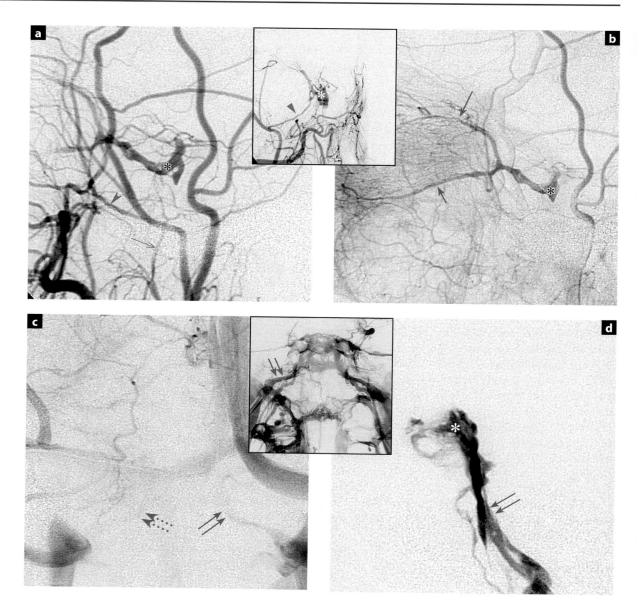

Fig. 8.19a–d. Case III: Approach through the thrombosed CS, initial DSA. Right ECA injection, lateral view early (**a**) and late (**b**) arterial phase: Very small arteriovenous shunt of the right CS (*asterisk*), supplied by branches of the ECA, such as a recurrent branch of the MMA (*arrowhead*, see inset: AP view) and a tiny pedicle from the AMA (*thin arrow*). This fistula could not be identified on MRI or MRA. Both the SOV (*arrow*) and the IOV (*short arrow*) appear partially thrombosed. No opacification of the IPS. Note: A rare case of a Type-C fistula. **c** Right ICA venogram, AP view: Faint opacification of the right IPS (fistula side) in AP view (*dotted double arrow*). The left IPS (*double arrow*) is better opacified. *Inset:* Jugular phlebogram: Clear visualization of the right (*double arrow*) and left IPS as a widely open vessels. This example demonstrates that a global angiogram (arteriogram and venogram) may be unreliable for selecting the most promising venous route to the CS. **d** Sinogram, lateral view: After successful passage of the right IPS (*double arrow*), a selective contrast injection into the posterior CS (*asterisk*) shows initially no connection with the fistulous compartment in the anterior CS. This can be due to anatomic compartmentalization, or more frequently thrombosis

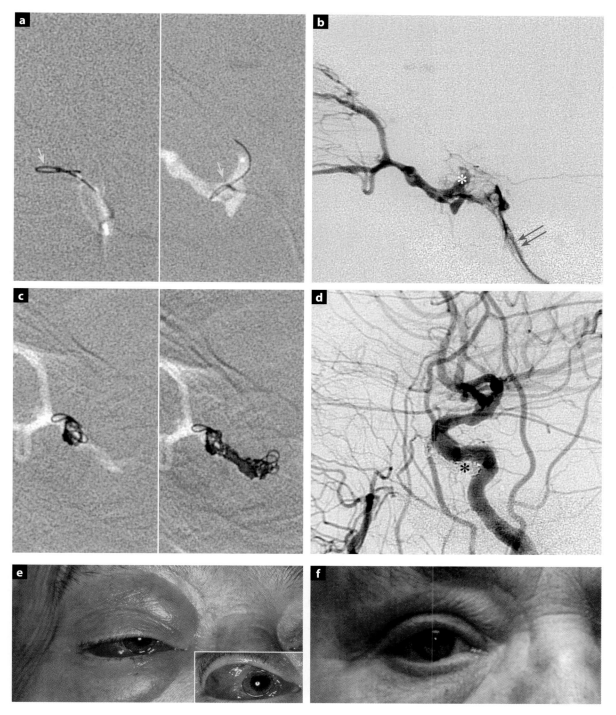

Fig. 8.20a–f. Case III: Transvenous occlusion and final result. a Road map, lateral view: As demonstrated for the IPS, the loop technique is helpful in navigating a guidewire (Headliner 0.012″) through a non-opacified (thus likely thrombosed) CS. **b** Sinogram, lateral view: When the anterior CS compartment (*asterisk*) is reached, the AV fistula becomes visible, draining into both ophthalmic veins. **c** Road maps, lateral view: Placement of the coils in the anterior CS proximal to the veins, disconnecting the anterior drainage from the AV shunt. **d** Control angiogram of the right CCA, lateral view: Complete occlusion of the arteriovenous fistula at the end of the procedure. **e** A 73-year-old patient with exophthalmos, eye redness, aggravated chemosis and decreased vision for several months. Various differential diagnoses included "tumoral lesion" (requiring a biopsy) and phlegmon (leading to nine teeth extractions). **f** Complete recovery within 4 months after occlusion of the fistula. (Benndorf 2002)

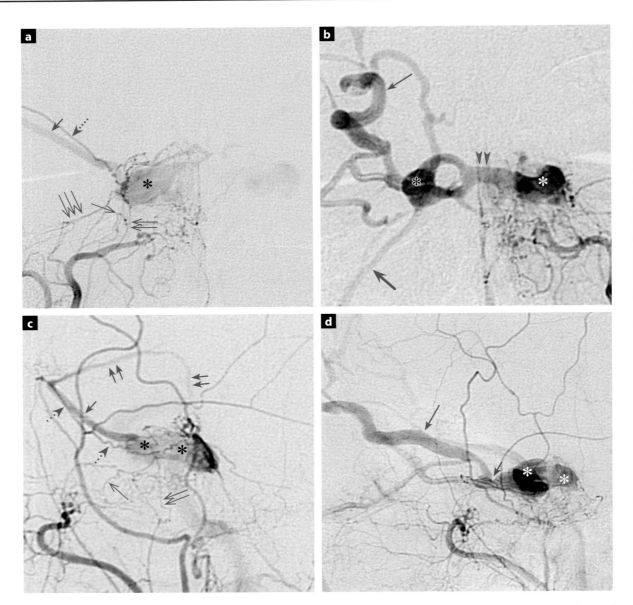

Fig. 8.21a–d. Case IV: Transfemoral SOV approach, initial DSA. a Right ECA injection, AP view: Arteriovenous shunt of the right lateral CS (*asterisks*), which drains mainly into the right SPPS (*short arrow*). The arterial supply is provided by network of small branches, including the AFR (*thin arrow*) and branches of MMA (*triple arrow*). No opacification of the right SOV. Note also the recurrent middle meningeal branch (*dotted arrows*). **b** Left ECA injection, AP view: Large arteriovenous shunt at the left CS (*white asterisk*) with filling of the intercavernous sinus (*arrowheads*) and the right CS (*b/w asterisk*), which drains via the SOV (*arrow*). Rare case of a true bilateral fistula. *Large arrow:* Right facial vein. **c** Right ECA injection, lateral view: Some of the small branches supplying the fistula on the right side such as the AFR (*thin arrow*), the AMA (*thin double arrow*) and the MMA (*short thin double arrow*) are better identifiable. The dominant venous drainage of the right CS fistula into the SPPS (*short arrow*) and via a paracavernous sinus (*short double arrow*) is seen. **d** Left ECA injection, lateral view: The enlarged right SOV (*arrow*) serves as sole draining vein of the left-sided arteriovenous shunt. Well visible is also the narrowing of the ophthalmic vein while passing through the supraorbital fissure (*short arrow*). It is interesting to note that AV both shunts appear to utilize different drainage routes

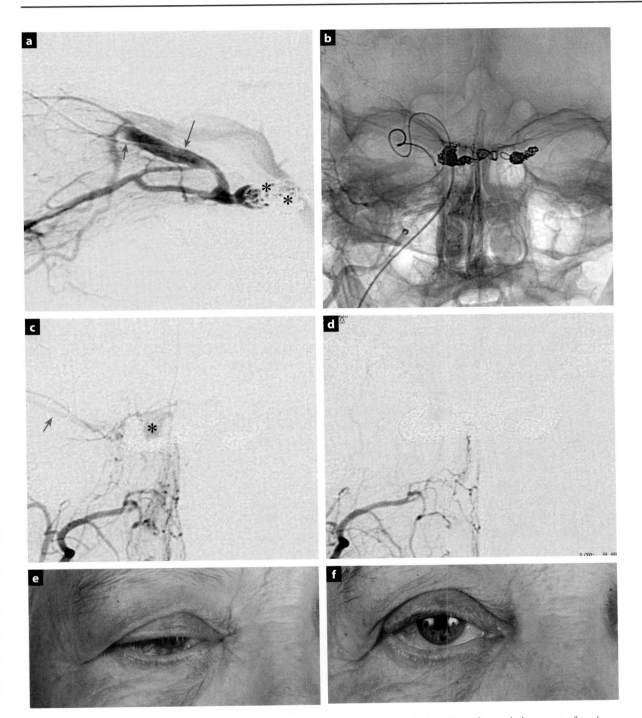

Fig. 8.22a–f. Case IV: Transvenous occlusion and final result. a Sinogram, lateral view: Transfemoral placement of a micro-catheter (*short arrow*) via the right IJV, facial vein and right SOV (*arrow*) into the left CS (cross-over approach). Decreased AV-shunting flow after placing the first coils (*asterisks*). **b** Non-subtracted view, in AP view: Packing of coils from the left CS and continued to the right side. Note: Pushing of some additional VortX coils through the tortuous anatomy caused considerable friction in the microcatheter, preventing a denser packing of the ICS. **c** Right ECA injection, AP view: Subtotal occlusion of the arteriovenous fistula at the end of the procedure with minimal residual AV-shunting flow in the CS (*asterisk*) and SPPS (*short arrow*). **d** Right ECA injection, AP view: Complete occlusion of the fistula during the follow-up exam 4.5 months later. **e** A 74-year-old patient with exophthalmos, ptosis, chemosis and diplopia. **f** Minimal residual conjunctival veins, otherwise resolved symptoms at follow-up (BENNDORF 2002)

DSA revealed an arteriovenous shunt at the right and left CS (true bilateral DCSF) draining into the right SOV and sphenoparietal sinus. An initial attempt to occlude the fistula remained unsuccessful, because the IPS could not be catheterized and the microcatheter was maneuverable only into the basilar plexus from which a passage into the CS was not possible. In the second session, a 4-F guiding catheter was placed in the right facial vein and then advanced until just proximal to the angular vein. Catheterization of the SOV from here was not possible at first, because different microcatheters (Tracker Excel, Tracker-18 and Tracker-10) did not have sufficient mechanical support to overcome tortuousities in the anterior SOV. Changing to a stiffer catheter type (Rapid Transit18) finally allowed for accessing the CS and navigating through the intercavernous sinus into the contralateral CS. Deployment of GDC-18 coils, starting with a 4 mm/10 cm, and some VortX18-coils resulted in a partial shunt reduction. Because the VortX coils exhibited noticeable friction, the occlusion was continued with GDCs-10. Despite several efforts, advancing the microcatheter to the connection between CS and sphenoparietal sinus was not possible due to the stiffness of the microcatheter. Therefore, coil packing was continued in the ICS. A subtotal occlusion with stagnating flow in the SOV was noted at the end of the procedure.

The patient recovered well within the next couple of days. She initially developed a postoperative swelling of the upper eyelid and complained about increased pain. The diplopia improved after 4 days, and her vision improved from 0.4 to 0.8 within 5 days. The patient was discharged under low molecular heparin (1 week) and 300 mg aspirin daily for 4 weeks. After 5.5 months, angiographic control documented a complete occlusion of the fistula while the symptoms had completely resolved.

8.3.3.5
Case Report V: Transophthalmic Approach (Cannulation) via the SOV (Figs. 8.23, 8.24)

A 56-year-old male (summer 1997), presented with exophthalmos, eye redness and a history of diplopia for 5 days. His IOP was elevated to 33 mm Hg. His arteriogram showed a small dural AVF on the right CS that primarily drained into the right SOV. Manual compression therapy was the initial therapeutic approach, but failed to show effect after 7 weeks. The patient experienced slight progression

of his symptoms. In order to occlude the fistula endovascularly, a transvenous IPS approach to the right CS was chosen. However, it was impossible to advance the microcatheter through an apparently occluded sinus or through the tortuous SOV. 48 following the unsuccessful catheterizations, the patient developed an increased IOP and decreased vision. Therefore, in a subsequent session, the SOV was surgically exposed and punctured with a 21-G needle (Terumo). This allowed the introduction of a Tracker-10 that reached the CS within a few minutes without difficulties. The fistulous compartment of the CS was densely packed with GDCs, which resulted in immediate occlusion of the fistula. After removal of catheter and cannula, the vein was manually compressed for about 20 min. The upper lid cut was closed with a suture. No postoperative bleeding or other complications were observed. A control angiogram after 5 min showed a stable result. The patient fully recovered and was able to pursue his work as a layout designer in a major newspaper. An angiographic control 18 months later confirmed stable occlusion of the fistula.

8.3.3.6
Case Report VI: Direct Puncture of the SOV (Figs. 8.25, 8.26)

A 59-year-old teacher (November 1996), reported an increasing bruit, diplopia, eye redness and prominence of his left eye. His cerebral angiogram revealed a small arteriovenous fistula at the supraorbital fissure that was supplied by meningeal branches of the ipsilateral ophthalmic and maxillary arteries and drained exclusively into the ipsilateral SOV. Transarterial embolization of the feeding pedicles from the ECA resulted in only partial occlusion. Because the symptoms of the patient did not improve, transvenous approaches were performed in February 1997. Due to thrombosis of the IPS, and a high-grade stenosis of the SOV, advancing a microcatheter into the CS was impossible by transfemoral techniques. The patient's condition deteriorated significantly over the following 48 h with secondary glaucoma and elevated uncontrollable IOPs of up to 76 mm Hg. Thus, the SOV was surgically exposed and cannulated with a 21-G venicath (Terumo). Unfortunately, the catheter navigation remained unsuccessful due to the highly stenotic SOV. Concerning the critical situation of the patient, direct puncture of the deep SOV posterior to the eyeball, was considered as

(Text continues on p.225)

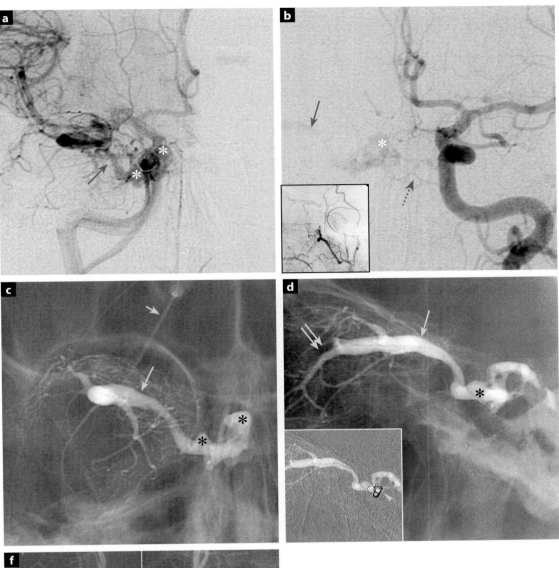

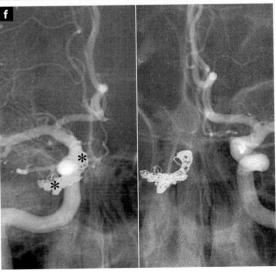

Fig. 8.23a–f. Case V: Transophthalmic SOV approach, initial DSA and transvenous occlusion. a Right and **b** left ICA injection AP views: Arteriovenous shunt at the right CS (*asterisks*) with supply from right and left MHT (*dotted arrow*). (*Inset:* Additional supply from right ECA). Drainage via SOV (*arrow*) only, no opacification of the IPS. **c** Sinogram AP and lateral (**d**): After exposure of the SOV by incision of the upper eye lid, cannulation using a 21-G needle (Terumo) and gentle navigation of a microcatheter (Tracker-10) through this vein, which is possible despite thrombosis in its anterior segment (*double arrow*). A previous attempt to catheterize the SOV by transfemoral approach failed due to significant tortuousities of the SOV and the angular vein. **e** Road map lateral: Placement of the first coil in the right CS. **f** ICA injection, non-subtracted AP view: Coils are densely packed in CS, conforming to the medial and inferior carotid wall

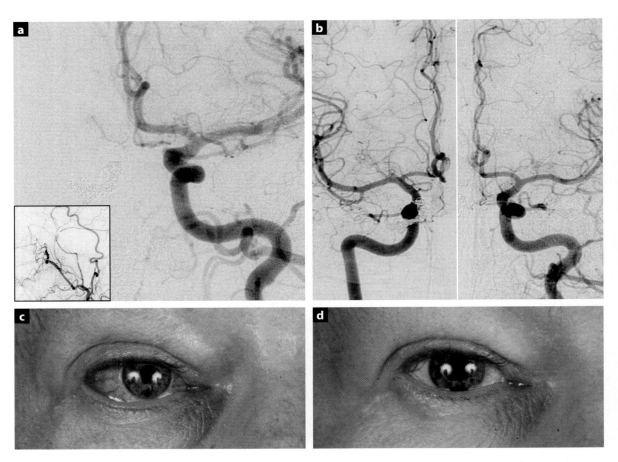

Fig. 8.24a–d. Case V: Final result and follow-up. Arteriogram of the left ICA (**a**) AP and ECA (*inset*). The control angiograms revealed complete occlusion of the arteriovenous fistula at the end of the procedure. **b** Bilateral ICA arteriogram confirmed this result 18 months later (BENNDORF et al. 2000b). **c** Before transvenous occlusion: A 56-year-old patient with mild exophthalmos, eye redness and diplopia due to 6th nerve palsy. This patient initially underwent manual compression therapy for 7 weeks that failed to show an effect. **d** At 3 months after treatment: Normalization of the intraocular pressure and resolution of the clinical symptoms, allowing the patient to resume his work as a layout designer with no cosmetic alterations). (BENNDORF 2002)

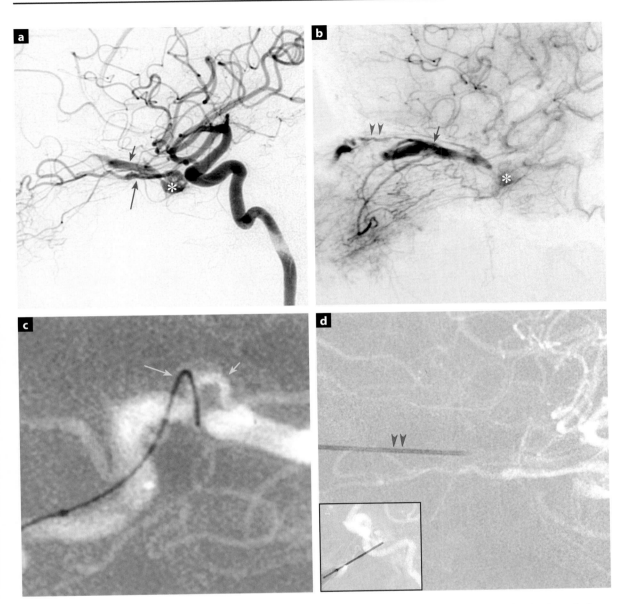

Fig. 8.25a–e. Case VI: Direct SOV puncture, initial DSA and transvenous occlusion. a,b Left ICA injection lateral views, early and late arterial phase: Small arteriovenous shunt at the left anterior CS (*asterisk*), supplied by a recurrent meningeal branch of the ipsilateral ophthalmic artery (*arrow*), draining exclusively into the SOV (*short arrow*). The SOV appears partiallly thrombosed in its anterior segment (*arrowheads*), possibly related to the previously attempted unsuccessful facial vein approach. No opacification of the IPS, the catherization of which failed as well. **c** Road map, lateral (magnified): After upper eye lid incision, a stenotic segment (*short arrow*) prevented advancement of the microguidewire (Transend 0.014″, *arrow*). Hence, no conventional access to the CS was feasible. **d,e** Considering the patient`s critical clinical condition with uncontrollable IOPs up to 76 mm Hg and imminent loss of visison, a direct deep intraorbital puncture of the SOV was performed: Using bi-plane road map, a 21G needle (*arrowheads*) was very slowly and gently advanced along the medial side of the globe until the SOV was reached in its posterior (intraconal) segment

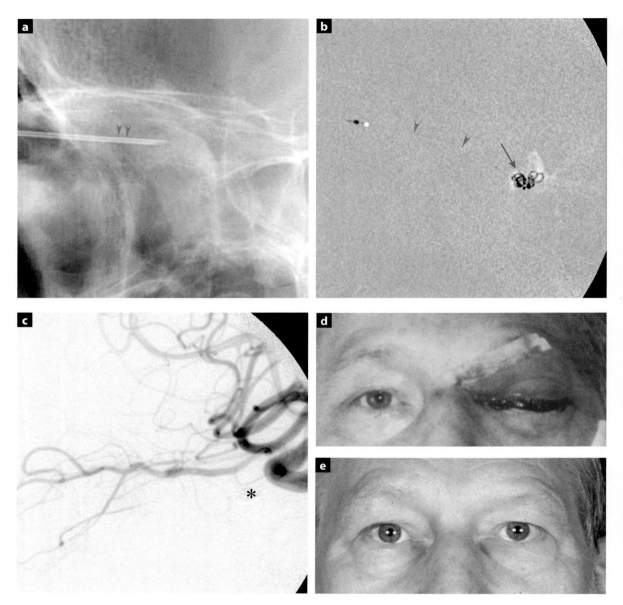

Fig. 8.26 a–e. Case VI: Transvenous occlusion and follow-up. a Non-subtracted lateral view: Documentation of the needle position in the posterior third of the orbit. **b** Road map, lateral view: After advancing a microcatheter (Tracker-10, *arrowheads*) to the fistula site, platinum coils were deployed (GDC) and densely packed in the venous compartment of the fistula. Control angiograms showed complete occlusion of the fistula by the end of the procedure. **c** Left ICA injection, lateral view: This result was confirmed stable after 3 months (*asterisk*=coils). **d, e** A 59-year-old teacher with exophthalmos, severe chemosis associated with an increased IOP (76 mm Hg). At 1 day after treatment (*E*), the eyelid is still swollen. (*F*), 3 months after treatment, the patient shows complete resolution of his symptoms (no cosmetic deformities) (BENNDORF et al. 2001).

a last resort. After thorough discussion of potentially associated risks with the ophthalmologist, neurosurgeon and maxillo-facial surgeon, a 21-G needle (Terumo) was very slowly advanced along the medial wall into the posterior third of the orbit using bi-plane road mapping. While approaching the SOV, the direction of the needle was controlled and corrected by carefully watching the fluoroscopy in both planes. The puncture was successful in the first attempt and allowed the introduction of a small microcatheter (Tracker-10) and its navigation to the fistula site. Detachable coils (GDCs-10) were gently deployed until a control injection showed a reduced filling of the AV shunt. After completing the occlusion, catheter and needle were removed and the incision was surgically closed. No postoperative complication occurred. The patient was discharged with normal IOP after 1 week and recovered completely within 3 months. A follow-up arteriogram after 12 months confirmed complete occlusion. 4 years later, the patient reported minimal tinnitus, but had no ophthalmological symptoms and IOP of 16 mm Hg. Another control angiogram showed minimal opacification in the area of the coil packing that was not interpreted as recanalization.

8.3.3.7
Case Report VII: Direct Puncture of the Sylvian Vein After Craniotomy (Figs. 8.27, 8.28)

A 57-year-old woman presented (May 1992) with painful exophthalmos and chemosis on the left side. There were no neurological deficits. Computed tomography revealed a dilated right SOV due to a dural AVF involving the left CS at the lower edge of the supraorbital fissure. The fistula was supplied by meningeal branches of ECA (MMA) and the ICA (ophthalmic artery and cavernous branches), while the venous drainage was directed posteriorly via the sphenoparietal sinus and the Sylvian vein into the vein of Labbé and the transverse sinus. A microcatheter was introduced first into the MMA and then the feeding pedicle was blocked by an injection of 40% NBCA/lipiodol mixture without occluding the AV shunt itself. Because of the tortuous anatomy of the ICA feeder and the ophthalmic artery, a distal position for another safe glue injection was not obtainable. None of the attempted venous approaches, such as the IPS and facial vein (SOV approach), proved successful, due to thrombosis and tortuousities. Because the patient devel-

oped progressive visual deterioration, emergency measures had to be considered. Because, surgical exposure of the angular vein or SOV was not an established practice in our institution at that time, an open surgical approach was chosen. In June 1992, following lateral craniotomy, the Sylvian vein was exposed by a neurosurgical colleague. The vein was clipped and punctured using an 18-G needle (plastic cannula). This veinicath was imbedded in Palacos® (methylmethacrylate, bone cement) and anchored at the skull for stabilization. After attaching a Y-connector, a Tracker-18 microcatheter could be advanced without any problems through the sphenoparietal sinus into the CS under fluoroscopic control. Placement of two small pushable fibered coils caused an immediate noticeable reduction of the AV shunting. After waiting a further 10 min, a second control angiogram showed complete disappearance of the AV shunt so that the cannula was removed and the procedure was finished. The clinical symptomatology resolved during the following 2 weeks and a control exam confirmed clinical and anatomic cure. The patient was seen for a follow-up exam 5 years later which confirmed stable occlusion.

8.3.4
Case Illustrations (Figs. 8.29–8.40)

Additional Case Illustrations show alternative venous routes, the use of liquid embolic agents, transarterial embolizations and other methods to treat DCSFs (Figs. 9.1–9.4).

(Text continues on p. 228)

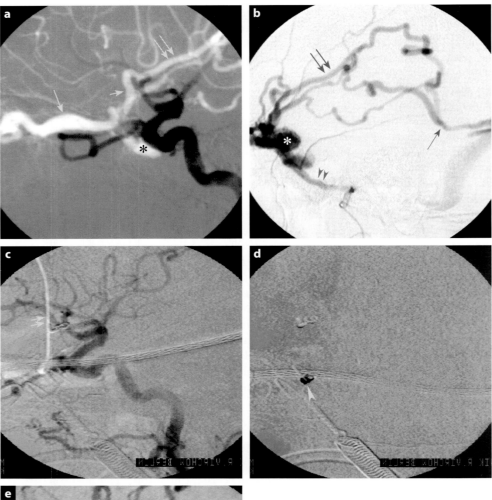

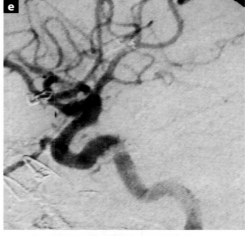

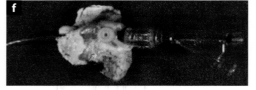

Fig. 8.27a–f. Case VII: Sylvian vein approach. Initial DSA, intraoperative transvenous occlusion and final result. (**a**), left ICA injection, lateral view (sequential subtraction, images were obtained using mobile C-arm used for intraoperative angiography): Arteriovenous shunt of the right CS (*asterisk*), supplied by a recurrent meningeal branch of the enlarged ophthalmic artery. Anterior drainage into the SOV (*arrow*) and cortical drainage via the SPPS (*short arrow*) into the Sylvian veins (*double arrow*). **b** Selective MMA injection left, lateral shows the enlarged MMA (*double arrowhead*) shunting directly into the CS (*asterisk*) and draining into dilated cortical veins: Sylvian veins (*double arrow*), vein of Labbé (*thin arrow*). **c,d** Intraoperative road map, lateral: After craniotomy, the arterialized Sylvian vein was carefully punctured using an 18-G needle. The needle was attached to a Y-connector and imbedded in Palacos® (methylmethacrylate) for stabilization. The microcatheter (Tracker®-18) could be easily advanced to the fistula site (*short double arrow*, **d**). After deploying only two 4/30 mm fibered coils (*arrowhead*), significant reduction of the AV-shunting flow was noted, which after 10 more min, resulted in complete occlusion of the fistula (**e**). Note that all attempts to occlude the fistula, including IPS and SOV approaches failed. **f** An 18-G needle with Y-connector (rotating hemostatic valve) imbedded in Palacos® (bone cement) as used for fixation at the skull, providing stabilization during advancement of the microcatheter into the CS

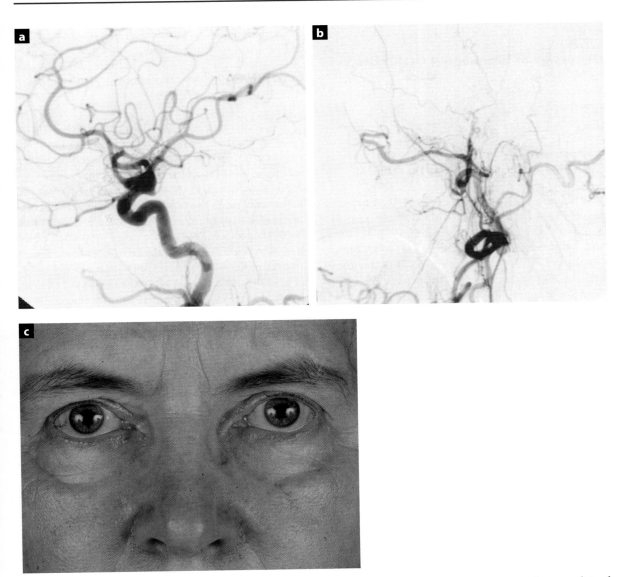

Fig. 8.28a–c. Case VII: Angiographic and clinical follow-up. a,b Left ICA and ECA 5-year follow-up arteriograms, lateral views: Persistent occlusion of the fistula. **c** A 57-year-old patient with complete resolution of her symptoms (left-sided exophthalmos and chemosis at the time of presentation in 1992) (Benndorf et al. 1997, 1999b)

Discussion of Transvenous Occlusions

8.4.1
Approaches

8.4.1.1
IPS Approaches
(Case Reports I–III, Case Illustrations III and XI)

The IPS approach was initially described as an access route to the cavernous sinus (CS) for treatment of direct CSFs (CCF) (DEBRUN et al. 1981; MANELFE and BERENSTEIN 1980). After its introduction as a venous route for embolization of indirect (dural) CSFs by HALBACH et al. (1989a) in 1989, the IPS has been increasingly used by numerous other groups (CHENG et al 2003; THEAUDIN et al. 2007; HALBACH et al. 1989a; GOBIN and GUGLIELMI 2000; KIYOSUE et al. 2004a; KIM et al. 2006; MEYERS et al. 2002; YAMASHITA et al. 1993; ANNESLEY-WILLIAMS et al. 2001, YU et al. 2007). Its frequent utilization as a venous approach to the CS is based on the following:

- The IPS represents the anatomically shortest, thus technically least complicated and safest route. Particularly in patients where this sinus is involved in the venous drainage, the IPS approach is fast and straightforward in the majority of cases. Anatomically, its course is relatively straight, with a horizontal and vertical segment forming a wide angle that does not cause luminal narrowing or catheter kinking with friction that hinders advancements of coils.
- Another advantage is the mechanical "stability" of the sinus. Its course along the petro-occipital suture (petroclival fissure), covered by the dura mater provides stability resembling a "pipe-like" structure. This stability is particularly important when a larger amount of coils need to be pushed through tortuous anatomy (e.g. like the SOV), eventually causing friction within the microcatheter, which may easily become a procedure-limiting factor. The IPS allows for advancing a guidewire or a microcatheter even when its lumen is narrowed, irregular or completely occluded due to thrombosis.
- The topographical anatomy of the IPS opening into the jugular vein allows a relatively stable positioning of a large guide catheter within the vein, or sometimes even into the IPS itself. This makes navigating a microcatheter into the ipsilateral or

contralateral CS considerably easier compared to the retrograde navigation through the SOV, where positioning of a guiding catheter is less stable (OISHI et al. 1999; HALBACH et al. 1989a, 1997; YAMASHITA et al. 1993).

It seems logical that the IPS was utilized early on as an alternative to transarterial balloon placement in direct CCFs with posterior drainage (MANELFE and BERENSTEIN 1980). Despite its obvious advantages, some operators prefer alternate venous routes, commonly when the IPS is angiographically not recognizable (GOLDBERG et al. 1996; HANNEKEN et al. 1989; HASUO et al. 1996), despite an increasing number of reported successful catheterization of such non-visualized IPSs (BENNDORF et al. 2000a; CHENG et al. 2003; HALBACH et al. 1989a; YAMASHITA et al. 1993; MALEK et al. 2000; ROY and RAYMOND 1997; QUINONES et al. 1997).

HALBACH et al. (1988) described first the successful catheterization of an angiographically occluded, but eventually passable IPS in two patients. Further, YAMASHITA et al. (1993) were able to successfully catheterize the sinus in two cases, despite it being "angiographically occult". QUINONES et al. (1997) reported on a 30% success rate for IPS catheterization, including angiographically occluded sinuses.

It is noteworthy that in those "unsuccessful cases" the venous drainage pattern was usually not analyzed in detail. A fistula that would not opacify the IPS during the early arterial phase was commonly referred to as "not angiographically demonstrated" (YAMASHITA et al. 1993; QUINONES et al. 1997), "angiographically invisible" (YU et al. 2007), "not opacified" (KLISCH et al. 2003; KUWAYAMA et al. 1998), "not patent" (GOLDBERG et al. 1996; MONSEIN et al. 1991; KRISHT and BURSON 1999), "not spontaneously opacified" (MONSEIN et al. 1991) or "hypoplastic" (MIZUNO et al. 2001). The question of whether or not the IPS was opacified during the venous phase of the angiogram was not addressed.

However, in my experience, it is helpful to clearly distinguish between two types of negative IPS drainage patterns: (1) non-opacification only during the early arterial phase (=not draining the fistula), but during the late venous phase (=draining the brain), and (2) no opacification at all. Cases with the former disposition may be considered not worth attempting by some operators, although they have a high chance of successful catheter navigation into the CS (Case Reports II–III). An IPS that does not serve as a venous outflow at all has likely undergone sub-total or complete thrombosis. As demonstrated in Case Report I and Fig. 8.3, this does not preclude the existence of anatomic communication, and thus the possibility of reaching the fistula site with a suitable tool.

The IPS may also serve as a draining pathway for the posterior fossa via the SPS; therefore, reading angiograms for decision-making must include the vertebral injections (Figs. 7.29 and 7.30). The only reliable proof of a thrombosed IPS is a direct sinogram via microcatheter, revealing an irregular, narrowed lumen, which nevertheless might be passable. A large volume jugular phlebogram, using several forceful injections from different levels of the proximal internal jugular vein, provides valuable additional anatomic information. It may reveal an either widely open IPS (Figs. 7.7 and 8.19), or a tiny residual portion of the thrombosed IPS, often visible as a small "notch", (Figs. 7.42, 8.3, 8.14). According to SHIU et al. (1968), four main variants of the IPS/IJV junction exist and may play a role in the overall success rate of retrograde IPS catheterizations. Because of its complex architecture and the lack of connection to the IJV, the IPS could not be catheterized in 31% of the cases. This rate may be lower today with advanced catheterization tools, improved imaging techniques and better anatomic understanding of this region. It can be assumed that some of the plexiform-like appearing connections between IPS and IJV in this early work, performed in the 1960s, represented in fact thrombosed IPSs. The chances of success when using this route in an individual case remain hard to predict. As illustrated in Chap. 7, the existence of an aberrant IPS needs to be considered since it may be used as an approach as well (BENNDORF and CAMPI 2001b; CALZOLARI 2002). Identifying such aberrant IPS (unusual deep termination) that enters as a small opening into a large vein, can be difficult if the catheter position is not at the right level, or not proximal enough to fill the IPS (Figs. 7.37 and 8.3). Several authors (HANNEKEN et al. 1989; HASUO et al. 1996; GUPTA et al. 1997; JAHAN et al. 1998) have stated that catheter navigation through the thrombosed IPS may carry an additional risk of rupture, causing subarachnoid hemorrhage (SAH). The current literature reveals 14 cases of IPS perforation, of which some resulted in SAH and others in cerebellar or extradural hematomas (see Table 8.3). Ten cases were successfully managed by endovascular means (KIM et al. 2006; HALBACH et al. 1991a; KING et al. 1989). HALBACH et al. (1988) observed a rupture with SAH in two patients with a direct CCF; both were suc-

cessfully treated by deployment of coils at the rupture site. This group also reported on a patient with a DCSF and intracerebellar hemorrhage after perforation of the IPS who partially recovered (HALBACH et al. 1991b). KING et al. (1989) published a rupture of the IPS during transvenous approach to a carotid cavernous fistula, causing a minor SAH that was subsequently managed by surgical exposure of the CS and injection of IBCA. YAMASHITA et al. (1993) described IPS rupture with extradural extravasation of contrast which stopped spontaneously without clinical consequences. INAGAWA et al. (1986) reported a patient who deteriorated after an unsuccessful occlusion via IPS approach. This deterioration was attributed to thrombosis of the IPS, and the patient was treated transarterially by balloon occlusion.

KIM et al. (2006) recently presented a series of 56 patients with three IPS perforations. The rate of sinus perforation is higher than reported by others but was controlled in all three cases by coil deployment at the rupture site with no significant neurological sequelae. The authors emphasize that sinus rupture may occur even when using supple guidewires and microcatheters without providing details of the devices being used. It raises the question of how gently (or forcefully) have these tools been manipulated.

In the 45 patients with DCSFs studied here, one perforation during catheterization of the inferior petrosal sinus was observed (BENNDORF et al. 2004) that remained clinically silent.

Apart from transvenous embolization of DCSFs, IPS catheterizations have been used extensively as a diagnostic means for venous blood sampling (petrosal sampling) in patients with Cushings disease. The literature shows that this procedure may be associated with complications as well (SHIU et al. 1968; BONELLI et al. 1999; MILLER et al. 1992; STURROCK and JEFFCOATE 1997; SEYER et al. 1994; LEFOURNIER et al. 1999; GANDHI et al. 2008) (Table 8.4)

BONELLI et al. (1999) recently reported about a patient who developed elevated blood pressure, headache and confusion during the procedure due to sinus rupture causing severe SAH, after using a Tracker-18 microcatheter. The authors also describe headaches and nausea without sequelae in three other patients (BONELLI et al. 2000.)

SHIU et al. (1968) already documented the rupture of a pontine vein during cavernous sinography for diagnosis of a pituitary adenoma. As demonstrated in Tables 8.3 and 8.4, more serious complications are observed during petrosal sampling than during transvenous catheterization for CSF occlusion.

Table 8.3. Adverse events during IPS catheterization for endovascular treatment of CSFs (modified after BENNDORF et al. 2000a)

Nunber of Cases	Author	Pathology	Catheter/Wire	Complication	Therapy	Outcome
1	IANAGAWA et al. 1986	Type-A	5F	Deterioration[1]	Balloon	Improved
1	KING et al. 1989	Type-A	–	SAH	IBCA	0
1	HALBACH et al. 1988	Type-A	3F/5F	SAH	Coils	0
1	HALBACH et al. 1991b	Type-A	–	SAH	Coils	0
1	HALBACH et al. 1991b	DCSF	–	ICH	Coils	Recovered
1	YAMASHITA et al. 1993	DCSF	Tracker-18	EDH	Spontaneous	0
1	OISHI et al. 1999	DCSF	0.035″	Dissection of dura	Conservative	CN palsy
1	KLISCH et al. 2003	DCSF		SAH	Conservative	Improved
1	BENNDORF et al. 2004	DCSF	0.035″	EDH	Conservative	0
3	KIM et al. 2006	DCSF	–	SAH	Coils	0

0 = no deficit; "Recovered" = no details, remaining symptoms improved; "Improved" = patient showed improvement with residual minor diplopia.

[1] Symptoms progressed, but resolved after transarterial balloon occlusion partially.

SAH = subarachnoid hemorrhage; EDH = epidural hematoma; ICH = intracranial hemorrhage; IBCA = Isobutyl-2-cynoacrylate; F = French.

Type A = direct CSF (Barrow); DCSF = indirect CSF (Type B-D Barrow); – = no details reported.

Table 8.4. Adverse events during IPS catheterization for petrosal sampling (modified after BENNDORF et al. 2000a)

N	Author	Catheter/Wire	Complication	Therapy	Outcome
1	SHIU et al. (1968)	0.05/0.031″	EDH	Conservative	0
4	MILLER et al. (1992)	5 F	Brain stem lesion	Conservative	0
			Pons hematoma	Conservative	Remaining deficit
			Medulla infarction	Conservative	Remaining deficit
			Brain stem lesion	Conservative	0
1	SEYER et al (1994)	5 F	Hemiparesis, CN paresis	Conservative	Remaining deficit
1	STURROCK and JEFFCOATE (1997)	5 F	Brain stem lesion	Conservative	Remaining defici
1	BONELLI et al. (1999)	Tracker-18	SAH, Hydrocephalus	VD	Remaining deficit
1	LEFOURNIER et al. (1999)	4 F/6 F	6th nerve palsy	Conservative	0
3	BONELLI et al. (2000)	–	Headaches, nausea	Conservative	0
1	GANDHI et al. (2008)	4 F	Brain stem lesion	Conservative	Remaining deficit

SAH = subarachnoid hemorrhage; VD = ventricular drainage; EDH = epidural hematoma; CN = cranial nerve; 0 = no residual deficit; F = French.

While SAH occurs here less frequently, brain stem infarction due to compromised venous drainage is observed more often. The reason for that may be the use of (relatively large) 5-F diagnostic catheters, especially when placed bilaterally as is often the case for diagnostic sampling in patients with Cushings disease. GANDHI et al. (2008) observed a patient who developed a partially reversible brainstem infarction, requiring intubation and tracheostomy. The authors discuss whether a variant venous drainage pattern or an outflow obstruction, induced by the diagnostic catheters, could have been the cause. Un-

fortunately, their figures are not supportive of either theory and appear misinterpreted with regard to the venous anatomy. However, it seems quite plausible that placement of a 4-F catheter becomes occlusive, forcing not only contrast into the pontine and mesencephalic veins, but also compromising normal venous circulation (Fig. 1b there).

Overall, the risk of venous ischemia due to catheter manipulation during endovascular therapy is relatively low, since small catheters (2- to 3-F microcatheters) are employed and are commonly used unilaterally. Consequences may be serious though when a 5-F catheter is introduced into the IPS block-ing the posterior venous outflow (THEAUDIN et al. 2007).

Furthermore, it can probably be assumed that in case of a thrombosed IPS, the normal venous circu-lation of the pons and brain stem has already accom-modated and uses collateral circulation. Thus, the blockage of this sinus by a guidewire or a microcath-eter will less likely cause a relevant compromise of the normal venous drainage with subsequent venous infarction. A rupture of the IPS causing a clinically significant intracranial hemorrhage may only occur if this sinus also drains an arteriovenous fistula and is thus exposed to increased intravascular pressure (KING et al. 1989).

Two possible mechanisms may cause hemorrhagic complications during endovascular manipulations (HALBACH et al. 1991b): First, a sudden increase in intravenous pressure during contrast injections; second, perforation of the thin venous wall during advancement of the sharp guidewire tip, stiffened by the catheter and narrow vascular structure. The first can be avoided by performing careful injections as a "test" under a blank road map to control cath-eter position (BENNDORF et al. 2000a). The second should remain extremely rare if a microguidewire is advanced very slowly under bilateral fluoroscopy. Under these circumstances, the use of a loop at the tip while advancing the wire within the thrombosed IPS was found to be very helpful. The softness of smaller devices such as 0.010″ or the 0.012″ guide-wires, provides better conformability to the specific anatomy of the IPS and prevents entanglement in an irregular, trabeculated or even thrombosed ve-nous lumen (BENNDORF et al. 2000a). Advancing a supple 0.012″ wire that can easily be formed into a loop is less traumatic than using a straight tip, par-ticularly if the catheter is already wedged. Because the IPS is mainly located in the extradural space, or is at least partially covered by the dura, rupture of the IPS resulting in a hemorrhage is hard to imagine unless the dura mater is perforated. Perforation of the dura mater requires a critical level of mechani-cal stress, as pointed out by SHIU et al. (1968), who found it almost impossible to perforate the dura ad-jacent to the IPS in studies performed on post mor-tem material. To reduce the risk of perforation, the author prefers not to use a stiff 0.035″ wire stiff as suggested by GOTO et al. (1999) and others (OISHI et al. 1999; KIRSCH et al. 2006). As reported by OISHI et al. (1999), this may cause dissection of clival dura and result in permanent 6th CN palsy, due to damage

of the nerve when passing Dorello's canal or due to direct injury by the guidewire. A 0.035″ wire cannot be used as a loop and has to be advanced in "Kuru-Kuru technique," like a "drill", to recanalize the IPS. This technique, although advocated by some au-thors (OISHI et al. 1999; GOTO and GOTO 1997; NEM-OTO et al. 1997), may carry the risk of perforation or damage to the 6th CN, especially when its lumen is narrowed and the wire tip becomes a small spear. A so-called "microcatheter pull-up technique" using a second microcatheter with a snare has been recently suggested by HANAOKA et al. (2006) as an alterna-tive. GOBIN et al. (2000) used a left IPS-ICS approach to place a microcatheter in the right IPS facilitating catheter navigation from the right IJV into the CS in a bilateral DCSF.

Case Illustration II (Fig. 8.31) shows that in some cases, even two microcatheters can be navigated through a thrombosed IPS. Such a "dual IPS ap-proach" can be very useful in cases with multidirec-tional venous drainage. It enables one to selectively disconnect one venous drainage (e.g. leptomenin-geal, cortical) while securing catheter position in another (anterior) compartment and help to avoid compartmentalization of the fistula.

Case Illustration X (Fig. 8.38) shows the staged management of a complex AVF involving the bi-lateral CS and the clivus. The CS AV shunts were approached and obliterated utilizing the (throm-bosed) IPS approach. The intraosseous lesion was successfully occluded in a second session using an intraosseous venous channel 3 months later.

8.4.1.2
Thrombosed Cavernous Sinus (Case Report III)

As demonstrated, standard 2D-DSA may easily fail to opacify the IPS or the CS. Beside hemodynamic factors, thrombotic processes within the CS or the IPS may play a role in the failure to visualize the sinus as well (HALBACH et al. 1997). Highly flexible, supple microcatheters and guidewires are not only useful when navigating through a thrombosed IPS, but also when passing intracavernous trabeculae or thrombi that may not be easy to identify, but are often present in DCSFs. The CS can be divided into anteroinferior and posterosuperior compartments, separated by the intracavernous ICA. Despite in-tracavernous septi, manipulation and advancement of microcatheters is usually not very difficult in most directions, ipsi- to contralateral or anterior to posterior. Despite the importance of modern angiographic equipment, profound knowledge of the complex anatomic structures and a good three-dimensional understanding of the CS are required for optimal use of tools and devices. Traditional cross-sectional imaging techniques, although improved over the last years (SCHUKNECHT et al. 1998), still do not provide satisfactory spatial resolution. Even currently available high-resolution DSA that enables depiction of the smallest AV shunts with certainty is limited in its capability to display small venous structures. Angiographic computed tomography (ACT, DynaCT) may improve CS visualization and will likely contribute to a better understanding of such complex vascular structures (see Chap. 7).

The reasons for incomplete CS visualization by 2D-DSA are threefold. First, non-opacified blood draining from other tributaries via the same venous structures, causing washout effects. This becomes obvious in cases where a CS that is angiographically "silent" (after arterial contrast administration) becomes clearly visible in a jugular phlebogram. Second, thrombotic processes, frequently associated with DCSFs (50%) (MIRONOV 1994), may be responsible for non-opacified CS compartments in the same way they are for a non-opacified IPS. It has been suggested that thrombosis of the IPS is one cause for acute progression of the ophthalmological symptoms (HALBACH et al. 1992, 1997), as the blood draining here is rerouted towards the SOV (SATOMI et al. 2005). Acute thrombosis of the IPS is the main reason for most angiographically "not-visualizable" sinuses that are still passable with a microcatheter (HALBACH et al. 1997). Third, local hemodynamics play a role, since the fistulous compartment, usually with higher pressure, is more difficult to fill using a manual intravenous contrast injection, even when performed via microcatheter placed in the CS (HALBACH 1997). Finally, although some authors doubt that a true trabecular structure exists (TAPTAS 1982; BEDFORD 1966), separation by intracavernous filaments and septi causing compartmentalization (DEBRUN et al. 1981; INAGAWA et al. 1986; CHALOUPKA et al. 1993; MULLAN 1979; BUTLER 1957; RIDLEY 1695; WINSLOW 1734; TENG et al. 1988a) may influence angiographic appearance of the CS as well. Thus, manipulation and navigation of microcatheters inside the CS can be difficult in some cases. Placement of a microcatheter into the desired location via one single approach may be impossible (YAMASHITA et al. 1993). If more than one fistula site exists that cannot be reached using one venous route, two or more approaches may be used simultaneously in one session (Case Illustration II and III).

CHALOUPKA et al. (1993) reported a CS compartmentalization in a patient with a DCSF in whom the fistula site in the anterior compartment was not reachable from the posterior CS. This particular disposition was called "true anatomical compartmentalization", since no communication was seen either in the angiograms or in the selective venograms via microcatheter placed within the CS. However, this situation resembles the one described in Case Report III, where catheter advancement was eventually possible indicating intracavernous thrombosis rather than anatomic separation. Thus, it appears doubtful that such a conclusion can be made based on contrast injections and guidewire resistance only. QUINONES et al. (1997) reported one case (Figure 2 therein) in which a petrosal venogram did not show a direct connection between the IPS and the CS and that subsequently underwent SOV embolization. Taking into account the limitations of angiographic appearance due to local hemodynamics and thrombotic processes, catheter navigation into seemingly "occluded CS compartments" may be feasible and is justified if gently performed, especially when more aggressive endovascular or surgical techniques can be avoided.

8.4.1.3
Transfemoral Facial Vein/Superior Ophthalmic Vein Approach (Case Report IV)

The transfemoral approach through the facial vein or the SOV was introduced by KOMIYAMA et al. (1990) and has been used by various groups with different success rates since (CHENG et al. 2003; THEAUDIN et al. 2007; KIM et al. 2006; ANNESLEY-WILLIAMS et al. 2001; BIONDI et al. 2003). It may be an effective alternative route and is indicated when the SOV is significantly enlarged due to anterior drainage, and the IPS cannot be passed. This approach is usually feasible when the SOV is dilated enough and allows even cross-over and packing of the contralateral CS. It may be technically challenging though, if the SOV is tortuous, stenosed or thrombosed (Case Report V).

Two aspects seem important. First, the SOV approach is in general less feasible than the IPS approach, due to the less favorable anatomy. There is a longer distance to be catheterized combined with tortuousities of the angular and superior ophthalmic veins. Furthermore, the guiding catheter usually has a mechanically less stable position within the IJV or the facial vein than for the IPS approach. Unstable position of the guiding catheter may easily become a procedure-limiting factor in cases where catheter advancement is already difficult due to the friction in the loops of the SOV. Thus, it is advantageous to place a 4-F guiding catheter in the facial vein, close to its connection with the angular vein. In contrast, some operators recommend positioning the guiding catheter in the IJV to avoid impairment or stasis of the venous outflow that may cause ophthalmic or neurological complications (BIONDI et al. 2003). CHENG et al. (2003) suggested "rubbing" over the patient's face toward the orbit to support advancement of the microcatheter.

The transfemoral SOV approach appears particularly feasible in patients with enlarged ophthalmic and facial veins. It may be technically challenging or even impossible in cases with low-flow fistulas and significant elongations of the angular and ophthalmic veins, or when associated with stenotic segments or thrombosis (MILLER et al. 1995; TENG et al. 1988b). BIONDI et al. (2003), in the first series of seven patients, achieved anatomic cure in six cases (85.7%), clinical cure in four (57%) and improvement in two (28.5%). In one patient catheterization of an occluded SOV failed. It was emphasized to remember the two anatomic roots of the SOV origin for full understanding of the angioarchitecture (Figs. 3.9, 3.10 and 7.31). Although the inferior SOV root should be easier to catheterize from the facial vein because of its relatively straight course, in most cases successful navigation is performed through the superior route. The reason for this may be that the inferior root is often poorly visualized (BIONDI et al. 2003), in addition to valves that have been reported by some authors (BIONDI et al. 2003; TESTUT and JACOB 1977; HOU 1993).

The author's personal experience confirms the one already made by MULLAN et al. (1979) and HALBACH et al. (1989a), who struggled with technical difficulties when navigating through the loops of the angular and ophthalmic veins. Although this has become technically easier with improved catheterization tools, the SOV anatomy not only remains tortuous compared to the IPS, but also may show an abrupt angle or narrowing at the level of the superior orbital fissure (HANAFEE et al. 1968). Manipulation of catheters and guidewires in the SOV may lead to temporary venous outflow restriction, thrombosis associated with transient aggravation of exophthalmos and vision loss (GUPTA et al. 1997;

BIONDI et al. 2003; DEVOTO et al. 1997). When the CS cannot be reached or the fistula is not occluded in the same procedure , a serious clinical condition may develop.

This latter observation was made by other operators (HALBACH et al. 1989a; DEVOTO et al. 1997), and in two of the author's patients, who experienced transient aggravation (Cases V and VI), and represents a clear disadvantage of this approach. Another potential complication of the approach through the SOV is the rupture of the vein with intraorbital bleeding and vision loss (WLADIS et al. 2007; LEIBOVITCH et al. 2006; HAYASHI et al. 2008). UFLACKER et al. (1986) emphasized that the age of the AV shunting plays an important role for the development of a thickened venous wall. Although animal experiments have shown that histological changes of a reactive wall hypertrophy start to develop approximately 7–10 days after establishment of an AV shunt, catheterizing the SOV in cases with longer-standing AV shunts may be safer. Interestingly enough, SATTLER (1905) already pointed out that the thickness of the venous wall may increase four times and numerous elastic fibers develop due to the elevated pressure. DCSFs are often longstanding shunts, and fresh arterialized veins are to be found more often in direct CCF fistulas with short history. WLADIS et al. (2007) reported recently an acute intraorbital hemorrhage during transfemoral SOV approach that led to an orbital compartment syndrome with vision loss due to transient flow arrest in the ophthalmic artery. This complication, erroneously called "obstruction" by the authors, was most likely caused by acute increase in intraocular pressure, exceeding the perfusion pressure of the orbit. Stagnation of ophthalmic artery flow may result in central retinal artery occlusion, which can cause significant irreversible retinal damage when exceeding 240 min (HAYREH et al. 2004).

In cases, where the facial vein cannot be reached by transfemoral approach, direct puncture at the mandible has been suggested as an alternative route (NAITO et al. 2002). SCOTT et al. (1997) reported five patients undergoing ultrasound-guided direct stick of the facial vein (transcutaneous approach).

8.4.1.4
Approaches via the Middle Temporal Vein or the Frontal Vein (Case Illustration I)

Basically all afferent and efferent veins connected to the angular or ophthalmic vein, or directly to the

CS (depending on their size), may be used as either transfemoral or direct percutaneous approaches. Catheterization of an enlarged draining middle temporal vein, that communicates with the angular vein for example, is not difficult (KOMIYAMA et al. 1990; KAZEKAWA et al. 2003; AGID et al. 2004, YU et al. 2009). AGID et al. (2004) divided the facial venous drainage into medial and lateral (representing the middle temporal vein), using the latter in one case after transfemoral catheterization. KAZEKAWA et al. (2003) recently reported on two cases successfully embolized with such an approach after direct puncture with an 18-G needle.

The communications between the SOV and the supraorbital and frontal veins were used extensively in the past for orbital phlebograms (BRISMAR and BRISMAR 1976a,b; CLAY et al. 1972). Catheter manipulations are not different from other approaches, with the exception of the direct puncture itself being a technical challenge. However, this puncture is usually successful when the vein is involved in the fistula drainage. When difficult to palpate, an additional tourniquet may help and has been used by the author on several occasions. VENTURI et al. (2003) used this transcutaneous approach in one patient, emphasizing the usefulness of this technique adapted from traditional diagnostic exams of the 1960s. The authors distended the frontal vein by posterior flexion of the head and compression of the jugular vein in the neck, and cannulated with an 18-G needle to allow for introduction of a 0.010″ guidewire and microcatheter. In the group of patients studied by the author, TVO has been performed using this approach in one case.

8.4.1.5
Transfemoral Superior Petrosal Sinus Approach
(Case Illustration II)

The use of the SPS was mentioned by MULLAN in 1979 as surgical access to the CS for treatment of CSFs.

As described first by MOUNAYER et al. (2002), transfemoral approach of the SPS may be successfully used for catheter navigation into the CS and is an alternative to IPS or SOV approach. The authors used jugular stick, a 5-F sheath and a 0.016″ guidewire (Radiofocus; Terumo, Tokyo, Japan) in combination with an Excelsior microcatheter (BSC), supported by a 5-F hydrophilic guiding catheter (Terumo). After reaching the CS, the fistula site was packed with mechanically detachable coils. The SPS is, although rarely opacified, usually not difficult to catheterize,

even when it is not involved in the drainage of the fistula. If not accessible from the ipsilateral side because of the acute angle between transverse sinus and SPS, navigation from the contralateral side may be another option and sometimes easier. This alternative has been communicated by ANDREOU et al. (2007) in a patient where the AV shunt drained primarily via the contralateral SPS.

THEAUDIN et al. (2007) reported the use of the SPS in two patients of which one procedure was successful. The authors emphasize the fact that the SPS should be patent for catheterization because recanalization may become hazardous due to anatomic proximity to the vein of Labbé. Case Illustration II shows the simultaneous catheter navigation to the CS by using the IPS approach from one side and the SPS from the other, allowing effective occlusion of a bilateral DCSF.

8.4.1.6
Transfemoral Pterygoid Plexus Approach
(PP Approach)

This approach has been described by DEBRUN (1993) for management of a direct CCF, and by JAHAN et al. (1998) for treatment of a DCSF. The PP can be used like any other femoral route if favorable anatomy is present. Catheterization of the pterygoid plexus may technically be more difficult than of the IPS, but when successful, it may provide a stable positioning for microcatheters, even when a contralateral approach is necessary. KLISCH et al. (2003) reported on two successful catheterizations of the CS via the PP in three cases with direct CCF, which may show venous drainage through this efferent pathway more frequently (29%) than DCSFs.

8.4.1.7
Transfemoral Cortical Vein Approach

Although reported for DAVFs in the transverse sinus (MIRONOV 1998), the transfemoral catheterization of a cortical draining vein is extremely rare in DCSFs. BELLON et al. (1999) reported a case in which a Prowler-14 microcatheter was successfully advanced from the IJV through the anterior SSS, into a cortical vein and into the CS via the sphenoparietal sinus. This allowed packing with GDCs, leading to complete obliteration of the fistula. The potential risks include perforation or rupture of the fragile arterialized cortical vein, pressure changes due to catheterization or inadvertent thrombosis.

Even if possibly lowered by the use of modern small and supple tools, these risks should be of serious concerns when choosing such an approach.

Although as for the SOV, cases with long-standing cortical venous drainage may have developed thickened and less fragile walls (KUWAYAMA et al. 1998), it is currently unknown whether such transformation is a regular process and involves the entire vein or only certain vessels segments.

8.4.1.8
Transcutaneous SOV Approach
(SOV Cannulation, Case Report V)

In 1969, PETERSON et al. reported the direct cannulation of the SOV after upper eyelid or sub-brow cut reported for treatment of a traumatic CCF. This was one of the first venous approaches to the CS ever described. TRESS et al. (1983) published most likely the first DCSF treated using this approach, which was the repeated by UFLACKER et al. (1986) and LABBÉ et al. (1987) and used by several groups in the 1990s with increasing success (OISHI et al. 1999; GOLDBERG et al. 1996; MILLER et al. 1995). TENG et al. (1988b) reported on the treatment of five patients with DCSFs using this approach. MONSEIN et al. (1991) described successful treatment of four patients using detachable coils via surgically exposed SOV with no complications. MILLER (1995) reported on two CCFs and 10 DCSFs, who were successfully treated via SOV approach. Detachable coils as well as thrombogenic coils were used, which was successful in nine cases. In one case, additional transarterial embolization had to be performed. Except for one patient, who developed persistent sixth nerve palsy, there were no complications in this series. GOLDBERG et al. (1996) published a series in which 9/10 fistulas were clinically and anatomically occluded using the direct SOV approach. In one patient in this group, severe intraorbital hemorrhage occurred during direct puncture of a small caliber vein. The same group of patients was expanded by two more patients and reported 1 year later by QUINONES et al. (1997) with 11/12 (91%) lesions permanently occluded.

The author has reported earlier on 4/5 patients (80%) managed successfully using this approach with complete occlusion of the fistula and resolution of their symptoms (BENNDORF et al. 2000b). The anterior cannulation and catheterization of the SOV was possible in two cases despite partial thrombosis of the anterior SOV (Fig. 8.23). Compared with transfemoral SOV catheterization, this technique is less time-consuming. The shorter distance to the CS causes less friction, which may be of importance when numerous coils have to be pushed, or when the fistula site has to be approached on the contralateral side. While the navigation of the catheter into the CS is usually a matter of only a few minutes, the surgical exposure and cannulation of the SOV, often performed in the angio-suite under sterile conditions (BENNDORF et al. 2004; GOLDBERG et al. 1996; MILLER et al. 1995), represents the actual technical challenge. For a successful procedure, a skilled surgeon (ophthalmic, maxillo-facial or neurosurgeon) with experience in performing microanastomoses is required. Some authors have even reported on bilateral SOV cannulation in either the same (MILLER et al. 1995; BERLIS et al. 2002) or a subsequent session (QUINONES et al. 1997). After successful puncture of the vein, coil placement should be performed using a high-resolution bi-plane system. This strategy differs from the one reported by GOLDBERG et al. (GOLDBERG et al. 1996), who suggested the embolization be performed in the ophthalmological operating room. Although, in general, a feasible and simple technique, the transophthalmic SOV approach may be associated with complications such as infection, granuloma, damage to the trochlea and vessel rupture with intraorbital bleeding and subsequent vision loss (GOLDBERG et al. 1996; OISHI et al. 1999; HALBACH et al. 1989a; QUINONES et al. 1997; MILLER et al. 1995).

Intraorbital bleeding was also observed by GIOULEKAS et al. (1997) who treated five patients with DCSF and observed major intraorbital bleeding caused by a control injection that ruptured the distal SOV. The same case, in which an 8-F sheath and a 5-F catheter were advanced into the SOV and CS, had been reported earlier by this group (TRESS et al. 1983).

GUPTA et al. (1997) reported on a patient with unilateral vision loss and neovascular glaucoma after attempted embolization of a DCSF via the SOV. The fistula could not be occluded and the vein was ligated at the end of the procedure, which resulted in uncontrollable elevated intraocular pressure. OISHI et al. (1999) observed in three out of eight patients (37%), whose fistulae were occluded using the SOV approach, persistent complications with forehead dysesthesia ($n=1$) and blepharoptosis ($n=2$) due to injury of the levator palpebrae muscle after prolonged surgical SOV exposure. These complications were not seen in the material studied by the author.

In a recent retrospective analysis of 25 patients undergoing the SOV approach, LEIBOVITCH et al. (2006) found significant difficulties in six (24%), among which three had a fragile or a very small vein that could not be cannulated. In two other patients, catheter navigation was impossible due to clotting or the small size of the vein and embolization could not be performed, but the patients recovered over 2–3 months. In one patient with a tortuous and clotted SOV, ligation of the distal vein was performed that also resulted in resolution of the symptoms. It is interesting to note that this group, which is among the most experienced at using this technique has recently recommended considering alternate transfemoral techniques because of the potential risks associated with SOV cannulation (intraorbital hemorrhage, 8%).

Difficulties in cannulation with subsequent uncontrollable bleeding has also been observed by others (HAYASHI et al. 2008). Perforating the SOV can be associated with potential loss of vision, and can only be controlled by emergent canthotomy (WLADIS et al. 2007). Because of its associated risks, the transfemoral or transophthalmic SOV approach should probably not, as suggested by some operators (MILLER 2007), be considered the method of choice, but probably more as an alternative strategy after consequently using the much easier and safer IPS approach first.

8.4.1.9
Transorbital SOV Approach
(Direct Puncture, Case Report VI)

The decision for this more aggressive approach in one of the patients was made only as a last resort after all other approaches failed. The increased risk of a direct puncture was discussed in detail with colleagues from ophthalmology, maxillo-facial and neurosurgery and had been carefully balanced against the potential risks associated with open surgery. The patient's significantly elevated intraocular pressure and his imminent risk of complete vision loss justified the SOV puncture in the deep orbit. In cases where surgical exposure and cannulation of the SOV is not an option, or additional mechanical obstacles prevent catheter navigation, retrobulbar puncture of the SOV has been suggested (GOLDBERG et al. 1996; TENG et al. 1988b). Currently small caliber microcatheters are available, which accommodate the use of small 21-G needles to facilitate such an invasive approach (BENNDORF et al. 2001a). How-

ever, even though the degree of vessel trauma is minimized, the risk of causing a major complication such as an intraorbital hemorrhage is nevertheless higher than using any other approach (GOLDBERG et al. 1996; LEIBOVITCH et al. 2006; UFLACKER et al. 1986; TENG et al. 1995). GOLDBERG et al. (1996) observed a massive intraorbital hemorrhage after attempting to puncture an apparently fragile SOV in the center of the orbit (see LEIBOVITCH et al. 2007).

Transcutaneous puncture of the SOV was pioneered by TENG et al. (1988b) who treated five patients without complications. The authors used steel spring coils, gel foam strips and IBCA for fistula occlusion. According to the authors, among transfemoral routes, only the IPS was attempted. If surgical dissection of the anterior SOV failed, the vein was punctured. Although the authors need to be congratulated on this early work, it is interesting to note that in at least one case (Case 3), the IPS appeared widely open in their angiogram and thus would have been a suitable route for safer transfemoral occlusion. It is also not really clear where exactly the vein was punctured, in the anterior orbit or deeper (intraconal) as bi-plane high-resolution fluoroscopy or road mapping was not yet available. Also, the use of 16-G or 18-G needles, 0.035-inch guidewires and 5-F catheters, appears relatively invasive as it may easily cause serious vessel trauma. Despite the advantage of deploying larger coils and reducing time and costs, choosing smaller needles, guidewires, microcatheters and coils appears advisable today (ONG et al. 2009).

CHAN et al. (2006) reported recently on a "novel" approach by performing a puncture of the intraconal SOV using an 18-G needle after failed attempts of femoral access and anterior SOV cannulation. This technique is however similar to the deep orbital puncture reported previously by the author (BENNDORF et al. 2001a)

WHITE et al. (2007) recently described a patient in whom the inferior ophthalmic vein was transorbitally punctured with an 18-G needle and successfully used for accessing the CS. The anatomy of the IOV may vary and the vein may occur not as a singular vein, but rather a plexus of veins (RHOTON 2002).

KUETTNER et al. (2006) treated two patients using cannulation of the SOV with a 16-G needle after palpebral incision. The fistulas were successfully occluded and symptoms resolved within several weeks. Both patients developed a persistent moderate blepharoptosis.

Modern high-resolution fluoroscopy and bi-plane road mapping, provide excellent visual control of needle positioning and advancement and have improved the feasibility and safety of intraorbital puncture techniques. Nevertheless, precautions considered for transfemoral catheter and wire manipulations in arterialized veins are even more important when directly puncturing an arterialized SOV (UFLACKER et al. 1986). The risk of lacerating, dissecting and rupturing this vein by a sharp needle is certainly greater and must not be neglected (WLADIS et al. 2007). Even when exposed to arterial pressure for longer periods of time, an AV shunting vein is a fragile structure. The risk of perforation by even minor and gentle needle or guidewire manipulations remains unpredictable, and thus should be minimized by using the smallest possible devices for this technique (20- to 21-G needles and 2.5- to 3-F microcatheters).

8.4.1.10
Direct Puncture of the Foramen Ovale

This approach is performed on another efferent vein from the CS: the emissary vein of the foramen ovale (foramen ovale plexus). A direct puncture of the CS through the foramen ovale to deflate a detachable balloon in the CS was reported by JACOBS et al. (1993). Using an 18-G needle that was guided into the CS, a 21-G Chiba spinal needle was introduced and used to puncture latex balloons. The technique of puncturing Meckel's cave through the foramen ovale under fluoroscopy for treatment of trigeminal neuralgia is a well known procedure.

The successful use of this approach for coil occlusion of a DCSF has been performed recently by E. HOUDART (personal communication).

8.4.1.11
Direct Puncture of the CS via the SOF
(Case Illustration XI)

The case described herein refers to a technique that was initially reported by TENG et al. (1988a) as an ultimate treatment option for a direct CCF with multiple (10×) recurrences. The same group later published a series of 11 patients, successfully treated using this technique, and reported transient ptosis in two patients as the only complications (TENG et al. 1995). All patients had undergone previous treatment by either carotid ligation or balloon de-

tachment; some of them had already lost their vision (see above). An 18-G needle and a 5-F catheter were used, while 2/11 patients developed ptosis and in 1/11 intraorbital bleeding had to be managed by immediate placement of a balloon in the ICA. The authors emphasized that this approach should be used as a last option, and in cases where alternative methods have failed, the ICA is occluded or the patient has vision loss. It is interesting to note that the angiograms of some of the patients showed an apparently patent IPS (Figs. 1 and 3 there), and thus this cases have actually been candidates for a less aggressive transfemoral approach.

TENG et al. (1995) argued that puncture of the CS is technically easier than that of the SOV because of better orientation using anatomic landmarks under fluoroscopy such as the supraorbital fissure (SOF), sella turcica and anterior clinoid processes. Such justification, as well as the fact that the SOV can only be visualized by repeated angiograms, appear lesser valid reasons today with the availability of high-resolution bi-plane road map on all modern angiographic systems. It could be argued whether or not the risk of an intraorbital puncture is higher than that of an intracranial puncture. The former may cause a manageable intraorbital hemorrhage with potential vision loss, while the latter may lead to a life-threatening subarachnoid or intracranial hemorrhage.

WORKMAN et al. (2002) more recently described a long-standing, direct CCF due to a gunshot wound, that reoccurred after 26 years of unsuccessful ligations and was treated with an intraocular trans-SOF approach. A 16-G angiocath was used to deploy 20 Gianturco 0.018″ coils. The authors discuss in detail the anatomic basis for this approach and its potentially associated complications.

Case Illustration III is an example of the use of the transorbital CS puncture in a DCSF. This patient was referred from another institution where transvenous access through the IJV had failed. Direct CS puncture was performed as a last treatment resort. Even though performed successfully, subarachnoid hemorrhage due to transgression of the subarachnoid space, intraorbital hematoma and vision loss, direct injury of the optic nerve, ophthalmic artery or intracavernous cranial nerves, globe puncture and infection are potential serious complications (WHITE et al. 2007; WORKMAN et al. 2002).

Furthermore, when the ICA is patent, as is commonly the case in DCSFs, the risk of lacerating or

(Text continues on p. 251)

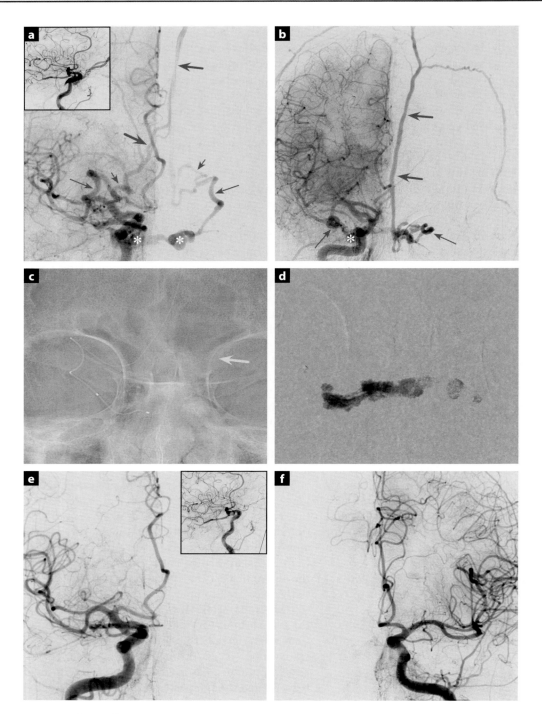

Fig. 8.29a–f. Case Illustration I: Frontal vein approach and TVO with NBCA. a,b Right ICA injections, AP views: Arteriovenous shunt of the right CS (*asterisks*) supplied by branches of the MHT. Venous drainage via the right and left SOV (*arrows*), both supraorbital (*short arrows*) and both frontal veins (FrV, *thick arrows*). No opacification of the IPS or the facial vein. **c** Percutaneous puncture of the FrV using a 18-G needle allows navigation of a microcatheter (*arrow*) to the cavernous sinus and subsequent occlusion of the fistula with intravenous injection of 20% NBCA (**d**). **e,f** Right and left CCA injection at the end of the procedure demonstrating complete occlusion of the fistula. *Insets* in **a** and **e** Lateral ICA projections pre- and postembolization. Note: Attempts to catheterize the CS using IPS and SPS approaches failed. (Courtesy: J. Moret, Paris)
Author: Puncture of frontal or supraorbital veins was a widely used technique in the days of orbital phlebography (1960s–1970s). The use of a torniquet can be helpful to get access

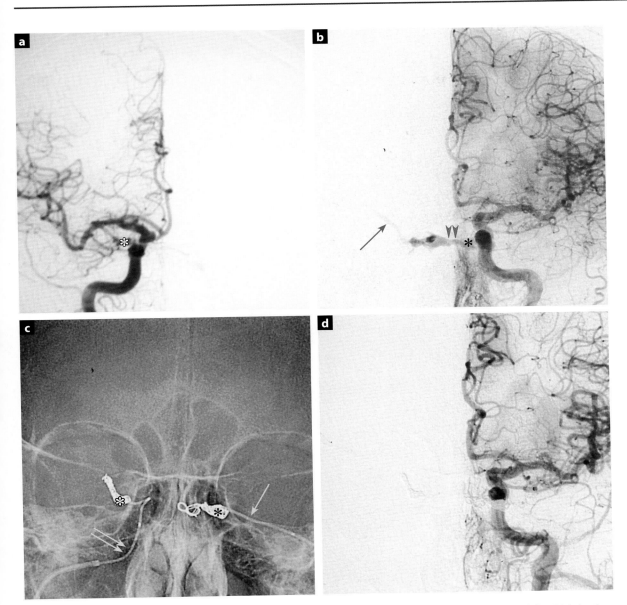

Fig. 8.30a–d. Case Illustration II: Simultaneous IPS and SPS approach in a bilateral fistula. a,b Right and left CCA injection, AP view: Arteriovenous shunt at the right (*white asterisk*) and left CS (*black asterisk*), supplied by ICA and ECA branches. Venous drainage via ICS (*arrowheads*) into the right SOV (*arrow*) **c** Non-subtracted AP view. Coilpacking of the right and left fistula site (*asterisks*) after catherization of both CSs using the right IPS (*double arrow*) and the left SPS (*single arrow*). **d** Left CCA injection, AP view: Complete occlusion of the fistula at the end of the procedure. The patient recovered fully. (Courtesy: J. Moret, Paris)

Author: In cases where a bilateral occlusion is necessary (usually bilateral fistulas, although rare) and cross-over navigation is not possible, different venous approaches can be used during the same session to achieve complete occlusion. The SPS may be difficult to catheterize when not draining the fistula and not clearly opacified. If not accessible ipsilaterally due to an acute angle between SPS and transverse sinus, navigation from the contralateral side may be another option

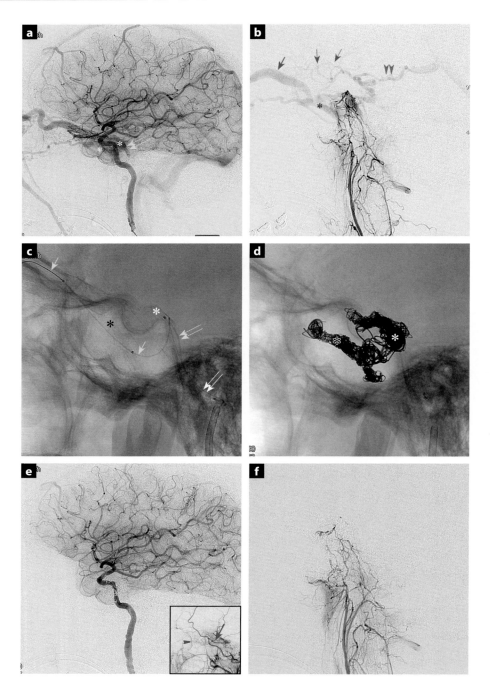

Fig. 8.31a–f. Case Illustration III: Dual IPS approach, TVO using coils. A 48-year-old woman presenting in March 2009 with eye redness and diplopia. a,b ICA and APA injection, lateral views show a fistula with anterior and posterior drainage. The IPS is tapered and partially occluded. The anterior/inferior CS compartment drains into the SOV (*arrow*) and cortical veins (*thin arrows*). The posterior/superior compartment drains into the leptomeningeal and deep veins (*double arrowheads*). **c,d** In order to block the anterior and posterior drainage independently, two microcatheters (Excelsior™ SL-10, Echelon™) were advanced into the CS using the IPS approach (thrombosed IPS). This allowed packing of the posterior compartment (*white asterisk, double arrows*), while keeping access to the anterior CS and SOV (*black asterisk, single arrows*). **e,f** Complete occlusion of the AV shunt at the end of the procedure. Note, the missing ophthalmic artery in **e** that appeared hemodynamically "occluded", but was spontaneously reconstituted through the ECA (*inset, arrowhead*: choroidal blush, *arrow*: OA). This phenomenon was reversed in the 3 months FU. The patient's vision was not affected. A dual approach to the CS can be useful to avoid rerouting or worsening of venous drainage into leptomeningeal or cortical veins

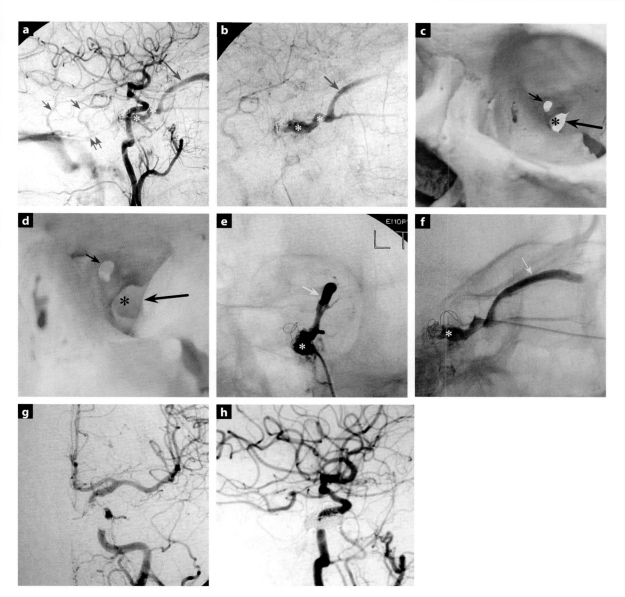

Fig. 8.32a–h. Case Illustration IV: Direct puncture of the cavernous sinus through the SOF. A 42-year-old woman with rapid left visual deterioration following transarterial and transvenous embolization in another institution that remained incomplete due to technical issues. The patient was urgently transferred; upon arrival, no light perception. Attempted access via facial vein failed due to thrombosis. **a** Left CCA injection lateral view early and late (**b**) phase: Arteriovenous shunt at the left CS (*asterisks*), supplied by branches from the ICA and ECA. Drainage mainly via SOV (*arrow*), no opacification of the IPS, but drainage via SPS (*thin double arrow*) and leptomeningeal veins (*thin arrows*). **c,d** Left orbit (dry skull) AP view: View onto the the SOF (*arrow*) through which the SOV courses to reach the CS region (*asterisk*); *short arrow:* Optic canal. **e,f** Control injection directly into the CS (*asterisk*), after direct puncture using a 16-G needle, introducing a catheter and placement of the first Gianturco 0.018"coils, shows partial occlusion with residual drainage into the SOV (*arrow*). **g,h** Final control, left ICA injection, lateral (**g**) and AP (**h**) views: Control arteriograms revealing complete occlusion of the fistula at the end of the procedure. The patient never recovered her vision; fundoscopic exam revealed venous infarction of the retina, probably caused by prolonged venous hypertension following the initial unsuccessful embolization. (Courtesy: J. Dion, Atlanta)

Author: Direct puncture of the CS through the SOF is a feasible but relatively agressive approach, associated with an incresaed risk of intraorbital or intracranial hemorrhage, and thus should remain a technique of last resort. Courtesy: J. Dion, Atlanta

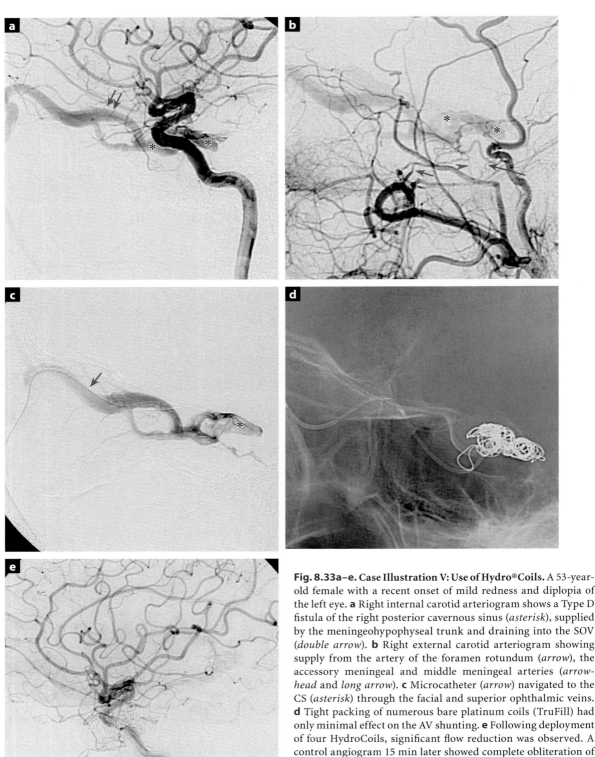

Fig. 8.33a–e. Case Illustration V: Use of Hydro®Coils. A 53-year-old female with a recent onset of mild redness and diplopia of the left eye. **a** Right internal carotid arteriogram shows a Type D fistula of the right posterior cavernous sinus (*asterisk*), supplied by the meningeohypophyseal trunk and draining into the SOV (*double arrow*). **b** Right external carotid arteriogram showing supply from the artery of the foramen rotundum (*arrow*), the accessory meningeal and middle meningeal arteries (*arrowhead* and *long arrow*). **c** Microcatheter (*arrow*) navigated to the CS (*asterisk*) through the facial and superior ophthalmic veins. **d** Tight packing of numerous bare platinum coils (TruFill) had only minimal effect on the AV shunting. **e** Following deployment of four HydroCoils, significant flow reduction was observed. A control angiogram 15 min later showed complete obliteration of the fistula. (Courtesy: M.E. Mawad, Houston)

Author: Because it reduces the total amount of coils, the radiation exposure and possibly the risk of secondary CN deficits, additional use of HydroCoils for indirect (and direct) CSFs can be a very useful adjunct

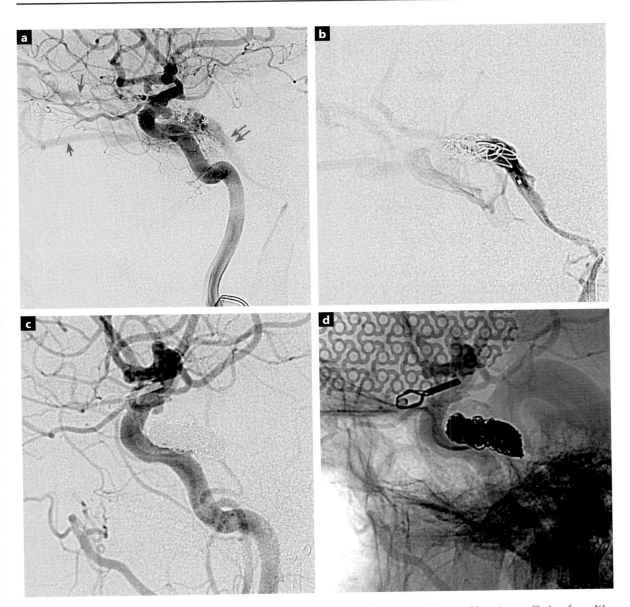

Fig. 8.34a–d. Case Illustration VI: Use of HyperSoft coils. High-flow fistula in a 64-year-old patient suffering from Wegener's granulomatosis with a 6-month history of eye redness and proptosis on the left side. **a** Right ICA injection, lateral view shows a fistula at the posterior CS, supplied mainly by the TMH, shunting into the left CS and draining into the left SOV (*arrow*), IOV (*short arrow*) and IPS (*double arrow*). **b** Left IPS approach using an Echelon™ microcatheter and placement of the first coils. **c,d** Complete occlusion of the AV shunt by extremely dense packing with a total of 51 HyperSoft coils (MicroVention)

Author: The use of softer coils has the advantage of creating a very dense packing, reducing the risk of compartmentalization as well as of secondary CN deficits, potentially caused by increased mechanical pressure of the coils. (Courtesy: R. Klucznik, Houston)

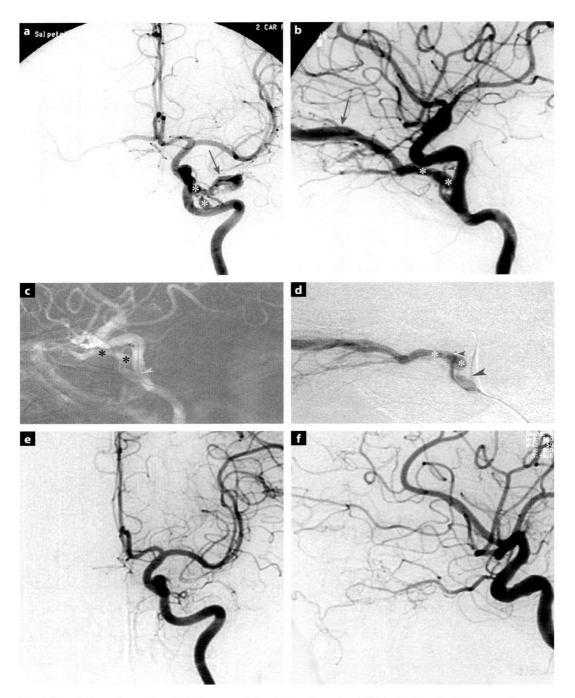

Fig. 8.35a–f. Case Illustration VII: Transarterial embolization using NBCA (Glubran®). A 55-year-old woman presenting with exophthalmos and chemosis of 6 months' standing, increased ocular pressure and decreased visual acuity for 2 days prior to the procedure (transvenous attempts failed). **a,b** Left ICA injection AP and lateral views, showing a small AV shunt (*asterisks*), fed by the ILT (*arrowhead*) draining into the SOV (*arrow*). **c** Road map during selective catheterization. *Small arrowhead*: Tip of microcatheter (*arrowhead*) at the origin of the ILT. **d** Selective sinogram after navigation of a Magic 1.2 (Balt Extrusion) using a 0.008″ Mirage (EV3). *Small arrowhead*: Tip of the microcatheter 3 mm inside the ILT (*arrowhead*: Microcatheter in the ICA lumen). **e,f** Control arteriograms after injection of 20% Glubran (NBCA) mixed with Lipiodol® showing complete obliteration of the AV shunt. (Courtesy: A. Biondi, Paris)

Author: Because the microcatheter is only a few mm inside the ILT, the risk of reflux is quite high and glue injection should be performed only by an experienced operator. A lower glue concentration is advisable

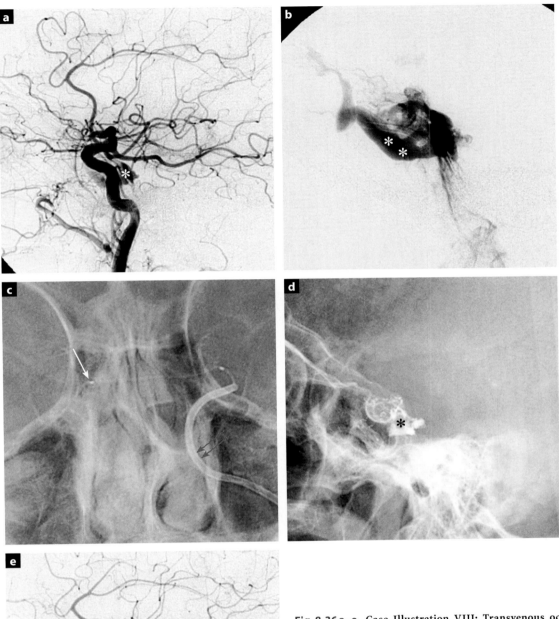

Fig. 8.36 a–e. Case Illustration VIII: Transvenous occlusion using NBCA. A 90-year-old female with significant exophthalmos and red eye. **a** Right CCA injection, lateral view: Arteriovenous shunt at the right CS (*asterisk*), supplied by branches from both ICA and ECA territories. **b** Venogram of the cavernous sinus (sinogram), lateral view: Because the right IPS could not be passed, an approach from the contralateral side through the ICS was performed, allowing for placement of a microcatheter at the fistula site (*white arrow*) (**c**). Note that a 4-F guide is advanced into the left IPS (*double arrow*). **d** Injection of 1 cc of glue (*asterisk*, 50% Glubran/lipiodol mixture) resulted in complete occlusion of the AV shunt (*E*). (Courtesy: J. Moret, Paris) *Author:* Intravenous injection of NBCA into the CS can be very effective, but carries the risk of untoward migration into pial veins. A higher concentration of the glue is recommended

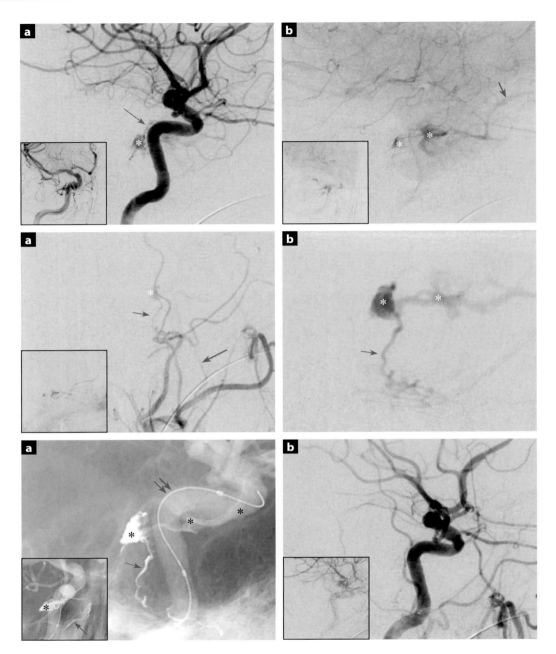

Fig. 8.37 a–f. Case Illustration IX: Transarterial Onyx injection using flow control. A 76-year-female presenting with right exophthalmus, chemosis and glaucoma, of 2 months' standing. **a, b** Right ICA injection, lateral-oblique views, early arterial and venous phase shows a small Type D fistula of the right posterior cavernous sinus (*asterisk*), supplied by the MHT (*thin arrow*) and draining into the SOV (*arrow*). *Insets:* RAO views, early and late phase. **c** Right ECA injection, lateral view showing a feeding pedicle (*arrow*) from the AMA (*long arrow*). *Insets:* Late arterial phase. **d** Superselective injection after microcatheter navigation into the AMA (*arrow*) shows fistula supply via the posteromedial ramus of the ILT (*thin arrow*). **e** Control arteriogram after a single transarterial Onyx injection (0.3 cc) into the AMA pedicle, during which an occlusion balloon (4×20 mm HyperGlide EV3, *double arrow*) was inflated across the MHT origin. Onyx cast seen in the posterior CS; less dense in the anterior CS (*asterisks*). Note that some reflux is seen in the feeding pedicle (*thin arrow*). The balloon was inflated for a short period of time, only when the Onyx® reached the CS to prevent reflux into the ICA via the TMH. The injection was stopped as soon as angiographic controls showed fistula occlusion. **f** Final control angiogram showing complete obliteration of the AV shunt. *Insets:* Late arterial phase. (Courtesy: G. Gal, Würzburg)
Author: Such indirect flow control can be very helpful to avoid Onyx® migration into the cerebral circulation

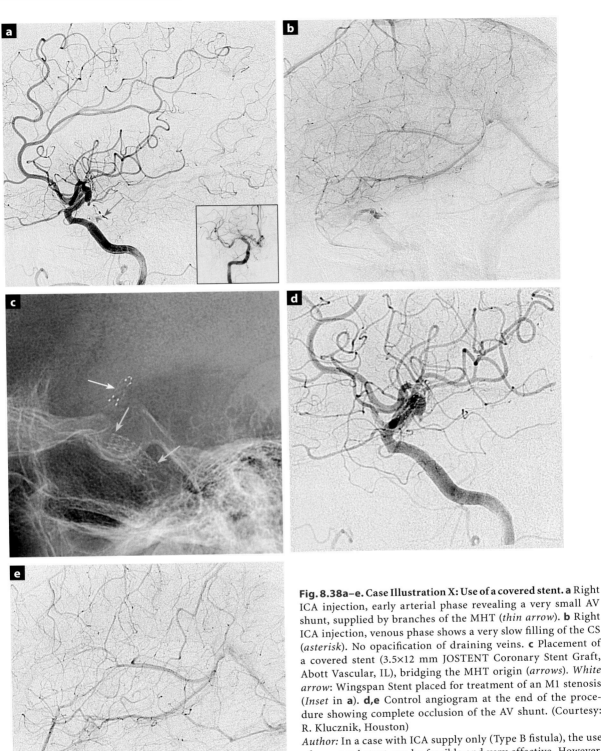

Fig. 8.38a–e. Case Illustration X: Use of a covered stent. a Right ICA injection, early arterial phase revealing a very small AV shunt, supplied by branches of the MHT (*thin arrow*). **b** Right ICA injection, venous phase shows a very slow filling of the CS (*asterisk*). No opacification of draining veins. **c** Placement of a covered stent (3.5×12 mm JOSTENT Coronary Stent Graft, Abott Vascular, IL), bridging the MHT origin (*arrows*). *White arrow*: Wingspan Stent placed for treatment of an M1 stenosis (*Inset* in **a**). **d,e** Control angiogram at the end of the procedure showing complete occlusion of the AV shunt. (Courtesy: R. Klucznik, Houston)

Author: In a case with ICA supply only (Type B fistula), the use of a covered stent can be feasible and very effective. However, because this device (JOSTENT) is relatively stiff and requires a 7 F or 8 F guiding catheter, its application is currently limited to favorable anatomy. A dedicated covered stent suitable for neurovascular anatomy is needed. Long-term dual antiplatelet therapy is required and represents another disadvantage

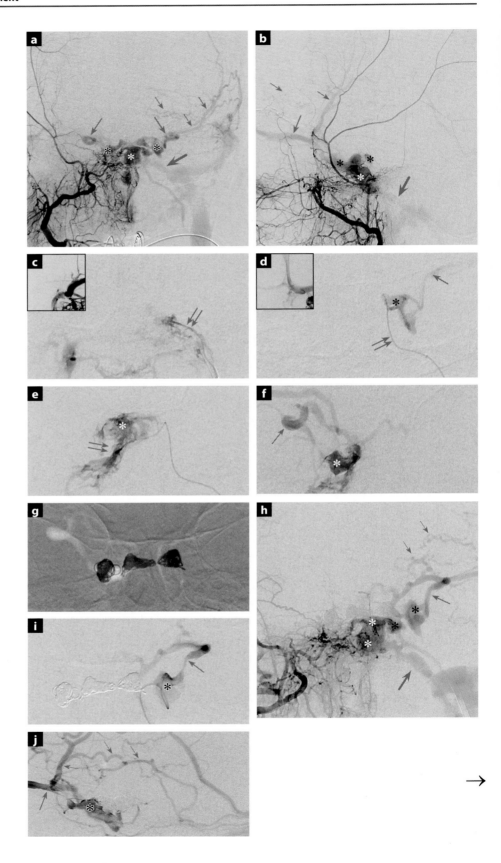

→

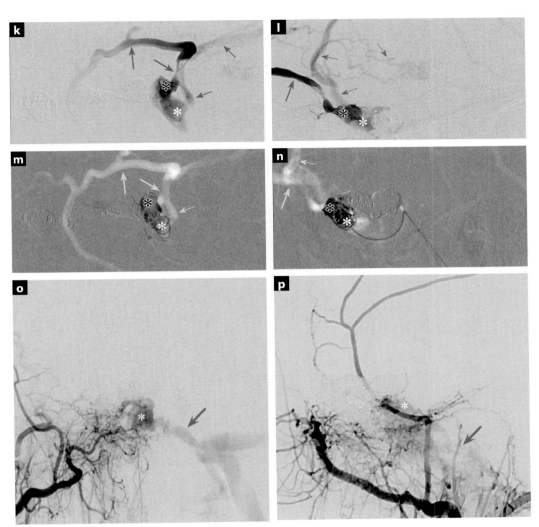

Fig. 8.39 a–p. Case Illustration XI: Staged TVO of a complex fistula with intraosseous compartment (perfomed together with Dr. A. Biondi in 10/2008 and 01/2009 at Pitié-Salpêtrière Hospital, Paris). A 72-year-old woman presented in March 2008 with intracranial bruit, bilateral chemosis, paresis of left 3rd cranial nerve and palsy of the right VIth nerve. **a,b** Right ECA injection AP and lateral views show a complex AV shunting lesion, involving both CSs (*black asterisks*) and a midline compartment that appears to be located withing the clivus (*white asterisk*). There is venous drainage into both SOVs (*arrows*), leptomeningeal and cortical veins on the left side (*small arrows*) and into a larger channel mimicking the left IPS (*thick arrow*). *Insets:* Left jugular phlebogram reveals that the IPS (*double arrows*) is in fact occluded (thrombosed), but can be passed using the loop technique (**c,d**). *Asterisk:* Left CS, *arrow:* Left SOV. **e** Superselective injection via microcatheter after crossing the midline (AP view) shows the thrombosed right IPS (*double arrow*) and right CS (*asterisk*). No fistula drainage is identified. **f** Repositioning of the microcatheter reveals the fistulous communication with the right SOV (*arrow*). Dense coil packing (**g**) resulted in occlusion of the AV shunt at the right CS. **h** The midline lesion (*white asterisks*) was not affected and continued to drain (*thick arrow*) directly into the IJV as well as into the left CS (*black asterisk*), the SOV (*arrow*) and leptomeningeal veins (*thin arrows*). **i,j** Catheter navigation into the left anterior CS shows the fistula drainage into the SOV (*arrows*) and cortical veins (*small arrows*). Caudal-oblique angulation in AP (**k**) and cranial-caudal angulation in lateral views (**l**) help to better visualize the relationship between the CS-SOV junction and the exiting cortical veins. This is difficult in standard views, but may be crucial to find a working projection for disconnection of these veins from the AV shunting. **m,n** In this case, the cortical veins enter the CS slightly posterior (*white asterisk*) to the CS-SOV junction (*black asterisk*). For disconnection of cortical and leptomeningeal drainage see also Figure 8.4. **o,p** Right and left ECA injections AP and lateral views: Complete occlusion of the AV shunt involving the CS on both sides. Note also the disappearance of the cortical venous drainage on the left side. There is persistent AV shunting involving the midline lesion and draining via a separate venous channel (*thick arrow*) directly into the IJV

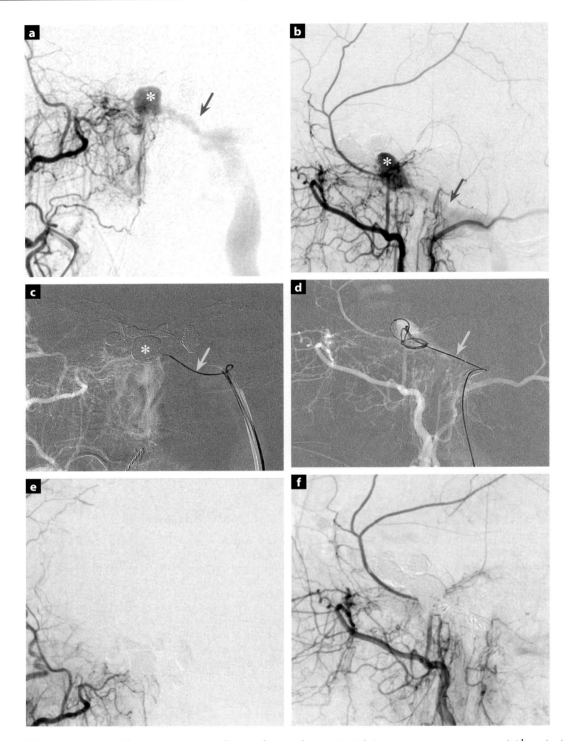

Fig. 8.40 a–e. Case Illustration XI: Staged TVO of a complex DCSF with intraosseous compartment (2nd session). a,b Right ECA injection, AP and lateral views prior to the 2nd procedure in 01/09 shows some diminshed flow, but otherwise unchanged residual AV shunting within the clivus. **c, d** Catheterization of the intraosseus venous pouch in the midline and subsequent coilpacking. **e, f** Final control demonstrating complete occlusion of the AV shunt at the end of the procedure. *Thick arrow*: Venous channel draining the intraosseus AV shunt into the jugular vein that was used as approach in **c,d** (not to be mistaken as IPS). The 3-months FU exam confirmed stable occlusion and recovery of the patient. (See the ACT imaging of this case in Fig. 7.78)

perforating the artery within the CS and creating a direct CCF is always present. As stated above, the risks associated with the use of a 16-G needle need to be weighed against the advantage of pushing 0.038″ coils allowing for a fast packing of the CS, reducing the overall radiation exposure and duration of the procedure.

Another recent paper summarizes the experience of the same group with this particular approach in a total of seven patients in whom complete occlusion was accomplished in a single session with one transient decrease in visual acuity that improved markedly after 48 h (WHITE et al. 2007). No other complications have been reported, and no further details of the patients or procedures are communicated. This technique was recently applied in three cases by ONG et al. (2009) without periprocedural or delayed complications. The authors used a 22-G spinal needle for puncture under biplane fluoroscopy that was exchanged for a 5-F sheath and used to inject Onyx-34. The importance of avoiding withdrawal of needle or catheter before the AV shunt is fully occluded is particularly stressed.

8.4.1.12
Sylvian Vein Approach: Combined Surgical/Endovascular Treatment (Case Report VII)

The puncture of the Sylvian vein following craniotomy was first described in 1997 by the author (BENNDORF et al. 1997, 1999b) and repeated by others (KRISHT and BURSON 1999). Although puncturing a cerebral vein is technically not difficult for an experienced vascular neurosurgeon, performing open surgery to gain this particular access carries its inherent risks and should be avoided whenever possible.

SCHMIDBAUER et al. (2001) reported on two patients, who were successfully managed using cannulation of the Sylvian vein following pterional craniotomy. Previous attempts of TAE and TVO failed to control the AV shunts. Both fistulas were occluded; one patient recovered well, the other suffered from thrombembolic stroke due to postoperative angiography with residual hemiparesis.

Cannulation of a cortical vein after craniotomy was successfully performed in one of the author's patients. This combined surgical-endovascular approach was chosen as an ultimate option after all transarterial and transvenous attempts of treatment repeatedly failed. In exceptional cases, where

indeed all possible transvenous routes have been attempted, surgical exploration of an arterialized vein with subsequent puncture and catheterization of the CS can become an alternate option. KUWAYAMA et al. (1998) described the case of a 48-year-old man who suffered from ICH caused by a DCSF draining only via the Sylvian vein, which was intraoperatively punctured, allowing for complete occlusion. Even though reports on such an approach are scarce, it represents a valuable technique in otherwise hopeless cases. The case presented here (BENNDORF et al. 1997) is also a good example of interdisciplinary team work in a difficult-to-treat lesion.

The use of similar approaches for treatment of cerebrovascular diseases was reported early by MULLAN (1979) and TRESS et al. (1983) for management of DCSFs. In a case with limited endovascular options due to anatomical variants of the CS, CHALOUPKA et al. (1993) discussed the need for combined neuroradiological and neurosurgical treatment options. As an alternative, KRISCHT et al. (1999) suggest a pretemporal extradural approach, through which the anterior CS can be punctured to place coils. BARKER et al. (1994) described a similar technique using a transsphenoidal, transethmoidal microsurgical approach, through which a successful embolization was performed. KLISCH et al. (2001) reported on a transnasal-transsphenoidal approach to the posterior CS.

HARA et al. (2002) reported an interesting surgical approach via the petrosal vein in two patients. Previous incomplete EVT had resulted in dangerous rerouting of leptomeningeal venous drainage causing hemiparesis in one. Both patients underwent suboccipital craniectomy and a combined surgical endovascular approach to the CS. The AV shunts were occluded using GDC packing of the CS leading to recovery in both patients.

In order to cannulate the deep SOV, BADILLA et al. (2007) recently suggested a temporal, extended superior eye-lid incision combined with lateral marginectomy of the orbital rim. This approach was eventually successful after transfemoral IPS and SOV catheterization failed due to compartmentalization of the CS and tortuousities of the ophthalmic veins. Although still associated with less morbidity than unroofing the orbit, this technique appears also relatively invasive.

DCSFs without cortical drainage are considered benign vascular lesions and should be managed with the least invasive approach first. While seldom seen, cases of persistent cortical drainage in DSCFs can be associated with neurological symptoms and severe hemorrhage, justifying more aggressive treatment options. Besides other potential complications such as seizure or infection, puncture and catheterization of an arterialized cortical vein carries a considerable risk, remains a last resort procedure and should be carried out only by an experienced neuroradiological-neurosurgical team. It should be reserved for patients in whom clinical symptoms are progressing and every possible alternate approach (transarterial, transvenous, transophthalmic, etc.) was indeed attempted and clearly failed. Choosing aggressive ("heroic") procedures other than as an ultimate option in an otherwise hopeless case is not acceptable and to be abandoned.

The case shown here was actually treated very early in the authors' experience (1992) and reported a few years later. In the early 1990s, catheter technology as well as angiographic equipment were in a less developed stage, thus limiting operators' capabilities. It is hard to imagine that with endovascular armamentarium and modern high resolution imaging of 2009 such an aggressive approach would still be necessary or justified.

In order to understand preferences for certain approaches advocated by other operators, one must also consider their clinical background. Operators with a surgical background may be in favor of operative or combined operative/endovascular techniques (Miller 2007; Goldberg et al. 1996; Hanneken et al. 1989; Kuwayama et al. 1998; Leibovitch et al. 2006; Barker et al. 1994; Badilla et al. 2007; Debrun et al. 1989).

It is presumably no coincidence that the larger series of TVO in DCSFs reported by interventional neuroradiologists recommend using transfemoral routes, in the vast majority the IPS approach (Cheng et al. 2003; Oishi et al. 1999; Theaudin et al. 2007; Wakhloo et al. 2005; Benndorf et al. 2004; Kim et al. 2006; Meyers et al. 2002; Klisch et al. 2003; Kirsch et al. 2006). This is owing to their extensive experience in transvenous catheterizations and occlusion techniques for dural arteriovenous lesions.

In conclusion, transfemoral catheterizations of the IPS, or direct IJV stick, are currently considered the techniques of choice for transvenous occlusions of DCSFs. Only when attempts of ipsi- and contralateral IPSs remain unsuccessful, transfemoral SOV approach, or SOV cannulation after surgical exposure, should be performed. Depending on the drainage pattern, less invasive approaches such as trans-

femoral catheter navigation through the MTV, PP or FV may be attempted. As shown in the treatment algorithm in Table 8.5, more aggressive techniques, such as direct puncture of the SOV, the IOV or even the CS, as well as combined neurosurgical-endovascular approaches should be considered only after all other options have truly been exploited. This rationale is based first on safety and second on efficacy of the various techniques of navigating a microcatheter, veinicath or a needle into the CS.

Table 8.5. Treatment algorithm for TVO in DCSFs [modified after Benndorf et al. (1999a)]

Transfemoral
- Inferior petrosal sinus (IPS, also via puncture of IJV)
- Facial vein (FV)/superior ophthalmic vein (SOV)
- Pterygoid plexus (PP)[a]
- Middle temporal vein (MTV)[a]
- Cortical vein[a]

Transcutaneous
- Puncture of frontal vein[a]
- Puncture of facial vein (US-guided)
- Surgical exposure and cannulation of SOV
- Puncture of CS through the foramen ovale

Transorbital
- Puncture of SOV or IOV
- Puncture of CS through the orbital fissure

Craniotomy
- Surgical exposure and puncture of a cortical (Sylvian) vein

[a]Depending on the dominant venous drainage.

8.4.2
Embolic Materials

8.4.2.1
Particles

PVA particles have been used to a limited degree by the author for transarterial embolizations (TAE). Their additional use prior or after TVO has not been found necessary in the vast majority of cases, including the ones showing subtotal occlusion at the end of the procedure.

8.4.2.2
Coils

Case Reports I–VI and Case Illustrations II, IV, V demonstrate how proper choice of coils may allow a dense packing that results in subtotal or complete occlusion by the end of the procedure (BENNDORF et al. 2000a). Various embolic materials have been used in the past for occlusion of CSFs, including cellulose, cotton, silk threads, Gianturco coils and balloons (MULLAN 1974; HALBACH et al. 1989a; TRESS et al. 1983; DEBRUN et al. 1975; SERBINENKO 1974). MULLAN (1974) initially used bronze-phosphor wire, which he inserted directly into the CS. HOSOBUCHI (1975), using direct insertion of copper wire into the CS was able to induce electrothrombosis in four patients with CSF. The concept of electrothrombosis for occlusion of CSFs was initially described by PETERSON et al. (1969), who were able to cure a direct CCF by introducing copper wires and applying 2 mA positive current. Serial angiograms demonstrated a progressive occlusion of the fistula over a 4-h period. TAKAHASHI et al. (1989) reported on the successful treatment of five patients in whom copper wires were introduced into the CS via transvenous approaches. By advancing copper wires using a microcatheter, the authors accomplished complete occlusion of the fistula in three cases (60%) and disappearance after 8 months in two (40%).

TRESS et al. (1983) occluded a DCSF with Gianturco steel coils. In the late 1980s, platinum was discovered as a new embolic material (YANG et al. 1988) and introduced to replace the commonly used Gianturco coils (ANDERSON et al. 1977, 1979; CHUANG et al. 1980; GIANTURCO et al. 1975). YANG et al. (1988) first described the use of platinum wires for occlusion of arteriovenous fistulas and achieved a complete occlusion in 6/9 cases. The ability to deliver these thin platinum wires through microcatheters with a size of 2.2 F into the desired territory pushed their intravascular use. HALBACH et al. (1989a) reported on the first large series using Gianturco coils and coils made of gold and platinum. In 9/13 patients (69.2%) angiographic occlusion could be documented, in five of these (38.5%) only coils were used, and in four (30.8%), coils were combined with IBCA. Coils with thrombogenic fibers have been increasingly utilized for transvenous fistula occlusions. However, the use of pushable, fibered coils may be problematic if they are not correctly placed at the fistula site or at the connection between the CS and its tributaries, or if a sufficiently dense packing of coils cannot be achieved. The latter may result in an incomplete occlusion, requiring subsequent treatment attempts with a more difficult anatomic access. Therefore, despite higher costs, it has become increasingly more acceptable to use mainly, or even exclusively detachable coils. Electro-

lytic detachable platinum coils are the most widely used embolic material in the endovascular therapy of cerebrovascular diseases. For occlusion of an AV shunt, the fact that platinum is about 3–4× more thrombogenic than stainless steel may be more important than the actual "electrothrombosis" itself. Electrothrombosis is thought to be caused by the negative charge of white and red blood cells, platelets and fibrinogen, attracted by the positive charge of the electrode (QURESHI et al. 2000). In addition to the fibrotic reaction that replaces the intraluminal clot, an inflammatory process can be observed in the granulation tissue, consisting of neutrophil, polymorphs, eosinophile granulocytes and lymphocytes (BYRNE et al. 1997).

The use of electrothrombosis for treatment of vascular lesions is not new. The induction of intraluminal clot by introducing metallic needles was documented in the 19th century (VELPEAU 1831; PHILIPS 1832). It is quite interesting to note that electrothrombosis for occlusion of CSFs had probably already been used by PETREQUIN in 1846, although at that time with an unfavorable outcome for the patient.

As early as 1880, SATTLER mentioned "*related to the pulsating exophthalmus, our expectations are that in the anterior tumor like segment of the ophthalmic vein an extensive, firm thrombus, and by slow progression of the thrombosis towards the cavernous sinus, occlusion of the ruptured wall of the carotid will occur.*" Later, in 1930, SATTLER again described electrolysis, called "galvanopuncture" that was performed in the following manner: "*In the unipolar electrolysis, a needle, connected to the positive pole is introduced into the pulsating tumor, while the wet, negative large indifferent needle [is] placed onto the body of the patient. In the bipolar electrolysis, both needles connected to the different poles are introduced and the current is increased up to 1–5 Milliampere. Because of the occurring pain, anesthesia is necessary*". Permanent healing by galvanopuncture was reported by several authors at that time (EVERSBUSCH 1897; MENACHO 1907) with three sessions of 15 min each in 2-week intervals being sufficient, such as in EVERSBUSCH's case (1897).

A number of authors have reported the results of endovascular treatment of CSFs with GDC (NESBIT and BARNWELL 1998; MAWAD et al. 1996; GUGLIELMI et al. 1995; BAVINZSKI et al. 1997; SINILUOTO et al. 1997) or other detachable coils (OISHI et al. 1999; YOSHIMURA et al. 1995; TERADA et al. 1996).

GUGLIELMI et al. (1992) were the first to report on a direct CSF that was treated using GDCs after failed transarterial balloon occlusion. The authors discussed occlusive factors and emphasized electrothrombosis as an important one, particularly when a patient is heparinized.

Whether or not electrothrombosis indeed plays a promoting role in the thrombotic transvenous occlusion of the AV shunt is open to question (GUGLIELMI et al. 1995). Some DCSFs may occlude immediately after placement of a few bare platinum coils. In other cases, the AV shunting remains partially open (subtotally occluded), even after pushing numerous coils or additional fibered coils and show an occlusion only in the follow-up examination (BENNDORF et al. 2000a). Blood thinning due to heparinization during the embolization procedure, (normalization can take hours post procedure) may affect this process (GUGLIELMI et al. 1995). Nevertheless, heparinization throughout transvenous embolization appears reasonable, because it helps not only to avoid thromboembolic complications on the arterial side, but also to prevent untoward progressive thrombosis on the venous side, especially inside the SOV that may cause visual deterioration. The complete interruption of the fistulous communication by dense mechanical coil packing appears more important than electrothrombotic effects. Mechanical blockage obtained with less thrombogenic but softer bare platinum coils likely compensates for the lower thrombogenicity. This assumption is supported by the fact that in four patients who were treated with material more thrombogenic than GDC, none showed an immediate complete occlusion (BENNDORF 2002).

Although there is no study allowing for direct comparison of different coil systems, and apart from the author's opinion, it appears justified to state that dense mechanical packing is more effective than loosely packed thrombogenic material. The fact that the effective mass per deployed coil unit is higher thans compared to fiber coils is considered another contributing factor (TOMSICK 1997a).

The key advantage of all detachable coils is the possibility to correct their positioning, avoiding untoward migration into venous compartments, where occlusion can cause clinical problems. Even unintentionally, premature occlusion of the IPS may cause access problems or rerouting of venous drainage. During TVO of a fistula with anterior drainage, the aim is to interrupt the communication between SOV and CS without dislodging coils deep into the ophthalmic vein, thus preventing an impairment of the normal orbital and ocular venous drainage.

The early experience of GUGLIELMI et al. (1995) has been confirmed by several other investigators (NESBIT and BARNWELL 1998; BAVINZSKI et al. 1997; SINILUOTO et al. 1997) who were able to effectively occlude direct CSFs using transarterial coil placement. In four cases of small to medium fistulas (3 mm), SINOLUTO et al. (1997) achieved complete occlusion in two at the end of the treatment, and in two others at follow-up. BAVINSKY et al. (1997) treated six patients with Type A fistulas and achieved complete occlusion in all cases, including one patient embolized transvenously. The authors observed a serious complication due to massive thrombosis leading to unilateral visual impairment and increased sixth nerve palsy that was explained by overpacking of the CS. NESBIT and BARNWELL (1998) were able to occlude 12 high-flow fistulas, including three Type A CCF. There was no coil migration requiring repositioning of the coil, as seen when using mechanically detachable coils (YOSHIMURA et al. 1995).

Initially, only a few series described the use of GDCs in DCSFs (JANSEN et al. 1999; OISHI et al. 1999; MAWAD et al. 1996; NAKAMURA et al. 1998). MAWAD et al. (1996) reported their results in eight patients (87%), in whom complete occlusion was accomplished, while in one case treatment failed due to intracavernous septae.

The advantages of all detachable coil systems are obvious in the transvenous treatment of DCSFs, where the critical task is the precise placement of the coils at the beginning of the procedure (BENNDORF et al. 2000a; OISHI et al. 1999). This can be achieved by deploying coils that are slightly larger (2–3 mm) than the targeted venous compartment (Fig. 8.4). For the SOV-CS junction, helical coils with approximately 5 mm diameter, or with a spherical configuration, proved helpful in creating a small basket with sufficient apposition to the venous wall. In order to achieve a most effective blockage of the fistulous flow in the SOV early during the procedure, this basket should be immediately filled with small and soft coils. The rationale behind this strategy has already been pointed out by HALBACH et al. (1997).

Using coils with a complex shape helps avoid overpacking the sinus, which may result in cranial nerve deficits. Further, in order to prevent venous infarction, selective occlusion is of importance in cases where the normal venous drainage via the Sylvian vein or the SPPS needs to be maintained (NAKAMURA et al. 1998). Such targeted compartmental embolization of DCSFs has been suggested by AGID et al. (2004).

The softness of today's platinum coils produced by various manufacturers is advantageous because it allows denser packing even in small interstices and trabecular compartments. To create such dense coil mesh may be more difficult using fibered coils, especially in small fistulas or when the CS is additionally thrombosed.

Despite its higher costs, the use of softer and more pliable coils minimizes the risk of creating small pockets in the CS that could complicate the procedure by rerouting the venous drainage and causing venous cortical hypertension (OISHI et al. 1999). Softer coils also minimize undesirable catheter buckling or kickback and guarantee a more stable access throughout the procedure. Unstable position of the microcatheter in the CS may lead to loose coil packing and compartmentalization. Finally, the use of softer coils lowers the overall risk of CN irritations caused by locally increased mechanical pressure (ROY and RAYMOND 1997). Because the CS is embedded in radiographically dense bony structures of the skull base and the middle cranial fossa, good fluoroscopic visualization of platinum coils is another advantage compared to stainless steel coils (OISHI et al. 1999). The safety and reliability of modern detachable systems is very high. Premature detachments are seldom, and secondary coil migration usually does not occur (BENNDORF et al. 2000a; OISHI et al. 1999; JAHAN et al. 1998; NESBIT and BARNWELL 1998; MAWAD et al. 1996; GUGLIELMI et al. 1995; BAVINZSKI et al. 1997). The use of soft and pliable coils in combination with improved braided microcatheters reduces friction, so that catheter damage or unraveling of coils occurs less often. An unraveled coil may be difficult to break, necessitating a catheter exchange that can be problematic in cases with difficult anatomy (e.g. cross-over approaches). Changing catheters may even lead to a complete loss of access to the fistula site, especially if some coils have already been deployed. If a catheter dislodges (e.g. during an IPS approach), coils may get deployed too early into the posterior CS compartment or within the IPS itself. This should be avoided, in particular when the CS-SOV junction is not yet occluded and the AV shunting is still open.

Although the largest experience in coiling of DCSFs probably exists with GDCs, all of the aforementioned advantages are equally true for other coil types with controlled detachment such as Micro-Plex coils (MicroVention, Terumo), TruFill™ DCS

Orbit Detachable Coil (Cordis Neurovascular, Miami Lakes), Detach-18/-11; (William Cook Europe, Bjaerverskov, Denmark) and others.

Bare platinum coils can be combined with more thrombogenic coils (NESBIT and BARNWELL 1998; JANSEN et al. 1999), as well as with liquid embolic agents such as NBCA (TROFFKIN and GIVEN 2007; WAKHLOO et al. 2005; ROY and RAYMOND 1997) or Onyx™ (SUZUKI et al. 2006). Such combination of GDCs and VortX coils has been in several early cases aiming to accelerate thrombosis in larger CS compartments (BENNDORF et al. 2000a). Whether or not fibered coils accelerated the fistulas' occlusion remained difficult to assess. One should also keep in mind that the compatibility between various coil types and microcatheters could be problematic. Pushing fibered coils through a small microcatheter may cause friction to a degree that the subsequent use of bare platinum coils can be compromised.

The additional injection of Onyx requires the use of DMSO compatible catheters from the beginning of the procedure, while endovenous injection of acrylic glue should be performed at the end of the coiling because it necessitates immediate catheter removal.

In the early TVO experience, mechanically detachable coils made of tungsten (MDS, Balt Extrusion, Montmorency, France) have been used as well. Tungsten has a slightly higher thrombogenicity than platinum (BYRNE et al. 1997); however, it is softer than platinum and thus cannot be as densely packed. This and the less reliable detachment system make these coils less suitable for targeted embolizations including DCSFs. In addition, coil corrosion has been reported (WEILL et al. 1998) and the material has meanwhile been replaced by platinum.

Newer mechanical systems such as the Detach-18 and Detach-11 coils (William Cook, Europe) showed satisfactory performance as demonstrated by KIYOSUE et al. (2004b) in five patients with DCSFs. In particularly, the J-shaped coil of this system appeared useful for occluding the trabeculated CS.

HydroCoils (Hydrogel)

The case shown in this monograph (Case Illustrations V), demonstrates the usefulness of this coil system when applied to venous occlusions. MORSI et al. (2004) were first to report the use of Hydro-Coils in addition to bare platinum coils for transvenous occlusion of a DCSF. Numerous platinum coils (TruFill, Cordis) tightly packed in the CS did not show noticeable effects on the AV shunting.

After placement of four HydroCoils™, significant flow reduction was evident. A control angiogram obtained 15 min later confirmed complete occlusion of the fistula that likely would have taken longer using only bare platinum coils. Longer procedure time can be associated with higher radiation dose (GABA et al. 2006), which may be particularly important for lengthy TVO procedures. KLURFAN et al. (2006) recently reported on a series of 10 patients with DAVFs, including five DCSFs, treated with a combination of bare platinum and HydroCoils, achieving complete anatomical cure in all. Angiographic follow-up was performed using MRA in two patients; two underwent DSA and one was lost to follow-up. In one (20%) patient, persistent 6th nerve palsy was seen after 10 months. Although data are currently limited, it can be assumed that HydroCoils will likely cause less CN deficits than bare platinum coils. The total amount of coils could be reduced, thereby decreasing costs, procedure time and radiation dose.

8.4.2.3
NBCA (Histoacryl™, Glubran™, Trufill™)

The use of liquid adhesives is well established in the treatment of AV shunting lesions, mainly for transarterial embolization of brain AVMs and DAVFs (LIU et al. 2000a; HENKES et al. 1998). The use of acrylic glue for embolizations of DCSFs has been mostly limited to transarterial injections for occluding feeding ECA pedicles, IMA or the cavernous ICA (LIU et al. 2000b; VINUELA et al. 1984; DEBRUN et al. 1988; HALBCH et al. 1987). Isobutyl-2-cyanoacrylate (IBCA) and later N-butyl-2-cyanoacrylate (NBCA) are liquid adhesives, primarily used in early TAE series (VINUELA et al. 1984; PICARD et al. 1987; KUPERSMITH etal. 1988). Limited experience and less advanced imaging and catheter technology in the 1970s and 1980s led to serious complications caused by passage of the glue through ECA/ICA collateral branches in the dural cavernous network.

A few reports describe the use of intravenous injections of NBCA directly into the cavernous sinus (WAKHLOO et al. 2005; ROY and RAYMOND 1997).

In 1979, KERBER et al. were the first to use acrylic glue (IBCA) for the treatment of a direct carotid artery fistula with the help of a calibrated leak balloon catheter. The authors observed temporary neurological disturbances but no permanent cranial nerve deficit despite the intercavernous deposition around cranial nerves in all three patients.

In 1988, TENG et al. (1988a) mentioned the endovenous injection of IBCA to promote occlusion of a direct CCF. The adjunctive use of glue during TVO has also been described by ROY and RAYMOND (1997), who injected NBCA into the coil basket in two high-flow DCSFs without complications, recommending the simultaneous compression of the eye bulb to avoid glue migration into the SOV.

In the group of patients studied, only a few (*n*=3) patients were treated with either additional or sole injection of glue. Case Illustrations VII and VIII show that glue can be injected either transarterially or transvenously with very good results and lead to an immediate occlusion of the fistula due to the thrombogenic effect of NBCA. The high thrombogenicity of glue is the major contributing factor in occlusions of AVFs, where coil occlusion alone is insufficient to induce thrombosis and occlusion. In particular, when no occluding effect occurs despite the deployment of a critical coil mass in the CS, adding glue may be a valuable option.

When injected transarterially, flow control may be achieved by navigating a microcatheter into a so-called wedged position. Flow control is unlikely achieved in the CS, except when placing an occlusion balloon on the arterial side (GAL et al. 2008). As a venous collector, the cavernous sinus is anatomically and hemodynamically open in various directions, depending on incoming and outgoing flow according to the AV shunting. The latter may change at any time during the injection. The flux of a liquid embolic agent is difficult to predict.

In some cases with partial occlusion by coils, small amounts of additional glue may be enough to induce thrombosis and achieve complete occlusion. A coil basket formed initially may help to avoid spillage of glue into the SOV or cortical veins (WAKHLOO et al. 2005).

Similar to other authors (ROY and RAYMOND 1997; TENG et al. 1995), CN irritations have not been observed in the studied material. Nevertheless, this potential complication may occur and needs to be considered before injecting Histoacryl directly into the CS.

In my early personal experience, one patient developed persistent pain around his lower nose (maxillary division of 5th cranial nerve) after NBCA injection into the artery of the foramen rotundum supplying a CSF.

ROY and RAYMOND (1997) injected NBCA into the coil basket in two high-flow dural fistulas without complications and recommend the simultaneous compression of the eye bulb to avoid glue migration into the SOV. Shaibani et al. (2007) demonstrated that NBCA injection into a small compartment of the CS may close the AV shunt when an intracavernous stenosis does not provide catheter positioning for proper coil deployment.

Wakhloo et al. (2005) reported the largest experience so far with 14 patients; six treated with NBCA alone, seven with a combination of NBCA and coils, and one with a combination of transarterial PVA injection and intravenous NBCA. The authors achieved complete cure in all cases, observing two technical complications (14%) and one transient 6th nerve palsy (7%). There was one inadvertent glue migration into the MCA, another into the SOV; both without clinical sequelae. Intravenous glue injection should be performed with the greatest of care to avoid uncontrolled migration into the normal venous circulation or retrogradely via ILT and MHT into the carotid lumen, causing stroke. The latter has been observed by Meyers et al. (2002) who injected glue under pressure exceeding pressure in the small dural branches.

More recently, a modified type of acrylic glue (Glubran[TM], GEM, Viareggio Italy) has become available that consists of a monomer NBCA and a monomer MS (owned by GEM). It has a lower thermal polymerization temperature than NBCA and is thought to be better controllable (see case Illustration VII). Preliminary experience in the treatment of brain AVM and DAVFs has been reported in one single study so far (Raffi et al. 2007).

8.4.2.4
Ethylene-Vinyl Alcohol Copolymer (Onyx[TM])

The use of the liquid, non-adhesive embolic agent Onyx[TM], (EV3, Irvine CA), mixed with dimethyl sulphoxide (DMSO) and tantalum (Jahan et al. 2001), was initially targeted for brain AVMs (Weber et al. 2007a,b; Song et al. 2007; van Rooij et al. 2007) and has only recently been extended to DAVFs (Suzuki et al. 2006; Toulgoat et al. 2006; Cognard et al. 2008; Rezende et al. 2006; Nogueira et al. 2008).

Regardless of its location, DAVFs have been considered the most difficult lesions to treat, especially by transarterial approach, because of their often elongated, tortuous ECA feeders, preventing a distal catheterization for effective glue injections. Transarterial embolization with NBCA has been one main treatment modality for treating cranial DAVFs, but its efficacy remains limited to cases with favorable anatomy, in which either distal or wedged positions were obtainable, allowing for deposition of glue downstream at the desired location. The dependence on highly experienced operators for effective and safe use of liquid embolic agents has been widely overcome with the introduction of Onyx (Cognard et al. 2008).

After proper training, the flux of Onyx is, in general, easier to control, shortening the learning curve for its optimized handling. The anatomical results currently obtainable with Onyx appear superior to what can be accomplished with NBCA. Creating a so-called "embolic plug" ("reflux-hold-reinjection" technique, "reflux and push technique") mitigates too much proximal reflux, while the embolic material penetrates slowly antegrade to the targeted vascular area. After casting the nidus itself, retrograde ("transnidal") filling of adjacent feeding pedicles is possible, allowing for complete obliteration, not only of the nidus but also of a complete arterial network surrounding the AV shunt. Thus, the recruitment of new feeding vessels that form after partial or incomplete obliteration is minimized and will likely improve long-term results of embolizations in DAVFs, including DCSFs. Similarly, a direct endovenous application of Onyx[TM] is easier to control than that of acrylic glue, and can be used as an adjuvant technique to coils (Suzuki et al. 2006; Toulgoat et al. 2006; Rezende et al. 2006; Nogueira et al. 2008; Warakaulle et al. 2003; He et al. 2008; Lv 2009).

Toulgoat et al. (2006) treated six patients with DAVFs in various locations with Onyx[TM] 18, accomplishing complete occlusions in all patients with catheterization of a single feeder and one injection. Nogueira et al. (2008) reported on 12 consecutive patients with DAVFs embolized with Onyx[TM] 18 or a combination of Onyx[TM] 18 and Onyx[TM] 34, achieving complete obliteration in 11 patients (91.7%) with a total of 17 procedures. The authors observed no significant morbidity or mortality and saw one recurrence that required retreatment. Cognard et al. (2008) achieved complete closure in 80% of their patients (n=30), observing clinical complications in two (6.6%).

The combined use of coils and Onyx for endovenous occlusion of DCSFs in three patients has been described by Suzuki et al. (2006). The authors achieved complete occlusion and considered the controlled and excellent penetration of Onyx to be superior for blocking the intricate communications in these fistulas.

ARAT et al. (2004) performed transvenous injection of Onyx for treatment of a dural carotid-cavernous fistula following an unsuccessful embolization using detachable coils and liquid adhesive agents resulting in complete resolution of symptoms after 3 month. The intracavernous injection was performed using a total of 0.6 ml of 8% ethyl-vinyl-alcohol-copolymer (Onyx 34) in a single injection casting not only of the CS, but also part of the SOV (see Fig. 3 in ARAT et al. 2004). The latter should probably be avoided, since it may cause SOV thrombosis with possible loss of vision, the preservation of which is the goal of EVT in DCSFs.

A number of disadvantages and limitations should be considered when using this material (SUZUKI et al. 2006; JAHAN et al. 2001) including:

- It requires DMSO-compatible microcatheters
- Angiotoxicity with angionecrosis or vasospasm
- Microcatheter retention due to entrapment
- Costs exceed that of NBCA (in certain geographic regions, except US)
- Discomfort in patients when treated without general anesthesia

Another, more general issue related to the use of Onyx™ is that the relative ease of control may lead to an underestimation of its potential of untoward penetration into venous compartments or exits that should not be occluded. In particular, within the CS, the degree of occlusion of only a selected compartment or all connections to afferent and efferent veins, and overfilling of the SOV are difficult to predict.

Case Illustration IX depicts how elegantly Onyx™ can be used in a DCSF with only minimal arterial supply through the ipsilateral AMA and MHT, when supported by indirect flow control. A balloon placed across the MHT and inflated during the Onyx injection into the AMA pedicles allows targeted deposition of Onyx™ with the CS. This prevents distal migration of the embolic agent into the SOV or reflux into the ICA.

Transarterial embolization of DAVFs may be accompanied by clinical complication due to proximal reflux causing CN deficits, or overinjection and subsequent extensive venous thrombosis (COGNARD et al. 2008). Recent literature provides an increasing number of smaller series reporting the successful use of Onyx™ for both transvenous and transarterial embolization of DCSFs (ONG et al. 2009; LV et al. 2008; GANDHI et al. 2009; ELHAMMADY 2009;

BHATIA 2009; HE 2008). Although the achieved high rates of technical success and occlusion are promising, the use of Onyx™ in CSFs is not without potential hazards.

HE et al. (2008) treated six patients using Onyx and coils observing two transient 6th nerve palsies after TVO (33%) and one transient facial nerve palsy (17%) after TAE.

In another series, complete occlusion was achieved in 11 patients undergoing TVO using a combination of coils and Onyx (LV et al. 2009). Two patients (18%) developed a bradycardia during the DMSO injection; transient or permanent CN palsies were not observed.

BATHIA et al. (2009) reported five patients undergoing TVO using Onyx-34 and achieved complete occlusion with resolution of clinical symptoms in all. One patient (20%) showed persistent 6th cranial nerve palsy that resolved after 3 months. The risk of potential reflux into cavernous ICA branches is emphasized as a major disadvantage. It can be minimized to some degree by using a higher viscosity (Onyx-34), and pausing the injection whenever reflux occurs.

Similarly, ELHAMMADY et al. (2009) treated a group of 12 CSFs, with 11 DCSFs, using Onyx for arterial and endovenous injections. The authors used a combination of coils and Onyx in five and Onyx only in three patients for TVO, achieving complete occlusion in all. In three other patients, TAE was performed resulting in complete obliteration as well. The authors observed two transient CN palsies (18%) and one permanent facial nerve palsy (9%) in the patients undergoing transarterial embolizations. This relatively high morbidity may be caused by ischemia in the arterial territory supplying the cranial nerves in the CS, by aggravated CS thrombosis and swelling, or is possibly related to direct angiotoxic effects of DMSO.

These newer observations may tone down a bit the prevailing Onyx enthusiasm and illustrate several important aspects: First, caution is warranted before injecting DMSO and Onyx directly into the CS as it seems currently unclear to what degree the cranial nerve function may be affected. Second, the use of Onyx must be performed under the same rules used for injecting NBCA. This includes avoiding dangerous anastomoses and respecting the normal arterial supply to the cranial nerves. Third, larger series with long-term clinical and angiographic FU are needed to validate efficacy and procedural morbidity of Onyx embolizations (WAKHLOO 2009).

Murugesan et al. (2008) recently reported a severe adverse pulmonary reaction following embolization of a cerebral AVM. The patient developed acute respiratory distress syndrome with hypoxemia following extubation, necessitating mechanical ventilatory support for 44 h. This unusual complication may be related to the excretion of DMSO through the lungs.

Increased radiation exposure due to prolonged injection time [mean injection time 45 min (Cognard et al. 2008)] is another controversial issue, but must be counterbalanced against long fluoroscopy time, often necessary for more distal catheter navigation and repeated sessions in the use of NBCA (Nogueira et al. 2008). In DCSFs, procedure time and radiation exposure may actually be reduced compared to time-consuming coil packing (Gandhi et al. 2009; Bhatia et al. 2009). Catheter entrapment may cause clinical complications (Carlson et al. 2007), but will likely be solved by technological advancements, such as the recent introduction of a detachable tip for the Sonic catheter from Balt (Tahon et al. 2008).

Overall, the experience with Onyx is still limited but encouraging, as it allows for better and more controlled penetration of the complex network of an AV shunt as compared to NBCA, and can be considered a valuable adjunct to the EVT armamentarium for the management of DCSFs, either alone or in combination with detachable coils.

It should be mentioned here that among liquid embolic materials, the use of alcohol has also been reported (Koebbe et al. 2003). In a group of six patients, intraarterial alcohol injection was performed under temporary balloon inflation in the ICA. Technical success was achieved in all cases, clinical improvement in five. One patient experienced worsening of her sixth nerve palsy due to CS thrombosis. Although known as highly effective for vascular occlusion, this technique carries a high risk of damaging the ICA endothelium as well as the cranial nerves traversing the CS, and thus should be used only as a last resort.

8.4.2.5
Stents and Covered Stents

The use of stents in the treatment of CSFs has been reported in a limited number of cases (Moron et al. 2005; Archondakis et al. 2007; Felber etal. 2004; Gomez et al. 2007), mainly in association with direct CSFs. Moron et al. (2005) demonstrated that preservation of the parent artery was achieved using stent-assisted coiling in five patients. The actual benefit in using stents lies in the possible reduction of the arterial inflow when deploying stents with a low porosity, or ideally, covered stents. Angiographic follow-up in eight patients with traumatic CCFs treated with covered stents (JoStent Coronary Stent Graft) demonstrated improved symptoms or complete regression in all. In two, a residual filling of the AV shunt was found at the end of the procedure. Six patients showed good patency of the carotid lumen, while one presented with an asymptomatic occlusion (Arachnondakis et al. 2007).

For effective use of covered stents, good wall apposition is crucial to fully seal the defect in the carotid wall of a CCF, or the TMH/ILT origins in a DCSF. If the stent is malapposed, the AV shunt may stay open (Lv et al. 2008). Care is necessary when further expanding the stent in a CCF, since an injured arterial wall provides little resistance. Thus, when a stent graft is over-inflated, additional damage could potentially enlarge the defect in the wall (personal observation in one case). Lv et al. (2008) observed the development of a complex AVF 9 months after placement of a covered stent for occlusion of a traumatic CCF.

The use of covered stents in dural cavernous sinus shunts has been described in one case by Kim et al. (2006). Residual slow flow directed toward pontomesencephalic veins occurred after transvenous coil packing, resulting in brain stem congestion associated with dysarthria. Bilateral placement of a stent graft resulted in complete occlusion of the shunt. Although neurological deterioration after TVO certainly justifies such an aggressive approach, a number of potential disadvantages have to be considered.

First, no covered stent dedicated for intracranial circulation is currently available. The stiffness of the JoStent coronary graft is an inherent limitation that may not allow easy navigation and can cause spasm or even dissection (Archondakis et al. 2007). Second, as with any stent placement, dual antiplatelet therapy (aspirin and clopidogrel) 2–3 days prior to the stent placement and 2–3 months post stenting, then aspirin only for 12 months or even indefinitely, is recommended. The required large size of the guiding catheter (7 or 8 F) in combination with agressive anticoagulation may cause additional complications at the puncture site.

Third, the short- and long-term patency of these stents is unknown. The PTFE layer may cause acute inflammation and ingrowth of fibrous connective tissue (Geremia et al. 1997; Link et al. 1996). On the other hand, evidence suggests that PTFE might reduce the rate of intimal hyperplasia (REDEKOP et al. 2001; GERCKEN et al. 2002). Fourth and not least, placing a covered stent may be effective in CSFs with solely ICA supply (Type B fistulas, see Case Illustration XI), while in Type C and D fistulas subsequent recruitment of ECA feeders may develop and the treatment remains ineffective.

Longer follow-ups and the development of softer stent grafts dedicated for neurovascular use will show whether or not covered stents play a role in the future armamentarium of endovascular treatment for DCSFs. The VIABAHNN Endoprosthesis from Gore (Gore & Associates, Inc., Arizona) has been FDA approved and may represent an alternative to the JoStent.

8.4.3
Anatomic Results, Clinical Outcome and Complications of Transvenous Occlusions and Transarterial Embolizations

Due to the paucity of early reports on transvenous treatment of DCSF, the validity of achieved results in anatomic and clinical cures as well as complications rates has been limited. Table 8.6 provides an overview of the results achieved by various groups and shows that more data have become available in recent years.

While most groups reported series of between 10–20 patients in the 1980s, the number of series studying more than 20 patients has increased. Thus, statements about efficacy and procedure released complications associated with TVO have become more valid.

In 1989, the first relevant series reporting transfemoral venous approaches was published by HALBACH et al. (1989a) (n=13). The authors primarily used a transfemoral approach through the IPS, the SOV and the basilar plexus, achieving 90% angiographic cure and 77% clinical cure. They observed two complications; one patient developed a stroke after placement of a balloon, while another suffered from transient vision loss.

YAMASHITA et al. (1993) achieved complete angiographic cure in 14 of 16 (88%) cases, interpreting the failure in two cases with coils that were not optimally placed within the CS. This may have been caused by intracavernous trabeculae, thrombosis or unfavorable anatomy of the SOV. There were 12% transient and 6% permanent deficits.

GOLDBERG et al. (1996) presented the first larger series of SOV cannulation and achieved immediate improvement or clinical cure in 100% of their patients (n=10). They were unsuccessful in two additional patients and observed one case of severe intraorbital bleeding.

QUINONES et al. (1997) achieved a 92% occlusion rate in 12 successfully catheterized patients and a clinical recovery in all but two patients (83%). The authors observed two delayed complications. One patient developed a palpebral silk granuloma, another transient contralateral cavernous sinus syndrome (6th nerve palsy). With the exception of two additional cases (Case 11 and 12), the aforementioned represents the same series as the one published by GOLDBERG et al. (1996) 1 year earlier. It should be noted, however, that the 82-year-old female who suffered from severe intraorbital hemorrhage after attempted transorbital deep puncture was not included in their results, and has not been mentioned in the second report of this group (QUINONES et al. 1997). Identifiable on the angiographic images [Figs. 6 and 3, respectively, in LEIBOVITCH et al. (2006)], this patient was recently presented by LEIBOVITCH et al. (2006) as an 86-year-old female in more detail with an apparently more complicated post-craniotomy course suffering from permanent left hemiplegia and vision loss. Such an unfortunate outcome after TVO of a DCSF is rather unusual and will presumably remain an exception, if less invasive routes and means are considered first.

ROY and RAYMOND (1997) reported on 24 patients with DAVFs; 12 with DCSFs. Nine were treated using transvenous occlusions only; 89% demonstrated complete anatomic occlusion. In this series, transient CN deficits occurred relatively frequently (50%), and in one patient permanent sixth nerve palsy was seen (8%). The authors explained these complications with local thrombosis inside the CS that led to CN irritations, and considered mechanical pressure less likely the reason, since the symptoms were irreversible.

OISHI et al. (1999) reported results and complications that may occur when employing different venous approaches. They achieved complete angiographic cure in 89% of cases with a relatively high complication rate of 32%. These complications consisted of transient 6th nerve palsies (n=3), dissections of the IPS (n=1), blepharoptosis (n=2), as well as permanent dysesthesia of the forehead (n=1) due to upper lid incision for the SOV approach. The authors were able to reduce this complication rate with gained experience and more frequent use of the IPS approach.

Gobin et al. (2000) reported angiographic cure in 24 of 26 patients (92%) and a complete clinical cure in 25 patients (96%). The authors observed two complications (7%): one transient 6th nerve palsy (4%) and one case of visual loss due to thrombosed central retinal vein (4%).

Cheng et al. (2003) treated 27 patients with TVO achieving complete angiographic obliteration 89% (30% immediate) and clinical cure in 96%. Two patients presented with recurrent symptoms and underwent a second procedure. The authors observed transient 6th nerve palsy in three patients (11%), which occurred with delay in two, suggesting progressive thrombosis and inflammation inside the CS, as discussed by others (Roy and Raymond 1997).

Meyers et al. (2002) recently reiterated the UCSF experience in 135 patients followed over a period of 15 years. The majority (76%) of patients undergoing EVT were treated by transvenous approach, achieving angiographic and clinical cure rates of 90%. Eight patients (6%) experienced symptomatic complications, including infarction ($n=1$), visual deterioration ($n=2$), diabetes insipidus ($n=1$) and orbital ecchymosis ($n=1$), but it remains unclear if these occurred during TVO or TAE. The overall procedure-related permanent morbidity was 2.3%; however, the authors do not specify whether it was related to TVO or TAE. Angiographic follow-up was obtained in 54%; one third of the patients required more than one intervention.

More recently, Theaudin et al. (2007) reported on 27 consecutive patients undergoing transvenous occlusions ($n=16$) or transarterial embolizations ($n=4$). Complete occlusion was achieved in 14/16 patients (88%) with early-improved symptoms in 12 (75%). One patient (6%) developed a temporal lobe hemorrhage immediately following transvenous occlusion in a fistula with cortical venous drainage, possibly due to blockage of the fistula drainage by placement of the guiding catheter into the IPS. The patient fully recovered without permanent deficit when seen at 1 year follow-up.

Yu et al. (2007) reported a series of 61 patients undergoing 64 successful TVO procedures and achieved anatomical cure in 95%. In 38 patients the fistula was occluded immediately after the procedure, in 20 a mild residual fistula was documented and completely occluded in FU exams (3–16 months). Three patients showed persistent symptoms and underwent repeat TVO, while 16 patients showed cure within 2 weeks,

22 after 3 months. There were two patients with transient 6th nerve palsy. Using catheterization of the SOV either via the facial or the middle temporal veins the authors were successful in 11/11 cases. It is interesting to note that the authors' technical success rate increased from 71.6% to 86.5% after adapting this transfacial SOV approach. Furthermore, it is worth mentioning that in 7/8 patients with residual symptoms the IPS was used as initial route.

Kim et al. (2006) achieved an immediate 75% occlusion rate (complete or nearly complete) with cure or improvement of symptoms in 91% of patients. A total of 11 complications (20%) were observed, including six cranial nerve palsies, three venous perforations and two patients who developed brainstem congestion. Although this rate is relatively high, most of the adverse events were transient or clinically silent. These authors discuss in detail potential mechanisms and possible management strategies (Kim et al. 2006):

- First, transient CN palsies seen in six cases (10.7%) were likely due to overpacking of the cavernous sinus or extensive thrombosis within the CS. This was also observed by us in one case after coil packing the left and right CS with a total of 16 GDCs-10, and two GDCs-18-VortX. The patient presented with exophthalmos and chemosis and developed a new diplopia due to 6th nerve palsy the day after treatment. She was heparinized for 3 days and treated with corticosteroids for 1 week. The patient recovered completely within 8 weeks. A follow-up arteriogram after 6 months confirmed complete occlusion of the fistula. It can be assumed that the relatively stiff VortX-18 coil may have caused nerve compression.

- Second, venous perforations during IPS catheterizations were seen in 5.4% (three cases), none of which resulted in clinical sequelae due to immediate recognition and coil embolization. Extravasation during IPS catheterization occurred in one of our patients; however, it remained clinically silent. Rupture of an IPS may not cause serious clinical complications as most perforations occur when a catheter is advanced through a thrombosed or occluded IPS with minimal or no AV shunt flow.

- Finally, venous congestion in association with DCSFs has been reported by a number of authors (Iwasaki et al. 2006; Kai et al. 2004; Uchino et al. 1997; Teng et al. 1991). Kim et al. (2006) demonstrated a rate in 3.6%, attributed to rerouted venous drainage after coil packing within the CS.

Such rerouting of venous drainage towards the posterior fossa following TVO of DCSFs has not been observed in the material studied. In all cases with preexisting cortical or leptomeningeal drainage, it was possible to disconnect the communication between the CS and the efferent venous drainage at the beginning of the procedure.

However, venous rerouting after TVO of a direct high-flow CCF using coils without achieving complete occlusion has occurred and resulted in an intracranial hemorrhage several hours after the procedure.

In summary, the results achieved by the various groups (Tables 8.6 and 8.7) show anatomic cure rates ranging from 52%–100%, depending on whether or not immediate complete or near complete (subtotal) obliteration of the AV shunt is considered the endpoint. Similarly, the rate of clinical cure ranges from 63%–100%, with the majority of groups achieving more than 80%–90%. This is higher than what was accomplished in the early era of EVT and lies above results obtainable using transarterial embolizations (GOLDBERG et al. 1996; HALBACH et al. 1987; SONIER et al. 1995), thus reflecting the experience gained

Table 8.6. Anatomic and clinical results of TVO in DCSFs reported in the literature (600 patients)

Author	N	Approach	Result DSA (complete cure)	Partial	None	Result (clinical cure)	Improved	None
TENG et al. (1988)	5	SOV	4 (80%)	1	-	5 (100%)	-	-
HALBACH et al. (1989)	13	IPS	9[d] (90%)	1	-	10[e] (76%)	3	-
YAMASHITA et al. (1993)	16	IPS	14 (88%)	-	2	14 (88%)	1	1
MILLER et al. (1995)	10	SOV	9 (90%)	-	1[r]	10 (100%)	-	-
ROY and RAYMOND (1997)	9	IPS; -	8 (89%)	-	1	8 (89%)	1	-
QUINONES et al. (1997)	12[a]	SOV	11[s] (92%)	1	-	10 (83%)	-	2
OISHI et al. (1999)	19	IPS, SOV	17 (89%)	2	-	17 (89%)	2	-
GOBIN et al. (2000)	26	IPS, SOV, PP	24 (92%)	2	-	25 (96%)	2	-
ANNESLEY-WILLIAMS et al. (2001)	11	IPS, SOV	7[f] (64%)	5[g]	-	8 (73%) 5[j]	3	-
MEYERS et al. (2002)	101[t]	IPS, SOV	121/135 (90%)[o]	-	-	90%	-	4%
BIONDI et al. (2003)	7	FV, SOV	6 (100) [q]	-	-	4 (67%)	2	-
CHENG et al. (2003)	27	IPS, SOV, CV	24 (89%)	-	-	26 (96%)	-	-
KLISCH et al. (2003)	11	IPS, SOV, FV	-[h]	-	-	8 (72%)	3	-
BENNDORF et al. (2004)	45	IPS, SOV, SPS, SV, FrV	42 (93%) [100%][i]	-	-	41(91%)	-	-
WAKHLOO et al. (2005)	14	IPS, SOV	12 (86%)	2 (100%)[m]	-	14 (100%)	-	-
KIM et al. (2006)	56	IPS, FV, SOV	29 (52%)	13 (75%)[n]	14	42 (46%)[k] (91%)	-	-
KIRSCH et al. (2006)	141[u]	IPS, SOV	114 (81%)[u]	18 (13%)	6 (4%)	94%[l]	-	5%
YU et al. (2007)	61[b]	IPS, SOV, FV, MTV	58 (95%) 38[p]	20 (33%)	3 (5%)	58 16[w]	22 [x]	3
THEAUDIN et al. 2007	16[c]	IPS, SPS, SOV	14 (88%)	-	-	10 (63%)	6	

IPS = inferior petrosal sinus, SPS = superior petrosal sinus, SOV = superior ophthalmic vein, PP = pterygoid plexus, FrV = frontal vein, FV = facial vein, CV = clival venous plexus

– no angiographic result or FU reported

[a] successfully catheterized out of 13, [b] technical success out of 71, [c] patients undergoing TVO out of 27, [d] out of 10 seen for angiographic FU and occluded, [e] out of all 13 patients, [f] one bilateral fistula, [g] not specified if immediate or long term occlusion, [h] group mixed with direct CCFs, TCCD or MRPA for FU, [i] all patients seen for angiographic FU showed complete occlusion, [j] immediately improved, [k] FU available, [l] 55% of the patients seen for long term FU, [m] after 6mos FU, [n] complete and nearly complete occlusion together (n=42), [o] not specified for TVO or TAE, angiographic FU obtained in 54%, [p] immediately occluded, [q] out of 6 patients with technical success, [r] required TAE for complete occlusion, [s] 3 patients seen for angiographic FU, [t] undergoing TVO out of 135, [u] TVO failed in 3, TAE performed in 32 patients , [v] FU in 4 patients pending, [w] = cured in 2 weeks, [x] cured after 3 months

Table 8.7. Reported procedure-related complications during TVO in the literature

Author	N	Approach	Complications	Rate
Halbach et al. (1989)	13	IPS	S (1), *VL (1)*	15% [8%]
Yamashita et al. (1993)	16	IPS	*VI (2), III (1), W (3)*, VP (1)	44% [0]
Miller et al. 1995	10	SOV	VI (1)	10% [10%]
Roy and Raymond (1997)	9[i]	IPS ;-	VI (1) *VI (5)*	66% [11%]
Quinones et al. (1997)	12	SOV	*VI (1)*	8% [0]
Oishi et al. (1999)	19	IPS,SOV	*VI (3)*, D (1), BP (2), VP (1)[e]	32% [16%]
Gobin et al. (2000)	26	IPS,SOV,PP	*VI (1)*, TCRV (1)	8% [4%]
Annesley-Williams et al. 2001	11	IPS, SOV	*W (2)*	18% [0]
Meyers et al. (2002)	101	IPS	S (1) *VL (2)* OE (1) VP (1)	5% [1%][d]
Cheng et al. (2003)	27	IPS, SOV,CV	*VI (3) MND (1)*	15% [0]
Klisch et al. (2003)	11	IPS, SOV,FV	*S (1)[a] SAH (1)[a]*	9% [0]
Benndorf et al. (2004)	45	IPS,SOV, SPS,SV,FrV	*VI (1) W (2)* VP (1)[b]	9% [0]
Wakhloo et al. (2005)	14	IPS,SOV,	VP (1) *VI (1)[f]*	14% [0]
Kim et al. (2006)	56	IPS,FV,SOV	*CN (5)* VI (1)[c] VP (3)[b] *BC (2)*	20% [2%]
Kirsch et al. (2006)	141	IPS, SOV	W (4) VP (5)[b] AE (5) RH (2) PE (2)[g]	13% [0]
Leibovitch et al. (2007)	25	SOV	IOB (2)[j] S (1)[h], VL (1)[h]	12% [4%]
Yu et al. (2007)	61	SOV, FV	VI (2)	3% [0]
Theaudin et al. (2007)	16	IPS, SPS, SOV	ICH (1)	6% [0]

IPS = inferior petrosal sinus, SPS = superior petrosal sinus, SOV = superior ophthalmic vein, PP = pterygoid plexus, FrV = frontal vein, FV = facial vein, CV = clival venous plexus

S = stroke, VI = permanent 6th CN deficit (VI = transient), B = bleeding, BP = blepharoptosis, D = dysesthesia, TCRV = thrombosis of the central retinal vein, W/W = permanent/transient ophthalmological worsening, CN = cranial nerve palsy (CN = transient), VP = venous perforation, BC = brainstem congestion, ICH = intracranial hemorrhage, IOB = intraorbital bleeding, OE = orbital ecchymosis, VL = vision loss, AE = 5 arterial emboli detected by MRI, RH = retinal hemorrhage, MND = minor neurological deficit, PE = pulmonary embolism, TIA = transient ischemic attack

*[ ] = rate of procedure related permanent morbidity, [?] = not reported

Retroperitoneal hematomas, femoral artery pseudoaneurysms or deep venous thrombosis are not considered

[a] same patient, [b] clinically silent, [c] mild residue after 42 months FU in one of six patients, [d] not specified if caused by TVO or TAE, [e] dissected dura caused transient 6th CN palsy, [f] 2 patients with NBCA migration into SOV and ICA without sequelae, [g] causing non-life threatening dyspnoe, [h] same patient as reported by Goldberg et al., [i] undergoing TVO only out of 12 with DCSF, [j] unremarkable recovery in one case; stroke and vision loss in another

and the skill level in utilizing transvenous occlusion techniques.

When examining anatomic (angiographic) results, one should consider the following confounding aspects. First, criteria used for determining angiographic endpoints may vary. Second, in some series, TAE is used prior to or in combination with TVO, skewing results (CHENG et al. 2003; OISHI et al. 1999; WAKHLOO et al. 2005; KIM et al. 2006; GOLDBERG et al. 1996; QUINONES et al. 1997; KIRSCH et al. 2006). Third, in several series, complete occlusion was achieved after multiple "multi-channel" approaches were used, either in the same or sequential sessions (BENNDORF et al. 2004; KLISCH et al. 2003; CHENG et al. 1999; YU et al. 2009). This was emphasized by KLISCH et al. (2003) who studied 31 DAVFs including 11 DCSFs, whereby some were managed by either several transvenous occlusion steps or by a combination of EVT with surgical techniques.

The complication rate of TVO, as documented by some groups, appears relatively high (31%) (OISHI et al. 1999). However, one should note that serious complications, such as stroke or intraorbital/intracranial hemorrhage, seldom occur (HALBACH et al. 1988; THEAUDIN et al. 2007). Furthermore, many complications have been reported as anecdotal cases (Table 8.8) versus larger series, underlining the fact that with increasing experience and skills, their rate can be reduced considerably. This becomes clear when looking at overall transient and permanent complication rates reported in relevant studies (Table 8.9), revealing that the overall rate of transient and permanent complications is in fact very low (11.6% and 1.8%, respectively).

The perforation of the IPS, to date the most frequent complication (2.1%), often remains clinically silent and can be effectively managed with endovascular techniques (BENNDORF et al. 2004; KIM et al. 2006).

The majority of CN deficits consist of 6th nerve palsies (overall 4.1%), most of which are transient. The abducens nerve may be more exposed to mechanical pressure caused by overpacking of the CS as the only true intracavernous nerve. Another explanation of this predilection could be its embedment into the wall of the IPS that is mostly used as venous approach.

The relatively low rate of CN deficits in our series (2%) could be related to the more frequent use of soft coils (GDC Soft coils) that may create less mechanical pressure to neuronal structures. CN deficits due to overpacking may likely further de-

crease with increasing use of softer platinum coils (or HydroCoils™) and liquid embolic agents. A permanent CN is rarely seen (0.5%) and has not been observed in our group, despite using aggressive techniques such as deep puncture of the SOV, craniotomy and puncture of the Sylvian vein. Permanent neurological deficits due to stroke during or after TVO occurred in 0.5% of patients and are below the rate reported by TAE series in 75 patients (5.3%) (VINUELA et al. 1984; HALBACH et al. 1987; PICARD et al. 1987; KUPERSMITH et al. 1988). The reported complication rates also vary due to the fact that some investigators include femoral or retroperitoneal hematomas, femoral vein thromboses and pulmonary embolisms (MEYERS et al. 2002; KLISCH et al. 2003; KIRSCH et al. 2006). Furthermore, one of the largest series to date reporting on 101/135 treated patients using TVO does not spec-

Table 8.8. Reported anecdotal complications during TVO of DCSFs

Author	Event
TRESS et al. (1983)	Intraorbital hemorrhage
HALBACH et al. (1991a)	Diabetes insipidus after CS catheterization (n=1)[b]
HALBACH et al. (1991b)	Cerebellar hemorrhage after IPS (n=1)[b]
GOLNIK et al. (1991)	Angle-closure glaucoma after TVO
FUKAMI et al. (1996)	Central retinal vein occlusion after TAE/TVO
ARAKI et al. (1997)	Intracerebral extravasation during TVO
DEVOTO et al. (1997)	Acute exophthalmos during TVO
GUPTA et al. (1997)	Severe vision loss and neovascular glaucoma
GIOULEKAS et al. (1997)	Intraorbital bleeding during SOV cannulation[a]
AIHARA et al. (1999)	Deterioration of ocular motor dysfunction after TVO
WLADIS et al. (2007)	Intraorbital hemorrhage and vision loss during TVO
HAYASHI et al. (2008)	Intraorbital bleeding during SOV cannulation (n=2)

[a] Same case as Tress et al. (1983)
[b] Both cases reported in a large series of EVT (1200 cases) with a total of 15 arterial and venous perforations

Table 8.9. Overall complication rate in larger TVO series (from Table 8.7, total of 613 patients)

Complications	Transient	Permanent
Cranial nerve deficit	25 (4.1%)	3 (0.5%)
Venous perforation (IPS)	13 (2.1%)	-
Stroke	-	3 (0.5%)
Blepharoptosis	-	2 (0.3%)
Worsening of ophthalmic symptoms	11 (1.8%)	-
Visual loss	4 (0.7%)	1 (0.2%)
Intraorbital bleeding	2 (0.3%)	-
Subarachnoid hemorrhage	1 (0.2%)	-
Intracranial hemorrhage	1 (0.2%)	-
Transient ischemic attack	1 (0.2%)	-
Orbital ecchymosis	1 (0.2%)	-
Brainstem congestion	2 (0.2%)	-
Thrombosis of the central retinal vein CRV[a]	-	1 (0.2%)
Minor neurological deficit	1 (0.2%)	-
Pulmonary embolism	2 (0.3%)	-
Retinal hemorrhage	2 (0.3%)	-
Arterial emboli	5 (0.8%)	-
Dysesthesia	-	1 (0.2%)
TOTAL	71 (11.6%)	11 (2.0%)

[a] Untreated patient

ify whether the observed permanent neurological deficits were related to TVO or TEA (Meyers et al. 2002).

The discussion of transvenous embolizations must consider angiographic and clinical results of TAE, representing the traditional way of treating arteriovenous shunting lesions (Vinuela et al. 1984; Picard et al. 1987; Fermand 1982; Barrow et al. 1985). One of the first series was reported by Vinuela et al. (1984), describing 10 patients with Type D fistulas, of which seven were occluded by embolizing the ECA feeders using PVA particles or IBCA. Cure was documented in five patients (50%) after 5 months. One patient developed hemiplegia and aphasia due to reflux of IBCA through the FRA into the ICA and MCA. Another experienced acute deterioration of his vision. Barrow et al. (1985) achieved good results in three of five patients (60%) treated by embolizing the ECA supply. Grossman et al. (1985) reported complete resolution of symptoms after particulate embolization in five of seven patients.

Picard et al. (1987) communicated results in a group of 32 patients; 25 (78%) underwent superselective embolization, achieving complete clinical and anatomical cure in 18 (72%) and demonstrated clinical cure without anatomic cure in six (24%). One patient (4%) suffered from stroke due to IBCA migration into the cerebral circulation and died after 3 months.

Halbach et al. (1987) achieved clinical cure in 77% and an improvement in 18% (n=22) patients treated between 1978 and 1986 by TAE of ECA branches using IBCA. One permanent deficit (4.5%) was seen in a patient who developed a stroke due to clot formation in the guiding catheter, as well as transient deficits in three cases (13%). The group later reported (Halbach et al. 1992) a complete cure rate of 78%, improvement in 20%, and a complication rate of 4%.

In the earlier series published by Debrun et al. (1988), who treated 25 patients with either PVA or Histoacryl, complete occlusion was reported in 48%. In two cases (8%), enlargement of ECA feeders occurred; additional TVO had to be performed in two others (8%), and one patient (4%) required surgical exposure of the SOV. Sonier et al. (1995) reported a 61% success rate by particulate embolization of IMA branches. In two cases (25%), TAE had to be repeated to achieve a complete occlusion, and transient facial edema was observed in another.

Kupersmith et al. (1988) reported the successful embolization of ECA branches in 88% of their patients using PVA and IBCA with two recanalizations (12%) and four complications (25%), including hemiparesis and hemianopia, permanent 12th nerve palsy and persisting visual field defect.

Vinuela et al. (1997) reiterated their experience based on 74 patients, reporting complete cure in 31% and positive clinical response in 85%. The morbidity was 3.2%; in two patients untoward glue migration into the intracranial circulation occurred, leading to hemiparesis and aphasia in one.

Liu et al. (2001) communicated the only larger series (n=55) in patients who were followed prospectively. In a subgroup of 41 patients (75%), TAE was performed using PVA (150–250 μm) and Histoacryl, injected into the distal ECA branches. The involved ICA branches were not approached. A 70.9% complete clinical cure rate was achieved, with improved symptoms in 14.5%. The authors do not specify whether these results were any different in the embolized (41 patients), or the non-embolized group (14 patients). Further, in 24 of these patients (58.5%), a transient worsening was observed that might be considered a transient adverse event, or even a complication (BENNDORF et al. 2004; MEYERS et al. 2002). In four patients (9.7%) there was no improvement, while four demonstrated aggravation of symptoms (9.7%). It is not reported whether *procedure related transient or permanent neurological deficits* were seen. The authors suggest the use of TAE to convert Type D into Type B fistulas and to shorten the time to complete cure with "conservative management". This treatment strategy appears questionable, however, since no evidence exists to date demonstrating that changing a Type D into a Type B fistula improves the overall prognosis of a DCSF.

Furthermore, it is important to note that in some TVO series, patients initially underwent inefficient TAE. GOLDBERG et al. (1996) performed PVA embolization of the ECA feeders prior to the SOV approach. Although the patients benefited clinically from the treatment due to reduction of the AV shunt, or even transient occlusion of the fistula, all demonstrated recanalization at angiographic follow-up and underwent subsequent TVO. THEAUDIN et al. (2007) recently reported a success rate of only 25% (1/5 patients) in patients undergoing TAE with 300–500 μm, followed by 500–700 μm until flow in the internal maxillary artery stopped. It is emphasized that none of these patients became completely asymptomatic, although clinical improvement was seen. A relatively large particle size (>300 μm) is recommended by some operators for ECA embolizations to avoid cranial nerve damage (HALBACH et al. 1992), while others suggest 100–300 μm (VINUELA et al. 1997). Larger particles will more likely produce an occlusion proximal to the fistula site, triggering recruitment of collaterals and recanalization. It must be borne in mind that the dural branches feeding a DCSF may also be involved in the normal blood supply of CN (4th, 5th, 6th, 7th, 9th, 10th, 11th, 12th) (HALBACH et al. 1992). As eluded to in Chap. 2, detailed knowledge of arterial anatomy in the CS area, ECA-ICA collaterals and anatomic variants is essential for performing TAE effectively and safely.

GREGOIRE et al. (2002) recently published the interesting case of a 60-year-old female presenting with diplopia and gait disturbance 3 days after arterial embolization due to cerebellar dysfunction caused by reversible pontine venous congestion. It demonstrates that the thrombotic process within the CS, triggered by particle embolization, may also be unpredictable. Paradoxical worsening caused by SOV thrombosis may occur following TAE (SERGOTT et al. 1987), and has been

documented in a significant number (61.5 %) of patients (LIU et al. 2001).

Aside from passage of PVA particles or liquid embolic agents into the brain circulation via ECA-ICA anastomoses, a major risk associated with transarterial injections of embolic agents is reflux of the embolic agent from cavernous ICA branches. Due to their size (normal diameter approximately 0.3 mm), they can be difficult or impossible to catheterize, even when enlarged and supplying an AV shunt. Even when possible, due to tortuousities, only their most proximal segments are usually accessible, making safe and effective injection of particles or liquid adhesives difficult to control (GOBIN et al. 2000; PICARD et al. 1987; PHATOUROS et al. 1999; HALBACH et al. 1989b). The TMH give rise to the inferior hypophysial artery, thus injection of embolic agents may cause malfunction of the pituitary gland resulting in diabetes insipidus, as was observed in one case after injection of 50% dextrose and pure alcohol mixture (PHATOUROS et al. 1999).

The occlusion of dural ICA branches using GDCs has been suggested (VINUELA et al. 1997) as a safer alternative to particles or liquid adhesives and may be effective in selected cases, but may be followed by recanalization.

Although liquid adhesives have been largely replaced by PVA particles and microspheres for TAE, their use can be a feasible option under certain conditions. LIU et al. (2000b) injected 10%–15% mixtures of NBCA with lipiodol and tungsten into ECA branches, achieving complete resolution of symptoms after 1 month without definite neurological complication. If anatomy of the arterial supply is favorable, complete cure may be achieved by injecting even small amounts via an enlarged ILT or MHT. This technique, however, is not without risk and requires an experienced operator (Illustrative Case VII). Another elegant alternate solution for "difficult-to-treat" cases is demonstrated in Illustrative Case IX, where an occlusion balloon, inflated across the ipsilateral TMH supply, allows for controlled injection of Onyx™ via a single pedicle from AMA (indirect flow control), resulting in complete obliteration of the fistula (GAL et al. 2008).

GANDHI et al. (2009) recently communicated a case of a Type D fistula that was successfully managed by TAE via the distal IMA using Onyx-18 in a single injection. The patient showed significant immediate improvement, but developed a novel 6th nerve palsy that resolved over 12 weeks. The figures of this case show an extensive Onyx cast not only in the CS itself, but also in the proximal supplying pedicles of the IMA. Such proximal occlusion may lead to inadvertent migration of embolic material into dangerous ECA-ICA anastomoses or small arteries supplying the CN nerves in the CS. Such a mechanism is most likely responsible for the permanent facial nerve paralysis seen after TAE in the series of ELHAMMADY et al. (2009)

Based on the literature, the occlusion rate of TAE ranging from 31%–88% lies below the results obtainable today with transvenous occlusion techniques. Recanalization has been observed in 25%–100% of the cases, while approximately two thirds of the patients may experience transient worsening of the symptoms. Although improvement of symptoms can be achieved with a shunt reduction of about 50%–85% (VINUELA et al. 1997; GROSSMAN et al. 1985), the potential for recanalization (GOLDBERG et al. 1993; LASJAUNIAS and BERENSTEIN 1987), and migration of embolic material causing paresis, aphasia, CN deficits, intracranial hemorrhage (VINUELA et al. 1984; HALBACH et al. 1987), worsening of ophthalmological symptoms (GOLNIK et al. 1991) or thrombosis of cortical veins (COGNARD et al. 1999; TOMSICK 1997b), nevertheless remain significant deterrents. Modern endovascular tools and advanced angiographic visualization in the 1990s have improved results and outcomes of TAE (VINUELA et al. 1997; LIU et al. 2000b; MACHO et al. 1996; LANZAS et al. 1996; ROBINSON et al. 1999); however, even in experienced hands, the aforementioned residual risks must be taken into account. Thus, the role of TAE in the management of DCSFs has changed as it has become more an adjunctive treatment option, employed in cases where TVO cannot be utilized (VINUELA et al. 1997), or prior to radiosurgery.

Major advances in of angiographic imaging technology with three-dimensional and cross-sectional imaging capabilities contribute to a better understanding of complex angioarchitecture of the CS and its afferent and efferent draining veins.

Due to its anatomical topography, short length, straight course and attachment to the dura along the petroclival fissure, the IPS approach represents the most preferred access route to the CS, followed by the transfacial approach through the SOV.

Improved catheter and guidewire technology enables exploration of virtually every possible venous access route to the CS, increasing the technical success rate. High-resolution bi-plane fluoroscopy and road mapping facilitate direct percutaneous puncture of draining veins such as the SOV, the IOV, the frontal vein or other tributaries providing additional access.

Improved and novel embolic agents such as softer detachable platinum coils or HydroCoils further increase efficacy and safety of transvenous occlusions. Whether newer liquid embolic agents such as Onyx™ will further enhance the efficacy and safety of TVO and possibly replace mechanical coil packing needs to be shown in future studies.

In agreement with most centers, it can be concluded that there is currently little reason to devote significant time and effort to the technically challenging catheterizations of dural cavernous ICA branches.

More invasive techniques such as direct puncture of intraorbital veins, the cavernous sinus, or open surgery will play a decreasing role in the therapeutic management of DCSFs. They should be reserved for combined surgical-endovascular approaches in truly intractable cases.

8.5
Conclusion

In conclusion, results obtained today with TVO of DCSFs demonstrate that overall rates of anatomical and clinical cure have improved considerably over the last 15 years.

At the same time, complications and morbidity associated with TVO has become very low, particularly as seen in larger series and when treatment is performed by experienced operators with appropriate training and skills in catheterization techniques.

References

Agid R, Willinsky RA, Haw C, Souza MP, Vanek IJ, ter-Brugge KG (2004) Targeted compartmental embolization of cavernous sinus dural arteriovenous fistulae using transfemoral medial and lateral facial vein approaches. Neuroradiology 46:156–160

Ahn JY, Lee BH, Joo JY (2003) Stent-assisted Guglielmi detachable coils embolisation for the treatment of a traumatic carotid cavernous fistula. J Clin Neurosci 10:96–98

Aihara N, Mase M, Yamada K, et al. (1999) Deterioration of ocular motor dysfunction after transvenous embolization of dural arteriovenous fistula involving the cavernous sinus. Acta Neurochir (Wien) 141:707-709; discussion 709–710

Anderson JH, Wallace S, Gianturco C (1977) Transcatheter intravascular coil occlusion of experimental arteriovenous fistulas. AJR Am J Roentgenol 129:795–798

Anderson JH, Wallace S, Gianturco C, Gerson LP (1979) "Mini" Gianturco stainless steel coils for transcatheter vascular occlusion. Radiology 132:301–303

Andreou A, Ioannidis I, Psomas M (2007) Transvenous embolization of a dural carotid-cavernous fistula through the contralateral superior petrosal sinus. Neuroradiology 49:259–263

Angulo-Hervias E, Crespo-Rodriguez AM, Guillen-Subiran ME, Izquierdo-Hernandez B, Barrena MR, Guelbenzu S (2006) [Progression following the embolisation of 100 intracranial arteriovenous malformations]. Rev Neurol 42:8–16

Annesley-Williams DJ, Goddard AJ, Brennan RP, Gholkar A (2001) Endovascular approach to treatment of indirect carotico-cavernous fistulae. Br J Neurosurg 15:228–233

Araki K, Nakahara I, Taki W, et al. (1997) [A case of cavernous dural arteriovenous fistula resulting in intracerebral extravasation during transvenous embolization]. No Shinkei Geka 25:733–738

Arat A, Cekirge S, Saatci I, Ozgen B (2004) Transvenous injection of Onyx for casting of the cavernous sinus for the treatment of a carotid-cavernous fistula. Neuroradiology 46:1012–1015

Arat A, Cil BE, Vargel I, et al. (2007) Embolization of high-flow craniofacial vascular malformations with onyx. AJNR Am J Neuroradiol 28:1409–1414

Archondakis E, Pero G, Valvassori L, Boccardi E, Scialfa G (2007) Angiographic follow-up of traumatic carotid cavernous fistulas treated with endovascular stent graft placement. AJNR Am J Neuroradiol 28:342–347

Badilla J, Haw C, Rootman J (2007) Superior ophthalmic vein cannulation through a lateral orbitotomy for embolization of a cavernous dural fistula. Arch Ophthalmol 125:1700–1702

Barker FG, 2nd, Ogilvy CS, Chin JK, Joseph MP, Pile-Spellman J, Crowell RM (1994) Transethmoidal transsphenoidal approach for embolization of a carotid-cavernous fistula. Case report. J Neurosurg 81:921–923

Barrow DL, Spector RH, Braun IF, Landman JA, Tindall SC, Tindall GT (1985) Classification and treatment of spontaneous carotid-cavernous sinus fistulas. J Neurosurg 62:248–256

Bavinzski G, Killer M, Gruber A, Richling B (1997) Treatment of post-traumatic carotico-cavernous fistulae using electrolytically detachable coils: technical aspects and preliminary experience. Neuroradiology 39:81–85

Beaujeux R, Laurent A, Wassef M, et al. (1996) Trisacryl gelatin microspheres for therapeutic embolization, II: preliminary clinical evaluation in tumors and arteriovenous malformations. AJNR Am J Neuroradiol 17:541–548

Bedford MA (1966) The "cavernous sinus". Brit J Ophthal 50:41–46

Bellon RJ, Liu AY, Adler JR, Jr., Norbash AM (1999) Percutaneous transfemoral embolization of an indirect carotid-cavernous fistula with cortical venous access to the cavernous sinus. Case report. J Neurosurg 90:959–963

Bendszus M, Klein R, Burger R, Warmuth-Metz M, Hofmann E, Solymosi L (2000) Efficacy of trisacryl gelatin microspheres versus polyvinyl alcohol particles in the preoperative embolization of meningiomas. AJNR Am J Neuroradiol 21:255–261

Benndorf G (2002) Angiographic diagnosis and endovascular treatment of cavernous sinus dural arteriovenous fistulas by transvenous occlusion. Humboldt University, Berlin

Benndorf G, Campi A (2001b) The aberrant inferior petrosal sinus: an unusual approach to the cavernous sinus. Neuroradiology DOI 10.1007/s002340100659

Benndorf G, Molsen HP, Lanksch W (1997) Puncture of the superficial sylvian vein for embolisation of cavernous dural arteriovenous fistula. WFITN, New York (abstract)

Benndorf G, Bender A, Lehmann TN, Menneking H, Lanksch W (1999) Transophthalmic approach for treatment of dural cavernous sinus fistulas. In: Congress of European Skull Base Society, Erlangen

Benndorf G, Bender A, Lehmann R, Lanksch W (2000a) Transvenous occlusion of dural cavernous sinus fistulas through the thrombosed inferior petrosal sinus: report of four cases and review of the literature [In Process Citation]. Surg Neurol 54:42–54

Benndorf G, Bender A, Mennking H, Unterberg A (2000b) Superior ophthalmic vein approach for endovascular treatment of dural cavernous sinus fistulas. Clin Neuroradiol 10:101–107

Benndorf G, Bender A, Campi A, Menneking H, Lanksch WR (2001) Treatment of a dural cavernous sinus fistula by deep orbit puncture of the superior ophthalmic vein. Neuroradiology 43:499–502

Benndorf G, Kroppenstedt S, Campi A, Unterberg A (2002) Selective neck occlusion of a large complex aneurysm of the middle cerebral artery trifurcation with the UltraSoft coil. AJNR Am J Neuroradiol 23:965–969

Benndorf G, Mounayer C, Piotin M, Spelle L, Moret J (2004) Transvenous occlusion (TVO) of dural cavernous sinus fistulas: techniques and results in 45 patients. In: ASNR Seattle, 2004

Berenstein A, Graeb DA (1982) Convenient preparation of ready-to-use particles in polyvinyl alcohol foam suspension for embolization. Radiology 145:846

Berlis A, Klisch J, Spetzger U, Faist M, Schumacher M (2002) Carotid cavernous fistula: embolization via a bilateral superior ophthalmic vein approach. AJNR Am J Neuroradiol 23:1736–1738

Bhatia KD, Wang L, Parkinson RJ, Wenderoth JD (2009) Successful treatment of six cases of indirect carotid-cavernous fistula with ethylene vinyl alcohol copolymer (Onyx) transvenous embolization. J Neuroophthalmol 29:3–8

Biondi A, Milea D, Cognard C, Ricciardi GK, Bonneville F, van Effenterre R (2003) Cavernous sinus dural fistulae treated by transvenous approach through the facial vein: report of seven cases and review of the literature. AJNR Am J Neuroradiol 24:1240–1246

Bonelli FS, Huston J, 3rd, Meyer FB, Carpenter PC (1999) Venous subarachnoid hemorrhage after inferior petrosal sinus sampling for adrenocorticotropic hormone [see comments]. AJNR Am J Neuroradiol 20:306–307

Bonelli FS, Huston J, 3rd, Carpenter PC, Erickson D, Young WF, Jr., Meyer FB (2000) Adrenocorticotropic hormone-dependent Cushing's syndrome: sensitivity and specificity of inferior petrosal sinus sampling. AJNR Am J Neuroradiol 21:690–696

Braun IF, Hoffman JC, Jr., Casarella WJ, Davis PC (1985) Use of coils for transcatheter carotid occlusion. AJNR Am J Neuroradiol 6:953–956

Braun JP and Tournade A (1977) Venous drainage in the craniocervical region. Neuroradiol 13:155–158

Brismar G, Brismar J (1976a) Spontaneous carotid-cavernous fistulas: phlebographic appearance and relation to thrombosis. Acta Radiol Diagn (Stockh) 17:180–192

Brismar G, Brismar J (1976b) Orbital phlebography. Technique and clinical applications. Acta Ophthalmol (Copenh) 54:233–249

Brothers MF, Kaufmann JC, Fox AJ, Deveikis JP (1989) n-Butyl 2-cyanoacrylate – substitute for IBCA in interventional neuroradiology: histopathologic and polymerization time studies. AJNR Am J Neuroradiol 10:777–786

Butler H (1957) The development of certain human dural venous sinuses. J Anat Lond 91:510

Byrne JV, Hope JK, Hubbard N, Morris JH (1997) The nature of thrombosis induced by platinum and tungsten coils in saccular aneurysms. AJNR Am J Neuroradiol 18:29–33

Calzolari F (2002) Unusual termination of the inferior petrosal sinus. Neuroradiology 44:796–797

Canton G, Levy DI, Lasheras JC (2005) Changes in the intraaneurysmal pressure due to HydroCoil embolization. AJNR Am J Neuroradiol 26:904–907

Carlson AP, Taylor CL, Yonas H (2007) Treatment of dural arteriovenous fistula using ethylene vinyl alcohol (onyx) arterial embolization as the primary modality: short-term results. J Neurosurg 107:1120–1125

Chaloupka JC, Goller D, Goldberg RA, Duckwiler GR, Martin NA, Vinuela F (1993) True anatomical compartmentalization of the cavernous sinus in a patient with bilateral cavernous dural arteriovenous fistulae. Case report [see comments]. J Neurosurg 79:592–595

Chaloupka JC, Vinuela F, Vinters HV, Robert J (1994) Technical feasibility and histopathologic studies of ethylene vinyl copolymer (EVAL) using a swine endovascular embolization model. AJNR Am J Neuroradiol 15:1107–1115

Chaloupka JC, Huddle DC, Alderman J, Fink S, Hammond R, Vinters HV (1999) A reexamination of the angiotoxicity of superselective injection of DMSO in the swine rete embolization model. AJNR Am J Neuroradiol 20:401–410

Chan CC, Leung H, O'Donnell B, Assad N, Ng P (2006) Intraconal superior ophthalmic vein embolisation for carotid cavernous fistula. Orbit 25:31–34

Cheng KM, Chang CN, Cheung YL (1999) Transvenous embolization of spontaneous carotid cavernous fistulas by sequential occlusion of the cavernous sinus. Interventional Neuroradiology 5:225–234

Cheng KM, Chan CM, Cheung YL (2003) Transvenous embolisation of dural carotid-cavernous fistulas by multiple venous routes: a series of 27 cases. Acta Neurochir (Wien) 145:17–29

Chuang VP, Wallace S, Gianturco C (1980) A new improved coil for tapered-tip catheter for arterial occlusion. Radiology 135:507–509

Clay C, Theron J, Vignaud J (1972) [Value of jugulography and orbital phlebography in pathology of the cavernous sinus]. Arch Ophtalmol Rev Gen Ophtalmol 32:123–135

Cognard C, Herbreteau D, Pasco A (1999) Intracranial dural arteriovenous fistulas: clinical complications after successful treatment. Neuroradiology 41:44[Suppl]

Cognard C, Januel AC, Silva NA, Jr., Tall P (2008) Endovascular treatment of intracranial dural arteriovenous fistulas with cortical venous drainage: new management using onyx. AJNR Am J Neuroradiol 29:235–241

Cromwell LD, Kerber CW (1979) Modification of cyanoacrylate for therapeutic embolization: preliminary experience. AJR Am J Roentgenol 132:799–801

Debrun G (1993) Endovascular management of carotid cavernous fistulas. In: Valavanis A (ed) Interventional neuroradiology. Springer, Berlin Heidelberg New York, pp 23–34

Debrun G, Lacour P, Caron JP, Hurth M, Comoy J, Keravel J (1975) Inflatable and released balloon technique experimentation in dog application in man. Neuroradiology 9:267–271

Debrun G, Lacour P, Vinuela F, et al. (1981) Treatment of 54 traumatic carotid-cavernous fistulas. J Neurosurg 77:678–692

Debrun GM, Vinuela F, Fox AJ, Davis KR, Ahn HS (1988) Indications for treatment and classification of 132 carotid-cavernous fistulas. Neurosurgery 22:285–289

Debrun GM, Nauta HJ, Miller NR, Drake CG, Heros RC, Ahn HS (1989) Combining the detachable balloon technique and surgery in imaging carotid cavernous fistulae. Surg Neurol 32:3–10

Derdeyn CP, Graves VB, Salamat MS, Rappe A (1997) Collagen-coated acrylic microspheres for embolotherapy: in vivo and in vitro characteristics. AJNR Am J Neuroradiol 18:647–653

Deshaies EM, Bagla S, Agner C, Boulos AS (2005) Determination of filling volumes in HydroCoil-treated aneurysms by using three-dimensional computerized tomography angiography. Neurosurg Focus 18:E5

Devoto MH, Egbert JE, Tomsick TA, Kulwin DR (1997) Acute exophthalmos during treatment of a cavernous sinus-dural fistula through the superior ophthalmic vein. Arch Ophthalmol 115:823–824

Duffner F, Ritz R, Bornemann A, Freudenstein D, Wiendl H, Siekmann R (2002) Combined therapy of cerebral arteriovenous malformations: histological differences between a non-adhesive liquid embolic agent and n-butyl 2-cyanoacrylate (NBCA). Clin Neuropathol 21:13–17

Elhammady MS, Wolfe SQ, Farhat H, Moftakhar R, Aziz-Sultan MA (2009) Onyx embolization of carotid-cavernous fistulas. J Neurosurg

Eversbusch (1897) Pulsierender Exophthalmus. Münch med Wochenschr, p 1180

Felber S, Henkes H, Weber W, Miloslavski E, Brew S, Kuhne D (2004) Treatment of extracranial and intracranial aneurysms and arteriovenous fistulae using stent grafts. Neurosurgery 55:631–638; discussion 638–639

Fermand M (1982) Les fistules durales de la loge caverneuse. Paris

Fukami T, Isozumi T, Shiino A, Nakazawa T, Matsuda M, Handa J (1996) [Central retinal vein occlusion after embolization for spontaneous carotid cavernous sinus fistula]. No Shinkei Geka 24:749–753

Gaba RC, Ansari SA, Roy SS, Marden FA, Viana MA, Malisch TW (2006) Embolization of intracranial aneurysms with hydrogel-coated coils versus inert platinum coils: effects on packing density, coil length and quantity, procedure performance, cost, length of hospital stay, and durability of therapy. Stroke 37:1443–1450

Gal G, Schuetz A, Unterlauft J, Solimosy L, Benndorf G (in press) Transarterial onyx embolization of a DCSF using indirect flow control. AJNR Am J Neuroradiol

Gandhi CD, Meyer SA, et al. (2008). Neurologic complications of inferior petrosal sinus sampling. AJNR Am J Neuroradiol 29(4):760–765.

Gercken U, Lansky AJ, Buellesfeld L, et al. (2002) Results of the Jostent coronary stent graft implantation in various clinical settings: procedural and follow-up results. Catheter Cardiovasc Interv 56:353–360

Geremia G, Bakon M, Brennecke L, Haklin M, Silver B (1997) Experimental arteriovenous fistulas: treatment with silicone-covered metallic stents. AJNR Am J Neuroradiol 18:271–277

Gianturco C, Anderson JH, Wallace S (1975) Mechanical devices for arterial occlusion. Am J Roentgenol Radium Ther Nucl Med 124:428–435

Gioulekas J, Mitchell P, Tress B, McNab AA (1997) Embolization of carotid cavernous fistulas via the superior ophthalmic vein. Aust N Z J Ophthalmol 25:47–53

Gobin P, Duckwiler G, Guglielmi G (2000) Endovascular techniques in the treatment of carotid-cavernous fistulas. In: Eisenberg MB, Al-Mefty O (eds) The cavernous sinus. Lippincott, Philadelphia, pp 209–225

Goldberg RA, Goldey SH, Duckwiler G, Vinuela F (1996) Management of cavernous sinus-dural fistulas. Indications and techniques for primary embolization via the superior ophthalmic vein. Arch Ophthalmol 114:707–714

Golnik KC, Newman SA, Ferguson R (1991) Angle-closure glaucoma consequent to embolization of dural cavernous sinus fistula. AJNR Am J Neuroradiol 12:1074–1076

Gomez F, Escobar W, Gomez AM, Gomez JF, Anaya CA (2007) Treatment of carotid cavernous fistulas using covered stents: midterm results in seven patients. AJNR Am J Neuroradiol 28:1762–1768

Goto K, Goto K (1997) The "Kuru-Kuru-Technique" for catheterization of the cavernous sinus. In: WFITN-Meeting, Val d`Isere, France, 1997

Goto K, Sidipratomo P, Ogata N, Inoue T, Matsuno H (1999) Combining endovascular and neurosurgical treatments of high-risk dural arteriovenous fistulas in the lateral sinus and the confluence of the sinuses. J Neurosurg 90:289–299

Gounis MJ, Lieber BB, Wakhloo AK, Siekmann R, Hopkins LN (2002) Effect of glacial acetic acid and ethiodized oil concentration on embolization with N-butyl 2-cyanoacrylate: an in vivo investigation. AJNR Am J Neuroradiol 23:938–944

Graves VB, Partington CR, Rufenacht DA, Rappe AH, Strother CM (1990) Treatment of carotid artery aneurysms with platinum coils: an experimental study in dogs. AJNR Am J Neuroradiol 11:249–252

Gregoire A, Portha C, Cattin F, Vuillier F, Moulin T, Bonneville JF (2002) [Symptomatic venous congestion of the brain stem after embolization for dural fistula of the cavernous sinus]. J Neuroradiol 29:183–188

Grossman RI, Sergott RC, Goldberg HI, et al. (1985) Dural malformations with ophthalmic manifestations: results of particulate embolization in seven patients. AJNR Am J Neuroradiol 6:809–813

Guglielmi G, Vinuela F, Briganti F, Duckwiler G (1992) Carotid-cavernous fistula caused by a ruptured intracavernous aneurysm: endovascular treatment by electrothrombosis with detachable coils. Neurosurgery 31:591–596; discussion 596-597

Guglielmi G, Vinuela F, Duckwiler G, Dion J, Stocker A (1995) High-flow, small-hole arteriovenous fistulas: treatment with electrodetachable coils. AJNR Am J Neuroradiol 16:325–328

Gupta N, Kikkawa DO, Levi L, Weinreb RN (1997) Severe vision loss and neovascular glaucoma complicating superior ophthalmic vein approach to carotid-cavernous sinus fistula [see comments]. Am J Ophthalmol 124:853–855

Halbach VV, Higashida RT, Hieshima GB, Reicher M, Norman D, Newton TH (1987) Dural fistulas involving the cavernous sinus: results of treatment in 30 patients. Radiology 163:437–442

Halbach VV, Higashida RT, Hieshima GB, Hardin CW, Yang PJ (1988) Transvenous embolization of direct carotid cavernous fistulas. AJNR Am J Neuroradiol 9:741–747

Halbach VV, Higashida RT, Hieshima GB, Hardin CW, Pribram H (1989a) Transvenous embolization of dural fistulas involving the cavernous sinus. AJNR Am J Neuroradiol 10:377–383

Halbach VV, Higashida RT, Hieshima GB, Hardin CW (1989b) Embolization of branches arising from the cavernous portion of the internal carotid artery. AJNR Am J Neuroradiol 10:143–150

Halbach VV, Higashida RT, Barnwell SL, Dowd CF, Hieshima GB (1991a) Transarterial platinum coil embolization of carotid-cavernous fistulas. AJNR Am J Neuroradiol 12:429–433

Halbach VV, Higashida RT, Dowd CF, Barnwell SL, Hieshima GB (1991b) Management of vascular perforations that occur during neurointerventional procedures. AJNR Am J Neuroradiol 12:319–327

Halbach VV, Higashida RT, Hieshima GB, David CF (1992) Endovascular therapy of dural fistulas. In: Vinuela F, Halbach VV, Dion JE (eds) Interventional neuroradiology. Raven Press, New York, pp 29–38

Halbach VV, Dowd CF, Higashida RT, et al. (1997) Transvenous coil Treatment of CCF. In: Tomsick T (ed) Carotid cavernous fistula. Digital Educational Publishing, Cincinnati, pp 163–176

Halbach VV, Dowd CF, Higashida RT, Balousek PA, Urwin RW (1998) Preliminary experience with an electrolytically detachable fibered coil. AJNR Am J Neuroradiol 19:773–777

Hanafee WN, Shiu PC, Dayton GO (1968) Orbital venography. Am J Roentgenol Radium Ther Nucl Med 104:29–35

Hanaoka M, Satoh K, Satomi J, et al. (2006) Microcatheter pull-up technique in the transvenous embolization of an isolated sinus dural arteriovenous fistula. Technical note. J Neurosurg 104:974–977

Hanneken AM, Miller NR, Debrun GM, Nauta HJ (1989) Treatment of carotid-cavernous sinus fistulas using a detachable balloon catheter through the superior ophthalmic vein. Arch Ophthalmol 107:87–92

Hara T, Hamada J, Kai Y, Ushio Y (2002) Surgical transvenous embolization of a carotid-cavernous dural fistula with cortical drainage via a petrosal vein: two technical case reports. Neurosurgery 50:1380–1383; discussion 1383–1384

Hasuo K, Mizushima A, Matsumoto S, et al. (1996) Type D dural carotid-cavernous fistula. Results of combined treatment with irradiation and particulate embolization. Acta Radiol 37:294–298

Hayashi K, Kitagawa N, Morikawa M, et al. (2008) [Difficult cannulation of the superior ophthalmic vein in the treatment of cavernous sinus dural arteriovenous fistula: two case reports]. No Shinkei Geka 36:165–170

Hayreh SS, Zimmerman MB, Kimura A, Sanon A (2004) Central retinal artery occlusion. Retinal survival time. Exp Eye Res 78:723–736

He HW, Jiang CH, Wu ZX, Li YX, Lu XL, Wang ZC (2008) Transvenous embolization with a combination of detachable coils and Onyx for a complicated cavernous dural arteriovenous fistula. Chin Med J (Engl) 121:1651–1655

Henkes H, Nahser HC, Berg-Dammer E, Weber W, Lange S, Kuhne D (1998) Endovascular therapy of brain AVMs prior to radiosurgery. Neurol Res 20:479–492

Henkes H, Kirsch M, Mariushi W, Miloslavski E, Brew S, Kuhne D (2004) Coil treatment of a fusiform upper basilar trunk aneurysm with a combination of „kissing" neuroform stents, TriSpan-, 3D- and fibered coils, and permanent implantation of the microguidewires. Neuroradiology 46:464–468

Heuser RR, Woodfield S, Lopez A (1999) Obliteration of a coronary artery aneurysm with a PTFE-covered stent: endoluminal graft for coronary disease revisited. Catheter Cardiovasc Interv 46:113–116

Hosobuchi Y (1975) Electrothrombosis of carotid-cavernous fistula. J Neurosurg 42:76–85

Hou Y (1993) Observations and measurements of the valves of the orbital veins. Chung Hua Yen 29:171–173

Hung RK, Loh C, Goldstein L (2005) Selective use of electrolytic detachable and fibered coils to embolize a wide-neck giant splenic artery pseudoaneurysm. J Vasc Surg 41:889–892

Inagawa T, Yano T, Kamiya K (1986) Acute aggravation of traumatic carotid-cavernous fistula after venography through the inferior petrosal sinus. Surg Neurol 26:383–386

Iwasaki M, Murakami K, Tomita T, Numagami Y, Nishijima M (2006) Cavernous sinus dural arteriovenous fistula complicated by pontine venous congestion. A case report. Surg Neurol 65:516–518; discussion 519

Jack CR, Jr., Forbes G, Dewanjee MK, Brown ML, Earnest F (1985) Polyvinyl alcohol sponge for embolotherapy: particle size and morphology. AJNR Am J Neuroradiol 6:595–597

Jacobs JM, Parker GD, Apfelbaum RI (1993) Deflation of detachable balloons in the cavernous sinus by percutaneous puncture. AJNR Am J Neuroradiol 14:175–177

Jahan R, Gobin YP, Glenn B, Duckwiler GR, Vinuela F (1998) Transvenous embolization of a dural arteriovenous fistula of the cavernous sinus through the contralateral pterygoid plexus. Neuroradiology 40:189–193

Jahan R, Murayama Y, Gobin YP, Duckwiler GR, Vinters HV, Vinuela F (2001) Embolization of arteriovenous malformations with Onyx: clinicopathological experience in 23 patients. Neurosurgery 48:984–995; discussion 995–987

Jansen O, Dorfler A, Forsting M, et al. (1999) Endovascular therapy of arteriovenous fistulae with electrolytically detachable coils. Neuroradiology 41:951–957

Jordan O, Doelker E, Rufenacht DA (2005) Biomaterials used in injectable implants (liquid embolics) for percutaneous filling of vascular spaces. Cardiovasc Intervent Radiol 28:561–569

Kai Y, Hamada JI, Morioka M, Yano S, Ushio Y (2004) Brain stem venous congestion due to dural arteriovenous fistulas of the cavernous sinus. Acta Neurochir (Wien) 146:1107-1111; discussion 1111–1112

Kazekawa K, Iko M, Sakamoto S, et al. (2003) Dural AVFs of the cavernous sinus: transvenous embolization using a direct superficial temporal vein approach. Radiat Med 21:138–141

Kerber CW, Bank WO, Horton JA (1978) Polyvinyl alcohol foam: prepackaged emboli for therapeutic embolization. AJR Am J Roentgenol 130:1193–1194

Kerber CW, Bank WO, Cromwell LD (1979) Cyanoacrylate occlusion of carotid-cavernous fistula with preservation of carotid artery flow. Neurosurgery 4:210–215

Kim DJ, Kim DI, Suh SH, et al. (2006) Results of transvenous embolization of cavernous dural arteriovenous fistula: a single-center experience with emphasis on complications and management. AJNR Am J Neuroradiol 27:2078–2082

King WA, Hieshima GB, Martin NA (1989) Venous rupture during transvenous approach to a carotid-cavernous fistula. Case report. J Neurosurg 71:133–137

Kirsch M, Henkes H, Liebig T, et al. (2006) Endovascular management of dural carotid-cavernous sinus fistulas in 141 patients. Neuroradiology 48:486–490

Kiyosue H, Hori Y, Okahara M, et al. (2004a) Treatment of intracranial dural arteriovenous fistulas: current strategies based on location and hemodynamics, and alternative techniques of transcatheter embolization. Radiographics 24:1637–1653

Kiyosue H, Mori H, Matsumoto S, et al. (2004b) Clinical use of a new mechanical detachable coil system for percutaneous intravenous embolization of cavernous sinus dural arteriovenous fistulas. Radiat Med 22:143–147

Kiyosue H, Hori Y, Matsumoto S, et al. (2005) Shapability, memory, and luminal changes in microcatheters after steam shaping: a comparison of 11 different microcatheters. AJNR Am J Neuroradiol 26:2610-2616

Klisch J, Schipper J, Husstedt H, Laszig R, Schumacher M (2001) Transsphenoidal computer-navigation-assisted deflation of a balloon after endovascular occlusion of a direct carotid cavernous sinus fistula. AJNR Am J Neuroradiol 22:537–540

Klisch J, Huppertz HJ, Spetzger U, Hetzel A, Seeger W, Schumacher M (2003) Transvenous treatment of carotid cavernous and dural arteriovenous fistulae: results for 31 patients and review of the literature. Neurosurgery 53:836–856

Klurfan P, Gunnarsson T, Shelef I, terBrugge KG, Willinsky RA (2006) Transvenous treatment of cranial dural AVFs with hydrogel coated coils. Interventional Neuroradiology 12:319–326

Kocer N, Kizilkilic O, Albayram S, Adaletli I, Kantarci F, Islak C (2002) Treatment of iatrogenic internal carotid artery laceration and carotid cavernous fistula with endovascular stent-graft placement. AJNR Am J Neuroradiol 23:442–446

Koebbe CJ, Horowitz M, Jungreis C, Levy E, Pless M (2003) Alcohol embolization of carotid-cavernous indirect fistulae. Neurosurgery 52:1111–1115; discussion 1115–1116

Komiyama M, Morikawa K, Fu Y, Yagura H, Yasui T, Baba M (1990) Indirect carotid-cavernous sinus fistula: transvenous embolization from the external jugular vein using a superior ophthalmic vein approach. A case report. Surg Neurol 33:57–63

Krisht AF, Burson T (1999) Combined pretemporal and endovascular approach to the cavernous sinus for the treatment of carotid-cavernous dural fistulae: technical case report. Neurosurgery 44:415–418

Kuettner C, Goetz F, Kramer FJ, Brachvogel P (2006) Interdisciplinary treatment of carotid cavernous fistulas via the superior ophthalmic vein. Mund Kiefer Gesichtschir 10:56–62

Kupersmith MJ, Berenstein A, Choi IS, Warren F, Flamm E (1988) Management of nontraumatic vascular shunts involving the cavernous sinus. Ophthalmology 95:121–130

Kuwayama N, Endo S, Kitabayashi M, Nishijima M, Takaku A (1998) Surgical transvenous embolization of a cortically draining carotid cavernous fistula via a vein of the sylvian fissure. AJNR Am J Neuroradiol 19:1329–1332

Labbe D, Courtheoux P, Rigot-Jolivet M, Compere JF, Theron J (1987) [Bilateral dural carotid-cavernous fistula. Its treatment by way of the superior ophthalmic vein]. Rev Stomatol Chir Maxillofac 88:120–124

Lanzas MG, Maravi E, Maso J, Hernandez-Abenza J (1996) [Low flow cavernous sinus fistula. Treatment by highly selective embolization]. Rev Neurol 24:452–455

Lasjaunias P, Berenstein A (1987) Dural arteriovenous malformation. Springer, Berlin Heidelberg New York

Laurent A, Wassef M, Chapot R, et al. (2005) Partition of calibrated tris-acryl gelatin microspheres in the arterial vasculature of embolized nasopharyngeal angiofibromas and paragangliomas. J Vasc Interv Radiol 16:507–513

Lee CY, Yim MB, et al. (2008) Mechanical detachment of Guglielmi detachable coils after failed electrolytic detachment: rescue from a technical complication. Neurosurgery 63(4 Suppl 2):293–294; discussion 294.)

Leibovitch I, Modjtahedi S, Duckwiler GR, Goldberg RA (2006) Lessons learned from difficult or unsuccessful cannulations of the superior ophthalmic vein in the treatment of cavernous sinus dural fistulas. Ophthalmology 113:1220–1226

Li T, Duan C, Wang Q, et al. (2002) [Endovascular embolization of cerebral arteriovenous malformation]. Zhonghua Yi Xue Za Zhi 82:654–656

Link J, Feyerabend B, Grabener M, et al. (1996) Dacron-covered stent-grafts for the percutaneous treatment of carotid aneurysms: effectiveness and biocompatibility – experimental study in swine. Radiology 200:397–401

Liu HM, Huang YC, Wang YH (2000a) Embolization of cerebral arteriovenous malformations with n-butyl-2-cyanoacrylate. J Formos Med Assoc 99:906–913

Liu HM, Huang YC, Wang YH, Tu YK (2000b) Transarterial embolisation of complex cavernous sinus dural arteriovenous fistulae with low-concentration cyanoacrylate. Neuroradiology 42:766–770

Liu HM, Wang YH, Chen YF, Cheng JS, Yip PK, Tu YK (2001) Long-term clinical outcome of spontaneous carotid cavernous sinus fistulae supplied by dural branches of the internal carotid artery. Neuroradiology 43:1007–1014

Lv X, Jiang C, et al. (2008) Results and complications of transarterial embolization of intracranial dural arteriovenous fistulas using Onyx-18. J Neurosurg 109(6):1083–1090

Lv X, Jiang C, Li Y, Wu Z (2009) Percutaneous transvenous packing of cavernous sinus with Onyx for cavernous dural arteriovenous fistula. Eur J Radiol 71:356–362

Lv XL, Li YX, Liu AH, et al. (2008) A complex cavernous sinus dural arteriovenous fistula secondary to covered stent placement for a traumatic carotid artery-cavernous sinus fistula: case report. J Neurosurg 108:588–590

Macho JM, Guelbenzu S, Barrena R, Valles V, Ibarra B, Valero P (1996) [Carotid cavernous fistula: endovascular therapy]. Rev Neurol 24:59–64

Malek AM, Halbach VV, Higashida RT, Phatouros CC, Meyers PM, Dowd CF (2000) Treatment of dural arteriovenous malformations and fistulas. Neurosurg Clin N Am 11:147–166, ix

Manelfe C, Berenstein A (1980) [Treatment of carotid cavernous fistulas by venous approach. Report of one case]. J Neuroradiol 7:13–19

Manelfe C, Djindjian R, Picard L (1976) [Embolization by femoral catheterization of tumors supplied by the external carotid artery. 40 cases]. Acta Radiol Suppl 347:175–186

Marden FA, Sinha Roy S, Malisch TW (2005) A novel approach to direct carotid cavernous fistula repair: Hydro-Coil-assisted revision after balloon reconstruction. Surg Neurol 64:140–143; discussion 143

Mawad M, Klucznik R, Boniuk M (1996) Endovascular treatment of dural arteriovenous malformations of the cavernous sinus with GDC (abstract). Neuroradiology 38:319

Men S, Ozturk H, Hekimoglu B, Sekerci Z (2003) Traumatic carotid-cavernous fistula treated by combined transarterial and transvenous coil embolization and associated cavernous internal carotid artery dissection treated with stent placement. Case report. J Neurosurg 99:584–586

Menacho (1907) Ann. d` oculist. In: Soc. opth. hispano-americ.; 1907 15.-16. April; Madrid, p 295

Meyers PM, Halbach VV, Dowd CF, et al. (2002) Dural carotid cavernous fistula: definitive endovascular management and long-term follow-up. Am J Ophthalmol 134:85–92

Miller DL, Doppman JL, Peterman SB, Nieman LK, Oldfield EH, Chang R (1992) Neurologic complications of petrosal sinus sampling. Radiology 185:143–147

Miller NR (2007) Diagnosis and management of dural carotid-cavernous sinus fistulas. Neurosurg Focus 23:E13

Miller NR, Monsein LH, Debrun GM, Tamargo RJ, Nauta HJ (1995) Treatment of carotid-cavernous sinus fistulas using a superior ophthalmic vein approach. J Neurosurg 83:838–842

Mironov A (1994) Pathogenetical consideration of spontaneous dural arteriovenous fistulas (DAVFs). Acta Neurochir (Wien) 131:45–58

Mironov A (1998) Selective transvenous embolization of dural fistulas without occlusion of the dural sinus. AJNR Am J Neuroradiol 19:389–391

Mizuno T, Kai Y, Todaka T, Morioka M, Hamada J, Ushio Y (2001) [Treatment of spontaneous carotid-cavernous fistula by the transvenous approach via the facial and angular route]. No Shinkei Geka 29:961–964

Monsein LH, Debrun GM, Miller NR, Nauta HJ, Chazaly JR (1991) Treatment of dural carotid-cavernous fistulas via the superior ophthalmic vein. AJNR Am J Neuroradiol 12:435–439

Moron FE, Klucznik RP, Mawad ME, Strother CM (2005) Endovascular treatment of high-flow carotid cavernous fistulas by stent-assisted coil placement. AJNR Am J Neuroradiol 26:1399–1404

Morse SS, Clark RA, Puffenbarger A (1990) Platinum microcoils for therapeutic embolization: nonneuroradiologic applications. AJR Am J Roentgenol 155:401–403

Morsi H, Benndorf G, Klucznik R, Mawad M (2004) Transvenous occlusion of a dural cavernous sinus fistula using a new expandable hydrogel-platinum coil (Hydrocoil®). Interventional Neuroradiology 10:151–154

Mounayer C, Piotin M, Spelle L, Moret J (2002) Superior petrosal sinus catheterization for transvenous embolization of a dural carotid cavernous sinus fistula. AJNR Am J Neuroradiol 23:1153–1155

Mounayer C, Hammami N, Piotin M, et al. (2007) Nidal embolization of brain arteriovenous malformations using Onyx in 94 patients. AJNR Am J Neuroradiol 28:518–523

Mullan S (1974) Experiences with surgical thrombosis of intracranial berry aneurysms and carotid cavernous fistulas. J Neurosurg 41:657–670

Mullan S (1979) Treatment of carotid-cavernous fistulas by cavernous sinus occlusion. J Neurosurg 50:131–144

Murugesan C, Saravanan S, Rajkumar J, Prasad J, Banakal S, Muralidhar K (2008) Severe pulmonary oedema following therapeutic embolization with Onyx for cerebral arteriovenous malformation. Neuroradiology 50:439–442

Naesens R, Mestdagh C, Breemersch M, Defreyne L (2006) Direct carotid-cavernous fistula: a case report and review of the literature. Bull Soc Belge Ophtalmol (299):43–54

Naito I, Magarisawa S, Wada H (2002) Facial vein approach approach by direct puncture at the base of the mandible for dural carotid cavernous fistula. Interventional Neuroradiology 8:67–70

Nakamura M, Tamaki N, Kawaguchi T, Fujita S (1998) Selective transvenous embolization of dural carotid-cavernous sinus fistulas with preservation of sylvian venous outflow. Report of three cases. J Neurosurg 89:825–829

Nemoto S, Mayanagi Y, Kirino T (1997) Endovascular treatment of the cavernous dural arterio-venous fistula. Interventional Neuroradiology 3[Suppl1]:136

Nesbit GM, Barnwell SL (1998) The use of electrolytically detachable coils in treating high-flow arteriovenous fistulas. AJNR Am J Neuroradiol 19:1565–1569

Nogueira RG, Dabus G, Rabinov JD, et al. (2008) Preliminary experience with onyx embolization for the treatment of intracranial dural arteriovenous fistulas. AJNR Am J Neuroradiol 29:91–97

Oishi H, Arai H, Sato K, Iizuka Y (1999) Complications associated with transvenous embolisation of cavernous dural arteriovenous fistula. Acta Neurochir (Wien) 141:1265–1271

Ong CK, Wang LL, Parkinson RJ, Wenderoth JD (2009) Onyx embolisation of cavernous sinus dural arteriovenous fistula via direct percutaneous transorbital puncture. J Med Imaging Radiat Oncol 53:291–295

Peterson E, Valberg J, Whittingham D (1969) Electrically induced thrombosis of the cavernous sinus in the treatment of carotid-cavernous-fistula. In: Drake C, Duvoisin R (eds) Fourth International Congress of Neurological Surgery. Ninth International Congress of Neurology; 1969; Amsterdam, New York, London: Excerpta Medica

Petrequin (1845) Anevrisme de l'artere opthalm. etc. In: Comptes rendu de l'academie de science. Paris, p 994

Phatouros CC, Higashida RT, Malek AM, Smith WS, Dowd CF, Halbach VV (1999) Embolization of the meningohypophyseal trunk as a cause of diabetes insipidus. AJNR Am J Neuroradiol 20:1115–1118

Phillips B (1832) A series of experiments performed for the purpose of showing that arteries may be obliterated without ligature, compression or the knife. In: Longman. London, p 66

Picard L, Bracard S, Mallet J (1987) Spontaneous dural arteriovenous fistulas. Semin Intervent Radiol 4:210–240

Piotin M, Liebig T, Feste CD, Spelle L, Mounayer C, Moret J (2004) Increasing the packing of small aneurysms with soft coils: an in vitro study. Neuroradiology 46:935–939

Quinones D, Duckwiler G, Gobin PY, Goldberg RA, Vinuela F (1997) Embolization of dural cavernous fistulas via superior ophthalmic vein approach. AJNR Am J Neuroradiol 18:921–928

Qureshi AI, Luft AR, Sharma M, Guterman LR, Hopkins LN (2000) Prevention and treatment of thromboembolic and ischemic complications associated with endovascular procedures: Part II – Clinical aspects and recommendations. Neurosurgery 46:1360-1375; discussion 1375–1366

Raffi L, Simonetti L, Cenni P, Leonardi M (2007) Use of Glubran 2 acrylic glue in interventional neuroradiology. Neuroradiology 49:829–836

Redekop G, Marotta T, Weill A (2001) Treatment of traumatic aneurysms and arteriovenous fistulas of the skull base by using endovascular stents. J Neurosurg 95:412–419

Rezende MT, Piotin M, Mounayer C, Spelle L, Abud DG, Moret J (2006) Dural arteriovenous fistula of the lesser sphenoid wing region treated with Onyx: technical note. Neuroradiology 48:130–134

Rhoton A (2002) The cavernous sinus, the cavernous venous plexus and the carotid collar. Neurosurgery 51:375–410

Ridley (1695) The anatomy of the brain. Smith and Walford, London

Robinson DH, Song JK, Eskridge JM (1999) Embolization of meningohypophyseal and inferolateral branches of the cavernous internal carotid artery. AJNR Am J Neuroradiol 20:1061–1067

Roy D, Raymond J (1997) The role of transvenous embolization in the treatment of intracranial dural arteriovenous fistulas. Neurosurgery 40:1133-1141; discussion 1141–1134

Sadato A, Wakhloo AK, Hopkins LN (2000) Effects of a mixture of a low concentration of n-butylcyanoacrylate and ethiodol on tissue reactions and the permanence of arterial occlusion after embolization. Neurosurgery 47:1197-1203; discussion 1204–1195

Satomi J, Satoh K, Matsubara S, Nakajima N, Nagahiro S (2005) Angiographic changes in venous drainage of cavernous sinus dural arteriovenous fistulae after palliative transarterial embolization or observational management: a proposed stage classification. Neurosurgery 56:494-502; discussion 494–502

Sattler H (1880) Pulsirender Exophthalmus. In: Graefe A, Saemisch T (eds) Handbuch der Gesamten Augenheilkunde. Engelmann, Leipzig, pp 745–948

Sattler H (1905) Ueber ein neues Verfahren bei der Behandlung des pulsierenden Exophthalmus. Klin Monatsbl f Augenheilk 4:1–6

Sattler H (1930) Pulsirender Exophthalmus. In: Graefe A, Saemisch T (eds) Handbuch der Gesamten Augenheilkunde. Springer, Berlin, pp 745–948

Schmidbauer JM, Voges M, Schwerdtfeger K, Ruprecht KW (2001) Embolization of dural carotid cavernous sinus fistulas via the sylvian vein in 2 patients. Ophthalmologe 98:766–770

Schuknecht B, Simmen D, Yuksel C, Valavanis A (1998) Tributary venosinus occlusion and septic cavernous sinus thrombosis: CT and MR findings. AJNR Am J Neuroradiol 19:617–626

Scialfa G, Scotti G (1985) Superselective injection of polyvinyl alcohol microemboli for the treatment of cerebral arteriovenous malformations. AJNR Am J Neuroradiol 6:957–960

Scott JA, De Nardo AJ, Horner T, Liepzig T, Payner T (1997) Facial venous access to the cavernous region AV-fistulas: a safe and reliable technique. In: ASITN/WFITN Scientific Conference; Sept.13-16; New York, p 99

Serbinenko FA (1974) Balloon catheterization and occlusion of major cerebral blood vessels. J Neurosurg 41:125–145

Sergott RC, Grossman RI, Savino PJ, Bosley TM, Schatz NJ (1987) The syndrome of paradoxical worsening of dural-cavernous sinus arteriovenous malformations. Ophthalmology 94:205–212

Seyer H, Honegger J, Schott W, et al. (1994) Raymond's syndrome following petrosal sinus sampling. Acta Neurochir (Wien) 131:157–159

Shaibani A, Rohany M, Parkinson R, et al. (2007) Primary treatment of an indirect carotid cavernous fistula by injection of N-butyl cyanoacrylate in the dural wall of the cavernous sinus. Surg Neurol 67:403–408; discussion 408

Shiu PC, Hanafee WN, Wilson GH, Rand RW (1968) Cavernous sinus venography. Am J Roentgenol Radium Ther Nucl Med 104:57–62

Siniluoto T, Seppanen S, Kuurne T, Wikholm G, Leinonen S, Svendsen P (1997) Transarterial embolization of a direct carotid cavernous fistula with Guglielmi detachable coils. AJNR Am J Neuroradiol 18:519–523

Song DL, Leng B, Xu B, Wang QH, Chen XC, Zhou LF (2007) [Clinical experience of 70 cases of cerebral arteriovenous malformations embolization with Onyx, a novel liquid embolic agent]. Zhonghua Wai Ke Za Zhi 45:223–225

Sonier CB, De Kersaint-Gilly A, Viarouge MP, Auffray-Calvier E, Cottier JP, Laffont J (1995) [Dural fistula of the cavernous sinus. Clinical and angiographic aspects. Results of particulate intravascular treatment]. J Neuroradiol 22:289–300

Stoesslein F, Ditscherlein G, Romaniuk PA (1982) Experimental studies on new liquid embolization mixtures (histoacryl-lipiodol, histoacryl-panthopaque). Cardiovasc Intervent Radiol 5:264–267

Strother C (2001) Electrothrombosis of saccular aneurysms via endovascular approach: part 1 and part 2. AJNR Am J Neuroradiol 22:1011–1012

Sturrock ND, Jeffcoate WJ (1997) A neurological complication of inferior petrosal sinus sampling during investigation for Cushing's disease: a case report. J Neurol Neurosurg Psychiatry 62:527–528

Suzuki S, Lee DW, Jahan R, Duckwiler GR, Vinuela F (2006) Transvenous treatment of spontaneous dural carotid-cavernous fistulas using a combination of detachable coils and Onyx. AJNR Am J Neuroradiol 27:1346–1349

Szwarc IA, Carrasco CH, Wallace S, Richli W (1986) Radiopaque suspension of polyvinyl alcohol foam for embolization. AJR Am J Roentgenol 146:591–592

Tahon F, Salkine F, Amsalem Y, Aguettaz P, Lamy B, Turjman F (2008) Dural arteriovenous fistula of the anterior fossa treated with the Onyx liquid embolic system and the Sonic microcatheter. Neuroradiology 50:429–432

Takahashi A, Yoshimoto T, Kawakami K, Sugawara T, Suzuki J (1989) Transvenous copper wire insertion for dural arteriovenous malformations of cavernous sinus. J Neurosurg 70:751–754

Takazawa H, Kubo M, Kuwayama N, et al. (2005) [Dural arteriovenous fistula involving the cavernous sinus as the cause of intracerebral venous hemorrhage: a case report]. No Shinkei Geka 33:143–147

Taki W, Yonekawa Y, Iwata H, Uno A, Yamashita K, Amemiya H (1990) A new liquid material for embolization of arteriovenous malformations. AJNR Am J Neuroradiol 11:163–168

Taptas JN (1982) The so-called cavernous sinus: a review of the controversy and its implications for neurosurgeons. Neurosurgery 11:712–717

Teng MM, Guo WY, Lee LS, Chang T (1988a) Direct puncture of the cavernous sinus for obliteration of a recurrent carotid-cavernous fistula. Neurosurgery 23:104–107

Teng MM, Guo WY, Huang CI, Wu CC, Chang T (1988b) Occlusion of arteriovenous malformations of the cavernous sinus via the superior ophthalmic vein. AJNR Am J Neuroradiol 9:539–546

Teng MM, Chang T, Pan DH, et al. (1991) Brainstem edema: an unusual complication of carotid cavernous fistula. AJNR Am J Neuroradiol 12:139–142

Teng MM, Lirng JF, Chang T, et al. (1995) Embolization of carotid cavernous fistula by means of direct puncture through the superior orbital fissure. Radiology 194:705–711

Terada T, Nakamura Y, Nakai K, et al. (1991) Embolization of arteriovenous malformations with peripheral aneurysms using ethylene vinyl alcohol copolymer. Report of three cases. J Neurosurg 75:655–660

Terada T, Kinoshita Y, Yokote H, et al. (1996) Clinical use of mechanical detachable coils for dural arteriovenous fistula [see comments]. AJNR Am J Neuroradiol 17:1343–1348

Testut I, Jacob O (1977) Apparato della vista. In: Trattoria di Anatomia Topografica. Utet, Torino, pp 377–478

Theaudin M, Saint-Maurice JP, Chapot R, et al. (2007) Diagnosis and treatment of dural carotid-cavernous fistulas: a consecutive series of 27 patients. J Neurol Neurosurg Psychiatry 78:174–179

Tomsick TA (1997a) Treatment of CCF via the superior ophthalmic vein: coil occlusion. In: Tomsick TA (ed) Carotid cavernous fistula. Digital Educational Publishing, pp 183–188

Tomsick TA (1997b) Types B, C, D (dural) CCF: etiology, prevalence and natural History. In: Tomsick TA (ed) Carotid cavernous fistula. Digital Educational Publishing, Cincinnati, pp 59–73

Toulgoat F, Mounayer C, Tulio Salles Rezende M, et al. (2006) [Transarterial embolisation of intracranial dural arteriovenous malformations with ethylene vinyl alcohol copolymer (Onyx18)]. J Neuroradiol 33:105–114

Tress BM, Thomson KR, Klug GL, Mee RR, Crawford B (1983) Management of carotid-cavernous fistulas by surgery combined with interventional radiology. Report of two cases. J Neurosurg 59:1076–1081

Troffkin NA, Given CA, 2nd. (2007) Combined transarterial N-butyl cyanoacrylate and coil embolization of direct carotid-cavernous fistulas. Report of two cases. J Neurosurg 106:903–906

Uchino A, Kato A, Kuroda Y, Shimokawa S, Kudo S (1997) Pontine venous congestion caused by dural carotid-cavernous fistula: report of two cases. Eur Radiol 7:405–408

Uflacker R, Lima S, Ribas GC, Piske RL (1986) Carotid-cavernous fistulas: embolization through the superior ophthalmic vein approach. Radiology 159:175–179

van Rooij WJ, Sluzewski M, Beute GN (2007) Brain AVM embolization with Onyx. AJNR Am J Neuroradiol 28:172–177; discussion 178

Velpeau A (1931) Memoire sur la piqure ou làcupuncture des arteres dans le traitement desanevrisme. Gaz Med Paris 2:1–4

Venturi C, Bracco S, Cerase A, et al. (2003) Endovascular treatment of a cavernous sinus dural arteriovenous fistula by transvenous embolisation through the superior ophthalmic vein via cannulation of a frontal vein. Neuroradiology 45:574–578

Vinuela F, Fox AJ, Debrun GM, Peerless SJ, Drake CG (1984) Spontaneous carotid-cavernous fistulas: clinical, radiological, and therapeutic considerations. Experience with 20 cases. J Neurosurg 60:976–984

Vinuela F, Duckwiler G, Guglielmi G (1997) CCF: types B, C, and D arterial embolisation. In: Tomsick TA (ed) Carotid cavernous fistula. Digital Educational Publishing, Cincinnati, pp 155–163

Wakhloo AK, Perlow A, Linfante I, et al. (2005) Transvenous n-butyl-cyanoacrylate infusion for complex dural carotid cavernous fistulas: technical considerations and clinical outcome. AJNR Am J Neuroradiol 26:1888–1897

Wakhloo AK (2009) Endovascular treatment of dural carotid cavernous sinus fistulas. J Neuroophthalmol 29:1–2

Warakaulle DR, Aviv RI, Niemann D, Molyneux AJ, Byrne JV, Teddy P (2003) Embolisation of spinal dural arteriovenous fistulae with Onyx. Neuroradiology 45:110–112

Weber W, Henkes H, Berg-Dammer E, Esser J, Kuhne D (2001) Cure of a direct carotid cavernous fistula by endovascular stent deployment. Cerebrovasc Dis 12:272–275

Weber W, Kis B, Siekmann R, Jans P, Laumer R, Kuhne D (2007a) Preoperative embolization of intracranial arteriovenous malformations with Onyx. Neurosurgery 61:244-252; discussion 252–244

Weber W, Kis B, Siekmann R, Kuehne D (2007b) Endovascular treatment of intracranial arteriovenous malformations with onyx: technical aspects. AJNR Am J Neuroradiol 28:371–377

Weill A, Ducos V, Cognard C, Piotin M, et al. (1998) Corrosion of Tungsten spirals: a disturbing finding. Intervent Neuroradiol 4:337–340

White JB, Layton KF, Evans AJ, et al. (2007) Transorbital puncture for the treatment of cavernous sinus dural arteriovenous fistulas. AJNR Am J Neuroradiol 28:1415–1417

Winslow JB (1734) Exposition Anatomique de la Structure du Corpus Humain. London

Wladis EJ, Peebles TR, Weinberg DA (2007) Management of acute orbital hemorrhage with obstruction of the ophthalmic artery during attempted coil embolization of a dural arteriovenous fistula of the cavernous sinus. Ophthal Plast Reconstr Surg 23:57–59

Workman M, Dion J, Tong FC, Cloft HJ (2002) Treatment of trapped CCF by direct puncture of the caversnous sinus by infraocular trans-SOF approach. Interventional Neuroradiology 8:299–304

Wright KC, Anderson JH, Gianturco C, Wallace S, Chuang VP (1982) Partial splenic embolization using polyvinyl alcohol foam, dextran, polystyrene, or silicone. An experimental study in dogs. Radiology 142:351–354

Yamashita K, Taki W, Nishi S, et al. (1993) Transvenous embolization of dural caroticocavernous fistulae: technical considerations. Neuroradiology 35:475–479

Yang PJ, Halbach VV, Higashida RT, Hieshima GB (1988) Platinum wire: a new transvascular embolic agent. AJNR Am J Neuroradiol 9:547–550

Yoshimura S, Hashimoto N, Kazekawa K, Nishi S, Sampei K (1995) Embolization of dural arteriovenous fistulas with interlocking detachable coils. AJNR Am J Neuroradiol 16:322–324

Yu SC, Cheng HK, Wong GK, Chan CM, Cheung JY, Poon WS (2007) Transvenous embolization of dural carotid-cavernous fistulae with transfacial catheterization through the superior ophthalmic vein. Neurosurgery 60:1032-1037; discussion 1037–1038

Zink WE, Meyers PM, Connolly ES, Lavine SD (2004) Combined surgical and endovascular management of a complex posttraumatic dural arteriovenous fistula of the tentorium and straight sinus. J Neuroimaging 14:273–276

Alternative Treatment Options

With regard to the relatively high rate of spontaneous thrombosis of dural cavernous sinus fistulas (DCSFs) in some studies, a number of investigators consider conservative management the first line of treatment, especially if symptoms are mild, no cortical venous drainage is present and the angiographic evaluation reveals a low-flow shunt. This may include observing and following patients, while they are regularly examined by an ophthalmologist to monitor their visual acuity and IOP. Retroorbital pain may be treated with standard analgesics, diplopia may be coped with by using prism therapy and elevated IOP (if necessary) by administrating topical agents such as Latanoprost for a few weeks (MILLER 2007). Worsening of symptoms may indicate an increase in AV shunting flow, but can be also part of the healing process that is accompanied by thrombosis of the CS and may involve the SOV to some degree. Administration of corticosteroids may help to cope with these symptoms and lessen their severity (SERGOTT et al. 1987). This management may also be useful until elective endovascular treatment is scheduled.

If IOP continues to increase, exophthalmos progresses or chemosis develops, definite occlusion of the AV shunt becomes inevitable. Although conservative management with or without manual compression therapy is recommended by numerous investigators (MILLER 2007; GROVE 1984; PHELPS et al. 1982; DE KEIZER 2003), glaucoma treatment may be insufficient and IOP can be difficult to control (KUPERSMITH et al. 1988).

While anticoagulation is used by some investigators to avoid postoperative thrombosis of the SOV and the central retinal vein, heparin is administered by others to control the thrombosis as part of the natural history of DCSFs. BIANCHI-MARZOLI et al. (1996) recently reported improvement in four patients after low-dose heparin administration, and deterioration in two other patients in whom the heparin was stopped. YOUSRY et al. (1997) observed an interesting case in which the AV shunt completely disappeared following systemic anticoagulation for 3 months. Other viable non-invasive options for conservative management include manual compression and controlled hypotension (see below).

9.1
Spontaneous Thrombosis

Early reports on spontaneous occlusion of CSFs include the monographs from SATTLER (1930), DANDY (1937) and HAMBY (1966), which reported 5.6%–10% occlusion rates. These relatively low numbers are presumably due to the inclusion of a large number of high-flow direct CCFs (PARKINSON 1965, 1987).

SATTLER (1930) reported that although he found occlusion in 18/322 cases (5.6%), this may be an underestimation, because in many treated and untreated cases, the outcome remained unknown. In two traumatic fistulas (0.6%), a slow regression of symptoms was seen without any therapeutic measure. The remaining 16 patients (10 traumatic and six spontaneous) underwent spontaneous thrombosis of the orbital veins, accompanied by severe inflammatory reactions.

Some data suggest that about 30% of the patients in all series show a spontaneous occlusion of the AV shunt, although the published material is quite heterogeneous (TOMSICK 1997). For example, NUKUI et al. (1984) and SASAKI et al. (1988) studied 20 and 26 patients, respectively, who were conservatively followed between 4 and 108 months (9 years). A regression of symptoms was noted in 18/20 (90%) and 19/26 (73%) cases, respectively, and was delayed in patients older than 60 years of age, in slow-flow fistulas and in cases with multiple draining veins. There was unfortunately no information on the anatomical outcome and whether disappearance of the symptoms correlated with complete angiographic occlusion. It appeared in these data that closure of the fistulas followed a pattern with a half-life of 18 months (BARCIA-SALORIO et al 2000).

Data on the "natural history" of DCSFs are in general incomplete, because some "spontaneous" occlusions occurred following cerebral angiography (NUKUI et al. 1984; SASAKI et al. 1988; TAKAHASHI et al. 1989; NEWTON and HOYT 1970; VOIGT 1978; SEEGER et al. 1980), manual compression therapy (KAI et al. 2007), or in groups of patients undergoing transarterial embolizations (KURATA et al. 1998; SATOMI et al. 2005).

Angiography-triggered occlusion was likely the underlying cause in the case of an AVF involving the IPS with symptoms mimicking a CSF, observed by the author. Following a bagatelle trauma, the 72-year-old gentleman developed right eye redness, chemosis and increasing diplopia due to 6th and 4th CN palsy. The DSA revealed a small arteriovenous shunt at the posterior CS, but mainly involving the IPS and exclusively supplied by bilateral dural branches of the APA. This patient, shown in Case Illustration XII, is one of the rare cases I have observed with a possibly related trauma in their history (see Sect. 5.2.5.). Due to a respiratory infection on initial admission, endovascular therapy had to be postponed and was rescheduled 6 days later. The angiogram at the beginning of this endovascular procedure showed a partial occlusion of the AV shunt, while the symptoms had regressed (Fig. 9.1). This occlusion was confirmed by a second control angiogram 3 months later, when the clinical exam demonstrated complete resolution of conjunctival engorgement and diplopia.

Such "spontaneous" occlusions of CSFs that follow intravascular contrast administrations have been described by several investigators (SEEGER et al. 1980; NISHIJIMA et al. 1985; ISFORT 1967; VOIGT et al. 1971; YAMAMOTO et al. 1995; POTTER 1954; PARSONS et al. 1954; FROMM and HABEL 1965; TOENNIS and SCHIEFER 1959).

VOIGT et al. (1971) reported the spontaneous occlusion of a bilateral DSCF associated with cerebral angiography. The authors questioned the role of vasoconstrictor effect of the contrast medium triggering local thrombosis. They favored a theory of stasis following changes in pressure gradients during angiography. The role of general anesthesia was explained usually accompanied by a lowered systemic blood pressure. The latter theory has been considered by others as well (POTTER 1954; PARSONS et al. 1954) and reveals some evidence in fistula occlusions achieved by induced hypotension (see below) (DE MIQUEL et al. 2005; ORNAQUE et al. 2003).

In 1980, SEEGER et al. presented six patients with spontaneous occlusions. They discussed the role of contrast medium that likely induces thrombosis by direct interaction with the endothelium that causes aggregation of platelets and white blood cells, accelerating the clumping of erythrocytes and thrombosis.

PHELPS et al. (1982), reporting the red eye shunt syndrome, observed six (32%) fistula occlusions. In this group, 7/19 patients (37%) underwent angiography, three of them (43%) obliterated soon after the exam. Spontaneous occlusions may be accompanied by exacerbation or regression of the symptoms, because a fresh thrombus in the CS may redirect AV shunting flow towards the SOV, increasing IOP. That is why a paradoxical increase of symptoms due to ongoing thrombosis can be seen in some of the patients (SEEGER et al. 1980; HAWKE et al. 1989; GROSSMAN et al. 1985). HAWKE et al. (1989) documented that a patient with initially isolated posterior drainage developed new ophthalmological symptoms after the IPS thrombosed. KURATA et al. (1993) emphasized that patients with singular SOV drainage and likely existing IPS thrombosis, demonstrated more significant chemosis and exophthalmos than those with more open efferent veins.

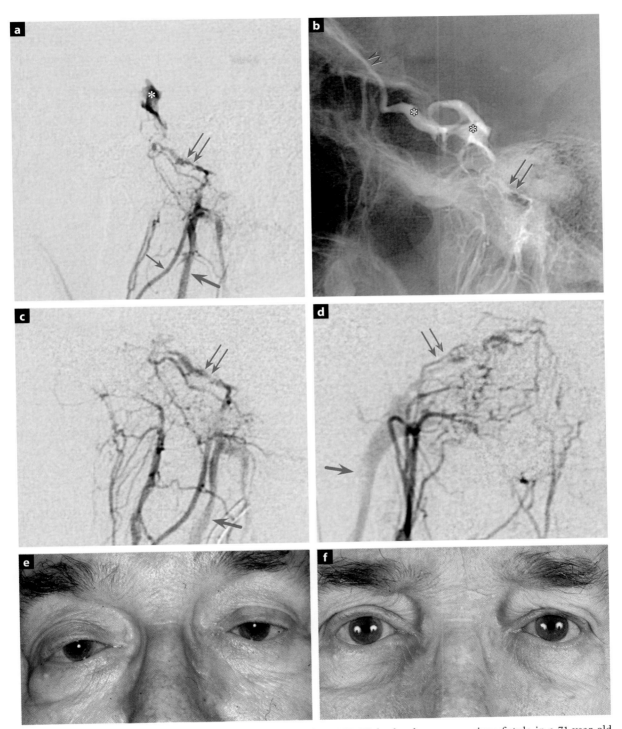

Fig. 9.1 a–f. Case Illustration XII: Spontaneous occlusion of a DCSF. Right dural cavernous sinus fistula in a 71-year-old male who presented 10/98 with eye redness and diplopia due to 4th and 6th nerve palsy. **a, b** The initial DSA (selective APA injection, lateral view) revealed a small AV shunt mainly involving the right IPS (*double arrow*), supplied exclusively by the APA (*arrow*) and draining into the ipsilateral CS (*asterisk*) and SOV (*arrowheads*) as well as into the IJV (*thick arrow*) **c, d** EVT had to be postponed due to a respiratory infection and was rescheduled 6 days later. At that time, the DSA showed an occlusion of the CS and a residual AV shunting into the IJV (lateral and AP views). His symptoms had improved. **e** Diplopia due to 4th and 6th nerve palsies on admission that resolved completely over a 3-month FU period (**f**)

As already discussed by Sattler (1930), spontaneous occlusion of a CSF, if caused by thrombosis of the ophthalmic and the retinal veins, may cause visual loss when the fistula "heals" (Sergott et al. 1987; Knudtzon 1950; Miki et al. 1988; Suzuki et al. 1989). Choroidal effusion with increasing orbital congestion and cranial neuropathy due to uncontrolled spontaneous thrombosis may occur, leading to dramatic worsening of the symptoms.

When patients undergo TVO, transient aggravation of symptoms due to induced CS thrombosis affecting orbital veins may also occur. However, the amount of thrombus forming within the CS and potentially causing pseudoinflammatory deleterious effects is much larger during spontaneous occlusions. In addition, the elevated venous pressure is at least partially reduced as long as coils are effectively blocking the AV shunting flow. While aiming for this reduction of the venous pressure has priority during endovascular management, excessive thrombosis of the SOV and the central retinal vein must be avoided. Thus, anticoagulation for 48 h, even after complete transvenous coil packing of the CS, may be required (Kupersmith et al. 1988; Tomsick 1997).

The author utilized an anticoagulation regimen if embolization visibly accelerated thrombosis, or when a patient developed progressive symptoms or increasing intraocular pressure post procedure.

9.2
Manual Compression Therapy

The most widely used non-invasive conservative management of CSF patients is intermittent manual compression therapy (MCT). This involves a simple maneuver to reduce the arterial inflow and the venous outflow of CSF and was used by Scott in 1834 for diagnostic purposes. In 1846, Vanzetti from Padua communicated verbally a simple digital compression between heart and tumor, and taught the same from 1853 onwards.

Gioppi, one of Vanzetti's peers and a professor of ophthalmology in Padua, reported in 1856 a more defined technique (Gioppi 1858). He described a 42-year-old female with pulsating exophthalmos that developed after pregnancy, who was treated with 15 min of intermittent external compression. After 4 days, pulsation and bruit were diminished. After 6 days, a slight recovery of the complete vision loss was observed.

Gioppi suggested four different compression techniques: (1) from anterior to posterior between the two heads of the sternocleidomastoid muscles, (2) using the 2nd, 3rd, and 4th finger of the left hand along the lateral margin and the thumb along the medial margin of the sternocleidomastoid muscle, while the right hand pushes the head to the involved side, (3) using the second finger at the anterior margin of the sternocleidomastoid muscle posteriorly and slightly lateral, and (4) slight compression against the larynx or trachea. While performing part of the compression therapy herself, Gioppi's patient was not always able to grab the carotid and had to use his third technique.

Two years later, in Verona, Scaramuzza treated a patient using intermittent digital compression for no longer than 4–5 min, 5–6 times per day over 18 days. After the 3rd day, partial regression was noted. After 16 days, complete regression of the exophthalmus occurred, and after 26 days complete "healing" of the fistula was observed [reported by Vanzetti (1858)].

Sattler (1880) mentioned that carotid compression might be less effective in traumatic fistulas than in idiopathic cases (spontaneous CSFs). In 29 patients in which digital or instrumental carotid compression was performed, only four (14%) showed success. Despite these somewhat discouraging results, he suggested beginning treatment of pulsating exophthalmus with a compression method, either digital, using a mechanical instrument (Fig. 2.7) or via a tourniquet, as was utilized by Nelaton. In spontaneous ("idiopathic") cases, such intermittent compression may already be sufficient to achieve improvement or cure. Bed rest and other measures to lower systemic blood pressure were also recommended. In 1924, Locke mentioned a rate of cure or improvement of 37% in 27 patients and 26.4% in 106 patients, respectively.

Manual compression therapy as a treatment option for CSFs has been advocated by numerous investigators as a minimally invasive procedure since. It was further supported by the encouraging experience reported by Halbach et al. in 1987. Patients with DCSFs were asked to compress their carotid arteries and jugular veins with their opposite hands while sitting for 10s several times per hour. When tolerated, the compression was increased 30s over a total of 4–6 weeks. Patients with angiographic evidence of cortical venous drainage were excluded. The authors achieved complete cure in 7/23 (30%) patients undergoing carotid jugular compression, while the

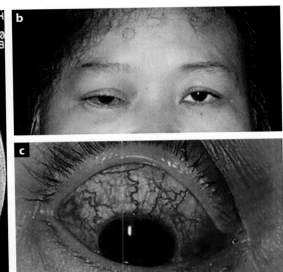

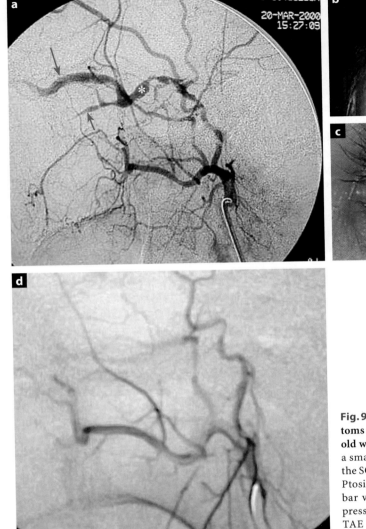

Fig. 9.2 a–d. Case Illustration XIII. Worsening symptoms after manual compression of the SOV in a 53-year-old woman. a ECA injection, lateral view demonstrates a small AV shunt at the CS (*asterisk*), filling very slowly the SOV (*arrow*) and partially the IOV (*short arrow*). **b, c** Ptosis and significant eye redness with dilated epibulbar veins indicating deterioration caused by the compression of the SOV. **d** ECA injection, lateral view after TAE with PVA particles shows complete occlusion of the AV shunt. (Courtesy: W. Lim, Singapore)

same group (HIGASHIDA et al. 1986) achieved occlusion of direct CCFs in eight of 48 patients (17%).

Since then, this occlusion rate (approximately one third) has been cited in numerous publications. Thus, manual compression therapy has been recommended as an adjunct or even alternate treatment option. In 1992, complete cure was reported in 34% of 53 patients (HALBACH et al. 1992). Quite surprisingly, in the most recent report on DCSF patients from the same investigators, including all patients from 1986–2000, manual compression therapy was curative in only one patient (0.74%), while it was used as an adjunctive technique to endovascular treatment in 34%. This raises questions about its true efficacy. Unfortunately, no validation of its actual treatment effects exists to date.

KAI et al. (2007) studied a group of 23 patients, achieving complete resolution of symptoms in eight cases (35%). The authors identified lower ocular pressure, a shorter interval between symptom onset and compression treatment and venous drainage solely via the superior ophthalmic vein without involvement of the inferior petrosal sinus as factors that would favor a complete occlusion achievable by this technique. Because the patients in this group underwent MRI/MRA for FU, it is not clear in how many cases anatomical occlusions were indeed achieved. It is also known that resolution of ophthalmological symptoms may occur while the venous drainage is rerouted posteriorly towards cortical veins, in fact creating, a more dangerous lesion.

Manual compression therapy was performed in only four of the author's patients, who were considered compliant. The therapy was performed as described previously. Although all patients reported some improvement over this period of time, none showed a notable reduction of the shunt flow in the control angiogram. In one patient, after 3 weeks compressing the SOV in the eye angle, an increase in symptoms occurred. All patients underwent subsequent endovascular therapy, which lead to complete anatomical and clinical cure.

The effect of compression therapy appears unpredictable, as there is no control on the change in the venous pressure or flow during this treatment. In fact, aggravation of symptoms such as retinal hemorrhage, induced by central retinal vein occlusion and hypoxic retinopathy preceding the spontaneous regression of spontaneous cavernous sinus fistulas has been reported (MIKI et al. 1988).

One factor that may possibly influence the efficacy of manual compression therapy is the dependence of the cerebral venous drainage on the posture of the patient. Recent studies have shown that the internal jugular vein serves as a main drainage vessel only in the supine position. When standing, this function is mainly taken over by the vertebral venous plexus (GISOLF et al. 2004). Consequently, compression of the IJV when standing or sitting will likely be less effective.

Thus, until controlled data become available, it remains doubtful whether or not manual compression therapy is in fact effective as a single treatment modality. There is otherwise no question that reducing the flow and pressure within the AV shunting communication is a useful adjunctive therapy to both transarterial and transvenous occlusion techniques. If consequently performed by a cooperative patient, it may even be effective as a single (conservative) treatment modality in direct CCF (SPINNATO et al. 1997).

Some investigators recommend the external compression of the SOV at the inner eye angle before the vein joins the angular vein (LOCKE 1924) or direct ocular compression (ISAMAT et al. 2000). Blocking the venous outflow in a case with anterior drainage may have similar untoward effects, causing either aggravation of ophthalmic symptoms or rerouting the venous flow and inducing cortical drainage.

Case Illustration XIII is an example in which manual SOV compression resulted in worsening of the symptoms (Fig. 9.2). The patient had to undergo subsequent transarterial embolization with particles to reduce the AV shunting.

9.3
Controlled Hypotension

Case Report VIII (Fig. 9.3.)

A 72-year-old woman presented with right chemosis, exophthalmos, glaucoma and loss of visual acuity of 0.05 in the right eye (09/17/1999). Performing manual carotid compressions, she felt subjectively better and had a visual acuity of 0.2 (09/29/1999). An angiogram was performed on 10/11/99, revealing a dural AVF of the left CS fed by the left meningohypophyseal trunk and draining into the right SOV. Ophthalmologically, there was a suspicion of a superior ophthalmic vein thrombosis and thus, low-molecular heparin was prescribed. Two weeks later, left retinal hemorrhages were found, and anticoagulation was suspended. Treatment of the AVF became necessary. Since embolization of the small ICA pedicle was considered dangerous, controlled hypotension was proposed. Her BP was lowered from 160/100 to 80/45, while the mean arterial pressure was maintained around 60 mmHg using propofol and nitroglycerine. After 8 min of hypotension, the patient suddenly noticed that her vision was clearer and better. In fact, her visual acuity improved over several days and was 0.4 in the RE and 0.5 in the LE at ophthalmologic FU 3 weeks later. The glaucoma treatment was stopped. The patient remained symptom free until 5 years later at the end of 2004.

The induction of controlled hypotension for occlusion of DCSFs is a new approach, which has not been widely communicated (DE MIQUEL et al. 2001; 2005; ORNAQUE et al. 2003). The first description was from DE MIQUEL et al. (2001), who reported eight consecutive patients with DAVFs, including two DCSFs who underwent 30 min of controlled hypotension using sodium nitroprussiate, esmolol and nitroglycerine. In four patients, the symptoms lessened; in two, angiography confirmed occlusion.

In 2003, ORNAQUE et al. reported a DAVF of the transverse sinus for which controlled hypotension was performed by lowering the blood pressure under general anesthesia utilizing propofol. The authors discovered the possible influence of low blood pressure on DAVF thrombosis and occlusion in a patient with hypovolemic shock due to massive hematoma after unsuccessful transfemoral embolization. A total of 13 patients were treated without general anesthesia using various blood pressure lowering drugs, including nitroglycerin, urapidil and nitroprussi-

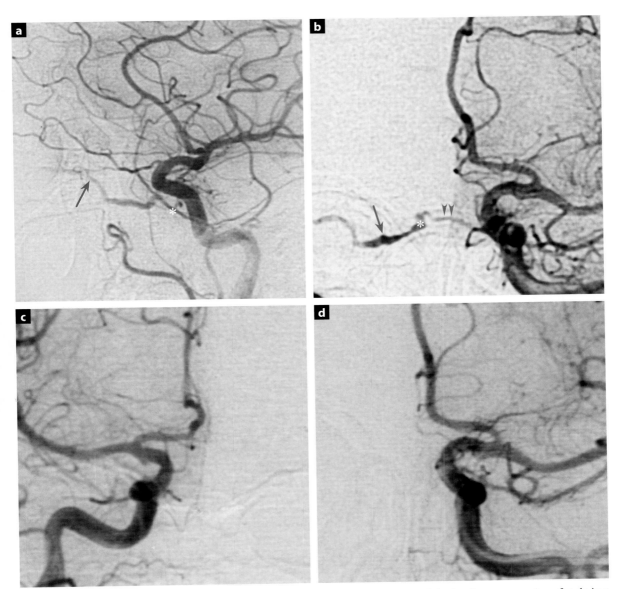

Fig. 9.3 a–d. Case Report VIII: Occlusion of a DCSF using controlled hypotension. Right dural cavernous sinus fistula in a 72-year-old woman who presented with chemosis and high intraocular pressure. The fistula evolved over several weeks and lead to a partial superior ophthalmic vein thrombosis. **a, b** Left ICA injection, lateral view shows a small transsellar branch (*arrowheads*) that supplies an AV shunt at the right CS (*asterisk*). The fistula drains only anteriorly leading to a sluggish filling of the right SOV (*arrow*). **c, d** Right and left ICA injection, AP view: Complete resolution of the AV shunt after a total of 30 min of controlled hypotension. (Courtesy: M. des Angeles de Miquel, Barcelona)

ate. This group included spinal AVFs ($n = 3$), DAVFs ($n = 2$) and DCSFs ($n = 8$). In four patients (31%), complete occlusion was accomplished, in four others the symptoms improved, in five (over 38%), there were no changes. The mean arterial pressure was lowered to 50–60 mmHg for a duration of 30–45 min. The patient reported by the authors was a 48-year-old male with a DAVF of the right transverse sinus initially undergoing partial embolization and was planned for surgery. Controlled hypotension during the general anesthesia using propofol for 90 min resulted in complete occlusion prior to surgical exploration. An arteriogram confirmed that the fistula remained closed for 15 days and during the following 6 months.

Propofol (Diprivan) is a short-acting anesthetic agent with minimal side effects commonly used for induction or maintenance of general anesthesia and for sedation of ICU patients. It is very feasible to induce short periods of controlled hypotension.

Recently, the same group reported on the long-term outcome in 14 patients with DAVFs in different locations (DE MIQUEL et al. 2005). Five patients (36%) had very low-flow DAVFs and four (28.5%) resolved completely. In one patient, the procedure could not be completed due to hemodynamic instability of the patient. Out of three patients (21.4%) with low AV shunt flow, two (14.3%) occluded and one (7%) significantly improved. In five cases (35.7%) where flow was considered medium, two (14.3%) occluded, one (7%) improved and one remained unchanged. In one high-flow fistula, the flow changed only slightly and the patient had to be treated by coil occlusion. The authors concluded that controlled hypotension is a good adjuvant tool in low-flow DAVFs and may lead to long-term occlusions.

The Case Report (Fig. 9.3) shown here depicted that induced hypotension can be effective, and thus should be considered in cases with small or residual AV shunting. The pathophysiological mechanism is still not fully understood and the role of venous pressure in the pathogenesis of DAVF is discussed in more detail in Chap. 5. Pressure changes, atmospheric or systemic blood pressure, especially when combined with intraarterial contrast application, may possibly promote thrombosis and occlusion in DCSFs, particularly in low-flow cases.

KUPERSMITH et al. (1988) reported two cases where occlusion of DCSF occurred following air travel. One patient developed choroidal detachment and 3rd nerve palsy; the angiogram performed the next day showed complete thrombosis of the DCSF, ipsilateral CS and SOV. Another patient demonstrated complete resolution of the bruit and bilateral 6th nerve paresis after a plane flight confirming angiographic occlusion the next day.

It is noteworthy that the role of lowered systemic blood pressure has been considered a causative factor in cases that developed "spontaneous" occlusion following angiographic procedures performed under general anesthesia (POTTER 1954; PARSONS et al. 1954). ECHOLS and JACKSON (1959) observed occasional success with bilateral carotid compression under hypothermia. They reported a 25-year-old patient with a traumatic CCF who underwent hypothermia with a body temperature reaching 85.5°F, leading to unattainable blood pressure and peripheral pulsation for 45 min. During this period, the bruit could not be heard, but returned after 1 h, although to a lesser degree. POTTER (1954), who observed a case of spontaneous cure after a period of severe hemorrhage and syncope, also discussed the role of hypotension for occlusion of CCFs.

Due to the general risks of adverse reactions associated with anesthetic drugs, the use of controlled hypotension under general anesthesia as a single means for therapeutic management is probably not justified. It appears, however, reasonable as an adjuvant measure in patients undergoing endovascular treatment, excluding those with cerebrovascular, renal or cardiac insufficiency.

9.4
Radiotherapy

Irradiation for treatment of a dural cavernous sinus fistula was introduced by BARCIA-SALORIO et al. in 1979 in a 65-year old patient suffering from chemosis, exophthalmos and diplopia. After stereotactic radiosurgery using a single cobalt source delivering 40 Gy, the patient was reported to be symptom free 2 months later. In 1982, BITOH et al. (1982), successfully treated two patients with ^{60}Co (Cobalt) using 32 Gy and 30 Gy achieving complete occlusion, documented by angiography. Radiotherapy of DCSFs has been advocated ever since as an alternate treatment option for DCSFs by several groups (BITOH et al. 1982; SODERMAN et al. 2006; HIRAI et al. 1998; YASUNAGA et al. 1987; YAMADA et al. 1984; PIEROT et al. 1992; MIZUNO et al. 1989; HASUO et al. 1996; GUO et al. 1998; MORIKI et al. 1993; ONIZUKA et al. 2003; POLLOCK et al. 1999). Conventional fractionated irradiation via linear accelerator (BARCIA-SALORIO et al. 2000; HIRAI et al. 1998; YASUNAGA et al. 1987), and more recently, a ^{60}Co source (BITOH et al. 1982; YAMADA et al. 1984) via gamma knife radiosurgery (GUO et al. 1998; MORIKI et al. 1993; POLLOCK et al. 1999; LINK et al. 1996) have been suggested.

In some series, radiotherapy has been combined with pre- or post-procedure embolization (HIRAI et al. 1998; PIEROT et al. 1992; HASUO et al. 1996; POLLOCK et al. 1999; LINK et al. 1996).

In 1982, BARCIA-SALORIO et al. described gamma knife radiosurgery in four patients as a "bloodless operation without anesthesia, with no surgical risk that can be applied independent of age and general condition of the patient".

Twelve years later, the same group (BARCIA-SALORIO et al. 1994a), reported 25 patients treated with a modified ^{60}Co therapy, applying an estimated dose of 30–40 Gy. In all, 22 patients had DCSFs, of which 20 (90%) could be completely obliterated during an average post-treatment period of 7.5 months (2–20). In Type B fistulas, a 100% occlusion rate was achieved, compared to 75% and 86% in Type C and D fistulas, respectively. In two cases, retreatment was required to achieve complete occlusion. The same group later reported an improved overall occlusion rate in DCSFs of 91.6% (Type B: 100%, Type C: 90%) in 24 patients, after a mean follow-up interval of 7.2 months (BARCIA-SALORIO et al. 2000). There were no post-irradiation injuries to the optical or ocular motor nerves. The occlusive effect is explained by early endothelial swelling that may evolve to partial or complete thrombosis associated with basal membrane rupture, necrosis, interstitial exudates and leukocyte invasion. This leads to fibroblastic and endothelial cell proliferation resulting in intimal hyperplasia that can be observed after application of doses between 30–40 Gy (JOANES et al. 1991). Hyaline degeneration may occur after 60 Gy (JOANES et al. 1998).

LINK et al. (1996) reported on results of gamma knife therapy in 29 patients with DAVFs, among which 10 were located at the CS. In 17 (59%) of these patients who had either pial or cortical drainage, additional transarterial embolization within 48 h after radiotherapy was performed. A reduction of the AV shunting by transarterial embolization may decrease the risk of bleeding in the latency period (post-treatment period) in these high-risk patients. By using this combined approach, complete occlusion was accomplished in 75% and a partial occlusion in 29.5% of cases. One of the patients with DCSF developed a mild transient expressive aphasia after the embolization.

HASUO et al. (1996) reported on nine patients with type D fistulas, who were treated with 30 Gy after particulate embolization, achieving immediate improvement and complete resolution of the symptoms over 4–19 months. The authors recommend this treatment as the therapy of choice in type D fistulas with only mild symptoms. GUO et al. (1998) recently published a series of 18 patients with DCSFs (B: $n = 1$, C: $n = 7$, D: $n = 10$), who were treated primarily with gamma knife surgery (22–38 Gy). Target levels were kept at 50%–90% isodose, while neural structures such as the optic nerve were kept at 8 Gy. Complete occlusion was achieved in 15 patients (83%). The remaining three showed partial obliteration with no complications or worsening of symptoms observed over a period of 27 months. The authors concluded that gamma knife treatment is a feasible and safe alternative for patients with DCSFs.

HIRAI et al. (1998) reported the use of multifractionated radiation, performed via a linear accelerator administering a total dose of 30 Gy over 15 sessions (2 Gy per session) in all but one patient, who received 40 Gy over 20 sessions. In 12 patients undergoing irradiation alone, cure was achieved in 75% of cases. Two cases with fast-flow fistulas showed no change; one demonstrated occlusion. In all, 14 patients underwent TAE or TVO. In six of these patients, endovascular treatment was combined with irradiation, achieving cure in 12 patients (86%). Two patients with fast-flow type fistulas demonstrated either no change or improvement of symptoms despite undergoing combined treatment. One patient suffered from ischemic stroke after TAE and recovered within 1 year, while another presented with transient epilation following TVO.

POLLOCK et al. (1999) treated 20 DCSFs with either radiosurgery alone ($n = 7$), or radiosurgery followed by particulate transarterial embolization ($n = 13$), achieving improvement of symptoms in 19 (95%), and total angiographic occlusion in 87%. Two patients who did not show initial angiographic occlusion experienced recurrence of the symptoms and underwent repeated TAEs. One patient underwent TVO. None of the patients who demonstrated angiographic occlusion (14/15) showed recurrent symptoms. Three patients (15%) in this group experienced complications: one patient developed a stroke during stereotactic angiography, one developed venous ischemia and another a permanent 6th nerve palsy due to acute CS thrombosis as a consequence of the embolization procedure.

SODERMAN et al. (2006) recently reported on 53 patients with 58 DAVFs treated with gamma knife surgery achieving total occlusion in 68% (angiographically proven obliteration) and significant flow reduction in 24%. Five patients (9%) with DCSFs were included receiving a minimal dose of either 10 Gy or 12 Gy resulting in complete obliteration (Case Illustration XIV). One patient (18.8%) with preexisting 6th nerve palsy received a maximal dose of 50 Gy and developed transient worsening of his symptoms. The entire series also contained a case of late reaction (10 years) with hemorrhage (1.9%), one patient with focal alopecia and two angiography related minor complications.

It is emphasized that DAVFs with cortical venous drainage may not respond to radiation, which is a disadvantage, as these patients have an increased risk of intracranial hemorrhage during the post-treatment period. DCSFs in general may have a lower risk of intracranial hemorrhage than DAVFs in other locations; neurological deficits due to venous congestion may develop during this latency period. Some investigators see this as a major downside of radiosurgery and favor embolization therapy instead (COGNARD et al. 2008). It should also be mentioned that in some cases of DCSFs, the time to occlusion is relatively short compared to the time required for obliteration of cerebral AVMs (HEROS 2006). In one of the largest series to date, 100% of Type B fistulas closed after a mean period of 5.9 months, 75% of Type C fistulas closed after 12.6 months and 85.7% of Type D fistulas closed after 8.16 months (BARCIA-SALORIO et al. 1994a). SODERMAN et al. (2008) reported the same phenomenon, assuming that the location within the dura mater and the usually narrow vessels may play a role in this relatively faster obliteration.

Although complications directly related to radiosurgery of DCSFs are rare, side effects may occur. LAU et al. (2006) reported on paradoxical worsening in a patient with DCSF undergoing radiotherapy who developed signs of SOV thrombosis and central retinal vein occlusion. As the radiation target includes not only the dura mater, but also the venous CS compartments, progressive obliteration in an unpredictable manner might be of general concern. As stressed for other indirect treatment modalities, a benign DCSF may transform into a more aggressive lesion, exposing the patient to increased risk of neurological deficit or intracranial hemorrhage and death. Such an untoward change may occur during the relatively long follow-up period, especially when radiosurgery is used as a single treatment option. To monitor changes in direction of the SOV flow, intermittent imaging follow-up using Doppler ultrasound may be recommended (CHIOU et al. 1998).

Definite occlusion of the AV shunt should be affirmed by intra-arterial DSA rather than MRA, as was recently reported by CHIOU et al. (1998), who successfully treated four patients, one with cortical venous drainage. Small remaining fistulous compartments are not detectable using MR angiography. Although stated otherwise by some investigators relying on symmetric diameters of the SOVs or appearance of the orbital fat tissue (STRUFFERT et al. 2007), MRA was completely unreliable to rule out small AV shunts, especially when draining posteriorly in several of my own cases.

Non-invasive imaging follow-up, if at all, should rather be used for patients undergoing TVO, in whom complete occlusion is mostly achieved at the end of the procedure or will occur within days or weeks post procedure in the majority of cases.

Although undue effects of radiation on the optic or oculomotor nerves have not been reported in patients with DCSFs, they may occur at a rate of 6.3% following radiosurgery of CS tumors (TISHLER et al. 1993). A dose limit of 8–10 Gy appears to be accepted for the optic nerve and the brain stem (GUO et al. 1998; TISHLER et al. 1993; BARCIA-SALORIO et al. 1994b), while such limits for intracavernous cranial nerves remain to be determined (BARCIA-SALORIO et al. 2000).

In summary, radiotherapy of DCSF represents an effective alternative (up to 90%) (BARCIA-SALORIO et al. 2000) and should be considered a valuable complement of the therapeutic spectrum for DCSFs. In selected cases in which endovascular means remain unsuccessful, ineffective, contraindicated or considered too risky, irradiation using a linear accelerator or gamma knife should be considered. In elderly patients with comorbidities, lengthy endovascular procedures under general anesthesia could be avoided, especially when they have already failed in previous sessions. Radiosurgery should focus primarily on small, low-flow shunts and, if possible, be combined with transarterial embolization or manual compression. The efficacy in high-flow lesions or direct CCF appears questionable (BARCIA-SALORIO et al. 2000). Newer data on the natural history seem to indicate that hemorrhage rates for DAVFs with cortical drainage may be lower than previously expected (SODERMAN et al. 2008). Nevertheless, radiotherapy should probably not be considered in those cases, or when neurological manifestation is already evident.

Although not seen by the author, so-called "intractable" cavernous sinus fistulas have been reported by others (LINK et al. 1996; GUERRO et al. 2006). Due to continuous advancement of endovascular tools and devices, improved visualization techniques and enhanced anatomic understanding, their number will also remain relatively small in the future.

9.5
Surgery

Direct surgical treatment of CSFs was the primary treatment modality in the pre-endovascular era; however, it was associated with significant morbidity and mortality (DANDY 1937; SATTLER 1930; LOCKE 1924; HAMBY and GARDNER 1933). Ligation of the ophthalmic veins was successfully performed by Lansdown in 1874 (LANDSDOWN 1875) and repeated by others (SATTLER 1880; LOCKE 1924) during subsequent years. LOCKE (1924) reported a 68.4% cure or improvement rate with this treatment, with a mortality of 5.3%. About 100 years after Ashley Cooper performed the first CCA ligation, De Schweinitz and Holloway reviewed 114 patients communicated in the literature to that date, and found a good outcome in 56%, no improvement in 17.5% and a recurrence rate of 20%. The overall mortality rate was 11.7%. LOCKE (1924) documented cure or improvement in 61.9% of the patients undergoing carotid ligations for treatment of pulsating exophthalmus and a mortality of 14.3%. Because of such high recurrence rates and poor, or even fatal outcomes, ligation of intracranial carotid arteries was proposed by HAMBY and GARDNER in 1933.

The introduction of microsurgical techniques enables direct surgical approaches to the CS for obliteration of direct and indirect CSFs (PARKINSON 1965, 1987; DOLENC 1990; ISAMAT et al. 1986; FRANCIS et al. 1995; VINUELA et al. 1984). ISAMAT et al. (1986) described four patients (three traumatic, one spontaneous), whose CS was exposed via pterional craniotomy allowing the introduction of muscle fragments and/or fibrin sealant. The same authors reported on seven additional patients treated by transmural injection of fibrin sealant into the CS achieving complete occlusion in all, preservation of the ICA in 4/4 cases and observing one transient postoperative hemiparesis (14.2%) (ISAMAT et al. 2000). It is emphasized that control of the hemodynamic condition by placing a temporary clip on the supraclinoid carotid and transient occlusion of the cervical ICA using manual compression or a rubber band can be a useful adjunct.

With the onset of transarterial embolization techniques, several investigators pioneered their use of direct and indirect CSFs (HALBACH et al. 1987; KERBER et al. 1979; MANELFE and BERENSTEIN 1980; BANK et al. 1978; PICARD et al. 1987; CHERMET et al. 1977). Particularly since SERBINENKO's introduc-

tion of balloons for occlusion of direct CCFs in 1974 (SERBINENKO 1974), direct surgical obliteration of CSFs has been increasingly abandoned.

Despite the establishment of EVT as a primary treatment modality today for direct fistulas and indirect fistulas, open surgery of the CS is still considered useful in certain cases (ISAMAT et al. 2000; TU et al. 1997; DAY and FUKUSHIMA 1997; VAN LOVEREN et al. 1991).

In the TU et al. (1997) series, 19/78 (24.3%) patients with type A–D CSFs who initially underwent EVT were definitively treated by subsequent microneurosurgery. The authors reported an occlusion rate of 100% and an ICA patency rate of 94%. Among these 19 patients, three (15.8%) had a DCSF in which either the small fistula size or multiple ECA branches were reported as reasons for failure of endovascular techniques. Interestingly enough, no transvenous techniques were attempted in any of these patients. Eight patients (42%) experienced transient 3rd nerve palsy, while in one patient (5.2%) permanent 6th nerve palsy was noted.

VAN LOEVEREN et al. (1991) performed direct surgery in eight patients with Type A fistulas between 1979 and 1996, achieving complete occlusion in 75% and reduction of the fistulas in 25%. There were immediate postoperative CN deficits in five patients (63%), among whom two were permanent (one patient was lost to long-term FU).

DAY et al. (1997) published a series of nine Type D fistulas treated by a combined extra-intradural approach to the CS and consecutive obliteration of the fistulous communication. In this group, endovascular treatment had been attempted using TAE (DE KEIZER 2003) and transvenous approaches (PHELPS et al. 1982), but failed. It is stated that Type D fistulas represented a "challenge" for endovascular treatment. This may be true for transarterial embolization, but is not for transvenous occlusion techniques using all available routes. It remains unclear to what extent endovascular treatment options were fully explored in some of the cases (Illustrative Case 1). While resolution of the symptoms and angiographic occlusion were complete in 100% of patients, transient diplopia and trigeminal hypoesthesia developed in each patient, resolving over 6 months. In addition, there was a high procedure-related morbidity of 22% [transient hemiparesis in one (11%) and permanent hemiparesis in another (11%)]. The success of this method, which was originally described by MULLAN (1979), relies on superb knowledge of the cavernous triangles while "sensing" how to avoid

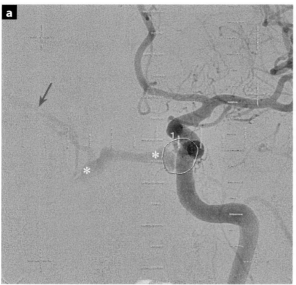

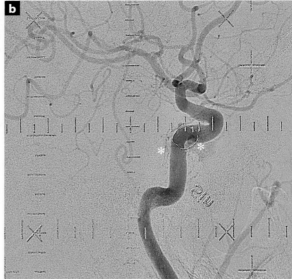

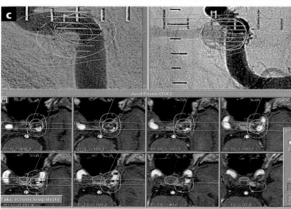

Fig. 9.4 a–e. Case Illustration XIV: Occlusion of a DCSF using radiosurgery. a, b DSA of an 80-year-old gentleman with a red eye on the right side caused by a left DCSF, draining over the midline towards the right CS (*asterisk*) and secondarily into the right Sylvian vein (*red arrow*). A previous endovascular treatment attempt had failed due to technical difficulties to catheterize the IPS and SOV on either side. The target volume was delineated in *white* and indexed with "*1*". **c** Dose planning for gamma knife radiosurgery: The prescription dose was 20 Gy with a maximum dose of 40 Gy (50% isodose), which is a common dose plan. The gamma knife collimators were "plugged" for optimal coverage of the target volume while the radiation dose to the optic nerve was kept below 8 Gy, and thus should not affect the vision of the patient. **d, e** At 24-month follow-up showing occlusion of the AV shunt. The patient had fully recovered from his eye redness within a few months. (Courtesy: M. Soederman, Stockholm)

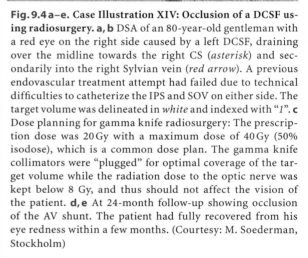

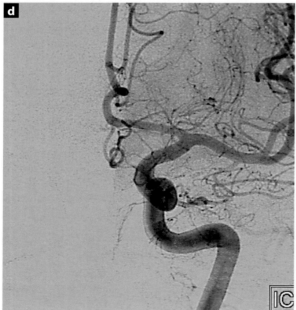

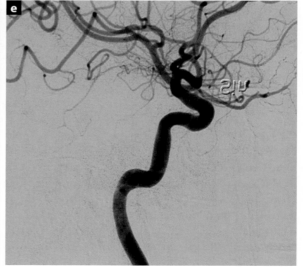

overpacking. The latter can be a problematic matter and appears even in experienced surgical hands not to be completely under control. To prevent overpacking is no less important than avoiding underpacking that will result in persistence of the fistula. These concerns appear to be an inherent problem of direct surgical treatment for DCSFs.

KRISHT et al. (1999) described a pretemporal approach to the anterior cavernous sinus for treatment of an "intractable" CS fistula that could not be treated by transvenous approach because of "thrombosis or absence of the petrosal sinuses". The authors used an extended pterional approach, dissecting the dura in the pretemporal region and drilling the posterior orbital roof to gain access to the anterior extension of the cavernous sinus, where they were able to introduce an atraumatic intravenous cannula. Intraoperative angiography demonstrated complete fistula obliteration after introduction of thrombogenic coils.

The same group (GUERRERO et al. 2006) recently reported another case of an "intractable" Type D fistula using a pretemporal direct approach combined with assisted coiling. The patient was reported to have undergone seven unsuccessful attempts at transarterial and transvenous embolization. The authors' approach represents an elegant surgical technique to overcome the complex anatomy in this region as well as block the fistula flow provided by the ECA branches. In this particular case, however, details of the fistula's angioarchitecture and why attempts at transvenous catheterizations remained unsuccessful are not reported. The only preoperative image shows an early arterial phase instead of a drainage pattern as erroneously mentioned in the text. All other figures show a stepwise increase of the coil packing. The final arteriogram does not allow one to determine whether complete or subtotal occlusion was achieved with any certainty. No follow-up arteriogram was provided. Thus, it remains somewhat questionable whether such "direct open embolization" was indeed indicated, and whether the performed coil packing was sufficient to achieve complete obliteration. Although it is advantageous to be able to target different CS compartments with coils, dense packing may be less easy to achieve while the CS is in fact open and its walls cannot be used as a buttress for the coils.

It can be stated that today so-called "technical challenges" in the EVT of Type D fistulas are mostly manageable with modern transvenous catheterization techniques and sophisticated bi-planar imaging. State-of-the-art endovascular techniques must not be neglected when considering a direct surgical approach in a DCSF. Reported postoperative deficits, particularly with combined operative and technical efforts (general anesthesia, craniotomy, opening of the CS, etc.), have contributed to the current trend of endovascular management (VAN LOVEREN et al. 1991) and recently invalidated the need for direct surgical treatment of DCSFs.

In summary, direct surgery, if at all necessary, should be applied in selected cases only to facilitate endovascular approaches. Cooperation between operating and endovascular colleagues is essential for achieving optimal clinical and anatomical results. Current endovascular tools and high-resolution imaging capabilities have minimized the need for direct surgery in the therapeutic management of DCSFs.

References

Bank WO, Kerber CW, Drayer BP, Troost BT, Maroon JC (1978) Carotid cavernous fistula: endarterial cyanoacrylate occlusion with preservation of carotid flow. J Neuroradiol 5:279–285

Barcia-Salorio JL, Broseta J, Herandez G, Ballester B, Masbout G (1979) Radiosurgical treatment of a carotid-cavernous fistula. Case report. In: Szikla G (ed) Stereotactic cerebral irradiations. Elsevier, Amsterdam, pp 251–256

Barcia-Salorio JL, Herandez G, Broseta J, Gonzalez-Darder J, Ciudad J (1982) Radiosurgical treatment of carotid-cavernous fistula. Appl Neurophysiol 45:520–522

Barcia-Salorio JL, Soler F, Barcia JA, Hernandez G (1994a) Stereotactic radiosurgery for the treatment of low-flow carotid-cavernous fistulae: results in a series of 25 cases. Stereotact Funct Neurosurg 63:266–270

Barcia-Salorio JL, Soler F, Barcia JA, Hernandez G (1994b) Radiosurgery of carotid-cavernous fistulae. Acta Neurochir Suppl 62:10–12

Barcia-Salorio JL, Barcia JA, Soler F (2000) Radiosurgery for Carotid-Cavernous Fistulas. In: M.B. E, Al-Mefty O, eds. The Cavernous Sinus. Philadelphia: Lipincott 227–240

Bianchi-Marszoli S, Righi C, Ciasca P (1996) Low dose heparin therapy for dural cavernous sinus fistulas. Neuroradiology 38:15 (Suppl.)

Bitoh S, Hasegawa H, Fujiwara M, Nakao K (1982) Irradiation of spontaneous carotid-cavernous fistulas. Surg Neurol 17:282–286

Chermet M, Cabanis EA, Debrun G, Haut J (1977) [Carotidocavernous fistula treated with inflatable balloons]. Bull Soc Ophtalmol Fr 77:903–908

Chiou HJ, Chou YH, Guo WY et al. (1998) Verifying complete obliteration of carotid artery-cavernous sinus fistula: role of color Doppler ultrasonography. J Ultrasound Med 17:289–295

Cognard C, Januel AC, Silva NA Jr, Tall P (2008) Endovascular treatment of intracranial dural arteriovenous fistulas with cortical venous drainage: new management using onyx. AJNR Am J Neuroradiol 29:235–241

Dandy W (1937) Carotid-cavernous aneurysms (pulsating exophthalmos). Zentralbl Neurochir 2:77–206

Day JD, Fukushima T (1997) Direct microsurgery of dural arteriovenous malformation type carotid-cavernous sinus fistulas: indications, technique, and results. Neurosurgery 41:1119–1124; discussion 1124–1116

de Keizer R (2003) Carotid-cavernous and orbital arteriovenous fistulas: ocular features, diagnostic and hemodynamic considerations in relation to visual impairment and morbidity. Orbit 22:121–142

de Miquel MA, Mayoral V, Ornaque I, Souto JM, Arruga J, Cambra R (2001) Controlled hypotension as a co-adjuvant treatment in dural very low flow dural fistulae. In: ASNR. Boston 303

de Miquel MA, Cambra R, Ornaque I et al. (2005) Controlled hypotension as an adjuvant treatment for closure of very low flow dural fistulae. Long term outcome. Neuroradiology 47:36–37

Dolenc VV (1990) Surgery of vascular lesions of the cavernous sinus. Clin Neurosurg 36:240–255

Echols DH, Jackson JD (1959) Carotid-cavernous fistula: a perplexing surgical problem. J Neurosurg 16:619–627

Francis PM, Khayata MH, Zabramski JM, Spetzler RF (1995) Carotid cavernous fistulae. Part I: presentation and features. In: Carter LPS, Spetzler RF, Hamilton MG (eds) Neurovascular surgery. McGraw-Hill, NewYork, pp 1049–1059

Fromm H, Habel J (1965) Angiographischer Nachweis eines sackfoermigen Aneurysmas. Nervenarzt 56:170

Gioppi G (1858) Aneurisma dell' arteria oftalmica. Giornale d'oftalmoogia Italiano. Aprile e Maggio

Gisolf J, van Lieshout JJ, van Heusden K, Pott F, Stok WJ, Karemaker JM (2004) Human cerebral venous outflow pathway depends on posture and central venous pressure. J Physiol 560:317–327

Grossman RI, Sergott RC, Goldberg HI et al. (1985) Dural malformations with ophthalmic manifestations: results of particulate embolization in seven patients. AJNR Am J Neuroradiol 6:809–813

Grove AS Jr (1984) The dural shunt syndrome. Pathophysiology and clinical course. Ophthalmology 91:31–44

Guerrero CA, Raja AI, Naranjo N, Krisht AF (2006) Obliteration of carotid-cavernous fistulas using direct surgical and coil-assisted embolization: technical case report. Neurosurgery 58:E382; discussion E382

Guo WY, Pan DH, Wu HM et al. (1998) Radiosurgery as a treatment alternative for dural arteriovenous fistulas of the cavernous sinus. AJNR Am J Neuroradiol 19:1081–1087

Halbach VV, Higashida RT, Hieshima GB, Reicher M, Norman D, Newton TH (1987) Dural fistulas involving the cavernous sinus: results of treatment in 30 patients. Radiology 163:437–442

Halbach VV, Higashida RT, Hieshima GB, David CF (1992) Endovascular therapy of dural fistulas. In: Vinuela F, Halbach VV, Dion JE (eds) Interventional Neuroradiology. Raven Press, New York, pp 29–38

Hamby W (1966) Carotid-cavernous fistula. Springfield, Illinois

Hamby W, Gardner W (1933) Treatment of pulsating exophthalmos with report of 2 cases. Arch Surg 27:676–685

Hasuo K, Mizushima A, Matsumoto S et al. (1996) Type D dural carotid-cavernous fistula. Results of combined treatment with irradiation and particulate embolization. Acta Radiol 37:294–298

Hawke SH, Mullie MA, Hoyt WF, Hallinan JM, Halmagyi GM (1989) Painful oculomotor nerve palsy due to dural-cavernous sinus shunt. Arch Neurol 46:1252–1255

Heros RC (2006) Gamma knife surgery for dural arteriovenous fistulas. J Neurosurg 104:861–863; discussion 865–866

Higashida RT, Hieshima GB, Halbach VV, Bentson JR, Goto K (1986) Closure of carotid cavernous sinus fistulae by external compression of the carotid artery and jugular vein. Acta Radiol Suppl 369:580–583

Hirai T, Korogi Y, Baba Y et al. (1998) Dural carotid cavernous fistulas: role of conventional radiation therapy – long-term results with irradiation, embolization, or both. Radiology 207:423–430

Isamat F, Ferrer E, Twose J (1986) Direct intracavernous obliteration of high flow carotid-cavernous fistulas. J Neurosurg 65:770–775

Isamat F, Twose J, Conesa G (2000) Surgical management of cavernous-carotid fistulas. In: Eisenberg MB, Al-Mefty O (eds) The cavernous sinus. Acomprehensive text. Lipincott, Philadelphia, pp 201–208

Isfort A (1967) [Spontaneous healing of a traumatic carotid artery-cavernous sinus fistula in a child during angiography]. Klin Monatsbl Augenheilkd 150:821–827

Joanes V, Barcia-Salorio JL, Ciudad J (1991) Narrow-beam gamma irradiation used in stereotactic radiosurgery for arteriovenous fistulae. Research in Surgery 3:67–73

Joanes V, Cerda-Nicolas M, Ciudad J, Barcia-Salorio JL (1998) Experimental arterial lesions after narrow-beam gamma irradiation used in stereotactic radiosurgery. Acta Neurochir (Wien) 140:1077–1081

Kai Y, Hamada J, Morioka M, Yano S, Kuratsu J (2007) Treatment of cavernous sinus dural arteriovenous fistulae by external manual carotid compression. Neurosurgery 60:253–257; discussion 257–258

Kerber CW, Bank WO, Cromwell LD (1979) Cyanoacrylate occlusion of carotid-cavernous fistula with preservation of carotid artery flow. Neurosurgery 4:210–215

Knudtzon A (1950) A remarkable case of pulsating exophthalmos in an old patient who recovered spontaneously after bilateral aseptic thrombosis of the cavernous sinus. Acta Ophthalmol 28:363–369

Krisht AF, Burson T (1999) Combined pretemporal and endovascular approach to the cavernous sinus for the treatment of carotid-cavernous dural fistulae: technical case report. Neurosurgery 44:415–418

Kupersmith MJ, Berenstein A, Choi IS, Warren F, Flamm E (1988) Management of nontraumatic vascular shunts involving the cavernous sinus. Ophthalmology 95:121–130

Kurata A, Takano M, Tokiwa K, Miyasaka Y, Yada K, Kan S (1993) Spontaneous carotid cavernous fistula presenting only with cranial nerve palsies. AJNR Am J Neuroradiol 14:1097–1101

Kurata A, Miyasaka Y, Kunii M, et al. (1998) The value of long-term clinical follow-up for cases of spontaneous carotid cavernous fistula. Acta Neurochir (Wien) 140:65–72

Lansdown F (1875) A case of varicose aneurism of the left orbit, cured by ligature of the diseased vessels. Brit M J 1:736&846

Lau LI, Wu HM, Wang AG, Yen MY, Hsu WM (2006) Paradoxical worsening with superior ophthalmic vein thrombosis after gamma knife radiosurgery for dural arteriovenous fistula of cavernous sinus: a case report suggesting the mechanism of the phenomenon. Eye 20:1426–1428

Link MJ, Coffey RJ, Nichols DA, Gorman DA (1996) The role of radiosurgery and particulate embolization in the treatment of dural arteriovenous fistulas. J Neurosurg 84:804–809

Locke C (1924) Intracranial arteriovenous aneurysm or pulsating exophthalmos. Ann Surg 80:1–24

Manelfe C, Berenstein A (1980) [Treatment of carotid cavernous fistulas by venous approach. Report of one case]. J Neuroradiol 7:13–19

Miki T, Nagai K, Saitoh Y, Onodera Y, Ohta H, Ikoma H (1988) [Matas procedure in the treatment of spontaneous carotid cavernous sinus fistula: a complication of retinal hemorrhage]. No Shinkei Geka 16:971–976

Miller NR (2007) Diagnosis and management of dural carotid-cavernous sinus fistulas. Neurosurg Focus 23:E13

Mizuno M, Takahara N, Matsumura H (1989) [Angiographic classification for the selection of treatment of spontaneous carotid-cavernous sinus fistula]. No Shinkei Geka 17:139–146

Moriki A, Mori T, Hirai T (1993) The successful treatment of two carotid cavernous fistula (CCF) cases using the gamma knife. Acta Neurochirurgica 122:140 (Suppl)

Mullan S (1979) Treatment of carotid-cavernous fistulas by cavernous sinus occlusion. J Neurosurg 50:131–144

Newton TH, Hoyt WF (1970) Dural arteriovenous shunts in the region of the cavernous sinus. Neuroradiology 1:71–81

Nishijima M, Iwai R, Horie Y, Oka N, Takaku A (1985) Spontaneous occlusion of traumatic carotid cavernous fistula after orbital venography. Surg Neurol 23:489–492

Nukui H, Shibasaki T, Kaneko M, Sasaki H, Mitsuka S (1984) Long-term observations in cases with spontaneous carotid-cavernous fistulas. Surg Neurol 21:543–552

Onizuka M, Mori K, Takahashi N et al. (2003) Gamma knife surgery for the treatment of spontaneous dural carotid-cavernous fistulas. Neurol Med Chir (Tokyo) 43:477–482; discussion 482–473

Ornaque I, Alonso P, Marti Valeri C et al. (2003) [Spontaneous closure of a intracranial dural arteriovenous fistula by controlled hypotension during a general anesthesia procedure. A case report]. Neurologia 18:746–749

Parkinson D (1965) A surgical approach to the cavernous portion of the carotid artery. Anatomical studies and case report. J Neurosurg 23:474–483

Parkinson D (1987) Carotid cavernous fistula, history and anatomy. In: Dolenc VV d, ed. The cavernous sinus: a multidisciplinary approach to vascular and tumorous lesions. Sprienger-Velag, Wien-New York: pp 3–29

Parsons TC, Guller EJ, Wolff HG, Dunbar HS (1954) Cerebral angiography in carotid cavernous communications. Neurology 4:65–68

Phelps CD, Thompson HS, Ossoinig KC (1982) The diagnosis and prognosis of atypical carotid-cavernous fistula (red-eyed shunt syndrome). Am J Ophthalmol 93:423–436

Picard L, Bracard S, Mallet J (1987) Spontaneous dural arteriovenous fistulas. Semin Intervent Radiol 4:210–240

Pierot L, Poisson M, Jason M, Pontvert D, Chiras J (1992) Treatment of type D dural carotid-cavernous fistula by embolization followed by irradiation. Neuroradiology 34:77–80

Pollock BE, Nichols DA, Garrity JA, Gorman DA, Stafford SL (1999) Stereotactic radiosurgery and particulate embolization for cavernous sinus dural arteriovenous fistulae. Neurosurgery 45:459–466; discussion 466–457

Potter JM (1954) Carotid-cavernous fistula; five cases with spontaneous recovery. Br Med J 4891:786–788

Sasaki H, Nukui H, Kaneko M et al. (1988) Long-term observations in cases with spontaneous carotid-cavernous fistulas. Acta Neurochir (Wien) 90:117–120

Satomi J, Satoh K, Matsubara S, Nakajima N, Nagahiro S (2005) Angiographic changes in venous drainage of cavernous sinus dural arteriovenous fistulae after palliative transarterial embolization or observational management: a proposed stage classification. Neurosurgery 56:494–502; discussion 494–502

Sattler H (1880) Pulsirender Exophthalmus. In: Graefe A, Saemisch T (eds) Handbuch der Gesamten Augenheilkunde. Engelmann, Leipzig, pp 745–948

Sattler H (1930) Pulsirender Exophthalmus. In: Graefe A, Saemisch T (eds) Handbuch der Gesamten Augenheilkunde. Springer-Verlag, Berlin Heidelberg New York, pp 745–948

Seeger JF, Gabrielsen TO, Giannotta SL, Lotz PR (1980) Carotid-cavernous sinus fistulas and venous thrombosis. AJNR Am J Neuroradiol 1:141–148

Serbinenko FA (1974) Balloon catheterization and occlusion of major cerebral blood vessels. J Neurosurg 41:125–145

Sergott RC, Grossman RI, Savino PJ, Bosley TM, Schatz NJ (1987) The syndrome of paradoxical worsening of dural-cavernous arteriovenous malformations. Ophthalmology 94:205–212

Soderman M, Edner G, Ericson K et al. (2006) Gamma knife surgery for dural arteriovenous shunts: 25 years of experience. J Neurosurg 104:867–875

Soderman M, Pavic L, Edner G, Holmin S, Andersson T (2008) Natural history of dural arteriovenous shunts. Stroke 39:1735–1739

Spinnato S, Talacchi A, Perini S, Dolenc V, Bricolo A (1997) Conservative treatment of a traumatic low-flow carotid-cavernous sinus fistula: a case report. Acta Neurochir (Wien) 139:1181–1184

Struffert T, Grunwald IQ, Mucke I, Reith W (2007) [Complex carotid cavernous sinus fistulas Barrow type D: endovascular treatment via the ophthalmic vein, imaging control with standardized MRI, long-term results]. Rofo 179:401–405

Suzuki Y, Kase M, Yokoi M, Arikado T, Miyasaka K (1989) Development of central retinal vein occlusion in dural carotid-cavernous fistula. Ophthalmologica 199:28–33

Takahashi A, Yoshimoto T, Kawakami K, Sugawara T, Suzuki J (1989) Transvenous copper wire insertion for dural arteriovenous malformations of cavernous sinus. J Neurosurg 70:751–754

Tishler RB, Loeffler JS, Lunsford LD et al. (1993) Tolerance of cranial nerves of the cavernous sinus to radiosurgery. Int J Radiat Oncol Biol Phys 27:215–221

Toennis W, Schiefer H (1959) Zirkulationstoerungen des Gehirns im Serien Angiogram. Springer, Berlin-Goettingen-Heidelberg

Tomsick TA (1997) Typ B,C, & D CCF: etiology, prevalence and natural history. In: Tomsick TA (ed) Carotid cavernous fistula. Digital Educational Publishing 59–73

Tu YK, Liu HM, Hu SC (1997) Direct surgery of carotid cavernous fistulae and dural arteriovenous malformations of the cavernous sinus. Neurosurgery 41:798–805; discussion 805–796

van Loveren H, Keller J, Fl-Kalliny M, Scodary DJ, Jr TJ (1991) The Dolenc technique for cavernous sinus exploration (cadaveric prosection). Technical note. J Neurosurg 74:837–844

Vanzetti (1858) Secondo caso di aneurisma dell' arteria oftalmica guarito colla compressione digitali della carotide, e cenni pratici intorno a questo metodo di curare gli aneurismi. Padova, and Annali universali di medicina. CLXV:151

Vinuela F, Fox AJ, Debrun GM, Peerless SJ, Drake CG (1984) Spontaneous carotid-cavernous fistulas: clinical, radiological, and therapeutic considerations. Experience with 20 cases. J Neurosurg 60:976–984

Voigt K (1978) [Neuroradiological diagnosis and treatment of dural carotid-cavernous sinus fistulae (author's transl)]. Arch Psychiatr Nervenkr 225:359–377

Voigt K, Sauer M, Dichgans J (1971) Spontaneous occlusion of a bilateral caroticocavernous fistula studied by serial angiography. Neuroradiology 2:207–211

Yamada F, Fukuda S, Matsumoto K, Yoshii N (1984) [Effect of radiotherapy on dural arteriovenous malformation. Long-term follow-up study and clinical evaluation]. Neurol Med Chir (Tokyo) 24:591–599

Yamamoto T, Asai K, Lin YW et al. (1995) Spontaneous resolution of symptoms in an infant with a congenital dural caroticocavernous fistula. Neuroradiology 37:247–249

Yasunaga T, Takada C, Uozumi H et al. (1987) Radiotherapy of spontaneous carotid-cavernous sinus fistulas. Int J Radiat Oncol Biol Phys 13:1909–1913

Yousry TA, Kuhne I, Straube A, Bruckmann H (1997) [An unusual combination of carotid artery-cavernous sinus fistula and sinus thrombosis. Successful therapy with anticoagulation]. Nervenarzt 68:135–138

Hemodynamic Aspects of DCSFs

10

CONTENTS

ments of regional blood flow (FEINDEL et al. 1967; HAEGGENDAL et al. 1965; INGVAR and LASSEN 1972; LASSEN et al. 1963).

NORNES (1979, 1980) pioneered the use of Doppler ultrasound to measure flow velocity in cerebral arteries and measured intraoperatively elevated perfusion pressures up to 50%. The use of Doppler techniques for more detailed assessment of blood flow in AVMs is extensively described in the monograph by HASSLER (1986). He studied flow characteristics in AVMs using transcranial Doppler sonography (TCD) as well as intravascular probes by measuring flow and pressure intraoperatively before and after removal. NORNES (1972) also used Doppler measurements in the management of five patients with CSFs (four traumatic, one spontaneous). He found "steal flow" ranging from 90–975 ml/min, forward flow rates in the ICA between 40–170 ml/min and reverse flow between 35–60 ml/min. Nornes used the ratio of reverse flow/forward flow as an indicator of sufficient collateral capacity of the cerebral circulation in the case of permanent ICA occlusion.

Many studies on hemodynamics of CSFs utilized transophthalmic ultrasound for detecting and monitoring patients with AV fistulas (KAWAGUCHI et al. 2002; DE KEIZER 1982, 1986) or duplex sonography of the ICA and ECA flow (LIN et al. 1994; CHEN et al. 2000). Lack of proper imaging tools is a reason for the scarce literature on AV shunting flow in CSFs that mainly focused on flow pattern on the arterial side pre- and post embolization. Very little is known about arteriovenous shunt flow and pressure in DAVFs in general, or in DCSFs in particular. Data on intrasinus flow and pressure is mostly lacking. Criteria for hemodynamic classifications are mainly based on the speed of contrast filling in angiograms, and thus are to a large degree subjective and impossible to quantify (see Sect. 4.3).

10.1
Introduction

The study of blood flow in arteriovenous shunting lesions goes back to SHENKIN et al. (1948), who were able to demonstrate a flow velocity elevated by a factor of three from the ICA into the IJV in patients with arteriovenous malformations (AVMs). MURPHY (1954) defined the "steal phenomenon" associated with clinical findings in AVMs such as seizures or psychic alterations. He concluded that the AVM shunt perfusion works at the expense of cerebral tissue perfusion. Further research by several investigators focused mainly on measure-

Basic Hemodynamic Principles

Blood flow through vessels follows the laws and principles of fluid dynamics, whose key parameters are as follows:

Vessel radius: r
Vessel cross-sectional area: A
Velocity: ν
Flux of fluid: Q
Viscosity: μ
Density: ρ
Resistance: R_s
Pressure gradient: ΔP
L = Tube length: L

Reynolds number: $R_e = \dfrac{\rho \nu L}{\mu}$

The flow rate Q depends on the difference in pressure between both ends of a tube and the resistance to that flow. Only 2% of the heart action is transformed into kinetic energy, while 98% is used to overcome frictional force (NORNES and GRIP 1980).

$$Q = \Delta P / R_s \tag{1}$$

Conservation of mass embodied in the continuity equation is one of the most basic concepts in fluid dynamics and thus in hemodynamics (SECCA and GOULAO 1998). To maintain constant flow, when the diameter of the tube gets smaller, the velocity will increase. More precisely,

$$Q = A\nu = \text{constant in a tube} \tag{2}$$

Conservation of energy is another key concept in the physics of flow and can be expressed in *Bernoulli's equation:*

$$P = \frac{1}{2}\rho v^2 \tag{3}$$

This equation is valid only for fluids without viscosity, and therefore does not directly apply to blood flow. However, it has been usefully applied to the estimation of pressure drops in larger arteries (carotid, aorta). Viscosity of blood is inversely related to temperature.

Hagen-Poiseuille's law is a third cornerstone law and is written as:

$$Q = \frac{\Delta P \pi r^4}{8L\mu} \tag{4}$$

The flow rate varies with the fourth power of its radius and is inversely proportional to its length and to the viscosity. Thus, the vessel's diameter is a critical factor for regulating blood flow in the human body. This law, however, is only strictly applicable to rigid, straight tubes with constant diameter and homogenous fluids under laminar (as opposed to turbulent) flow conditions. In reality blood is inhomogeneous and flows through compliant vessels with changing diameters and curvatures. It has a variable viscosity changing with shear rate and the concentration of red blood cells (hematocrit). Under normal temperatures and pressures and a 40% hematocrit, blood viscosity is approximately four times that of water. Very low flow shear rates may result in relative values of more than 1000 or "prestasis" (HASSLER 1986).

Flow and resistance (*Rs*) are inversely proportional to each other (Eq. 2) and for Hagen-Poiseuille's flow, *the resistance to the flow* is written as:

$$R_s = \frac{8L\eta}{\pi r^4} \tag{5}$$

In a closed vessel under constant pressure gradient, the flow will increase with a larger radius, decreasing length and a lower viscosity (SECCA and GOULAO 1998).

In arteriovenous shunting lesions velocity is increased and the flow may become unsteady or turbulent, especially when the Reynolds number R_e exceeds 400. The flow becomes less laminar and develops marginal swirls; laminar flow completely disappears for a R_e above 2,000 (HASSLER 1986). While studies on hemodynamics in brain AVMs have been of interest for a number of investigators (NORNES and GRIP 1979, 1980; MIYASAKA et al. 1994; NORBASH et al. 1994; HASSLER and THRON 1994; DUCKWILER et al. 1990), there is only scant research of this type in DAVFs or DCSFs.

Invasive Assessment of Hemodynamics

In order to study hemodynamics in intracranial arteriovenous shunting lesions, direct invasive measurements of arterial and venous flow velocities were performed by the author during embolizations of AVMs, DAVFs and DCSFs (BENNDORF et al. 1994a,b, 1995). In addition, simultaneous pressure measurements in draining sinuses of AVMs (BENNDORF et al. 1994b) or DCSFs (BENNDORF and WELLNHOFER 2002) were recorded.

For assessments of flow and pressure, two different sensor-tipped micro-guidewires were used:

1. The FloWire system from Cardiometrics (Mountain View, CA) was developed in the 1990s for invasive studies of coronary blood flow velocities, pre- and post angioplasty (SERRUYS et al. 1993; DI MARIO et al. 1995; LABOVITZ et al. 1993; WELLNHOFER et al. 1997). A few investigators utilized this technology for hemodynamic studies in other vascular territories, mainly the cerebrovascular circulation (BENNDORF et al. 1994a, 1995, 1997; MURAYAMA et al. 1996; HENKES et al. 1993).

This Doppler guidewire consists of a 0.014″ (0.036 mm) micro-guidewire, onto which a Doppler probe is mounted with a sample volume of 5 mm, provided by a 10-MHz transducer. The "SmartWire" was initially a modified version of the FloWire (Doppler Wire) with a more flexible tip for use in the tortuous cerebral circulation (Fig. 10.1). The SmartMap enabled real-time display and recording of flow velocity and flow pattern. The system is currently manufactured by Volcano (Laguna Hill, CA) and meanwhile offers a new Smart-II Wire for pressure measurements and a ComboWire (ComboMap) for assessment of coronary flow reserve (CFR) and fractional flow reserve (FFR). The latest wire versions have a special core for better trackability, a PTFE coating and are compatible with standard 18-microcatheters. The following parameters can be recorded:

- MPV = Maximum (over pulsatile cycle) peak velocity
- APV = Average (over pulsatile cycle) peak velocity
- PI (CPI) = Pulsatility index (PI) = (IPV max-IPV mean) / APV
- IPV = Instantaneous peak velocity

2. The PressureWire (Radi Medical Systems AB, Uppsala Sweden) is a guidewire-mounted high-fidelity fiberoptic pressure sensor, located 3 cm proximal to the shapeable radiopaque tip (Fig. 10.1). Similar to the FloWire the PressureWire was also initially developed for intracoronary use (DI MARIO et al. 1993, 1995; GORGE et al. 1993) and applied to other territories to only some degree (BENNDORF et al. 1994b; ABILDGAARD et al. 1995). It was intended for use with a PGA interface that provided pressure values, but no curve. The latest version (*Certus*) comes as a hydrophilic-coated 0.014″ (0.036 mm) guidewire in 175 cm/300 cm length and measures pressures between 30 and 300 mmHg. Using the principle of thermodilution, monitoring intravascular temperature is possible and flow velocities can be calculated, although a waveform is not obtained. The wire can also be advanced through various standard microcatheters (e.g. Tacker-Excel). The initial version of Radi's PressureWire was relatively stiff compared to the FloWire and could not be advanced through the carotid siphon. Flexibility may be improved with the latest versions, but has not been tested by the author for this purpose.

The above described wire configurations with two sensors have only recently become available. In earlier studies, two separate wires (one for flow, another for pressure) had to be used. Both systems are employed to measure pressure gradients, intracoronary flow and the fractional flow reserve (FFR) that is currently used as a standard diagnostic tool in cardiac catheterization laboratories (WELLNHOFER et al. 1997; ABILDGAARD et al. 1995; MARQUES et al. 2002; NISANCI et al. 2002; ALFONSO et al. 2000; BRIGUORI et al. 2001).

A few reports describe non-coronary interventions (MAHMUD et al. 2006; CAVENDISH et al. 2008) measurements of carotid artery pressure during angiography (KANAZAWA et al. 2008) and even assessment of cerebrospinal fluid pressure in Chiari I animal models (TURK et al. 2006).

In order to obtain data on venous flow and pressure in AV shunting lesions, the author used the two sensor-tipped guidewires, which were simultaneously or alternatingly advanced into the great dural cerebral sinuses, such as the sigmoid sinus (SS), transverse sinus (TS), straight sinus (StS), superior sagittal sinus (SSS) or the CS.

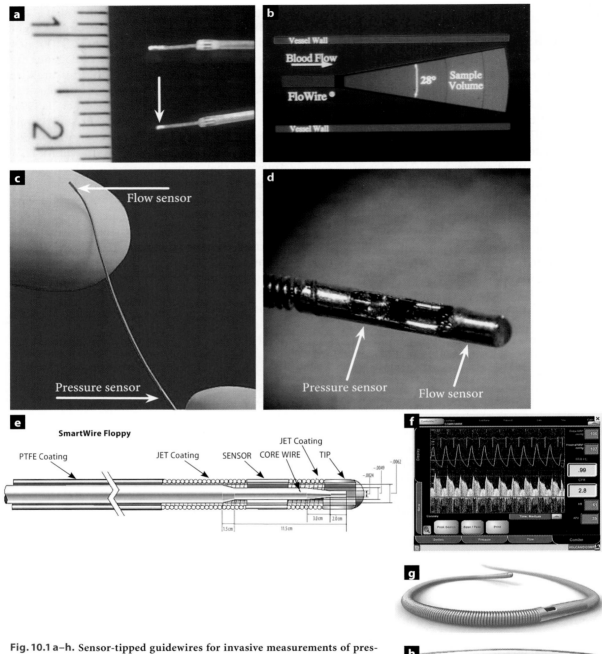

Fig. 10.1 a–h. Sensor-tipped guidewires for invasive measurements of pressure and flow. a Original 0.014″ FloWire®/SmartWire® (*arrow*, Cardiometrics) carrying a miniaturized 10 Mhz Doppler probe next to a standard 0.014″ guidewire, here introduced into 0.018″ microcatheters as used by the author. **b** A 5 mm sample volume of the Doppler probe. **c, d** Magnified views of the currently available ComboWire® with two sensors: Doppler probe at the tip and pressure sensor either with 1.5 cm offset or next to the flow sensor (*arrows*, Volcano Therapeutics Inc., Laguna Hills, CA). **e, f** Scheme of the current SmartWire® Floppy and the SmartMap® (ComboMap®) for real time monitoring of pressure and flow. **g, h** Recent version of the 0.014″ (0.36 mm) PressureWire® (Radi Medical Systems AB, Sweden) with the opening for the sensor 3 cm proximal to the tip, and the RadiAnalyzer. Using thermodilution, flow data can also be estimated

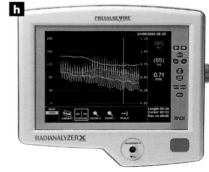

Flow Velocity and Pressure Measurements in Brain AVMs and DAVFs

These studies were conducted by the author between 1993 and 1997 at Charité, Berlin (BENNDORF et al. 1994a,b, 1995, 1997). A total of 24 patients with intracranial AVMs and DAVFs were included, undergoing 42 measurements during endovascular treatment. The FloWire was usually advanced via a 5-F or 6-F coaxial catheter system into the dural sinuses of interest, such as the superior sagittal sinus, transverse sinus or straight sinus.

In this series, maximum flow velocities up to 166 cm/s were measured in arterialized sinuses (directly draining the arteriovenous shunt), indicating disturbed or even turbulent flow (HASSLER 1986), while a maximum of 57 cm/s was found in non-arterialized sinuses. The pulsatility index was found to be similar in arterialized and non-arterialized sinuses with a trend to somewhat lower values in the latter (Fig. 10.2)

In DAVFs, increased pulsatility was found not only in the region of the fistula itself (transverse sinus PI = 3.5), but also upstream in the parietal superior sagittal sinus (PI = 1.86). Disturbed flow was found in AV shunt draining sinuses only when the Doppler probe was positioned close to the nidus, or where the main draining vein entered a larger sinus. In four patients without AV shunt a clear pulsatile flow pattern was recorded as well. Pressure measurements revealed values between 6–16 mm Hg in non-arterialized versus 19–41 mmHg in arterialized sinuses.

Major changes in flow pattern were found in DAVFs. In one patient, who suffered from a distressing bruit, the DSA showed a partial retrograde opacification of the transverse sinus in the early arterial phase, which caused a contrast "wash out" of the normal antegrade flow in this sinus during the venous phase of the angiogram. This sinus segment remained non-opacified during the late venous phase, mimicking possible thrombosis or even occlusion. Retrograde catheterization, however, demonstrated a patent sinus that exhibited extremely disturbed flow (Fig. 10.3). This flow turbulence was apparently caused by two opposing flow components: the normal antegrade flow from the SSS and the AV shunting retrograde flow. It can be considered a point of "reversal", which position depends on the degree of AV shunting and may shift up- or downstream by either the natural course of the fistula or by inter-

vening endovascular treatment. In the case shown here, TAE of ECA feeders diminished the retrograde component and established normal antegrade flow in this sinus as was documented by continuous recording during the injection of glue. The patient's associated symptoms subsided.

Hemodynamics and Pathophysiology in CSFs

The ophthalmic artery mainly supplies the retinal and choroidal circulation. The retinal arteries supply the inner retinal layers and the choroidal arteries, which contain the main blood volume and supply the high metabolic demand of the outer retinal layers (SANDERS and HOYT 1969). Because both the retinal and choroidal vessels are subjected to the intraocular pressure, this circulatory system requires an intraluminal pressure that exceeds the intraocular pressure (normal between 10 and 20 mm Hg). The entire blood circulation of the eye depends on the arteriovenous pressure gradient that, if reduced, will impede the eye blood circulation. The pressure gradient may be lowered by either decreased arterial pressure (hypotension, arteriovenous shunt) or by increased venous pressure (glaucoma, arteriovenous shunt). Whenever this pressure gradient is reduced, the orbital circulation will adjust, mostly by lowering the peripheral resistance through the opening of precapillary shunts and dilatation of small venules (SANDERS and HOYT 1969). These compensatory mechanisms may be exhausted and the blood circulation will be insufficient to meet metabolic demands of the retina that then becomes hypoxic causing loss of visual acuity. If such a condition persists, intraretinal hemorrhages may follow.

An arteriovenous shunt at the CS will, especially when draining anteriorly, cause a significant elevation in the venous ophthalmic pressure that will retard normal antegrade flow in afferent tributaries or even cause flow reversal. It will increase flow in other efferent veins such as the IPS or the PP and may cause "steal effects" in small dural arteries supplying cranial nerves.

Most important for the clinical symptomatology of CSFs are the effects on the orbital venous circulation. Here the AV shunt may cause a drastic reduction in the normal arteriovenous

(Text continues on p. 300)

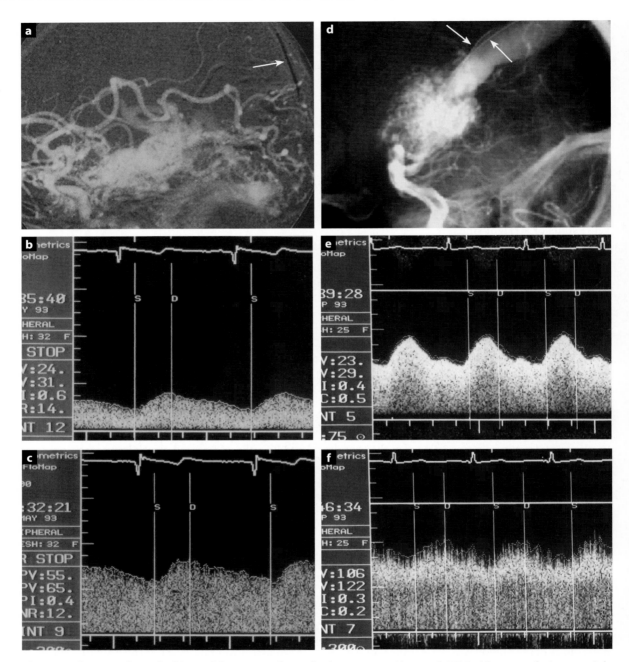

Fig. 10.2 a–f. Venous flow velocities and flow pattern in two brain AVMs. a–c Temporal AVM with venous drainage mainly via basal vein of Rosenthal, internal cerebral vein and straight sinus (SS). The APV in the arterialized straight sinus (**b**) was at 55 cm/s significantly elevated versus 24 cm/s in the non-arterialzed superior sagittal sinus (SSS, **c**). Note also the pulsatile flow in the SSS. *White arrow*: FloWire in the SSS. **d–f** Brain stem AVM draining exclusively into the vein of Galen. The average peak velocity in the SS was remarkably increased up to 106 cm/s, while the maximum peak velocity reaches 122 cm/s versus 29 cm/s (**e**). Interestingly, in both cases the pulsatility index (PI) in the arterialized straight sinus was reduced compared to that in the SSS (0.4 vs 0.6 and 0.3 vs 0.4). Note in **d**: Two sensor-tipped guidewires advanced into the SS (*arrows*) for simultaneous measurements of pressure and flow. The mean venous pressure in the SS was 40 mm Hg. (BENNDORF et al. 1994, 1995)

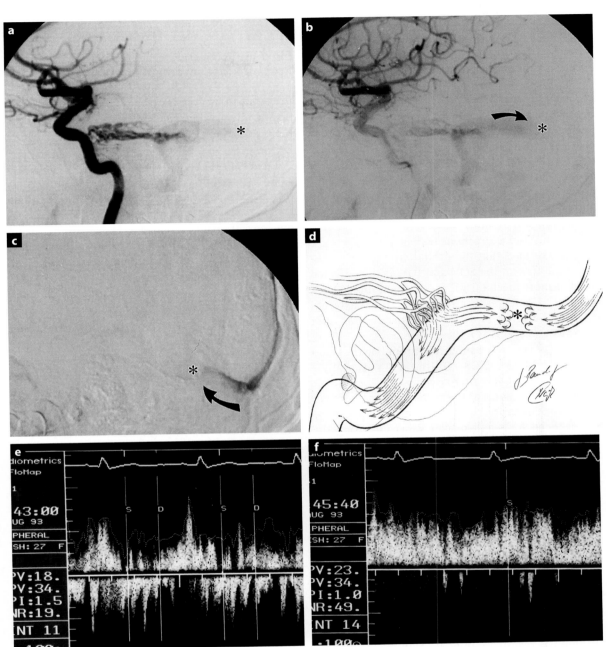

Fig. 10.3 a–f. Turbulent flow pattern in a DAVF of the sigmoid sinus. a, b ICA injection early and late arterial phase shows the filling of the sigmoid sinus and some retrograde opacification of the transverse sinus until a certain segment (*asterisk*). **c,** Late venous phase shows the washout of the normal anterograde venous flow in the transverse sinus causing a pseudo "filling defect" in the same region (*asterisk*). This sinus was not thrombosed or occluded. The antegrade flow of contrast was washed out (diluted) instead by the retrograde (non-opacified) AV shunting flow. Two opposing flows apparantly mix here: Upstream (retrograde) and downstream (anterograde) flow, causing a maximum of disturbance with secondary eddies (*asterisks* in **d**). FloWire measurements confirmed this phenomenon, demonstrating a very unstable, turbulent pattern at this "reversal point" (antegrade flow above, retrograde flow below baseline) (**e**). **f** Subsequent transarterial embolization diminished the retrograde AV shunting component and normalized the flow pattern in this sinus with dominating antegrade flow in the sinus, documented by continuous monitoring of venous flow (BENNDORF et al. 1995)

pressure gradient required to allow normal blood supply to the retina and other intraorbital tissues. As elaborated by SANDERS and HOYT (1969), the elevated venous pressure generates reduced perfusion pressure, which may be further raised by increased intraocular pressure. The eye will attempt to adapt to these changes by lowering the peripheral resistance through microcirculatory changes consisting of capillary shunting, dilatation and venous dilatation. These compensations of the ocular circulation become visible in conjunctival changes with tortuousities, dilatation and thickening of arterialized veins. Fluorescein angiography may show the development of microaneurysms and perivenous leakage.

It is assumed that the orbital circulation, especially the flow in the SOV and IOV, is less affected and has more mechanisms for compensation:

- Arterial collateral circulation from external carotid arteries to increase the arterial pressure (SANDERS and HOYT 1969).
- The SOV is widely connected through to the facial vein, through the CS with the IPS and multiple other efferent and afferent veins.
- Dilatation of some of these major veins will lower the overall venous pressure which is indirectly beneficial for small orbital veins including the central retinal vein.

These compensatory mechanisms explain why in some patients with moderate or high flow in the CS/SOV, the IOP is only moderately elevated and the vision may be normal.

The situation becomes entirely different when venous outflow restriction develops due to thrombosis, which is often associated with dural arteriovenous shunts of the CS. Therefore, in many DCSFs with "low-flow shunts", the venous pressure, and subsequently the IOP, may be significantly elevated, particularly if thrombosis of the SOV occurs. If this thrombosis results in an acute SOV occlusion, the venous system of the orbit may not be able to adapt fast enough and the IOP may rise to extreme levels as seen in one of our patients (76 mmHg, see Case Report VI). In such a fistula, the AV shunting volume plays a minor role in the pathophysiology, as it is the elevated venous pressure that causes the reduction in the normal arteriovenous gradient in the ocular circulation leading to reduced retinal perfusion.

10.6
Flow Velocity and Pressure Measurements in DCSFs

Venous flow velocity and pressure were assessed before, during and after TVO of the CS in three patients (Table 10.1).

Case #1: A Type D fistula with dominant posterior drainage into the SPS and leptomeningeal veins (Fig. 10.4). The opacification of the AV shunt on DSA images was relatively slow. The direct intrasinus measurements revealed 5–14 cm/s in the left CS that showed minimal drainage into a presumably thrombosed IPS; values are considered low for an AV shunting lesion.

- With up to 30 cm/s the flow velocity was more increased in the right CS, where posterior drainage into the SPS and leptomeningeal veins was present.
- Interestingly, these pressure values were inversed with lower values on the right (39 mm Hg) and higher values on the left side (28 mm Hg).

Case #2: A Type D fistula with venous outflow restriction due to thrombosis of both SOVs. The flow velocity reached maximal 18 cm/s, while the intrasinus pressure was measured at 30 mm Hg. During the coil packing the mean intrasinus pressures reached 60 mm Hg, then fluctuated and decreased again towards the end of the procedure, but remained above levels of adjacent sinuses (IPS).

Case #3: A Type D fistula, the flow was angiographically very low or stagnant due to thrombosis of the SOV and the CS itself (see also Case report III). The Doppler probe did not detect any measurable flow, while the PressureWire documented significantly elevated intrasinus pressure with 40 mmHg (Figs. 10.5).

Table 10.1. Measurement of venous flow velocity and pressure in three DCSFs

n	Fistula type	Flow (DSA)	Flow velocity (cm/s)	Pressure (mmHg)
1	D	Moderate	14/30	39/28
2	D	Low	18	30
3	C	Very low	0	40*

*Contralateral side in the CS.

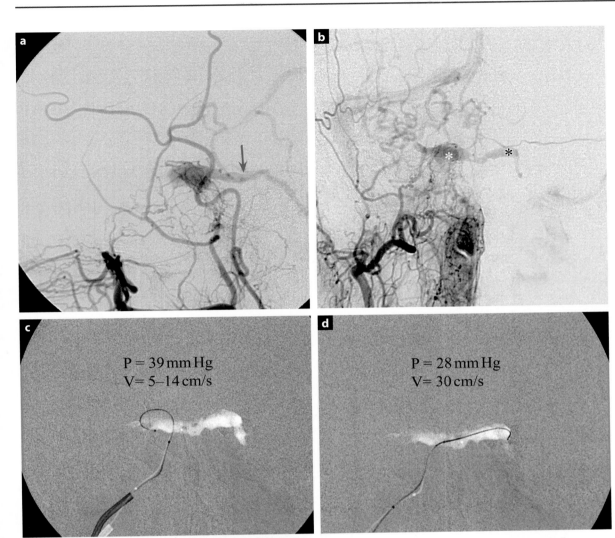

$$P = 39\,\text{mm Hg}$$
$$V = 5{-}14\,\text{cm/s}$$

$$P = 28\,\text{mm Hg}$$
$$V = 30\,\text{cm/s}$$

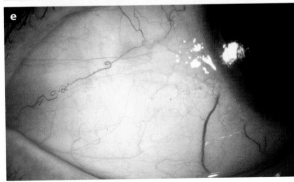

Fig. 10.4 a–d. Intracavernous measurements of pressure and flow (Case #1): a, b Type D fistula at the posterior right CS (*black asterisk*), no anterior drainage, but leptomeningeal venous drainage via the right SPS (*arrow*). Note the minimal drainage on the left side, indicating outflow restriction. **c,d** Road mapping of transvenous catheterization from right to left with assessment of intracavernous pressure and flow using sensor-tipped guidewires. The flow velocity in the left CS was 5–14 cm/s, the venous pressure reached 39 mm Hg. In the right CS, the velocity increased with 30 cm/s, while the pressure was lower with 28 mm Hg. This difference may be explained by the less restricted outflow in the right CS, where the AV shunt utilized the SPS and leptomeningeal veins for drainage. Note that there is no visible anterior drainage, corresponding with the patients minor dilataion of cunjunctival veins (**e**). Towards the end of the coil occlusion, pressure values slightly increased, likely due to the tight packing causing additional mechanical pressure. Following TVO, the patient fully recovered without cranial nerve dysfunction. (BENNDORF et al. 2001)

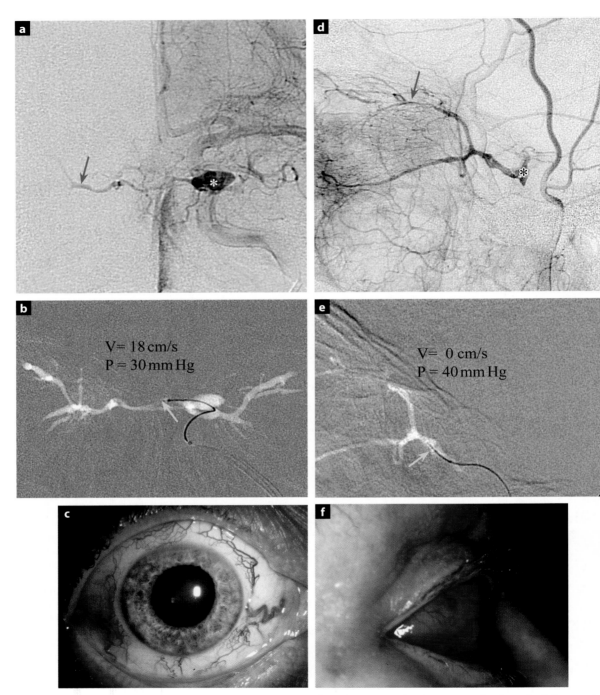

Fig. 10.5 a–d. Intracavernous measurements of pressure and flow (Cases #2 and #3): a Type D fistula at the left posterior CS (*asterisk*) without posterior drainage, but bilateral anterior drainage via a partially thrombosed SOV (*short arrow*). **b** After catheterization through the thrombosed IPS, measurements revealed flow velocities up to 18 cm/s and pressures up to 30 mm Hg, indicating a "low-flow/high-pressure" condition. During coil packing of the CS, transient elevated values of up to 60 mm Hg were noted. *Arrow*: FloWire within the CS. **c** This patient exhausted her compensatory venous dilatations and developed bilateral retinal hemorrhages, but fully recovered after treatment (for more details see Case Report I). **d** Type C fistula with faint opacification of the CS via ECA branches only. In this case, all venous exits appeared either thrombosed or occluded. **e** There was no measurable flow velocity, consistent with the contrast stagnation seen in the DSA. However, the intrasinus pressure was remarkably increased to 40 mm Hg, explaining the severe clinical symptoms of the patient with exophthalmos, aggravated chemosis and visual loss (**f,** for more details see Case Report III). *Arrow*: FloWire within the CS. (BENNDORF et al. 2001)

Comments

The CS represents a unique venous reservoir that receives and drains blood through multiple connecting veins and sinuses. The intracavernous venous flow is further characterized by major cerebral arteries, the internal carotids, whose pulse waves are transmitted throughout the sinus and thought to be responsible for the transport of venous blood toward the jugular vein. The complexity of this pump system has been experimentally studied in great detail already by RABISCHONG in 1974. Studies on hemodynamics of CSFs were conducted as early as 1958 by HEYCK, who used nitrous oxide to indirectly determine the AV shunt blood flow.

The interest in identifying distinct hemodynamic features of CSFs has lead to a limited number of studies on the subject using either intraarterial angiography (HAYES 1958; PHELPS 1982; BRASSEL 1983), transcranial Doppler ultrasound (NORNES 1972) or extracranial duplex sonography (LIN 1994). As discussed in more detail in Sect. 4.3, these attempts to better understand and classify arteriovenous shunts of the CS remain necessarily insufficient, as collected data are small, mostly focusing on flow velocities and are usually not assessed within the CS itself.

The usefulness of transophthalmic ultrasonic examinations to discriminate low-flow dural shunts from direct high-flow fistulas and other causes of proptosis, such as conjunctivitis or endocrine ophthalmopathy has been reported (DE KEIZER 1982, 1986). As this modality encompasses only AV shunts with anterior drainage, assessment of hemodynamics in DCSFs based on flow velocities in the SOV will remain limited in its clinical and prognostic value. Flow data on DCSFs with posterior drainage are completely lacking in the medical literature, thus flow velocity as a single parameter is an inaccurate indicator for the severity of ophthalmic symptoms in the individual patient. For example, as long as anterior flow is moderate, normal venous drainage of the ocular and ophthalmic organs may still function well. On the other hand, venous outflow restriction of the AV shunting due to developing stenosis or thrombosis of the SOV will cause immediate elevation of the venous pressure associated with aggravation of a patient's symptoms. The severity of symptoms is considered related to the flow rate in AV shunts (BARROW et al. 1985). However, depending on the individual angioarchitecture in a DCSF, draining routes and outflow restrictions, this may not be true at all and clinical assessment may be-

come more or less arbitrary (PHELPS et al. 1982). For an accurate hemodynamic classification of DCSFs with clinical or therapeutic implication for prognosis, assessment of intracavernous or even retinal vascular pressure and perfusion would be needed. Like in other DAVFs, data on intrasinus pressure are scarce in DCSFs, or non-existing and most assumptions made on CSFs hemodynamics are purely based on flow velocity and IOP measurements.

Different types of pressure associated with different flow conditions need to be considered to understand hemodynamics in fistulas with various degrees of AV shunting flow. A low-flow arteriovenous fistula is intuitively considered a benign fistula because of its frequent association with minor symptoms and spontaneous occlusion. As demonstrated in the cases presented here, this view may be somewhat misleading. Although shunt flow may be very low or even close to zero (not measurable as in Case 1, Table 10.1), even a small arterialized inflow into the CS can cause devastating ophthalmic and ocular symptoms if venous hypertension due to outflow restriction is present. Such elevation of static pressure may also lead to reversal of flow and redistribution into leptomeningeal veins, potentially changing the clinical prognosis.

High-flow fistulas, on the other hand, will cause major symptoms only if venous pressure increase occurs as well; in this case, dynamic pressure. It is also known that fistulas with unrestricted posterior venous drainage into the superior or inferior petrosal sinus may be completely asymptomatic. As explained above, the orbital circulation can compensate to some degree increased pressure with its collateral circulation so that the IOP will remain normal.

Elevations of mostly static pressures, as observed in Cases #1–3 with low-flow conditions, can be expected in many DCSFs with ongoing thrombosis of the SOV, IPS or the CS itself. The inverse relationship of pressure and flow velocity in Case #1 corresponds with the concept of CS outflow restriction causing venous hypertension. Redistribution of blood flow due to pressure changes in the CS and its connecting efferent and afferent veins is a main feature in the natural history of DCSFs. Case #2 emphasizes that venous hypertension in the orbital system may affect also the ocular systems when compensatory mechanisms are exhausted. This can eventually result in a reduction of the perfusion pressure which can lead to hypoxic changes and intraretinal hemorrhages (Chap. 10.5.). Case #3 revealed no measureable AV shunt flow while the patient suffered from advanced chemosis, exophthalmos and visual loss. It clearly demonstrates that the assumption that a "low-flow" fistula will have a mild clinical course, and thus does not require any therapeutic intervention, can be erroneous in some cases, leading to serious clinical deterioration.

Whether or not an elevated venous pressure in the CS will increase the intraocular pressure, or the pressure in draining leptomeningeal veins, depends to a large degree on the individual angioarchitecture. Thus, if a CS is anatomically isolated from the anterior venous drainage due to thrombosis, occlusion or anatomic compartmentalization, a CSF may not necessarily lead to orbital venous hypertension and subsequent increased IOP. On the other hand, it can probably be assumed that even in cases where the SOV is thrombosed, and appears "angiographically not involved" in the drainage of the CS AV shunt, some anatomic, hemodynamic or other biomechanic communication may still exist. Therefore, even though not perceivable by imaging information, elevated pressure in the CS may be very well transmitted into the ophthalmic venous system.

In Case #2, the left CS was exposed to higher pressure values than the right, whereas the patient's ophthalmic symptoms were dominant on the right side. On the contrary, in Case #3 the patient's symptoms were clearly caused by the elevated CS pressure evidencing that her SOV, although thrombosed and to a large degree angiographically occluded, transmitted significant pressure. The compromised ocular and orbital venous circulation due to thrombotic outflow restriction will be further aggravated by a residual AV shunt, even when very small and almost undetectable by angiography.

Some authors may classify Cases #2 and #3 as "restrictive" or "late restrictive" types, representing the final stage in the natural history that will undergo complete spontaneous occlusion and healing (SUH et al. 2005). However, as this classification is purely based on angiographic patterns, associated and potentially deleterious effects of hemodynamic parameters are not being considered. Only indirect conclusions with regard to impairment of cerebellar hemodynamics in cases with posterior drainage can be made (FUJITA et al. 2002). Lack of realistic data on flow and pressure and their changes during the natural course of these fistulas is the reason that questions, such as why DCSFs with leptomeningeal venous drainage tend to bleed less frequently than DAVFs with the same type of drainage, remain un-

answered to date. Full understanding of pathophysiology and assessment of prognosis and associated risks will become possible only if the forces inherent to the shunting flow can be measured accurately and interpreted properly in the context of individual anatomy. As the increased intraocular pressure is responsible for ophthalmological symptoms, venous hypertension in DCSFs is likely playing a more important role than flow velocity or shunt volume per se, especially in patients with partial or complete occlusion of draining veins. With regard to orbital symptoms, except for the pulsating exophthalmos, an elevated static pressure under low-flow conditions may have similar deleterious effects on the intraorbital pressure in patients with DCSFs as has a high dynamic pressure under high-flow conditions.

Although more data, including that of patients with high-flow shunts, are necessary to fully understand these relationships, it seems justified to suggest including venous pressure in hemodynamic classifications. "Low-flow" fistulas exhibiting venous hypertension might be more properly identified as "high-pressure" fistulas.

To the author's knowledge, the study of AIHARA et al. (1999) is the only one published that provides some venous pressure measurements in the CS before and after TVO. The authors reported three patients, observing a significant increase from 43 mmHg to 75 mmHg in one "high-flow" fistula, and discuss a possible causal relationship with a diplopia that developed after treatment and resolved within 4 months. In another patient with a "high-flow" fistula, a fall in intrasinus pressure from 93 mmHg to 48 mmHg was documented. This patient complained of temporary worsening of her symptoms. Flow measurements were not performed and the figures do not allow a clear judgment about the flow conditions. Assuming a high-flow situation with unrestricted venous outflow in these cases, the elevated pressure most likely is dynamic pressure caused by increased flow velocities.

Increase of intrasinus pressure occurring during coil packing and at the end of the coil occlusion was observed in two of my cases, with no clinical correlation such as CN deficits. As it has been suggested, increased local (mechanical) pressure due to the densely packed platinum coils may be an explanation (AIHARA et al. 1999). Such pressure elevation caused by mechanical stress may be difficult to differentiate from increased pressure due to rerouting of venous drainage or premature occlusion of venous exits such as the SOV. It may, however, explain the development of new CN deficits after overpacking the CS in cases of complete shunt occlusions (Roy and Raymond 1997). The influence of coil overpacking with CN deficits has recently been studied by Nishino et al. (2008), who found that the cumulative volume and specific location of coils correlate with CN deficits induced by TVO.

The small number of cases available and the lack of continuous and truly simultaneous assessment of both parameters, flow and pressure, is a limiting factor of the presented invasive studies of hemodynamics in DCSFs. It should also be noted that for invasive measurements, the type of measured pressure depends on the orientation of the probe relative to the local flow direction. If the probe is perpendicular to the flow, static pressure will be measured. If the probe is pointing upstream, dynamic pressure will also be assessed. Systematic collection of such data that may be facilitated using currently available devices with sensors for both pressure and flow are needed to gain sufficient insights into the hemodynamics of cavernous sinus arteriovenous shunts and their correlation with clinical presentations of DCSFs patients.

In summary, rather little is known about hemodynamics in DCSFs, except for flow in the SOV in cases with anterior drainage, and the flow in supplying carotid arteries. Sufficient data on flow and pressure within the CS itself, or its efferent and afferent veins, are lacking due to inaccessibility with clinical imaging modalities such as ultrasound and MRI. Invasive tools for measurements, such as improved sensor-tipped guidewires, currently remain the only reliable source for studying hemodynamics in vivo and may play an increasing role during endovascular treatment of these lesions. Hemodynamic classifications based on angiographic contrast filling pattern or ultrasound measurements remain inaccurate and incomplete. This is demonstrated by invasively recorded pressure and flow data revealing that some "low-flow fistulas" might be more properly named "high-pressure fistulas". Further studies of in vivo hemodynamics are needed for a complete understanding of the complex pathophysiology, clinical presentation, and natural course of DCSFs.

References

Abildgaard A, Klow NE (1995) A pressure-recording guidewire for measuring arterial transstenotic gradients: in vivo validation. Acad Radiol 2:53–60

Aihara N, Mase M, Yamada K, et al. (1999) Deterioration of ocular motor dysfunction after transvenous embolization of dural arteriovenous fistula involving the cavernous sinus. Acta Neurochir (Wien) 141:707–709; discussion 709–710

Alfonso F, Flores A, Escaned J, et al. (2000) Pressure wire kinking, entanglement, and entrapment during intravascular ultrasound studies: a potentially dangerous complication. Catheter Cardiovasc Interv 50:221–225

Barrow DL, Spector RH, Braun IF, Landman JA, Tindall SC, Tindall GT (1985) Classification and treatment of spontaneous carotid-cavernous sinus fistulas. J Neurosurg 62:248–256

Benndorf G, Boerschel M, Schneider GH, Unterberg A, Lanksch W, Fleck E (1994b) Measurement of pressure and flow velocity in dural sinuses in patients with arteriovenous malforamtions and fistulas with sensor-tipped microguide wires. In: RSNA, 1994

Benndorf G, Podrabsky P, Wellnhofer E, et al. (1994a) Measurement of blood flow velocity by Doppler-tipped guide wires in patients with arteriovenous malforamtions and fistulae. In: Takahashi M (ed) XVth Symposium Neuroradiologicum; Kumamato. Springer-Verlag, Berlin Heidelberg New York.

Benndorf G, Podrabsky P, Wellnhofer E, et al. (1995) Measurement of blood flow velocity by Doppler-tipped guide wires in patients with arteriovenous malforamtions and fistulae. Neuroradiology 37:489–491

Benndorf G, Singel S, Proest G, Lanksch W, Felix R (1997) The Doppler guide wire: clinical applications in neuroendovascular treatment. Neuroradiology 39:286–291

Benndorf G, Wellnhofer E (2002) Assessment of intracavernous pressure and flow in dural cavernous sinus fistulas (DCSF). In: XVIIth Symposium Neuroradiologicum; Paris: Masson;

Brassel F (1983) Haemodynamik und Therapie der Karotis-Kavernosus Fistel. Bonn

Briguori C, Nishida T, Adamian M, et al. (2001) Assessment of the functional significance of coronary lesions using a monorail catheter. J Invasive Cardiol 13:279–286

Cavendish JJ, Carter LI, Tsimikas S (2008) Recent advances in hemodynamics: noncoronary applications of a pressure sensor angioplasty guidewire. Catheter Cardiovasc Interv 71:748–758

Chen YW, Jeng JS, Liu HM, Hwang BS, Lin WH, Yip PK (2000) Carotid and transcranial color-coded duplex sonography in different types of carotid-cavernous fistula. Stroke 31:701–706

de Keizer R (1986) Carotid cavernous fistulas and Doppler flow velocity measurements. Neuo-ophthalmology 8:205–211

de Keizer R (2003) Carotid-cavernous and orbital arteriovenous fistulas: ocular features, diagnostic and hemodynamic considerations in relation to visual impairment and morbidity. Orbit 22:121–142

de Keizer RJ (1982) A Doppler haematotachographic investigation in patients with ocular and orbital symptoms due to a carotid-cavernous fistula. Doc Ophthalmol 52:297–307

Di Mario C, de Feyter PJ, Slager CJ, de Jaegere P, Roelandt JR, Serruys PW (1993) Intracoronary blood flow velocity and transstenotic pressure gradient using sensor-tip pressure and Doppler guidewires: a new technology for the assessment of stenosis severity in the catheterization laboratory. Cathet Cardiovasc Diagn 28:311–319

Di Mario C, Gil R, Krams R, De Feyter PJ, Serruys W (1995) New invasive techniques of assessment of the physiological significance of coronary stenoses in humans. Eur Heart J 16 Suppl I:104–114

Duan YY, Zhou XY, Liu X, et al. (2008) Carotid and transcranial color-coded duplex ultrasonography for the diagnosis of dural arteriovenous fistulas. Cerebrovasc Dis 25:304–310

Duckwiler G, Dion J, Vinuela F, Jabour B, Martin N, Bentson J (1990) Intravascular microcatheter pressure monitoring: experimental results and early clinical evaluation. AJNR Am J Neuroradiol 11:169–175

Feindel W, Yamamoto YL, Hodge P (1967) The human cerebral microcirculation studied by intra-arterial radioactive tracers, Coomassie Blue and fluorescein dyes. Bibl Anat 9:220–224

Fujita A, Nakamura M, Tamaki N, Kohmura E (2002) Haemodynamic assessment in patients with dural arteriovenous fistulae: dynamic susceptibility contrast-enhanced MRI. Neuroradiology 44:806–811

Gorge G, Erbel R, Niessing S, Schon F, Kearney P, Meyer J (1993) Miniaturized pressure-guide-wire: evaluation in vitro and in isolated hearts. Cathet Cardiovasc Diagn 30:341–347

Haeggendal E, Ingvar DH, Lassen NA, et al. (1965) Pre- and postoperative measurements of regional cerebral blood flow in three cases of intracranial arteriovenous aneurysms. J Neurosurg 22:1–6

Hassler W (1986) Hemodynamic aspects of cerebral angiomas. Acta Neurochirurgica Sppl 37:1–136

Hassler W, Thron A (1994) Flow velocity and pressure measurements in spinal dural arteriovenous fistulas. Neurosurg Rev 17:29–36

Hayes GJ (1958) Carotid cavernous fistulas: diagnosis and surgical management. Am Surg 24:839–843

Henkes H, Nahser HC, Klotzsch C, Diener HC, Kuhne D (1993) [Endovascular Doppler sonography of intracranial blood vessels. Technical indications and potential applications]. Radiologe 33:645–649

Heyck H (1958) [Hemodynamics of cerebral arteriovenous aneurysms & fistulae of the cavernous sinus; results of measurement of the cerebral circulation volume & oxygen difference in 15 cases.]. Dtsch Z Nervenheilkd 177:327–347

Ingvar DH, Lassen NA (1972) [Brain blood flow and its regulation. Actual Neurophysiol (Paris) 9:165–190

Kanazawa R, Ishihara S, Okawara M, Ishihara H, Kohyama S, Yamane F (2008) [A study of intraarterial pressure changing during cerebral angiography]. No Shinkei Geka 36:601–606

Kawaguchi S, Sakaki T, Uranishi R (2002) Color Doppler flow imaging of the superior ophthalmic vein in dural arteriovenous fistulas. Stroke 33:2009–2013

Labovitz AJ, Anthonis DM, Cravens TL, Kern MJ (1993) Validation of volumetric flow measurements by means of a Doppler-tipped coronary angioplasty guide wire. Am Heart J 126:1456–1461

Lassen NA, Hoedt-Rasmussen K, Sorensen SC, et al. (1963) Regional cerebral blood flow in man determined by krypton. Neurology 13:719–727

Lin HJ, Yip PK, Liu HM, Hwang BS, Chen RC (1994) Noninvasive hemodynamic classification of carotid-cavernous sinus fistulas by duplex carotid sonography. J Ultrasound Med 13:105–113

Mahmud E, Brocato M, Palakodeti V, Tsimikas S (2006) Fibromuscular dysplasia of renal arteries: percutaneous revascularization based on hemodynamic assessment with a pressure measurement guidewire. Catheter Cardiovasc Interv 67:434–437

Marques KM, Spruijt HJ, Boer C, Westerhof N, Visser CA, Visser FC (2002) The diastolic flow-pressure gradient relation in coronary stenoses in humans. J Am Coll Cardiol 39:1630–1636

Miyasaka Y, Kurata A, Tokiwa K, Tanaka R, Yada K, Ohwada T (1994) Draining vein pressure increases and hemorrhage in patients with arteriovenous malformation. Stroke 25:504–507

Murayama Y, Usami S, Hata Y, et al. (1996) Transvenous hemodynamic assessment of arteriovenous malformations and fistulas. Preliminary clinical experience in Doppler guidewire monitoring of embolotherapy. Stroke 27:1358–1364

Murphy J (1954) Cerebrovascular disease. Year Book Publishers, Chicago

Nisanci Y, Sezer M, Umman B, Yilmaz E, Mercanoglu S, Ozsaruhan O (2002) Relationship between pressure-derived collateral blood flow and diabetes mellitus in patients with stable angina pectoris: a study based on coronary pressure measurement. J Invasive Cardiol 14:118–122

Nishino K, Ito Y, Hasegawa H, et al. (2008) Cranial nerve palsy following transvenous embolization for a cavernous sinus dural arteriovenous fistula: association with the volume and location of detachable coils. J Neurosurg 109:208–214

Norbash AM, Marks MP, Lane B (1994) Correlation of pressure measurements with angiographic characteristics predisposing to hemorrhage and steal in cerebral arteriovenous malformations. AJNR Am J Neuroradiol 15:809–813

Nornes H (1972) Hemodynamic aspects in the management of carotid-cavernous fistula. J Neurosurg 37:687–694

Nornes H, Grip A (1980) Hemodynamic aspects of cerebral arteriovenous malformations. J Neurosurg 53:456–464

Nornes H, Grip A, Wikeby P (1979) Intraoperative evaluation of cerebral hemodynamics using directional Doppler technique. Part 2: Saccular aneurysms. J Neurosurg 50:570–577

Phelps CD, Thompson HS, Ossoinig KC (1982) The diagnosis and prognosis of atypical carotid-cavernous fistula (red-eyed shunt syndrome). Am J Ophthalmol 93:423–436

Rabischong P, Paleirac R, Vignaud J, et al. (1974) [Angiographic and experimental contributions to the hemodynamics of the cavernous plexus]. Ann Radiol (Paris) 17:285–292

Roy D, Raymond J (1997) The role of transvenous embolization in the treatment of intracranial dural arteriovenous fistulas. Neurosurgery 40:1133–1141; discussion 1141–1134

Sanders MD, Hoyt WF (1969) Hypoxic ocular sequelae of carotid-cavernous fistulae. Study of the caues of visual failure before and after neurosurgical treatment in a series of 25 cases. Br J Ophthalmol 53:82–97

Secca MF, Goulao A (1998) Hemodynamic experiments on AVMs. In: 8th Advanced Course of the ESNR; Lisbon: Centauro, Bologna, pp 41–47

Serruys PW, Di Mario C, Meneveau N, et al. (1993) Intracoronary pressure and flow velocity with sensor-tip guidewires: a new methodologic approach for assessment of coronary hemodynamics before and after coronary interventions. Am J Cardiol 71:41D–53D

Shenkin H, Spitz E, Grant F, Kety S (1948) Physiologic studies of arteriovenous malformation of the brain. J Neurosurg 5:165–172

Suh DC, Lee JH, Kim SJ, et al. (2005) New concept in cavernous sinus dural arteriovenous fistula: correlation with presenting symptom and venous drainage patterns. Stroke 36:1134–1139

Tsai LK, Jeng JS, Wang HJ, Yip PK, Liu HM (2004) Diagnosis of intracranial dural arteriovenous fistulas by carotid duplex sonography. J Ultrasound Med 23:785–791

Turk A, Iskandar BJ, Haughton V, Consigny D (2006) Recording CSF pressure with a transducer-tipped wire in an animal model of Chiari I. AJNR Am J Neuroradiol 27:354–355

Wellnhofer E, Finke W, Bernard L, Danschel W, Fleck E (1997) Improved assessment of intravascular Doppler coronary flow velocity profile. Int J Card Imaging 13:25–34

Summary

11

Complete understanding of the vascular anatomy of DCSFs has been compromised by the complexity of the supplying dural arterial network and by the nature of the cavernous sinus as a venous collector draining blood from cerebral and orbital venous circulation. Since its initial description, and despite numerous angiographic and cadaver studies, controversy concerning the true anatomic structure of the cavernous sinus (CS) persists to some extent still today. The CS is most likely not an unbroken trabeculated venous cavity, or a plexus of various-sized veins; rather it represents a complex venous compartment where numerous dural sinuses and veins converge to form larger venous spaces around the carotid artery, which could be termed *caverns* and whose angiographic appearance is influenced by hemodynamics and the existence of intracavernous thrombi.

More likely than the initially and erroneously assumed rupture of the thin-walled dural arteries, a spontaneous thrombosis within the cavernous sinus, seen in as many as 62% of DCSFs, is believed to play a major role in the etiology of the fistulas. Recanalization of thrombosed sinus compartments leads to functional enlargement of micro-AV shunts within the rich vascular network of the dura mater. Associated venous hypertension is considered an additional cause for the development of dural arteriovenous shunts, as it may stimulate angiogenic activity and DAVF formation. Other predisposing or triggering factors include pressure changes during air travel, bagatelle trauma, hormonal changes during pregnancy and menopause, systemic hypertension and arteriosclerotic diseases, basic fibroblast growth factor, vascular endothelial growth factor or resistance to activated protein C.

Several classifications of cavernous sinus fistulas have been developed over the years, either based on etiology (spontaneous versus traumatic), the type of the arteriovenous shunt (direct versus indirect), the type of venous drainage (anterior versus posterior) or hemodynamics (low-flow versus high-flow). The most widely applied classification groups spontaneous lesions into Type A–D, among which Type B–D are DCSFs based on the origin of their arterial supply. More recently, the type of venous drainage pattern and its role in the natural course of the fistulas has been considered. However, none of these attempts to classify DCSFs is unanimously accepted, or can fully satisfy the need for a guide in prognosis, clinical decision-making or treatment indications. As the arterial anatomy of these fistulas is of lesser importance in the era of occlusive transvenous treatment, simply dividing them into direct and indirect fistulas may be sufficient for practical purposes.

The signs and symptoms in patients with low-flow DCSFs are in principle similar to those with direct high-flow CCF, but commonly milder and less progressive. They are influenced by size, location of the AV shunt as well as by the type of venous drainage. Clinical presentation in the initial stage can be non-specific with retro-orbital headaches, mild conjunctival injection or isolated diplopia. Consequently, the disease may be overlooked or is mistaken as endocrine orbitopathy, conjunctivitis or ocular myositis. More advanced stages may present with proptosis, chemosis, retinal hemorrhages or even visual loss. Patients with dominant posterior drainage can present with so-called white-eyed cavernous shunt and may remain undiagnosed for months or even years. Rare differential diagnoses also include orbital tumors or phlegmon. Neglecting a DCSF in the clinical differential diagnoses causes progression of the disease with potentially serious deterioration of the patient's symptoms and the risk of vision loss. Neurological deficits or intracranial hemorrhage associated with DCSFs are seldom observed (1.5%), despite a relatively frequent occurrence of cortical venous drainage (31%).

Various non-invasive imaging tools are available to detect or rule out a cavernous arteriovenous shunt, including CT, CTA and MRA. Transorbital or transcranial Doppler sonography are useful modalities for screening and confirming an initial clinical diagnosis, or for follow-up. Some clinicians use a pneumotonometer to diagnose DCSFs. For definitive diagnosis and optimal treatment planning, intra-arterial bi-plane DSA remains the gold standard diagnostic test and is considered indispensable in most institutions. Up to the present time, some patients with DCSFs are misdiagnosed, experiencing a frustrating and unpleasant clinical course. Thus, any questionable case should undergo intra-arterial superselective angiography as early as possible. The risks of neurological complications associated with cerebral angiography in experienced hands are very low nowadays (1.3% transient, 0.5% permanent complications).

Modern high-resolution imaging including three-dimensional DSA and angiographic computed tomography (ACT) has revolutionized neurovascular imaging providing novel insights into complex anatomic structures such as the CS and its adjacent environment. The often complex arterial supply by numerous dural branches arising from the artery of the foramen rotundum, ascending pharyngeal artery, middle meningeal or accessory meningeal arteries can be visualized in high-resolution cross-sectional images providing a novel perspective as compared to traditional AP and lateral standard angiographic views. The arrangement of efferent CS veins that are obscured or difficult to identify in standard 2D angiograms, such as the inferior petroclival vein, the internal carotid venous plexus or the anterior condylar confluens can readily be depicted, complementing and expanding our existing anatomic understanding. Precise knowledge of venous anatomy and good three-dimensional understanding remains essential for safe and effective endovascular treatment of arteriovenous shunting lesions of the sellar and skull base region.

In addition to endovascular occlusion techniques, therapeutic options of DCSFs encompass conservative management or alternative treatment methods such as manual compression, controlled hypotension and radiosurgery. Although fistula occlusion using TAE with particles can be accomplished in 31%–88%, recanalization has been observed in 25%–100% of cases. Untoward embolization causing neurological deficits with paresis, aphasia, CN deficits or even intracranial hemorrhage as well as limited long-term durability remain major disadvantages. This has changed the role of TAE into a more adjunctive modality for cases where TVO cannot be utilized or is contraindicated. The reduction of AV shunt flow to increase the efficacy of radiosurgery in intractable cases is another indication. Recent advances in the endovascular armamentarium, such as the introduction of new liquid embolic agents (Onyx), have significantly improved safety and efficacy of TAE of DAVFs. This paradigm shift may also affect future treatment strategies in DCSFs.

Improved knowledge and understanding of the venous anatomy at the CS region and skull base, as well as the development of newer catheterization tools have resulted in the exploration of different venous access routes that can be employed either as alternatives or as complements to achieve definite cure. The establishment of various detachable coil systems contributes to the increase in anatomic occlusion rates up to 100%, while the rate of clinical cure ranges from 52%–100%, with the majority of groups achieving more than 90%. This is superior to results achieved during the early era of endovascular treatment and better than outcomes of TAE series, thus reflecting the level of experience and skill gained in utilizing transvenous occlusion techniques. Current complication rates derived from larger series ($n = 613$) is 11.6% for transient and 1.8% for permanent deficits (stroke 0.5%).

Key to successful, safe and effective transvenous treatment is the willingness to accept a "multiple-route" approach that eventually enables one to gain access to the CS. Beginning with the simplest and most straightforward IPS approach, only a stepwise increase towards technically more difficult and more aggressive methods, including the transcutaneous SOV approach, is reasonable. Premature utilization of more invasive techniques such as direct puncture of the SOV or CS, as well as combined surgical-endovascular techniques should be considered as a last resort with regard to the benign nature of the disease. In suitable cases with mild symptoms, conservative management and appropriate clinical follow-up may be indicated. Manual compression therapy can be applied in compliant patients without contraindications. Controlled hypotension or radiosurgery may be valuable alternatives, especially in patients with difficult anatomical access, contraindications for endovascular treatment or significant comorbidities. Direct surgery for treatment of DCSFs has a minor, complementary role in exceptionally intractable cases, and should be abandoned if at all possible.

To date, hemodynamic characterization of DCSFs is insufficient and mainly based on measurements of flow velocity in the SOV or in ECA branches using percutaneous Doppler ultrasound. Although data on intrasinus flow or pressure are scarce, they may be necessary to fully understand the pathophysiology and natural course of the disease. The characterization of a DCSF as benign, "low-flow" lesions may be too general and insufficient, especially if thrombosis and venous outflow restriction lead to venous hypertension. These types of fistulas may be more appropriately identified as *high-pressure AV shunts*.

In conclusion, modern radiologic imaging has remarkably improved diagnostic tests for patients with DCSFs. However, some fistulas are still diagnosed late in the course of the disease or remain unrecognized, leading to frustrating delays in the appropriate therapeutic management. The current status of angiographic equipment, as well as the quality of endovascular tools and devices available today, not only allow a timely and accurate diagnosis, but also demand an early, safe and effective therapeutic intervention whenever angiographically or clinically indicated.

Subject Index

MEDICAL RADIOLOGY Diagnostic Imaging and Radiation Oncology

Titles in the series already published

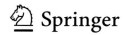

MEDICAL RADIOLOGY   Diagnostic Imaging and Radiation Oncology
Titles in the series already published

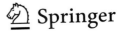 Springer

Printing and Binding: Stürtz GmbH, Würzburg